Guide to Clinical Preventive Services

An Assessment of the Effectiveness of 169 Interventions

Guide to Clinical Preventive Services

An Assessment of the Effectiveness of 169 Interventions

Report of the U.S.
Preventive Services
Task Force

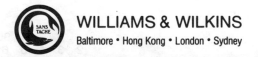
WILLIAMS & WILKINS
Baltimore • Hong Kong • London • Sydney

Editor: Michael Fisher
Associate Editor: Carol Eckhart
Design: Janis Oppelt
Production: Barbara J. Felton

William & Wilkins
428 East Preston Street
Baltimore, Maryland 21202, USA
800/638-4007 (in Maryland)
800/638-5198 (outside Maryland)

Accurate indications, adverse reactions, and dosage schedules for drugs are provided in this book, but it is possible that they may change. The reader is urged to review the package information data of the manufacturers of the medications mentioned.

Printed in the United States of America

Library of Congress Cataloging-in-Publication Data

U.S. Preventive Services Task Force.
    Guide to clinical preventive services: an assessment of the effectiveness of
169 interventions. Report of the U.S. Preventive Services Task Force.
      p.   cm.
    ISBN 0-683-08507-7
    1. Medicine, Preventive—Handbooks, manuals, etc. 2. Health promotion—Handbooks, manuals, etc.   I. Title.
    [DNLM: 1. Health Promotion—methods—United States. 2. Preventive
Health Services—United States. 3. Primary Prevention—standards—United
States. WA 108 U84g]
    RA427.2.U24   1989
    362.1—dc20
    DNLM/DLC
for Library of Congress   89-16599
                                CIP

90 91 92 93
2 3 4 5 6 7 8 9 10

Foreword

The publication of the U.S. Preventive Services Task Force *Guide to Clinical Preventive Services* is a significant event in the health of the Nation. The product of over four years of intensive effort by a panel of 20 experts from medicine and related fields, this important document establishes new priorities for medical care.

The Task Force advocates periodic health examinations tailored to and timed by the patient's age, sex, and other risk factors in place of annual "complete physical examinations" in which all patients receive the same routine battery of tests and procedures.

The *Guide* carefully reviews the evidence for and against screening tests, counseling procedures, and immunizations to promote health and prevent disease. In developing these guidelines, the Task Force employed an explicitly documented methodology, carefully evaluating the burden of suffering of the diseases considered as well as the efficacy and effectiveness of the interventions.

Documenting the effectiveness of medical care has become an important issue in both clinical and policy settings, and the *Guide* makes an important contribution to this process. Physicians and other medical providers are well advised to be more selective in ordering screening tests, since their inappropriate use is at best wasteful and at worst harmful.

Another major contribution of the *Guide* is its emphasis on personal behavior and therefore behavioral counseling. Behavior and health are strongly linked. Improved control of behavioral risk factors, such as use of tobacco, alcohol, and other drugs, lack of exercise, and poor nutrition, could prevent half of premature deaths, one-third of all cases of acute disability, and half of all cases of chronic disability. It is extraordinarily important that physicians and other providers educate their patients about these matters.

Although the main audience for the *Guide to Clinical Preventive Services* is primary care providers, it will also be of value to policymakers, researchers, employers, and those in the health care financing community. I commend this report and its important message to all of them.

EDWARD N. BRANDT, JR., M.D., PH.D.
Executive Dean, College of Medicine
University of Oklahoma Health Sciences Center
Oklahoma City, OK
Former Assistant Secretary for Health
Department of Health and Human Services
Washington, DC

Preface

The publication of the *Guide to Clinical Preventive Services* marks the beginning of an important new phase in the battle against premature death and disability. Abundant evidence documents that the majority of deaths among Americans under age 65 are preventable, many through interventions best provided in a clinician's office. The means are available to prevent many of these premature deaths, as well as many injuries and other types of morbidity. This *Guide*, resulting from the most comprehensive evaluation and synthesis of preventive interventions to date, offers the elements of an operational blueprint for their delivery.

Prepared under the supervision of the U.S. Preventive Services Task Force for presentation to the U.S. Department of Health and Human Services, the *Guide* rigorously reviews evidence for 169 interventions to prevent 60 different illnesses and conditions. The problems addressed in this report are common ones seen every day by primary care providers: cardiovascular and infectious diseases, cancers, injuries (both intentional and unintentional), alcohol and other drug abuse, and many others. Primary care clinicians have a key role in screening for many of these problems and immunizing against others. Of equal importance, however, is the clinician's role in counseling patients to change unhealthful behaviors related to diet, smoking, exercise, injuries, and sexually transmitted diseases.

The *Guide* is the culmination of over four years of literature review, debate, and synthesis of critical comments from expert reviewers. It offers the Task Force members' best judgment, based on the evidence, of the clinical preventive services that prudent clinicians should provide their patients in the course of routine clinical care. The recommendations are grouped by age, sex, and other risk factors. The quality of the evidence supporting each recommendation and the recommendations of other authorities are listed wherever possible, so that the reader may judge for him- or herself whether specific recommendations are appropriate.

Some will offer criticism that the recommendations go too far, expecting busy physicians and nurses to abandon their other clinical duties to become counselors or nutritionists. It is our belief that the "new morbidity" of injuries, infections, and chronic diseases demands a new paradigm for prevention in primary care—one that includes counseling about safety belt use and diet as well as giving immunizations and screening for cancer.

Others will find the Task Force recommendations too conservative. By limiting recommendations to those screening interventions, counseling maneuvers, and immunizations that have proven efficacy and effectiveness, the Task Force reaffirms the commitment to first do no harm. All possible preventive interventions have not been examined, of course; much remains to be done as research yields new data. Nonetheless, most will agree that as a result of this effort a compelling scientific case has been made for a core or basic level of key preventive services that should be made available to all Americans.

Though the recommendations presented are solely those of the Task Force, the *Guide* has benefited from unprecedented cooperation—between the U.S. and Canadian Task Forces, between the Federal Government and the private sector, and between the Task Force and literally hundreds of reviewers. This in itself is a gratifying accomplishment. But the real challenge lies ahead, in the offices and clinics of busy practitioners. It is our hope that the solid scientific base provided by the *Guide* will facilitate efforts to meet that challenge—to improve the health of the American people through the delivery of effective services for disease prevention and health promotion.

ROBERT S. LAWRENCE, M.D.
Chairman, U.S. Preventive Services
Task Force
Chief of Medicine, Cambridge
Hospital, and
Director, Division of Primary Care
Harvard Medical School
Cambridge, MA

J. MICHAEL MCGINNIS, M.D.
Deputy Assistant Secretary for Health
and
Director, Office of Disease Prevention
and Health Promotion
U.S. Department of Health and
Human Services
Washington, DC

U.S. Preventive Services Task Force

Robert S. Lawrence, M.D., Chairman
Chief of Medicine, Cambridge Hospital
Director, Division of Primary Care
Harvard Medical School
Cambridge, MA

Gordon H. DeFriese, Ph.D.
Director, Health Services Research
  Center
University of North Carolina
Chapel Hill, NC

E. Harvey Estes, M.D.
Professor, Department of Community
  and Family Medicine
Duke University Medical Center
Durham, NC

Jonathan E. Fielding, M.D., M.P.H.
Professor of Public Health and
  Pediatrics
UCLA School of Medicine
Vice President and Health Director
Johnson & Johnson Health
  Management, Inc.
Los Angeles, CA

Harvey V. Fineberg, M.D., Ph.D.
Dean, Harvard School of Public
  Health
Boston, MA

Suzanne W. Fletcher, M.D., M.Sc.
Professor of Medicine and
  Epidemiology
University of North Carolina
Chapel Hill, NC

Gary D. Friedman, M.D., M.S.
Assistant Director for Epidemiology
  and Biostatistics
Division of Research
Kaiser Permanente Medical Care
  Program
Oakland, CA

Lawrence W. Green, Dr.P.H.
Vice President and Director
Health Promotion Program
Henry J. Kaiser Family Foundation
Menlo Park, CA

John C. Greene, D.M.D., M.P.H.
Dean, School of Dentistry
University of California
San Francisco, CA

George A. Gross, D.O., M.P.H.
Professor, Community Health
  Sciences
Michigan State University
East Lansing, MI

M. Alfred Haynes, M.D., M.P.H.
Director, Drew/Meharry/Morehouse
  Consortium Cancer Center
Los Angeles, CA

Thomas E. Kottke, M.D.
Senior Associate Consultant
Cardiovascular Division
Mayo Clinic
Rochester, MN

F. Marc LaForce, M.D.
Physician-in-Chief
The Genesee Hospital
Rochester, NY

Jack H. Medalie, M.D., M.P.H.
Professor and Chairman
Department of Family Medicine
Case Western Reserve University
Cleveland, OH

Louise B. Russell, Ph.D.
Professor, Institute of Health, Health
  Care Policy, and Aging Research
Rutgers University
New Brunswick, NJ

Carol S. Scatarige, M.D., M.P.H.
NDC Medical Center
Norfolk, VA

Paul D. Stolley, M.D., M.P.H.
Professor of Medicine
University of Pennsylvania
Philadelphia, PA

Fernando M. Trevino, Ph.D., M.P.H.
Associate Professor
Department of Preventive Medicine
  and Community Health
University of Texas
Galveston, TX

William H. Wiese, M.D., M.P.H.
Director, Division of Community
  Medicine
Department of Family, Community,
  and Emergency Medicine
University of New Mexico
Albuquerque, NM

Carolyn A. Williams, R.N., Ph.D.
Professor and Dean, College of
  Nursing
University of Kentucky
Lexington, KY

Task Force Staff

Steven H. Woolf, M.D., M.P.H.
Scientific Editor and Writer

Douglas B. Kamerow, M.D., M.P.H.
Managing Editor and Project Director

Angela D. Mickalide, Ph.D.
Staff Coordinator

Acknowledgments

The *Guide to Clinical Preventive Services* was prepared under the supervision of the U.S. Preventive Services Task Force, which is solely responsible for its recommendations and whose members are listed on the preceding pages. Staff of the Task Force were based at and provided support by the Office of Disease Prevention and Health Promotion, U.S. Department of Health and Human Services.

Support from the following institutions for Task Force activities and staff is gratefully acknowledged: The Kellogg Foundation, the American College of Preventive Medicine, the Association of Teachers of Preventive Medicine, and the Johns Hopkins University School of Hygiene and Public Health. Appreciation is expressed to the members of the Canadian Task Force on the Periodic Health Examination for their collaboration, manuscript reviews, and support.

Project Director during early stages of preparation of the *Guide* was Robert A. Fried, M.D., now at the University of Colorado.

In addition to the numerous reviewers identified in Appendix B, appreciation is also expressed to the following:

Senior Advisors to the U.S. Preventive Services Task Force

H. David Banta, M.D., Gezondheidesraad, The Netherlands
Robert Berg, M.D., University of Rochester Medical Center, Rochester, NY
Lester Breslow, M.D., M P H , University of California, Los Angeles, CA
Kurt Deuschle, M.D., Mount Sinai School of Medicine, New York, NY
John Farquhar, M.D., Stanford University, Stanford, CA
Paul Frame, M.D., Tri-County Family Medicine, Dansville, NY
Steven Jonas, M.D., M.P.H., State University of New York, Stony Brook, NY
Sidney Katz, M.D., Case Western Reserve University, Cleveland, OH
Charles Kleeman, M.D., University of California, Los Angeles, CA
Alexander Leaf, M.D., Massachusetts General Hospital, Boston, MA
Donald Logsdon, M.D., Project INSURE, New York, NY
Sam Shapiro, Johns Hopkins University, Baltimore, MD
Anne Somers, Robert Wood Johnson Medical School, Princeton, NJ
Reuel Stallones, M.D., M.P.H., University of Texas, Houston, TX (deceased)
Jeremiah Stamler, M.D., Northwestern University Medical School, Chicago, IL
Irving Zola, Ph.D., Brandeis University, Waltham, MA

Coauthors of Task Force Background Papers

Renaldo N. Battista, M.D., Sc.D., McGill University, Montreal, Canada
David H. Bor, M.D., Harvard Medical School, Cambridge, MA
Milo L. Brekke, Ph.D., Brekke Associates, Minneapolis, MN
Carl J. Caspersen, Ph.D., M.P.H., Centers for Disease Control, Atlanta, GA
Christopher M. Coley, M.D., Harvard Medical School, Boston, MA
John M. Douglas, M.D., University of Colorado, Denver, CO
Marianne C. Fahs, Ph.D., M.P.H., Mount Sinai Medical Center, New York, NY
Lael C. Gatewood, Ph.D., University of Minnesota, Minneapolis, MN
Sally S. Harris, M.D., M.P.H., University of North Carolina, Chapel Hill, NC
David U. Himmelstein, M.D., Harvard Medical School, Cambridge, MA
Julie J. Hindmarsh, M.P.H., Baltimore County Family Resource Coordination Office, Towson, MD
Charles R. Horsburgh, Jr., M.D., Centers for Disease Control, Atlanta, GA

Sonja S. Hutchins, M.D., M.P.H., Centers for Disease Control, Atlanta, GA
Kevin K. Knight, M.D., M.P.H., University of California, Los Angeles, CA
Anthony L. Komaroff, M.D., Harvard Medical School, Boston, MA
Lawrence H. Kushi, Sc.D., University of Minnesota, Minneapolis, MN
Reginald Louie, D.D.S., M.P.H., U.S. Public Health Service, San Francisco, CA
Jeanne S. Mandelblatt, M.D., Albert Einstein College of Medicine, Bronx, NY
Mary F. Morrison, M.D., University of Pennsylvania, Philadelphia, PA
David M. Nathan, M.D., Harvard Medical School, Boston, MA
Michael S. O'Malley, M.S.P.H., University of North Carolina, Chapel Hill, NC
Hyeoun-Ae Park, Ph.D., University of Minnesota, Minneapolis, MN
Theodore M. Pass, Ph.D., Harvard School of Public Health, Boston, MA
Richard J. Pels, M.D., Harvard Medical School, Cambridge, MA
Michael R. Polen, M.A., Kaiser Permanente Medical Care Program, Oakland, CA
David N. Rose, M.D., Mount Sinai Medical Center, New York, NY
Jeffrey M. Samet, M.D., Harvard Medical School, Boston, MA
Clyde B. Schechter, M.D., Mount Sinai Medical Center, New York, NY
Joe V. Selby, M.D., Kaiser Permanente Medical Care Program, Oakland, CA
Donald S. Shepard, Ph.D., Harvard School of Public Health, Boston, MA
Alan Silver, M.D., M.P.H., Mount Sinai Medical Center, New York, NY
Daniel E. Singer, M.D., Harvard Medical School, Boston, MA
William C. Taylor, M.D., Harvard Medical School, Boston, MA
Steffie Woolhandler, M.D., M.P.H., Harvard Medical School, Cambridge, MA
Samuel J. Wycoff, D.M.D., M.P.H., University of California, San Francisco, CA

Staff Members and Others Who Assisted in the Preparation of the *Guide*

Office of Disease Prevention and Health Promotion
    James Harrell, M.A., Deputy Director
    David Adcock, M.D., M.P.H., Luther L. Terry Preventive Medicine Fellow
    John Bailar III, M.D., Ph.D., Science Advisor
    David Baker, Publications Manager
    Renee Curry, Medical Student Intern
    Mary Jo Deering, Ph.D., Director, Health Communication Staff
    Toni Goodwin, Secretary
    Linda Harris, Ph.D., Special Assistant to the Director
    Stephanie Maxwell, Research Assistant to the Director
    Sara White, M.S., Health Communication Advisor
Johns Hopkins University Preventive Medicine Residents
    Ling Chin, M.D., M.P.H.
    James Michael Crutcher, M.D., M.P.H.
    Gregory Dent, M.D., M.P.H.
    Ellen Frank, M.D., M.P.H.
    Marsha Guilford, M.D., M.P.H.
    Hugh McKinnon, M.D., M.P.H.
    Michael Parkinson, M.D., M.P.H.
    Marcel Salive, M.D., M.P.H.
    Jeanette Smith, M.D., M.P.H.
    Marilyn P. Wong, M.D., M.P.H.
Technical Resources, Inc. (Editorial support for production of the *Guide*)
    Joanna Fringer, M.A., Program Manager
    Dana Donofrio, Word Processor
    Margaret Leahy, Editor
    Laura Pancoast, Word Processor
    Kim Switlick, Word Processor
HCR (Logistical support for Task Force meetings and review process)
    Barbara Robinson, M.Ed., Vice President
    Michele Chang
    Susan Evett
    Donna Grande
    Kathleen Higgins
    Suzanne Schwartz
Triton, Inc. (Graphics support)
    John Borstel, Senior Graphics Editor

Contents

Metabolic Disorders

Infectious Diseases

Hematologic Disorders

Ophthalmologic and Otologic Disorders

Prenatal Disorders

Musculoskeletal Disorders

Mental Disorders and Substance Abuse

II. Counseling

III. Immunizations/Chemoprophylaxis

Appendices

Overview

i.

Introduction

This report is intended for primary care clinicians: physicians, nurses, nurse practitioners, physicians' assistants, other allied health professionals, and students. It provides recommendations for clinical practice on 169 preventive interventions—screening tests, counseling interventions, immunizations, and chemoprophylactic regimens—for the prevention of 60 target conditions. The patients for whom these services are recommended include asymptomatic individuals of all age groups and risk categories. Thus, the subject matter is relevant to all of the major primary care specialties: family practice, internal medicine, pediatrics, and obstetrics-gynecology. The recommendations in each chapter are based on a standardized review of current scientific evidence and include a summary of published clinical research regarding the clinical effectiveness of each preventive service. A listing of the relevant recommendations of major professional organizations and health agencies is also included for each preventive service.

Clinicians have always intuitively understood the value of prevention. Faced daily with the difficult and often unsuccessful task of treating advanced stages of disease, primary care providers have long sought the opportunity to intervene early in the course of disease or even before disease develops. The benefits of incorporating prevention into medical practice have become increasingly apparent over the past 20 to 30 years as previously common and debilitating conditions have declined in incidence following the introduction of effective clinical preventive services. Infectious diseases such as poliomyelitis, which once occurred in regular epidemic waves (over 18,300 cases in 1954), have become rare in the United States as a result of childhood immunization.[1] Only five cases of paralytic poliomyelitis were reported in the United States in 1987.[1] Before rubella vaccine became available, rubella epidemics occurred regularly in the United States every six to nine years; a 1964 pandemic resulted in over 12 million rubella infections, with over 11,000 fetal losses and about 20,000 infants born with congenital rubella syndrome.[2,3] The incidence of rubella has decreased 99% since 1969, when the vaccine first became available.[4,5] Similar trends have occurred with diphtheria, pertussis, and other once-common childhood infectious diseases.[1]

Preventive services for the early detection of disease have also been associated with dramatic reductions in morbidity and mortality. Age-adjusted mortality from strokes has decreased by more than 50% since 1972, a trend attributed in part to earlier detection and treatment of hypertension.[6,7] Cervical cancer mortality has fallen by 73% since 1950,[8] due in part to widespread Papanicolaou testing to detect cervical dysplasia.[9,10] Children with metabolic disorders such as phenylketonuria and congenital hypothyroidism, who once suffered severe irreversible mental retardation, now usually retain normal cognitive function as a result of routine newborn screening and treatment.[11-13]

Although immunizations and screening tests remain important preventive services, the most promising role for prevention in current medical practice may lie in changing the personal health behaviors of patients long before clinical disease develops. The importance of this aspect of clinical practice is demonstrated by a growing body of evidence linking a handful of personal health behaviors to the leading causes of death in the United States: heart disease, cancer, cerebrovascular disease, injuries, and chronic obstructive pulmonary disease.[14] Smoking alone contributes to one out of every six deaths in the United States,[15] including 130,000 deaths each year from cancer, 115,000 from coronary artery disease, 27,500 from cerebrovascular disease, and 60,000 from chronic obstructive pulmonary disease.[16] Failure to use safety belts and driving while intoxicated are major contributors to motor vehicle injuries, which accounted for over 47,000 deaths in 1987.[14] Physical inactivity and dietary factors contribute to coronary atherosclerosis, cancer, diabetes, osteoporosis, or other common diseases.[17-20] Certain sexual practices increase the risk of unintended pregnancy, sexually transmitted diseases, and acquired immunodeficiency syndrome.[21,22]

Although there are sound clinical reasons for emphasizing prevention in medicine, studies have shown that physicians often fail to provide recommended clinical preventive services.[23] This is due to a variety of factors, including lack of reimbursement for preventive services.[24] Also, busy clinicians often have insufficient time with patients to deliver the range of preventive services that are recommended. But even when these barriers to implementation are accounted for, clinicians fail to perform preventive services as recommended.[25] One reason for this is uncertainty among clinicians as to which services should be offered.

Part of the uncertainty among clinicians derives from the fact that recommendations come from multiple sources, and these recommendations are often different. Recommendations relating to clinical preventive services are issued regularly by Government health agencies,[6,26-28] medical specialty organizations,[29-35] professional and scientific organizations,[36-38] voluntary associations,[39-41] and individual experts.[42-47]

In addition, a major reason clinicians may be reluctant to perform preventive services is skepticism about their clinical effectiveness. It is often unclear whether performance of certain preventive interventions can significantly reduce morbidity or mortality from the target condition the clinician is attempting to prevent. It is also unclear how to compare the relative effectiveness of different preventive services, making it difficult for busy clinicians to decide which interventions are most important during a brief patient visit. A broader concern is that some maneuvers may ultimately result in more harm than good. While this concern applies to all clinical practices, it is especially important in relation to preventive services because the individuals who receive these interventions are often relatively healthy. Minor complications or rare adverse effects that would be tolerated in the treatment of a severe illness take on greater significance in the asymptomatic population and require careful evaluation to determine whether benefits exceed risks. Moreover, preventive services such as routine screening are often recommended for a large proportion of the population, and there are therefore potentially significant economic implications to implementation.

These uncertainties increasingly have raised questions about the value of the routine health examination of asymptomatic persons, in which the same battery of tests and physical examination procedures are performed as part of a routine checkup. The annual physical examination of healthy persons was first proposed by the American Medical Association in 1922.[48] For many years after, it was common practice among health professionals to recommend routine physicals and comprehensive laboratory testing as effective preventive medicine. It is now increasingly clear, however, that while routine visits with the primary care clinician are important, performing the same interventions on all patients and performing them as frequently as every year are not the most clinically effective approaches to disease prevention. Rather, both the frequency and the content of the periodic health examination need to be tailored to the unique health risks of the individual patient and should take into consideration the quality of the evidence that specific preventive services are clinically effective. This approach to the periodic visit was endorsed by the American Medical Association in 1983 in a policy statement that withdrew support for a standard annual physical examination.[36] Current thinking is that the individualized periodic health visit should place greater emphasis on evidence of clinical effectiveness, and thus increased attention is turning to the collection of reliable data on the effectiveness of specific preventive services.

One of the first comprehensive efforts to examine these issues systematically was undertaken by the Canadian government, which in 1976 convened the Canadian Task Force on the Periodic Health Examination. This expert panel adopted a highly organized approach to evaluating the effectiveness of clinical preventive services. Explicit criteria were developed to judge the quality of evidence from published clinical research, and uniform decision rules were used to link the strength of recommendations for or against a given preventive service to the quality of the underlying evidence (see Appendix A). These ratings were intended to provide the clinician with a means of selecting those preventive services supported by the strongest evidence of effectiveness. Using this approach, the Canadian Task Force examined preventive services for 78 target conditions, releasing its recommendations in a monograph published in 1979.[49] In 1982, the Canadian Task Force reconvened and applied its methodology to new evidence as it became available, publishing revised recommendations and evaluations of new topics in 1984, 1986, and 1988.[50-52]

A similar effort was launched in the United States in 1984, when Edward N. Brandt, M.D., Ph.D., the Assistant Secretary for Health of the Department of Health and Human Services, commissioned the U.S. Preventive Services Task Force. This 20-member non-Federal panel included 14 physicians with expertise in primary care medicine (family practice, internal medicine, and pediatrics), clinical epidemiology, and public health. The panel also included a dentist, a nurse, a health services researcher, a health educator, a health economist, and a medical sociologist. Like the Canadian panel, the U.S. Task Force was charged with developing recommendations for clinicians on the appropriate use of preventive interventions, based on a systematic review of evidence of clinical effectiveness.[53] A similar methodology was adopted at the outset of the project (see Chapter ii). This enabled the U.S. and Canadian panels to collaborate in a binational effort to review evidence and develop recommendations on preventive services.

The U.S. Task Force met 14 times between July 1984 and February 1988. Its objective was to develop comprehensive recommendations addressing preventive services for all age groups. The panel members and their scientific support staff, based at the Office of Disease Prevention and Health Promotion of the Department of Health and Human Services, reviewed evidence and developed recommendations on preventive services for 60 target conditions affecting patients from infancy to old age. This report, which summarizes the findings and clinical recommendations of the panel, was prepared by the scientific staff of the Task Force in the final year of the project (1988–1989). Both the meetings of the Task Force and the preparation of this work have been carried out in close collaboration with professional organizations throughout the United States and with U.S. Government agencies that share an interest in prevention.

Several important findings have emerged from the review of evidence in this report. First, the data suggest that among the most effective interventions available to clinicians for reducing the incidence and severity of the leading causes of disease and disability in the United States are those that address the personal health practices of patients. Primary prevention as it relates to such risk factors as smoking, physical inactivity, poor nutrition, and alcohol and other drug abuse holds generally greater promise for improving overall health than many secondary preventive measures such as routine screening for early disease. Although certain screening tests, such as mammography[54] and Papanicolaou smears,[55] can be highly effective in reducing morbidity and mortality, the Task Force found that many others are of unproven effectiveness. Screening tests with inadequate accuracy, when performed routinely without regard to risk factors, often produce large numbers of false-positive results that may result in unnecessary diagnostic testing and treatment. Many tests that lack evidence of improved clinical outcome have the additional disadvantage of being expensive, especially when performed on large numbers of persons in the population.

Thus, the second principal finding of this report is the need for greater selectivity in ordering tests and providing preventive services. In particular, the proper selection of screening tests requires careful consideration of the age, sex, and other individual risk factors of the patient if the clinician is to minimize the risk of adverse effects and unnecessary expenditures due to screening (see Chapter ii). An appreciation of the risk profile of the patient is also necessary to determine which interventions are most important during the clinical encounter. The need for evaluating risk factors underscores a time-honored principle of medical practice: the importance of a complete medical history and detailed discussion with patients regarding personal health practices.

The third principal finding of the Task Force report is that conventional clinical activities (e.g., diagnostic testing) may be of less value to patients than activities once considered outside the traditional role of the clinician (e.g., counseling and patient education). This suggests a new paradigm in defining the responsibilities of the primary care provider. In the past, the role of the clinician related primarily to the treatment of illnesses; the asymptomatic healthy individual did not need to see the doctor. In addition, personal health behaviors were often not viewed as a legitimate clinical issue. A patient's use of safety belts, for example, would receive less attention from the clinician than the results of a complete blood count (CBC) or a routine chest xray. A careful review of the data, however, suggests that different priorities are in order. Motor vehicle injuries affect nearly 4 million persons each year in the United States;[56] they account for over 45,000 deaths each year and are a leading cause of death in persons aged 5–44.[14] Proper use of safety belts can prevent 40–60% of motor vehicle injuries and deaths.[57,58] In contrast, there is little good evidence that performing routine CBCs or chest x-rays improves clinical outcome,[59,60] and these procedures are associated with increased health care expenditures.

The fourth finding is that the shifting responsibility of clinicians also implies a changing role for patients. The increasing evidence of the importance of personal health behaviors and primary prevention means that patients must assume greater responsibility for their own health. Whereas the clinician is often the key figure in the treatment of acute illnesses and injuries, the patient is the principal effector in primary prevention. In the traditional doctor-patient relationship, the patient adopts a passive role and expects the doctor to assume control of the treatment plan. One of the initial tasks of the clinician practicing primary prevention is shifting the locus of control to the patient. To achieve competence in this task, some clinicians may need to develop new skills in helping to empower patients and in counseling them to change certain health related behaviors (see Chapter iv).

Fifth, preventive services need not be delivered exclusively during visits devoted entirely to provention. While preventive checkups often provide more time for counseling and other preventive services, and although healthy individuals may be more receptive to such interventions than those who are sick, the illness visit is an equally important time to practice prevention. In fact, some individuals may see clinicians only when they are ill or injured. The illness visit may provide the only opportunity to reach such individuals who, due to limited access to care, would be otherwise unlikely to receive preventive services. For many conditions, the Task Force found that devising strategies to increase access to preventive services for such individuals is more likely to reduce morbidity and mortality than performing preventive services more frequently on those who are already regular recipients of preventive care and who are often in better health.

Sixth, the gaps in evidence identified by the Task Force underscore the size of the research agenda in preventive medicine. For most topics examined in this report, the Task Force found inadequate evidence to evaluate effectiveness or to determine the optimal frequency of a preventive service. In some cases, the necessary studies have never been performed. But for many other topics, studies have been performed—in some cases, large numbers of studies—but the findings are unreliable because of improper study design or systematic biases. Thus, while it is certainly important to perform more research in preventive medicine, there is an even greater need in prevention and other medical specialties for better quality research in evaluating effectiveness. The studies reviewed in this report suggest that clinical researchers evaluating effectiveness often fail to give adequate attention to potential flaws in the design of their studies. This observation confirms the findings of other reviewers regarding the need to improve the overall methodologic quality of clinical research.[61]

Finally, the process used by the U.S. and Canadian Task Forces to evaluate effectiveness may be as important a contribution to medical policy as are the recommendations themselves. Although only preventive services have been examined in this report, the techniques that have been developed by the U.S. Task Force for the standardized review of evidence and for developing clinical practice recommendations based on documented decision rules are equally applicable to many other medical practices. The availability of such techniques comes at a time when increasing attention is being focused on devising better methods for evaluating effectiveness in clinical practice.[62] The methodology presented in this report may be useful to others who share an interest in using systematic methods for reviewing published clinical research and assessing the overall health effects of clinical practices.

It is hoped that this report will help resolve some of the uncertainties among primary care clinicians regarding the effectiveness of preventive services. A comprehensive approach has been taken to explore issues of prevention for a wide range of disease categories and for patients of all ages. The systematic approach to the review of evidence for each topic should provide clinicians with the means to compare the relative effectiveness of different preventive services and to determine, on the basis of scientific evidence, what is most likely to benefit their patients. Basing such decisions on rigorous research will be an important step forward in the advancement of disease prevention and health promotion in the United States.

REFERENCES

1. Centers for Disease Control. Summary of notifiable diseases, United States, 1987. MMWR 1988; 36:1–59.

2. Witte JJ, Karchmer AW, Case G, et al. Epidemiology of rubella. Am J Dis Child 1969; 118:107–11.
3. Orenstein WA, Bart KJ, Hinman AR, et al. The opportunity and obligation to eliminate rubella from the United States. JAMA 1984; 251:1988–94.
4. Centers for Disease Control. Rubella and congenital rubella—United States, 1984–1986. MMWR 1987; 36:664.
5. Idem. Rubella and congenital rubella syndrome—New York City. MMWR 1986; 35: 770–9.
6. 1988 Joint National Committee. The 1988 Report of the Joint National Committee on Detection, Evaluation, and Treatment of High Blood Pressure. Arch Intern Med 1988; 148:1023–38.
7. Garraway WM, Whisnant JP. The changing pattern of hypertension and the declining incidence of stroke. JAMA 1987; 258:214–7.
8. National Cancer Institute. 1987 annual cancer statistics review, including cancer trends, 1950–1985. Washington, D.C.: Department of Health and Human Services, 1988. (Publication no. DHHS (NIH) 882789.)
9. Yu S, Miller AB, Sherman GJ. Optimising the age, number of tests, and test interval for cervical screening in Canada. J Epi Comm Health 1982; 36:1–10.
10. Miller AB, Visentin T, Howe GR. The effect of hysterectomies and screening on mortality from cancer of the uterus in Canada. Int J Cancer 1981; 27:651–7.
11. Berman PW, Waisman HA, Graham FK. Intelligence in treated phenylketonuric children: a developmental study. Child Develop 1966; 37:731–47.
12. Hudson FP, Mordaunt VL, Leahy I. Evaluation of treatment begun in first three months of life in 184 cases of phenylketonuria. Arch Dis Child 1970; 45:5–12.
13. Williamson ML, Koch R, Azen C, et al. Correlates of intelligence test results in treated phenylketonuric children. Pediatrics 1981; 68:161–7.
14. National Center for Health Statistics. Advance report of final mortality statistics, 1986. Monthly Vital Statistics Report [Suppl], vol. 37, no. 6. Hyattsville, Md.: Public Health Service, 1988. (Publication no. DHHS (PHS) 88–1120.)
15. Centers for Disease Control. Smoking-attributable mortality and years of potential life lost—United States, 1984. MMWR 1987; 36:6937.
16. Department of Health and Human Services. Reducing the health consequences of smoking: 25 years of progress. A report of the Surgeon General. Rockville, Md.: Department of Health and Human Services, 1989. (Publication no. DHHS (PHS) 89–8411.)
17. Bouchard C, Shephard RJ, Stephens T, et al., eds. Exercise, fitness, and health: research and consensus. Proceedings of the International Conference on Exercise, Fitness, and Health. Champaign, Ill.: Human Kinetics Publishers (in press).
18. Department of Health and Human Services. The Surgeon General's report on nutrition and health. Washington, D.C.: Government Printing Office, 1988. (Publication no. DHHS (PHS) 88–50210.)
19. The Lipid Research Clinics Coronary Primary Prevention Trial Results. I. Reduction in incidence of coronary heart disease. JAMA 1984; 251:351–64.
20. The Lipid Research Clinics Coronary Primary Prevention Trial Results. II. The relationship of reduction in incidence of coronary heart disease to cholesterol lowering. JAMA 1984; 251:365–74.
21. Hatcher RA, Guest F, Stewart F, et al. Contraceptive technology, 1988–1989. Atlanta, Ga.: Printed Matter, Inc., 1988.
22. Curran JW, Jaffe HW, Hardy AM, et al. Epidemiology of HIV infection and AIDS in the United States. Science 1988; 239:610–6.
23. Lewis CE. Disease prevention and health promotion practices of primary care physicians in the United States. Am J Prev Med [Suppl] 1988; 4:9–16.
24. Logsdon DN, Rosen MA. The cost of preventive health services in primary medical care and implications for health insurance coverage. J Ambul Care Man 1984; 46–55.
25. Lurie N, Manning WG, Peterson C, et al. Preventive care: do we practice what we preach? Am J Public Health 1987; 77:801–4.
26. National Cancer Institute. Working guidelines for early cancer detection: rationale and

supporting evidence to decrease mortality. Bethesda, Md.: National Cancer Institute, 1987.

27. Report of the National Cholesterol Education Program Expert Panel on Detection, Evaluation, and Treatment of High Blood Cholesterol in Adults. Arch Intern Med 1988; 148:36–69.

28. Immunization Practices Advisory Committee. New recommended schedule for active immunization of normal infants and children. MMWR 1986; 35:577–9.

29. American College of Physicians. Periodic health examination: a guide for designing individualized preventive health care in the asymptomatic patient. Ann Intern Med 1981; 95:729–32.

30. Idem. Common diagnostic tests: use and interpretation. Philadelphia: American College of Physicians, 1987.

31. American College of Obstetricians and Gynecologists. Standards for obstetric-gynecologic services, 6th ed. Washington, D.C.: American College of Obstetricians and Gynecologists, 1985:17–8.

32. Peter G, Giebink GS, Hall CB, et al., eds. Report of the Committee on Infectious Diseases, 20th ed. Elk Grove Village, Ill.: American Academy of Pediatrics, 1986:266–75.

33. American Academy of Pediatrics. Guide to implementing safety counseling. Elk Grove Village, Ill.: American Academy of Pediatrics, 1985.

34. Idem. Vision screening and eye examination in children. Committee on Practice and Ambulatory Medicine. Pediatrics 1986; 77:918–9.

35. American Academy of Ophthalmology. Infants and children's eye care. Statement by the American Academy of Ophthalmology to the Select Panel for the Promotion of Child Health, Department of Health and Human Services. San Francisco, Calif.: American Academy of Ophthalmology, 1980.

36. American Medical Association. Medical evaluations of healthy persons. Council on Scientific Affairs. JAMA 1983; 249:1626–33.

37. American Dental Association. Accepted dental therapeutics, 39th ed. Chicago, Ill.: American Dental Association, 1982.

38. National Academy of Sciences, Institute of Medicine. Ad Hoc Advisory Group on Preventive Services. Preventive services for the well population. Washington, D.C.: National Academy of Sciences, 1978.

39. American Cancer Society. Report on the cancer-related health checkup. CA 1980; 30:194–240.

40. American Heart Association. Cardiovascular and risk factor evaluation of healthy American adults: a statement for physicians by an ad hoc committee appointed by the steering committee. Circulation 1987; 75:1340A-62A.

41. American Diabetes Association. Physician's guide to non-insulin dependent (type II) diabetes. Diagnosis and treatment. Alexandria, Va.: American Diabetes Association, 1988.

42. Frame PS, Carlson SJ. A critical review of periodic health screening using specific screening criteria. J Fam Pract 1975; 2:283–9.

43. Frame PS. A critical review of adult health maintenance. Part 1. Prevention of atherosclerotic diseases. J Fam Pract 1986; 22:341–6.

44. Idem. A critical review of adult health maintenance. Part 2. Prevention of infectious diseases. J Fam Pract 1986; 22:417–22.

45. Idem. A critical review of adult health maintenance. Part 3. Prevention of cancer. J Fam Pract 1986; 22:511–20.

46. Idem. A critical review of adult health maintenance. Part 4. Prevention of metabolic, behavioral, and miscellaneous conditions. J Fam Pract 1986; 23:29–39.

47. Breslow L, Somers AR. The lifetime health-monitoring program: a practical approach to preventive medicine. N Engl J Med 1977; 292:601–8.

48. American Medical Association. Periodic health examination: a manual for physicians. Chicago, Ill.: American Medical Association, 1947.

49. Canadian Task Force on the Periodic Health Examination. The periodic health examination. Can Med Assoc J 1979; 121:1194–254.

50. *Idem*. The periodic health examination. 1984 update. Can Med Assoc J 1984; 130: 1278–85.
51. *Idem*. The periodic health examination. 1986 update. Can Med Assoc J 1986; 134: 721–9.
52. *Idem*. The periodic health examination. 1988 update. Can Med Assoc J 1988; 138: 617–26.
53. Lawrence RS, Mickalide AD. Preventive services in clinical practice: designing the periodic health examination. JAMA 1987; 257:2205–7.
54. Shapiro S, Venet W, Strax P, et al., eds. Periodic screening for breast cancer. Baltimore, Md.: Johns Hopkins Press, 1988.
55. International Agency for Research on Cancer Working Group on Evaluation of Cervical Cancer Screening Programmes. Screening for squamous cervical cancer: duration of low risk after negative results of cervical cytology and its implication for screening policies. Br Med J 1986; 293:659–64.
56. National Highway Traffic Safety Administration. National accident sampling system, 1986: a report on traffic crashes and injuries in the United States. Washington, D.C.: Department of Transportation, 1988:x. (Publication no. DOT HS 807–296.)
57. Department of Transportation. Final regulatory impact assessment on amendments to Federal Motor Vehicle Safety Standard 208, Front Seat Occupant Protection. Washington, D.C.: Department of Transportation, 1984. (Publication no. DOT HS 806–572.)
58. Campbell BJ. Safety belt injury reduction related to crash severity and front seated position. J Trauma 1987; 27:733–9.
59. Tape TG, Mushlin AI. The utility of routine chest radiographs. Ann Intern Med 1986; 104:663–70.
60. Shapiro MF, Greenfield S. The complete blood count and leukocyte differential count. Ann Intern Med 1987; 106:65–74.
61. Feinstein AR. Scientific standards in epidemiologic studies of the menace of daily life. Science 1988; 242:1257–63.
62. Institute of Medicine. Assessing medical technologies. Washington, D.C.: National Academy Press, 1985.

ii.

Methodology

This report presents a systematic approach to evaluating the effectiveness of clinical preventive services. The recommendations, and the review of evidence from published clinical research on which they are based, are the product of a methodology established at the outset of the project. The intent of this analytic process has been to provide clinicians* with current and scientifically defensible information about the relative effectiveness of different preventive services and the quality of the evidence on which these conclusions are based. This information can help clinicians who have limited time to select the most appropriate preventive services to offer in a periodic health examination for patients of different ages and risk categories. The critical appraisal of evidence is also intended to identify preventive services of uncertain effectiveness as well as those that could result in more harm than good if performed routinely by clinicians.

For the content of this report to be useful, and to clarify differences between the U.S. Preventive Services Task Force recommendations and those of other groups, it is important for the reader to be aware of the process by which this report was developed, as well as how it differs from the consensus development process used to derive most clinical practice guidelines. First, the objectives of the review process, including the types of preventive services to be examined and the nature of the recommendations to be developed, were carefully defined early in the process. Second, the Task Force adopted explicit criteria for recommending the performance or exclusion of preventive services and applied these "rules of evidence" systematically to each topic it studied. Third, literature searches and assessments of the quality of individual studies were conducted in accordance with rigorous, predetermined methodologic criteria. Fourth, guidelines were adopted for translating these findings into sound clinical practice recommendations. Finally, these recommendations were reviewed extensively by experts in the United States, Canada, and the United Kingdom. Each of these steps is examined in greater detail below.

Definition of Objectives

Systematic rules were used to select the target conditions and candidate preventive interventions to be evaluated by the Task Force.

---

*The provider of preventive services in primary care is often a physician. The term "clinician" is used in this report, however, to include other primary care providers such as nurses, nurse practitioners, physicians' assistants, and other allied health professionals. Although physicians may be better qualified than other providers to perform certain preventive services or to convince patients to change behavior, some preventive services are more effectively performed by nonphysicians with special training (e.g., nurses, dietitians, smoking cessation counselors, mental health professionals).

Selection of Target Conditions

The Task Force began by preparing a list of important diseases and injuries in the United States that might be preventable through clinical intervention. The 60 target conditions were selected on the basis of two important criteria:

Burden of Suffering from the Target Condition.   Conditions that are relatively uncommon in the United States or are of only minor clinical significance were not considered in this report. Thus, consideration was given to both the *prevalence* (proportion of the population affected) and *incidence* (number of new cases per year) of the condition. Conditions that were once common but have become rare because of effective preventive interventions (e.g., poliomyelitis) were included in the review.

Potential Effectiveness of the Preventive Intervention.   Conditions were excluded from analysis if the panel could not identify a potentially effective preventive intervention that could be performed by clinicians.

Selection of Preventive Services

For each target condition, the Task Force used two criteria to select the preventive services to be evaluated. First, in general, only preventive services carried out on *asymptomatic persons*** were reviewed. Thus, only primary and secondary preventive measures were addressed. *Primary preventive measures* involve entirely asymptomatic individuals (e.g., routine immunization of healthy children), whereas *secondary preventive measures* identify and treat asymptomatic persons who have already developed risk factors or preclinical disease but in whom the disease itself has not become clinically apparent. Obtaining a Papanicolaou smear to detect cervical dysplasia before the development of cancer is a form of secondary prevention. Preventive measures in symptomatic patients, such as antibiotic therapy to prevent postoperative wound infection or insulin therapy to prevent the complications of diabetes mellitus, are considered *tertiary prevention* and are outside the scope of this report.

The second criterion for selecting preventive services for review was that the maneuver had to be perfomed in the *clinical setting*. Only those preventive services that would be carried out by clinicians in the context of routine health care were examined. Findings should not be extrapolated to preventive interventions performed in other settings. Screening tests are evaluated in terms of their effectiveness when performed during the clinical encounter (i.e., *case-finding*). Screening tests performed at schools, worksites, health fairs, and other community locations

----

**The term "asymptomatic person" as used in this report differs from its customary meaning in medical practice. Although "asymptomatic" is often considered synonymous with "healthy," the term is used in this report to describe individuals who lack clinical evidence of the target condition. Signs and symptoms of illnesses unrelated to the target condition may be present without affecting the designation of "asymptomatic." Thus, a 70-year-old man with no genitourinary symptoms who is screened for prostate cancer would be designated asymptomatic for that condition, even if he were hospitalized for (unrelated) congestive heart failure. Preventive services recommended for "asymptomatic patients" therefore need not be delivered only during preventive checkups of healthy persons but apply equally to clinical encounters with patients being seen for other reasons. In fact, the illness visit may provide the clinician with the best opportunity for delivering some preventive services. Persons in need of preventive services who have limited access to care rarely visit clinicians unless they become ill.

are not within the scope of this report. Also, preventive interventions performed outside the clinical setting (e.g., health and safety legislation, mandatory screening, community health promotion) are not specifically evaluated, although clinicians can play an important role in promoting such programs and in encouraging the participation of their patients.

After the complete set of target conditions and preventive services were identified, they were divided into three categories: screening tests, counseling interventions, and immunizations and chemoprophylaxis. *Screening tests* are those preventive services in which a special test or standardized examination procedure is used to identify patients requiring special intervention. Nonstandardized historical questions, such as asking patients whether they smoke, and tests involving symptomatic patients are not considered screening tests. *Counseling* interventions are those in which the patient receives information and advice regarding personal behaviors (e.g., diet) to reduce the risk of subsequent illness or injury. Counseling regarding the health-related behaviors of persons who have already developed signs and symptoms is specifically excluded. *Immunizations* discussed in this report include vaccines and immunoglobulins (passive immunization) taken by persons with no evidence of infectious disease. *Chemoprophylaxis* refers to the use of drugs or biologics taken by asymptomatic persons as primary prevention to reduce the risk of developing a disease.

Criteria for Determining Effectiveness

Preventive services are required to meet predetermined criteria to be considered effective. The criteria of effectiveness for the three categories of preventive services (Table 1) provided the analytic framework for the evaluation of effectiveness in the 60 chapters in this report. Each of these criteria must be satisfied to evaluate the "causal pathway" of a preventive service, the chain of events that must occur for a preventive maneuver to influence clinical outcome.[1] Thus, a screening test is not considered effective if it lacks sufficient accuracy to detect the condition earlier than without screening or if there is inadequate evidence that early detection improves outcome. Similarly, counseling interventions cannot be considered effective in the absence of firm evidence that changing personal behavior can improve outcome and that clinicians can influence this behavior through counseling. Effective immunization and chemoprophylactic regimens require evi-

Table 1.
Criteria of Effectiveness

Screening Tests
- Efficacy of Screening Tests
- Effectiveness of Early Detection

Counseling Interventions
- Efficacy of Risk Reduction
- Effectiveness of Counseling

Immunizations
- Efficacy of Vaccine

Chemoprophylaxis
- Efficacy of Chemoprophylactic Agent
- Effectiveness of Counseling

dence of biologic efficacy; in the case of chemoprophylactic agents, evidence is also necessary that patients will comply with long-term use of the drug.

The methodologic issues involved in evaluating screening tests require further elaboration. As mentioned above, a screening test must satisfy two major requirements to be considered effective:

- The test must be able to detect the target condition earlier than without screening and with sufficient accuracy to avoid producing large numbers of false-positive and false-negative results (*efficacy of screening test*).

- Persons with disease who are detected early should have a better clinical outcome than those who are detected without screening (*effectiveness of early detection*).

These two headings appear in each of the 47 screening chapters in this report.

Efficacy of Screening Test.   In a departure from the conventional definition of "efficacy," the term "efficacy of a screening test" is used in this report to describe accuracy and reliability. *Accuracy* is measured in terms of four indices: sensitivity, specificity, and positive and negative predictive value (Table 2). *Sensitivity* refers to the proportion of persons with a condition who correctly test "positive" when screened. A test with poor sensitivity will miss cases (persons with the condition) and will produce a large proportion of *false-negative* results; true cases will be told incorrectly that they are free of disease. *Specificity* refers to the proportion of persons without the condition who correctly test "negative" when screened. A test with poor specificity will result in healthy persons being told they have the condition (*false positives*). An accepted reference standard ("gold standard") is essential to

Table 2.
Definition of Terms

Term	Definition	Formula*
Sensitivity	Proportion of persons with condition who test positive	$\dfrac{a}{a + c}$
Specificity	Proportion of persons without condition who test negative.	$\dfrac{d}{b + d}$
Positive Predictive Value	Proportion of persons with positive test who have condition.	$\dfrac{a}{a + b}$
Negative Predictive Value	Proportion of persons with negative test who do not have condition.	$\dfrac{d}{c + d}$

*Explanation of symbols:

	Condition Present	Condition Absent
Positive Test	a	b
Negative Test	c	d

Legend:
a = true positive
b = false positive
c = false negative
d = true negative

determining sensitivity and specificity, because it provides the means for distinguishing between "true" and "false" test results.

The use of screening tests with poor sensitivity and/or specificity is of special significance to the clinician because of the potentially serious consequences of false-negative and false-positive results. Persons who receive false-negative results may experience important delays in diagnosis and treatment. Some might develop a false sense of security, resulting in inadequate attention to risk reduction and delays in seeking medical care when warning symptoms become present. False-positive results can lead to follow-up testing that may be uncomfortable, expensive, and, in some cases, potentially harmful. If follow-up testing does not disclose the error, the patient may even receive unnecessary treatment. There may also be psychological consequences. Persons informed of an abnormal medical test that is falsely positive may experience unnecessary anxiety until the error is corrected. *Labeling* may affect behavior; for example, studies have shown that some persons with hypertension identified through screening may experience altered behavior and decreased work productivity.[2,3]

A proper evaluation of a screening test must therefore include a determination of the likelihood of producing false-positive results. This is done by calculating the *positive predictive value* (PPV) of the test (Table 2) in the population to be screened. The PPV of a screening test is the proportion of positive results that are correct (true positives). A test with low PPV can generate more false-positive than true-positive results, but this depends to a large extent on the type of population in which it is used. The PPV increases and decreases in accordance with the prevalence of the target condition in the screened population. Thus, unlike sensitivity and specificity, the PPV is not a constant performance characteristic of a screening test. If the target condition is sufficiently rare in the screened population, even tests with excellent sensitivity and specificity can have low PPV, generating more false-positive than true-positive results. This mathematical relationship is best illustrated by an example:

> A population of 100,000 in which the prevalence of a hypothetical cancer is 1% would have 1000 persons with cancer and 99,000 without cancer. A screening test with 90% sensitivity and 90% specificity would detect 900 of the 1000 cases, but would also mislabel 9900 healthy persons (Table 3). Thus, the PPV (the proportion of persons with positive test results who actually had cancer) would be 900/10,800, or 8.3%. If the same test were performed in a population with a lower cancer prevalence of 0.1%, the PPV would fall to 0.9%, a ratio of 111 false positives for every true case of cancer detected.

Reliability (reproducibility), the ability of a test to obtain the same result when repeated, is another important consideration in the evaluation of screening tests. An accurate test with poor reliability, whether due to differences in results obtained by different individuals or laboratories (*interobserver variation*) or by the same observer (*intraobserver variation*), may produce results that vary widely from the correct value, even though the average of the results approximates the true value.

Effectiveness of Early Detection.   Even if the test accurately detects early-stage disease, one must also question whether there is any benefit to the patient in having done so. Early detection should lead to the implementation of clinical interventions that can prevent or delay progression of the disorder. Detection of the disorder is of little clinical value if the condition is not treatable. Thus, *treatment efficacy* is fundamental for an effective screening test. Even with the availability

Table 3.
Positive Predictive Value (PPV) and Prevalence

Testing Conditions

Size of Population = 100,000
Sensitivity of Test = 90%
Specificity of Test = 90%

	Cancer Prevalence = 1%			Cancer Prevalence = 0.1%	
	Cancer Present	Cancer Absent		Cancer Present	Cancer Absent
Positive Test	900	9900	Positive Test	90	9990
Negative Test	100	89,100	Negative Test	10	89,910
	PPV = 8.3%			PPV = 0.9%	

of an efficacious form of treatment, *early detection* must offer added benefit over conventional diagnosis and treatment if screening is to improve outcome. The effectiveness of a screening test is questionable if asymptomatic persons detected through screening have the same clinical outcome as those who first present with symptoms.

Lead-Time and Length Bias.   It is often very difficult to determine with certainty whether early detection truly improves outcome. This is a common problem when evaluating cancer screening tests. For most forms of cancer, five-year survival is higher for persons with early-stage disease.[4] Such data are often interpreted as evidence that early detection of cancer is effective, because death due to cancer appears to be delayed as a result of screening and early treatment. Survival data do not constitute true proof of benefit, however, because they are easily influenced by *lead-time bias*: Survival can appear to be lengthened when screening simply advances the time of diagnosis, lengthening the period of time between diagnosis and death without any true prolongation of life.[5]

Length bias can also result in overestimation of the effectiveness of cancer screening. This refers to the tendency of screening to detect a disproportionate number of cases of slowly progressive disease and to miss aggressive cases that, by virtue of rapid progression, are present in the population only briefly. The "window" between the time a cancer can be detected by screening and the time it will be found because of symptoms is shorter for rapidly growing cancers, so they are less likely to be found by screening. As a result, persons with aggressive malignancies will be underrepresented in the cases detected by screening, and the cases found by screening may do better than average even if the screening itself does not influence outcome. Due to this bias, the calculated survival of persons detected through screening could overestimate the actual effectiveness of screening.[5]

Assessing Population Benefits.   Although these considerations provide necessary information about the clinical effectiveness of preventive services, other factors must often be examined to obtain a broader picture of the potential health impact on the population as a whole. Interventions of only minor effectiveness in terms of *relativo riok* may have significant impact on the population in terms of absolute risk if the target condition is common and associated with significant morbidity and mortality. Under these circumstances, a highly effective intervention (in terms of relative risk) that is applied to a small high-risk group may save fewer lives than one of only modest clinical effectiveness applied to large numbers of affected persons (see Table 4). Failure to consider these epidemiologic characteristics of the target condition can lead to misconceptions about overall effectiveness.

Potential adverse effects of interventions must also be considered in assessing overall health impact, but often these effects receive inadequate attention when effectiveness is evaluated. For example, the widely held belief that early detection of disease is beneficial leads many to advocate screening even in the absence of definitive evidence of benefit. Some may discount the clinical significance of potential adverse effects. A critical examination will often reveal that many kinds of testing, especially among ostensibly healthy persons, have potential adverse effects. Direct physical complications from a test procedure (e.g., colonic perforation during sigmoidoscopy), labeling and diagnostic errors based on test results (see above), and increased economic costs are all potential consequences of screening tests. Resources devoted to costly screening programs of uncertain effectiveness may consume time, personnel, or money needed for other more effective health care services. In this report, potential adverse effects are considered clinically relevant and are always evaluated along with potential benefits in determining whether a preventive service should be recommended.

Methodology for Reviewing Evidence

In evaluating effectiveness, the Task Force used a systematic approach to collect evidence from published clinical research and to judge the quality of individual studies.

Literature Retrieval Methods.   Studies were obtained for review by computerized literature search of MEDLARS. Keywords used for each topic are available on request. The reference list was supplemented by citations obtained from experts and from reviews of bibliographic listings, textbooks, and other sources. This report was completed in February 1989, and studies published subsequently are not addressed.

Exclusion Criteria.   Many preventive services involve tests or procedures that are not used exclusively in the context of primary or secondary prevention. Sigmoidoscopy, for example, is also performed for purposes other than screening. Thus, studies evaluating the effectiveness of procedures or tests involving patients

Table 4.
Effect of Morality Rate on Total Deaths Prevented

Reduction in Mortality with Intervention	Deaths per Year from Target Condition	Total Deaths Prevented with Intervention
50%	10	5
1%	100,000	1000

who are symptomatic or have a history of the target condition are not considered admissible evidence for evaluating effectiveness in asymptomatic persons. Such tests are instead considered *diagnostic tests*, even if they are described by investigators as "screening tests." Uncontrolled studies, comparisons between time and place (cross-cultural studies, studies with historical controls), descriptive data, and animal studies have also been excluded from the review process when evidence from randomized controlled trials, cohort studies, or case-control studies (see below) is available. *Etiologic evidence*, which demonstrates a causal relationship between a risk factor and a disease, was considered less persuasive than evidence from well-designed *intervention studies*, which measure the effectiveness of modifying the risk factor. As mentioned above, studies of preventive interventions not performed by clinicians were excluded from review.

Evaluating the Quality of the Evidence.   The methodologic quality of individual studies has received special emphasis in this report. Although all types of evidence were considered, increased weight was given to well-designed studies. Three types of study designs received special emphasis: randomized controlled trials, cohort studies, and case-control studies. In *randomized controlled trials*, participants are assigned in a randomized fashion to a study group (which receives the intervention) or a control group (which receives a standard treatment, which may be no intervention or a placebo). Randomization enhances the comparability of the two groups and provides a more valid basis for measuring statistical uncertainty. In this manner, differences in outcome can be attributed to the intervention rather than to other differences between groups. In a *blinded* trial, the investigators, the subjects, or both (*double-blind study*) are not told to which group subjects have been assigned, so that this knowledge will not influence their assessment of outcome. Controlled trials that are not randomized are subject to a variety of biases, including *selection bias*: Persons who volunteer or are assigned by investigators to study groups may differ in characteristics other than the intervention itself.

A *cohort study* differs from a clinical trial in that the investigators do not determine at the outset which persons receive the intervention or exposure. Rather, persons who have already been exposed and controls who have not been exposed are selected by the investigators to be followed *longitudinally* over time in an effort to observe differences in outcome. The Framingham Heart Study, for example, is a large ongoing cohort study providing longitudinal data on cardiovascular disease in residents of a Massachusetts community in whom potential cardiovascular risk factors were first measured over 30 years ago. Cohort studies are therefore *observational*, whereas clinical trials are *experimental*. Cohort studies are more subject to systematic bias than randomized trials because treatments, risk factors, and other covariables may be chosen by patients or physicians on the basis of important (and often unrecognized) factors that are related to outcome. It is therefore especially important for investigators to identify and correct for *confounding variables*, related factors that may be more directly responsible for clinical outcome than the intervention/exposure in question. For example, increased mortality among persons with low body weight can be due to the confounding variable of underlying illness.

Both cohort studies and clinical trials have the disadvantage of often requiring large sample sizes and/or many years of observation to provide adequate *statistical power* to measure differences in outcome. Failure to demonstrate a significant effect in such studies may be the result of statistical properties of the study design rather than a true reflection of poor clinical effectiveness. Both clinical trials and cohort studies have the advantage, however, of generally being *prospective* in design: the clinical outcome is not known at the beginning of the study and therefore is less likely to influence the collection of data.

Large sample sizes and lengthy follow-up periods are often unnecessary in *case-control studies*. This type of study differs from cohort studies and clinical trials in that the study and control groups are selected on the basis of whether they have the *disease* (cases) rather than whether they have been *exposed* to a risk factor or clinical intervention. The design is therefore *retrospective*, with the clinical outcome already known at the outset. In contrast to the Framingham Heart Study, a case-control study might first identify persons who have suffered myocardial infarction (cases) and those who have not (controls) and evaluate both groups to assess differences in risk factors preceding the onset of clinical disease. Principal disadvantages of this study design are that important confounding variables may be difficult to identify and adjust for, clinical outcome is already known and may influence the measurement and interpretation of data (*observer bias*), and participants may have difficulty in accurately recalling past medical history and previous exposures (*recall bias*).

Other types of study designs, such as cross-cultural studies, uncontrolled cohort studies, and case reports, provide useful data but do not generally provide strong evidence for or against effectiveness. Cross-cultural comparisons can demonstrate differences in disease rates between populations or countries, but these may be due to a variety of genetic and environmental factors other than the variable in question. Uncontrolled studies may demonstrate impressive treatment results or better outcomes than have been observed in the past (historical controls), but the absence of internal controls raises the question of whether the results would have occurred even in the absence of the intervention, perhaps as a result of other concurrent medical advances or case-selection. For further background on methodologic issues in evaluating clinical research, the reader is referred to several recent reviews.[5-7]

In summary, claims of effectiveness in published research must be interpreted with careful attention to the type of study design. Impressive findings, even if reported to be statistically significant, may be an artifact of measurement error, the manner in which participants were selected, or other design flaws rather than a reflection of a true effect on clinical outcome. In particular, p-values measure only random variability in results and do not account for bias; thus, even impressively low p-values are of little value when the data may be subject to substantial bias. Conversely, research findings suggesting ineffectiveness may result from low statistical power, inadequate follow-up, and other design limitations.

The quality of the evidence is therefore as important as the results. For these reasons, the U.S. Preventive Services Task Force established a hierarchy of evidence in which greater weight was given to those study designs that are, in general, less subject to bias and misinterpretation. The hierarchy ranked the following designs in decreasing order of importance: randomized controlled trials, nonrandomized controlled trials, cohort studies, case-control studies, comparisons between time and places, uncontrolled experiments, descriptive studies, and expert opinion. For many of the preventive services examined in this report, the Task Force assigned "evidence ratings" reflecting this hierarchy using a five-point scale (I, II-1, etc.) adapted from the scheme developed originally by the Canadian Task Force on the Periodic Health Examination (see Appendix A).[8-11]

Translating Science into Clinical Practice Recommendations

The strength of recommendations to perform or not perform a preventive service is based on the quality of the evidence that its performance will result in more good than harm. Interventions that have been proved effective in well-designed studies or have demonstrated consistent benefit in a large number of studies of weaker design are generally recommended in this report. Interventions that have been proved to be ineffective or harmful are generally not recommended. Some preventive services are described as "clinically prudent," even though convincing evidence of effectiveness is lacking. This occurs when performance of the maneuver is not associated with significant harm or cost but has the potential of reducing the incidence of a leading cause of death or suffering in the specified group for which it is recommended. Maneuvers are often recommended for high-risk groups even though there is no additional evidence of greater effectiveness in these individuals than in the general population. This policy is based on the recognition that the absence of evidence of effectiveness does not rule out effectiveness; if, in fact, the maneuver is effective, individuals at increased risk of developing the disease are most likely to benefit.

For some preventive services no recommendation is made, because the evidence is inadequate to support a recommendation for or against performing the maneuver. For example, there is generally little scientific evidence regarding the clinical effectiveness of teaching self-examination of the breast, testes, or skin. Under these circumstances, available data are so limited that the clinician is best advised to exercise individual judgment and discretion on a case-by-case basis. Similarly, there are often inadequate data to determine the optimal frequency for performing preventive services. Rather than suggesting an arbitrary interval for testing that is not scientifically defensible, the Task Force generally recommends that clinicians use individual judgment in choosing an appropriate interval based on the patient's medical history and personal circumstances.

Some preventive services are specifically not recommended even though there is no convincing evidence that they are ineffective. This position is taken with those interventions whose potential adverse effects are of clinical concern, as well as those procedures that could generate significant increases in health care costs were they to be performed on a large proportion of the population. For example, even though further research is needed to fully evaluate the effectiveness of ultrasound screening for cancer of the prostate, ovary, or pancreas, this test is specifically not recommended by the Task Force pending the results of these studies. In addition to the potential risks of false-positive labeling, routine ultrasound screening of the general population would be costly and could divert limited resources needed for other more effective health care services. Under these circumstances, the Task Force required evidence of effectiveness before recommending widespread implementation of the preventive service.

In selected situations, even preventive services of proven effectiveness may not be recommended due to concerns about feasibility and compliance. Benefits observed under carefully controlled experimental conditions may not be generalizable to normal medical practice. That is, the preventive service may have proven *efficacy* but may lack *effectiveness*. It may be difficult for clinicians to perform the procedure in the same manner as investigators with special expertise and a standardized protocol. Patients may be less willing than research volunteers to comply with interventions that lack widespread acceptability. The cost of the procedure and other logistical considerations may make implementation of the recommendation difficult for the health care system without compromising quality or the delivery of other health care services.

For some preventive services examined by the Task Force, recommendations to perform or exclude the maneuver from the periodic health examination have been assigned a rating from a five-point (A–E) scale developed originally by the Canadian Task Force on the Periodic Health Examination (see Appendix A).[8–11]

The rationale for these ratings is outlined in background papers available for review in a separate publication.[12] Background papers on selected preventive services have also been published in the *Journal of the American Medical Association*.[13-20] For the majority of topics examined in this report, which were not examined in this manner, scientific reviews and evaluations were conducted under Task Force supervision by scientific staff who were recruited by the Task Force and based at the Office of Disease Prevention and Health Promotion in Washington, D.C.

Outside Review Process

The Task Force recommendations have been reviewed by over 300 experts in Government health agencies, academic medical centers, and medical organizations in the United States, Canada, and the United Kingdom. The report has received extensive review by representatives of the U.S. Public Health Service. Recommendations were modified on the basis of reviewer comments if the reviewer identified relevant studies not examined in the report, misinterpretations of findings, or other issues deserving revision within the constraints of the Task Force methodology. The format of this report was designed in consultation with representatives of medical specialty organizations, including the American Medical Association, the American College of Physicians, the American Academy of Family Physicians, the American Academy of Pediatrics, the American College of Obstetricians and Gynecologists, the American College of Preventive Medicine, the American Dental Association, and the American Osteopathic Association.[21]

Recommendations appearing in this report are intended as guidelines, providing clinicians with information on the proven effectiveness of preventive services in published clinical research. Recommendations for or against performing these maneuvers should not be interpreted as standards of care but rather as statements regarding the quality of the supporting scientific evidence. Clinicians with limited time can use this information to help select the preventive services most likely to benefit patients in selected risk categories. However, sound clinical decisionmaking requires careful consideration of many variables; the science base must be examined along with other important aspects of the medical history and the clinical setting. Departure from these recommendations by clinicians familiar with a patient's individual circumstances is often appropriate and should not necessarily be interpreted by patients or others as compromising quality of care.

REFERENCES

1. Battista RN, Fletcher SW. Making recommendations on preventive practices: methodological issues. Am J Prev Med [Suppl] 1988; 4:5367.
2. Lefebvre RC, Hursey KG, Carleton RA. Labeling of participants in high blood pressure screening programs: implications for blood cholesterol screenings. Arch Intern Med 1988; 148:1993–7.
3. MacDonald LA, Sackett DL, Haynes RB, et al. Labelling in hypertension: a review of the behavioural and psychological consequences. J Chron Dis 1984; 37:933–42.
4. American Cancer Society. Cancer statistics, 1989. CA 1989; 39:332.
5. Sackett DL, Haynes RB, Tugwell P. Clinical epidemiology. Boston: Little, Brown, 1985.
6. Fletcher RH, Fletcher SW, Wagner EH. Clinical epidemiology: the essentials. Baltimore, Md.: Williams and Wilkins, 1988.
7. Bailar JC III, Mosteller F, eds. Medical uses of statistics. Waltham, Mass.: NEJM Books, 1986.
8. Canadian Task Force on the Periodic Health Examination. The periodic health examination. Can Med Assoc J 1979; 121:1193–254.

9. *Idem*. The periodic health examination. 1984 update. Can Med Assoc J 1984; 130: 1278–85.

10. *Idem*. The periodic health examination. 1986 update. Can Med Assoc J 1986; 134: 721–9.

11. *Idem*. The periodic health examination. 1988 update. Can Med Assoc J 1988; 138: 617–26.

12. Lawrence RS, Goldboom RB, eds. Preventing disease: beyond the rhetoric. New York: Springer-Verlag (in press).

13. O'Malley MS, Fletcher SW. Screening for breast cancer with breast self-examination: a critical review. JAMA 1987; 257:2197–203.

14. LaForce FM. Immunizations, immunoprophylaxis, and chemoprophylaxis to prevent selected infections. JAMA 1987; 257:2464–70.

15. Horsburgh CR, Douglas JM, LaForce FM. Preventive strategies in sexually transmitted diseases for the primary care physician. JAMA 1987; 258:815–21.

16. Kottke TE, Battista RN, DeFriese GH, et al. Attributes of successful smoking cessation interventions in medical practice: a meta-analysis of 39 controlled trials. JAMA 1988; 259:2882–9.

17. Polen MR, Friedman GD. Automobile injury: selected risk factors and prevention in the health care setting. JAMA 1988; 259:76–80.

18. Knight KK, Fielding JE, Battista RN. Occult blood screening for colorectal cancer. JAMA 1989; 261:587–93.

19. Selby JV, Friedman GD. Sigmoidoscopy in the periodic health examination. JAMA 1989; 261:595–602.

20. Harris SS, Caspersen CJ, DeFriese GH, et al. Physical activity counseling for healthy adults as a primary preventive intervention in the clinical setting: report for the US Preventive Services Task Force. JAMA 1989; 261:3590–8.

21. Centers for Disease Control. Chronic disease control activities of medical and dental organizations. MMWR 1988; 37:325–8.

iii.

The Periodic Health Examination: Age-Specific Charts

The periodic health visit is an important opportunity for the delivery of clinical preventive services. Determining the specific preventive services that are most appropriate for inclusion in the periodic health examination has been one of the principal objectives of the U.S. Preventive Services Task Force project. The process by which these determinations were made is discussed in detail in Chapter ii. This chapter explores the recommended *content* of the periodic health examination. It includes a series of eight tables that list the specific preventive services that should be considered for patients in different age groups.

The Task Force judged it especially important to tailor the content of the periodic health examination to the individual needs of the patient and to emphasize those preventive services that have proved to be effective in properly conducted studies. This approach is based on the recognition that the leading causes of illness and injury in an individual patient depend on age, sex, and other risk factors. The clinician whose time with patients is limited is therefore best advised to target preventive measures toward those conditions most likely to significantly influence the health and well-being of the patient being examined. The two most important factors to consider are the leading causes of morbidity and mortality in the patient and the potential effectiveness of clinical interventions in altering the natural history of those diseases.

Leading causes of morbidity and mortality are essential to consider with each patient if the clinician is to determine which conditions are most important to prevent. Failure to do so can lead to misplaced priorities when performing the periodic health examination. For example, a clinician wishing to include a preventive measure during the few remaining minutes of an office visit with an adolescent male might consider teaching the patient how to perform testicular self-examination. An estimated 350 persons will die from testicular cancer in the United States during 1989, and it is believed that early detection is an important means of improving survival.[1] However, a teenage male is considerably more likely to die from an injury than from cancer or any other disease. Of the 39,929 deaths among young persons (aged 15–24 years) in the United States during 1986, 19,975 were due to injuries (15,227 due to motor vehicles crashes), 5522 were due to homicides, and 5120 were the result of suicide.[2] All forms of cancer combined accounted for only 2115 deaths in this age group.[2] It seems likely on the basis of mortality data alone that a few minutes with an adolescent might be more productively spent by discussing the prevention of unintentional and intentional injuries. Leading causes of morbidity, such as unintended pregnancy, depression, and drug abuse, are also important target conditions.

Clinical efforts directed toward these important conditions may be of limited value, however, if the preventive intervention does not result in improved outcome.

Thus, the second major consideration in setting priorities is effectiveness. Although homicide and suicide are leading causes of death among adolescents, the effectiveness of efforts by clinicians to prevent deaths from intentional injuries has not been established (see Chapters 45 and 46). However, measures to reduce the risk of motor vehicle injuries, the leading cause of death in this age group, are well established. Proper use of safety belts has proved to reduce the risk of injury and death from motor vehicle crashes by as much as 40–60%.[3,4] Alcohol intoxication is associated with half of all injury fatalities.[5,6] With one out of three deaths among young persons occurring in motor vehicle crashes,[2] the busy clinician seeing young patients is best advised to direct attention to the use of safety belts and the dangers of driving while under the influence of alcohol.

Age is only one of many risk factors the clinician must consider in designing an appropriate periodic health examination. Among persons in special high-risk groups, the leading causes of morbidity and mortality may differ considerably from other individuals of the same age and sex. For example, although sexually transmitted diseases and unintended pregnancy are unlikely problems for sexually abstinent teenagers, they are important sources of morbidity among those who are sexually active. One out of four cases of gonorrhea (195,274 cases) reported in the United States during 1987 occurred among persons aged 10–19.[7] Intravenous drug use is also uncommon in the general population, but among individuals with this history, acquired immunodeficiency syndrome (AIDS) is the leading cause of death.[8] Thus, the most important preventive interventions in the periodic health examination of an intravenous drug user are counseling to obtain treatment for chemical dependency and education about measures to prevent transmission of infectious disease. These and other methodologic issues in establishing priorities for performing preventive services are discussed in greater detail in Chapter ii.

The differences in priorities among individuals in different age groups and risk categories and the effectiveness of some preventive services in only certain populations suggest that a uniform periodic health examination cannot be recommended for all persons. The reader will note that recommendations throughout this report are targeted toward individuals who meet specific risk factor criteria; only rarely do they apply universally to all patients. While it is therefore difficult to design a periodic health examination that accounts fully for differences among patients, the eight tables that follow identify those recommended preventive services that should be considered for patients in specific age groups.

The reader is urged to refer to appropriate chapters in this report to obtain more detailed information about the proper indications for specific preventive services than can be provided in the tables. The review of evidence in the text also provides the scientific rationale for the recommendations, which are based on a systematic methodology (see Chapter ii). The reader can also compare the Task Force recommendations with those of major organizations and Government agencies, which are listed in each chapter under the heading *Recommendations of Others*. In addition, all chapters include a detailed *Clinical Intervention* section that provides concise information for the clinician on currently recommended techniques, dosages, and other specifics for performing recommended preventive services.

The preventive services examined in this report and appearing in Tables 1–8 have been carefully defined. They include only those preventive services that would be performed by clinicians on asymptomatic persons in the context of routine health care (see Chapter ii). Preventive measures involving persons with signs or symptoms of disease and those performed outside the clinical setting are not within the scope of this report or its recommendations.

The tables are not intended to be a complete list of all preventive services that should be offered during the periodic health examination. Rather, these recommendations encompass only those preventive services that have been examined in the report and that have been chown to have satisfactory evidence of clinical effectiveness, based on the methodology discussed in Chapter ii. Since the evaluations were defined by specific preventive services, general procedures such as the medical history and the physical examination were not examined in their entirety. *The interventions listed are therefore not exhaustive.* The periodic health examination performed by most pediatricians, for example, includes a number of maneuvers that were not examined by the Task Force, such as screening for developmental disorders and anticipatory guidance. The interested reader should refer to the recommendations of other groups for futher information on such topics.[9,10] Similarly, recommendations relating to preventive services during pregnancy should not be interpreted as comprehensive guidelines for prenatal care.

Recommendations by the Task Force against performing certain preventive services are not intended to be unconditional. The clinician may judge such maneuvers to be appropriate in light of the medical history of the patient, local standards of care, or other individual circumstances.

Many of the preventive services appearing in Tables 1–8 are recommended only for members of high-risk groups and are not considered appropriate in the routine examination of all persons in the age group. The specific risk groups for which the maneuver is considered appropriate are identified by an annotated *high-risk* (HR) *code* accompanying each table. The reader should refer to appropriate chapters in the report for more detailed guidelines to help identify individuals at increased risk. Risk factors that are especially important for clinicians to identify at an early stage but that are not considered appropriate for routine screening are listed under the heading *Remain Alert For.* Many of the disorders appearing under this heading are often overlooked by clinicians due to failure to recognize suggestive signs or symptoms or the importance of early identification.

A frequency schedule for periodic health visits is recommended in each table. These intervals are considered clinically prudent; however, scientific data are lacking to determine the optimal frequency for such visits. Clinicians should exercise discretion in selecting an appropriate schedule, especially for patients with abnormal signs or symptoms and those with chronic illness. *The preventive services listed in each table are not necessarily recommended at every periodic visit.* For example, although thyroid function tests may be clinically prudent in elderly women, they are not recommended annually even though periodic visits in this age group are recommended once a year.

Although the preventive services listed in Tables 1–8 can serve as the basis for designing periodic checkups devoted entirely to disease prevention, they may also be performed during visits for other reasons (e.g., illness visits, chronic disease checkups) when indicated. For patients with limited access to care, the illness visit may provide the only realistic opportunity for the clinician to discuss prevention. It is recognized that busy clinicians may not be able to perform all recommended preventive services during a single clinical encounter. Indeed, it is not clear that such a grouping is either necessary or clinically effective. Patients suffering from an acute illness or injury may not be receptive to some preventive interventions. The clinician must therefore use discretion in selecting appropriate preventive services from these lists and may wish to give special emphasis to those preventive services aimed at the leading causes of illness and disability in the age group. Age-specific *leading causes of death* are listed in each table to aid the clinician in making this assessment. Recommended preventive services that cannot be performed by the clinician could be scheduled for a later health visit.

Immunizations appearing in Tables 1–8 are those recommended on a routine

Table 1.
Birth to 18 Months
Schedule: 2, 4, 6, 15, 18 Months*

Leading Causes of Death:
Conditions originating in
  perinatal period
Congenital anomalies
Heart disease
Injuries (nonmotor vehicle)
Pneumonia/influenza

SCREENING

Height and weight
Hemoglobin and hematocrit[1]
HIGH-RISK GROUPS
  Hearing[2] (HR1)
  Erythrocyte protoporphyrin
    (HR2)

This list of preventive services is not exhaustive.
It reflects only those topics reviewed by the U.S. Preventive Services Task Force. Clinicians may wish to add other preventive services on a routine basis, and after considering the patient's medical history and other individual circumstances. Examples of target conditions not specifically examined by the Task Force include:
  Developmental disorders
  Musculoskeletal malformations
  Cardiac anomalies
  Genitourinary disorders
  Metabolic disorders
  Speech problems
  Behavioral disorders
  Parent/family dysfunction

PARENT COUNSELING

Diet
Breastfeeding
Nutrient intake, especially iron-rich
  foods

Injury Prevention
Child safety seats
Smoke detector
Hot water heater temperature
Stairway gates, window guards, pool
  fence
Storage of drugs and toxic chemicals
Syrup of ipecac, poison control telephone number

Dental Health
Baby bottle tooth decay

**Other Primary
Preventive Measures**
Effects of passive smoking

IMMUNIZATIONS & CHEMOPROPHYLAXIS

Diphtheria-tetanus-pertussis
  (DTP) vaccine[3]
Oral poliovirus vaccine
  (OPV)[4]
Measles-mumps-rubella
  (MMR) vaccine[5]
Haemophilus influenzae
  type b (Hib) conjugate
  vaccine[6]
HIGH-RISK GROUPS
  Fluoride supplements
    (HR3)

FIRST WEEK
Ophthalmic antibiotics[7]
Hemoglobin electrophoresis
  (HR4)[7]
T4/TSH[8]
Phenylalanine[8]
Hearing (HR1)

Remain Alert For:
Ocular misalignment
Tooth decay
Signs of child abuse or
  neglect

*Five visits are required for immunizations. Because of lack of data and differing patient risk profiles, the scheduling of additional visits and the frequency of the individual preventive services listed in this table are left to clinical discretion (except as indicated in other footnotes).

1. Once during infancy. 2. At age 18-month visit, if not tested earlier. 3. At ages 2, 4, 6, and 15 months. 4. At ages 2, 4, and 15 months. 5. At age 15 months. 6. At age 18 months. 7. At birth. 8. Days 3 to 6 preferred for testing.

Table 1.   Birth to 18 Months   High-Risk Categories

HR1 Infants with a family history of childhood hearing impairment or a personal history of congenital perinatal infection with herpes, syphilis, rubella, cytomegalovirus, or toxoplasmosis; malformations involving the head or neck (e.g., dysmorphic and syndromal abnormalities, cleft palate, abnormal pinna); birthweight below 1500 g; bacterial meningitis; hyperbilirubinemia requiring exchange transfusion; or severe perinatal asphyxia (Apgar scores of 0–3, absence of spontaneous respirations for 10 minutes, or hypotonia at 2 hours of age).

HR2 Infants who live in or frequently visit housing built before 1950 that is dilapidated or undergoing renovation; who come in contact with other children with known lead toxicity; who live near lead processing plants or whose parents or household members work in a lead-related occupation; or who live near busy highways or hazardous waste sites.

HR3 Infants living in areas with inadequate water fluoridation (less than 0.7 parts per million).

HR4 Newborns of Caribbean, Latin American, Asian, Mediterranean, or African descent.

Table 2.
Ages 2–6
Schedule: See Footnote*

Leading Causes of Death:
Injuries (nonmotor vehicle)
Motor vehicle crashes
Congenital anomalies
Homicide
Heart disease

SCREENING

Height and weight
Blood pressure
Eye exam for amblyopia
  and strabismus[1]
Urinalysis for bacteriuria
HIGH-RISK GROUPS
  Erythrocyte protopor-
    phyrin[2] (HR1)
  Tuberculin skin test (PPD)
    (HR2)
  Hearing[3] (HR3)

This list of preventive services is not exhaustive. It reflects only those topics reviewed by the U.S. Preventive Services Task Force. Clinicians may wish to add other preventive services on a routine basis, and after considering the patient's medical history and other individual circumstances. Examples of target conditions not specifically examined by the Task Force include:
  Developmental disorders
  Speech problems
  Behavioral and learning
    disorders
  Parent/family dysfunction

PATIENT & PARENT COUNSELING

Diet and Exercise
Sweets and between-meal snacks,
  iron-enriched foods, sodium
Caloric balance
Selection of exercise program

Injury Prevention
Safety belts
Smoke detector
Hot water heater temperature
Window guards and pool fence
Bicycle safety helmets
Storage of drugs, toxic chemicals,
  matches, and firearms
Syrup of ipecac, poison control tele-
  phone number

Dental Health
Tooth brushing and dental visits

Other Primary Preventive Measures
Effects of passive smoking
HIGH-RISK GROUPS
  Skin protection from ultraviolet light
    (HR4)

IMMUNIZATIONS & CHEMOPROPHYLAXIS

Diphtheria-tetanus-pertussis
  (DTP) vaccine[4]
Oral poliovirus vaccine
  (OPV)[4]
HIGH-RISK GROUPS
  Fluoride supplements
    (HR5)

Remain Alert For:
Vision disorders
Dental decay, malalignment,
  premature loss of teeth,
  mouth breathing
Signs of child abuse or
  neglect
Abnormal bereavement

---

*One visit is required for immunizations. Because of lack of data and differing patient risk profiles, the scheduling of additional visits and the frequency of the individual preventive services listed in this table are left to clinical discretion (except as indicated in other footnotes).

1. Ages 3–4.   2. Annually.   3. Before age 3, if not tested earlier.   4. Once between ages 4 and 6.

Table 2. Ages 2–6   High-Risk Categories

HR1 Children who live in or frequently visit housing built before 1950 that is dilapidated or undergoing renovation; who come in contact with other children with known lead toxicity; who live near lead processing plants or whose parents or household members work in a lead-related occupation; or who live near busy highways or hazardous waste sites.

HR2 Household members of persons with tuberculosis or others at risk for close contact with the disease; recent immigrants or refugees from countries in which tuberculosis is common (e.g., Asia, Africa, Central and South America, Pacific Islands); family members of migrant workers; residents of homeless shelters; or persons with certain underlying medical disorders.

HR3 Children with a family history of childhood hearing impairment or a personal history of congenital perinatal infection with herpes, syphilis, rubella, cytomegalovirus, or toxoplasmosis; malformations involving the head or neck (e.g., dysmorphic and syndromal abnormalities, cleft palate, abnormal pinna); birthweight below 1500 g; bacterial meningitis; hyperbilirubinemia requiring exchange transfusion; or severe perinatal asphyxia (Apgar scores of 0–3, absence of spontaneous respirations for 10 minutes, or hypotonia at 2 hours of age).

HR4 Children with increased exposure to sunlight.

HR5 Children living in areas with inadequate water fluoridation (less than 0.7 parts per million).

Table 3.
Ages 7–12
Schedule: See Footnote*

Leading Causes of Death:
Motor vehicle crashes
Injuries (nonmotor vehicle)
Congenital anomalies
Leukemia
Homicide
Heart disease

SCREENING

Height and weight
Blood pressure
HIGH-RISK GROUPS
　Tuberculin skin test (PPD)
　(HR1)

This list of preventive services is not exhaustive. It
reflects only those topics reviewed by the U.S. Preventive Services Task Force.
Clinicians may wish to add
other preventive services on
a routine basis, and after
considering the patient's
medical history and other individual circumstances. Examples of target conditions
not specifically examined by
the Task Force include:
　Developmental disorders
　Scoliosis
　Behavioral and learning
　　disorders
　Parent/family dysfunction

PATIENT & PARENT COUNSELING

Diet and Exercise
Fat (especially saturated fat), choles-
　terol, sweets and between-meal
　snacks, sodium
Caloric balance
Selection of exercise program

Injury Prevention
Safety belts
Smoke detector
Storage of firearms, drugs, toxic
　chemicals, matches
Bicycle safety helmets

Dental Health
Regular tooth brushing and dental
　visits

Other Primary Preventive Measures
HIGH-RISK GROUPS
　Skin protection from ultraviolet light
　(HR2)

CHEMOPROPHYLAXIS

HIGH-RISK GROUPS
　Fluoride supplements
　(HR3)

Remain Alert For:
Vision disorders
Diminished hearing
Dental decay, malalignment,
　mouth breathing
Signs of child abuse or
　neglect
Abnormal bereavement

*Because of lack of data and differing patient risk profiles, the scheduling of visits and the frequency
of the individual preventive services listed in this table are left to clinical discretion.

Table 3.   Ages 7–12   High-Risk Categories

HR1   Household members of persons with tuberculosis or others at risk for close contact with the disease; recent immigrants or refugees from countries in which tuberculosis is common (e.g., Asia, Africa, Central and South America, Pacific Islands); family members of migrant workers; residents of homeless shelters, or persons with certain underlying medical disorders.

HR2   Children with increased exposure to sunlight.

HR3   Children living in areas with inadequate water fluoridation (less than 0.7 parts per million).

Table 4.
Ages 13–18
Schedule: See Footnote*

Leading Causes of Death:
Motor vehicle crashes
Homicide
Suicide
Injuries (nonmotor vehicle)
Heart disease

SCREENING

History
Dietary intake
Physical activity
Tobacco/alcohol/drug use
Sexual practices

Physical Exam
Height and weight
Blood pressure
HIGH-RISK GROUPS
Complete skin exam
(HR1)
Clinical testicular exam
(HR2)

Laboratory/Diagnostic Procedures
HIGH-RISK GROUPS
Rubella antibodies (HR3)
VDRL/RPR (HR4)
Chlamydial testing (HR5)
Gonorrhea culture (HR6)
Counseling and testing for
HIV (HR7)
Tuberculin skin test (PPD)
(HR8)
Hearing (HR9)
Papanicolaou smear
(HR10)[1]

COUNSELING

Diet and Exercise
Fat (especially saturated fat), cholesterol, sodium, iron,[2] calcium[2]
Caloric balance
Selection of exercise program

Substance Use
Tobacco: cessation/primary prevention
Alcohol and other drugs: cessation/ primary prevention
Driving/other dangerous activities while under the influence
Treatment for abuse
HIGH-RISK GROUPS
Sharing/using unsterilized needles and syringes (HR12)

Sexual Practices
Sexual development and behavior[3]
Sexually transmitted diseases: partner selection, condoms
Unintended pregnancy and contraceptive options

Injury Prevention
Safety belts
Safety helmets
Violent behavior[4]
Firearms[4]
Smoke detector

Dental Health
Regular tooth brushing, flossing, dental visits

Other Primary Preventive Measures
HIGH-RISK GROUPS
Discussion of hemoglobin testing (HR13)
Skin protection from ultraviolet light (HR14)

IMMUNIZATIONS & CHEMOPROPHYLAXIS

Tetanus-diphtheria (Td) booster[5]
HIGH-RISK GROUPS
Fluoride supplements (HR15)

This list of preventive services is not exhaustive. It reflects only those topics reviewed by the U.S. Preventive Services Task Force. Clinicians may wish to add other preventive services on a routine basis, and after considering the patient's medical history and other individual circumstances. Examples of target conditions not specifically examined by the Task Force include:
Developmental disorders
Scoliosis
Behavioral and learning disorders
Parent/family dysfunction

Remain Alert For:
Depressive symptoms
Suicide risk factors (HR11)
Abnormal bereavement
Tooth decay, malalignment, gingivitis
Signs of child abuse and neglect.

*One visit is required for immunizations. Because of lack of data and differing patient risk profiles, the scheduling of additional visits and the frequency of the individual preventive services listed in this table are left to clinical discretion (except as indicated in other footnotes).

1. Every 1–3 years. 2. For females. 3. Often best performed early in adolescence and with the involvement of parents. 4. Especially for males. 5. Once between ages 14 and 16.

Table 4.   Ages 13–18   High-Risk Categories

HR1 Persons with increased recreational or occupational exposure to sunlight, a family or personal history of skin cancer, or clinical evidence of precursor lesions (e.g., dysplastic nevi, certain congenital nevi).

HR2 Males with a history of cryptorchidism, orchiopexy, or testicular atrophy.

HR3 Females of childbearing age lacking evidence of immunity.

HR4 Persons who engage in sex with multiple partners in areas in which syphilis is prevalent, prostitutes, or contacts of persons with active syphilis.

HR5 Persons who attend clinics for sexually transmitted diseases; attend other high-risk health care facilities (e.g., adolescent and family planning clinics); or have other risk factors for chlamydial infection (e.g., multiple sexual partners or a sexual partner with multiple sexual contacts).

HR6 Persons with multiple sexual partners or a sexual partner with multiple contacts, sexual contacts of persons with culture-proven gonorrhea, or persons with a history of repeated episodes of gonorrhea.

HR7 Persons seeking treatment for sexually transmitted diseases; homosexual and bisexual men; past or present intravenous (IV) drug users; persons with a history of prostitution or multiple sexual partners; women whose past or present sexual partners were HIV-infected, bisexual, or IV drug users; persons with long-term residence or birth in an area with high prevalence of HIV infection; or persons with a history of transfusion between 1978 and 1985.

HR8 Household members of persons with tuberculosis or others at risk for close contact with the disease; recent immigrants or refugees from countries in which tuberculosis is common (e.g., Asia, Africa, Central and South America, Pacific Islands); migrant workers; residents of correctional institutions or homeless shelters; or persons with certain underlying medical disorders.

HR9 Persons exposed regularly to excessive noise in recreational or other settings.

HR10 Females who are sexually active or (if the sexual history is thought to be unreliable) aged 18 or older.

HR11 Recent divorce, separation, unemployment, depression, alcohol or other drug abuse, serious medical illnesses, living alone, or recent bereavement.

HR12 Intravenous drug users.

HR13 Persons of Caribbean, Latin American, Asian, Mediterranean, or African descent.

HR14 Persons with increased exposure to sunlight.

HR15 Persons living in areas with inadequate water fluoridation (less than 0.7 parts per million).

Table 5.
Ages 19–39
Schedule: Every 1–3 Years*

Leading Causes of Death:
Motor vehicle crashes
Homicide
Suicide
Injuries (nonmotor vehicle)
Heart disease

SCREENING

History
Dietary intake
Physical activity
Tobacco/alcohol/drug use
Sexual practices

Physical Exam
Height and weight
Blood pressure
HIGH-RISK GROUPS
Complete oral cavity exam (HR1)
Palpation for thyroid nodules (HR2)
Clinical breast exam (HR3)
Clinical testicular exam (HR4)
Complete skin exam (HR5)

Laboratory/Diagnostic Procedures
Nonfasting total blood cholesterol
Papanicolaou smear[1]
HIGH-RISK GROUPS
Fasting plasma glucose (HR6)
Rubella antibodies (HR7)
VDRL/RPR (HR8)
Urinalysis for bacteriuria (HR9)
Chlamydial testing (HR10)
Gonorrhea culture (HR11)
Counseling and testing for HIV (HR12)
Hearing (HR13)
Tuberculin skin test (PPD) (HR14)
Electrocardiogram (HR15)
Mammogram (HR3)
Colonoscopy (HR16)

COUNSELING

Diet and Exercise
Fat (especially saturated fat), cholesterol, complex carbohydrates, fiber, sodium, iron[2], calcium[2]
Caloric balance
Selection of exercise program

Substance Use
Tobacco: cessation/primary prevention
Alcohol and other drugs:
Limiting alcohol consumption
Driving/other dangerous activities while under the influence
Treatment for abuse
HIGH-RISK GROUPS
Sharing/using unsterilized needles and syringes (HR18)

Sexual Practices
Sexually transmitted diseases: partner selection, condoms, anal intercourse
Unintended pregnancy and contraceptive options

Injury Prevention
Safety belts
Safety helmets
Violent behavior[3]
Firearms[3]
Smoke detector
Smoking near bedding or upholstery
HIGH-RISK GROUPS
Back-conditioning exercises (HR19)
Prevention of childhood injuries (HR20)
Falls in the elderly (HR21)

Dental Health
Regular tooth brushing, flossing, dental visits

Other Primary Preventive Measures
HIGH-RISK GROUPS
Discussion of hemoglobin testing (HR22)
Skin protection from ultraviolet light (HR23)

IMMUNIZATIONS

Tetanus-diphtheria (Td) booster[4]
HIGH-RISK GROUPS
Hepatitis B vaccine (HR24)
Pneumococcal vaccine (HR25)
Influenza vaccine[5] (HR26)
Measles-mumps-rubella vaccine (HR27)

This list of preventive services is not exhaustive. It reflects only those topics reviewed by the U.S. Preventive Services Task Force. Clinicians may wish to add other preventive services on a routine basis, and after considering the patient's medical history and other individual circumstances. Examples of target conditions not specifically examined by the Task Force include:
Chronic obstructive pulmonary disease
Hepatobiliary disease
Bladder cancer
Endometrial disease
Travel-related illness
Prescription drug abuse
Occupational illness and injuries

Remain Alert For:
Depressive symptoms
Suicide risk factors (HR17)
Abnormal bereavement
Malignant skin lesions
Tooth decay, gingivitis
Signs of physical abuse

*The recommended schedule applies only to the periodic visit itself. The frequency of the individual preventive services listed in this table is left to clinical discretion, except as indicated in other footnotes.

1. Every 1–3 years.   2. For women.   3. Especially for young males.   4. Every 10 years.   5. Annually.

Table 5. Ages 19–39   High-Risk Categories

HR1 Persons with exposure to tobacco or excessive amounts of alcohol, or those with suspicious symptoms or lesions detected through self-examination.

HR2 Persons with a history of upper-body irradiation.

HR3 Women aged 35 and older with a family history of premenopausally diagnosed breast cancer in a first-degree relative.

HR4 Men with a history of cryptorchidism, orchiopexy, or testicular atrophy.

HR5 Persons with family or personal history of skin cancer, increased occupational or recreational exposure to sunlight, or clinical evidence of precursor lesions (e.g., dysplastic nevi, certain congenital nevi).

HR6 The markedly obese, persons with a family history of diabetes, or women with a history of gestational diabetes.

HR7 Women lacking evidence of immunity.

HR8 Prostitutes, persons who engage in sex with multiple partners in areas in which syphilis is prevalent, or contacts of persons with active syphilis.

HR9 Persons with diabetes.

HR10 Persons who attend clinics for sexually transmitted diseases; attend other high-risk health care facilities (e.g., adolescent and family planning clinics); or have other risk factors for chlamydial infection (e.g., multiple sexual partners or a sexual partner with multiple sexual contacts, age less than 20).

HR11 Prostitutes, persons with multiple sexual partners or a sexual partner with multiple contacts, sexual contacts of persons with culture-proven gonorrhea, or persons with a history of repeated episodes of gonorrhea.

HR12 Persons seeking treatment for sexually transmitted diseases; homosexual and bisexual men; past or present intravenous (IV) drug users; persons with a history of prostitution or multiple sexual partners; women whose past or present sexual partners were HIV-infected, bisexual, or IV drug users; persons with long-term residence or birth in an area with high prevalence of HIV infection; or persons with a history of transfusion between 1978 and 1985.

HR13 Persons exposed regularly to excessive noise.

HR14 Household members of persons with tuberculosis or others at risk for close contact with

the disease (e.g., staff of tuberculosis clinics, shelters for the homeless, nursing homes, substance abuse treatment facilities, dialysis units, correctional institutions); recent immigrants or refugees from countries in which tuberculosis is common; migrant workers; residents of nursing homes, correctional institutions, or homeless shelters; or persons with certain underlying medical disorders (e.g., HIV infection).

HR15 Men who would endanger public safety were they to experience sudden cardiac events (e.g., commercial airline pilots).

HR16 Persons with a family history of familial polyposis coli or cancer family syndrome.

HR17 Recent divorce, separation, unemployment, depression, alcohol or other drug abuse, serious medical illnesses, living alone, or recent bereavement.

HR18 Intravenous drug users.

HR19 Persons at increased risk for low back injury because of past history, body configuration, or type of activities.

HR20 Persons with children in the home or automobile.

HR21 Persons with older adults in the home.

HR22 Young adults of Caribbean, Latin American, Asian, Mediterranean, or African descent.

HR23 Persons with increased exposure to sunlight.

HR24 Homosexually active men, intravenous drug users, recipients of some blood products, or persons in health-related jobs with frequent exposure to blood or blood products.

HR25 Persons with medical conditions that increase the risk of pneumococcal infection (e.g., chronic cardiac or pulmonary disease, sickle cell disease, nephrotic syndrome, Hodgkin's disease, asplenia, diabetes mellitus, alcoholism, cirrhosis, multiple myeloma, renal disease, or conditions associated with immunosuppression).

HR26 Residents of chronic care facilities or persons suffering from chronic cardiopulmonary disorders, metabolic diseases (including diabetes mellitus), hemoglobinopathies, immunosuppression, or renal dysfunction.

HR27 Persons born after 1956 who lack evidence of immunity to measles (receipt of live vaccine on or after first birthday, laboratory evidence of immunity, or a history of physician-diagnosed measles).

Table 6.
Ages 40–64
Schedule: Every 1–3 Years*

Leading Causes of Death:
Heart disease
Lung cancer
Cerebrovascular disease
Breast cancer
Colorectal cancer
Obstructive lung disease

SCREENING

History
Dietary intake
Physical activity
Tobacco/alcohol/drug use
Sexual practices

Physical Exam
Height and weight
Blood pressure
Clinical breast exam[1]
HIGH-RISK GROUPS
Complete skin exam (HR1)
Complete oral cavity exam (HR2)
Palpation for thyroid nodules (HR3)
Auscultation for carotid bruits (HR4)

Laboratory/Diagnostic Procedures
Nonfasting total blood cholesterol
Papanicolaou smear[2]
Mammogram[3]
HIGH-RISK GROUPS
Fasting plasma glucose (HR5)
VDRL/RPR (HR6)
Urinalysis for bacteriuria (HR7)
Chlamydial testing (HR8)
Gonorrhea culture (HR9)
Counseling and testing for HIV (HR10)
Tuberculin skin test (PPD) (HR11)
Hearing (HR12)
Electrocardiogram (HR13)
Fecal occult blood/sigmoidoscopy (HR14)
Fecal occult blood/colonoscopy (HR15)
Bone mineral content (HR16)

COUNSELING

Diet and Exercise
Fat (especially saturated fat), cholesterol, complex carbohydrates, fiber, sodium, calcium[4]
Caloric balance
Selection of exercise program

Substance Use
Tobacco cessation
Alcohol and other drugs:
Limiting alcohol consumption
Driving/other dangerous activities while under the influence
Treatment for abuse
HIGH-RISK GROUPS
Sharing/using unsterilized needles and syringes (HR19)

Sexual Practices
Sexually transmitted diseases; partner selection, condoms, anal intercourse
Unintended pregnancy and contraceptive options

Injury Prevention
Safety belts
Safety helmets
Smoke detector
Smoking near bedding or upholstery
HIGH-RISK GROUPS
Back-conditioning exercises (HR20)
Prevention of childhood injuries (HR21)
Falls in the elderly (HR22)

Dental Health
Regular tooth brushing, flossing, and dental visits

Other Primary Preventive Measures
HIGH-RISK GROUPS
Skin protection from ultraviolet light (HR23)
Discussion of aspirin therapy (HR24)
Discussion of estrogen replacement therapy (HR25)

IMMUNIZATIONS

Tetanus-diphtheria (Td) booster[5]
HIGH-RISK GROUPS
Hepatitis B vaccine (HR26)
Pneumococcal vaccine (HR27)
Influenza vaccine (HR28)[6]

This list of preventive services is not exhaustive. It reflects only those topics reviewed by the U.S. Preventive Services Task Force. Clinicians may wish to add other preventive services on a routine basis, and after considering the patient's medical history and other individual circumstances. Examples of target conditions not specifically examined by the Task Force include:
Chronic obstructive pulmonary disease
Hepatobiliary disease
Bladder cancer
Endometrial disease
Travel-related illness
Prescription drug abuse
Occupational illness and injuries

Remain Alert For:
Depressive symptoms
Suicide risk factors (HR17)
Abnormal bereavement
Signs of physical abuse or neglect
Malignant skin lesions
Peripheral arterial disease (HR18)
Tooth decay, gingivitis, loose teeth

*The recommended schedule applies only to the periodic visit itself. The frequency of the individual preventive services listed in this table is left to clinical discretion, except as indicated in other footnotes.

1. Annually for women. 2. Every 1–3 years for women. 3. Every 1–2 years for women beginning at age 50 (age 35 for those at increased risk). 4. For women. 5. Every 10 years. 6. Annually.

Table 6.   Ages 40–64   High-Risk Categories

HR1 Persons with a family or personal history of skin cancer, increased occupational or recreational exposure to sunlight, or clinical evidence of precursor lesions (e.g., dysplastic nevi, certain congenital nevi).

HR2 Persons with exposure to tobacco or excessive amounts of alcohol, or those with suspicious symptoms or lesions detected through self-examination.

HR3 Persons with a history of upper-body irradiation.

HR4 Persons with risk factors for cerebrovascular or cardiovascular disease (e.g., hypertension, smoking, CAD, atrial fibrillation, diabetes) or those with neurologic symptoms (e.g., transient ischemic attacks) or a history of cerebrovascular disease.

HR5 The markedly obese, persons with a family history of diabetes, or women with a history of gestational diabetes.

HR6 Prostitutes, persons who engage in sex with multiple partners in areas in which syphilis is prevalent, or contacts of persons with active syphilis.

HR7 Persons with diabetes.

HR8 Persons who attend clinics for sexually transmitted diseases, attend other high-risk health care facilities (e.g., adolescent and family planning clinics), or have other risk factors for chlamydial infection (e.g., multiple sexual partners or a sexual partner with multiple sexual contacts).

HR9 Prostitutes, persons with multiple sexual partners or a sexual partner with multiple contacts, sexual contacts of persons with culture-proven gonorrhea, or persons with a history of repeated episodes of gonorrhea.

HR10 Persons seeking treatment for sexually transmitted diseases; homosexual and bisexual men; past or present intravenous (IV) drug users; persons with a history of prostitution or multiple sexual partners; women whose past or present sexual partners were HIV-infected, bisexual, or IV drug users; persons with long-term residence or birth in an area with high prevalence of HIV infection; or persons with a history of transfusion between 1978 and 1985.

HR11 Household members of persons with tuberculosis or others at risk for close contact with the disease (e.g., staff of tuberculosis clinics, shelters for the homeless, nursing homes, substance abuse treatment facilities, dialysis units, correctional institutions); recent immigrants or refugees from countries in which tuberculosis is common (e.g., Asia, Africa, Central and South America, Pacific Islands); migrant workers; residents of nursing homes, correctional institutions, or homeless shelters; or persons with certain underlying medical disorders (e.g., HIV infection).

HR12 Persons exposed regularly to excessive noise.

HR13 Men with two or more cardiac risk factors (high blood cholesterol, hypertension, cigarette smoking, diabetes mellitus, family history of CAD); men who would endanger public safety were they to experience sudden cardiac events (e.g., commercial airline pilots); or sedentary or high-risk males planning to begin a vigorous exercise program.

HR14 Persons aged 50 and older who have first-degree relatives with colorectal cancer; a personal history of endometrial, ovarian, or breast cancer; or a previous diagnosis of inflammatory bowel disease, adenomatous polyps, or colorectal cancer.

HR15 Persons with a family history of familial polyposis coli or cancer family syndrome.

HR16 Perimenopausal women at increased risk for osteoporosis (e.g., Caucasian race, bilateral oophorectomy before menopause, slender build) and for whom estrogen replacement therapy would otherwise not be recommended.

HR17 Recent divorce, separation, unemployment, depression, alcohol or other drug abuse, serious medical illnesses, living alone, or recent bereavement.

HR18 Persons over age 50, smokers, or persons with diabetes mellitus.

HR19 Intravenous drug users.

HR20 Persons at increased risk for low back injury because of past history, body configuration, or type of activities.

HR21 Persons with children in the home or automobile.

HR22 Persons with older adults in the home.

HR23 Persons with increased exposure to sunlight.

HR24 Men who have risk factors for myocardial infarction (e.g., high blood cholesterol, smoking, diabetes mellitus, family history of early-onset CAD) and who lack a history of gastrointestinal or other bleeding problems, and other risk factors for bleeding or cerebral hemorrhage.

HR25 Perimenopausal women at increased risk for osteoporosis (e.g., Caucasian, low bone mineral content, bilateral oophorectomy before menopause or early menopause, slender build) and who are without known contraindications (e.g., history of undiagnosed vaginal bleeding, active liver disease, thromboembolic disorders, hormone-dependent cancer).

HR26 Homosexually active men, intravenous drug users, recipients of some blood products, or persons in health-related jobs with frequent exposure to blood or blood products.

HR27 Persons with medical conditions that increase the risk of pneumococcal infection (e.g., chronic cardiac or pulmonary disease, sickle cell disease, nephrotic syndrome, Hodgkin's disease, asplenia, diabetes mellitus, alcoholism, cirrhosis, multiple myeloma, renal disease or conditions associated with immunosuppression).

HR28 Residents of chronic care facilities and persons suffering from chronic cardiopulmonary disorders, metabolic diseases (including diabetes mellitus), hemoglobinopathies, immunosuppression, or renal dysfunction.

Table 7.
Ages 65 and Over
Schedule: Every Year*

Leading Causes of Death:
Heart disease
Cerebrovascular disease
Obstructive lung disease
Pneumonia/influenza
Lung cancer
Colorectal cancer

SCREENING	COUNSELING	IMMUNIZATIONS
History Prior symptoms of transient ischemic attack Dietary intake Physical activity Tobacco/alcohol/drug use Functional status at home	**Diet and Exercise** Fat (especially saturated fat), cholesterol, complex carbohydrates, fiber, sodium, calcium[3] Caloric balance Selection of exercise program	Tetanus-diphtheria (Td) booster[5] Influenza vaccine[1] Pneumococcal vaccine *HIGH-RISK GROUPS* Hepatitis B vaccine (HR16)
Physical Exam Height and weight Blood pressure Visual acuity Hearing and hearing aids Clinical breast exam[1] *HIGH-RISK GROUPS* Auscultation for carotid bruits (HR1) Complete skin exam (HR2) Complete oral cavity exam (HR3) Palpation of thyroid nodules (HR4)	**Substance Use** Tobacco cessation Alcohol and other drugs: Limiting alcohol consumption Driving/other dangerous activities while under the influence Treatment for abuse **Injury Prevention** Prevention of falls Safety belts Smoke detector Smoking near bedding or upholstery Hot water heater temperature Safety helmets *HIGH-RISK GROUPS* Prevention of childhood injuries (HR12)	**This list of preventive services is not exhaustive.** It reflects only those topics reviewed by the U.S. Preventive Services Task Force. Clinicians may wish to add other preventive services on a routine basis, and after considering the patient's medical history and other individual circumstances. Examples of target conditions not specifically examined by the Task Force include: Chronic obstructive pulmonary disease Hepatobiliary disease Bladder cancer Endometrial disease Travel-related illness Prescription drug abuse Occupational illness and injuries
Laboratory/Diagnostic Procedures Nonfasting total blood cholesterol Dipstick urinalysis Mammogram[2] Thyroid function tests[3] *HIGH-RISK GROUPS* Fasting plasma glucose (HR5) Tuberculin skin test (PPD) (HR6) Electrocardiogram (HR7) Papanicolaou smear[4] (HR8) Fecal occult blood/Sigmoidoscopy (HR9) Fecal occult blood/Colonoscopy (HR10)	**Dental Health** Regular dental visits, tooth brushing, flossing **Other Primary Preventive Measures** Glaucoma testing by eye specialist *HIGH-RISK GROUPS* Discussion of estrogen replacement therapy (HR13) Discussion of aspirin therapy (HR14) Skin protection form ultraviolet light (HR15)	**Remain Alert For:** Depression symptoms Suicide risk factors (HR11) Abnormal bereavement Changes in cognitive function Medications that increase risk of falls Signs of physical abuse or neglect Malignant skin lesions Peripheral arterial disease Tooth decay, gingivitis, loose teeth

*The recommended schedule applies only to the periodic visit itself. The frequency of the individual preventive services listed in this table is left to clinical discretion, except as indicated in other footnotes.

1. Annually.   2. Every 1–2 years for women until age 75, unless pathology detected.   3. For women.   4. Every 1–3 years.   5. Every 10 years.

Table 7. Ages 65 and Over

High-Risk Categories

HR1 Persons with risk factors for cerebrovascular or cardiovascular disease (e.g., hypertension, smoking, CAD, atrial fibrillation, diabetes) or those with neurologic symptoms (e.g., transient ischemic attacks) or a history of cerebrovascular disease.

HR2 Persons with a family or personal history of skin cancer, or clinical evidence of precursor lesions (e.g., dysplastic nevi, certain congenital nevi), or those with increased occupational or recreational exposure to sunlight.

HR3 Persons with exposure to tobacco or excessive amounts of alcohol, or those with suspicious symptoms or lesions detected through self-examination.

HR4 Persons with a history of upper-body irradiation.

HR5 The markedly obese, persons with a family history of diabetes, or women with a history of gestational diabetes.

HR6 Household members of persons with tuberculosis or others at risk for close contact with the disease (e.g., staff of tuberculosis clinics, shelters for the homeless, nursing homes, substance abuse treatment facilities, dialysis units, correctional institutions); recent immigrants or refugees from countries in which tuberculosis is common (e.g., Asia, Africa, Central and South America, Pacific Islands); migrant workers; residents of nursing homes, correctional institutions, or homeless shelters; or persons with certain underlying medical disorders (e.g., HIV infection).

HR7 Men with two or more cardiac risk factors (high blood cholesterol, hypertension, cigarette smoking, diabetes mellitus, family history of CAD); men who would endanger public safety were they to experience sudden cardiac events (e.g., commercial airline pilots); or sedentary or high-risk males planning to begin a vigorous exercise program.

HR8 Women who have not had previous documented screening in which smears have been consistently negative.

HR9 Persons who have first-degree relatives with colorectal cancer; a personal history of endometrial, ovarian, or breast cancer; or a previous diagnosis of inflammatory bowel disease, adenomatous polyps, or colorectal cancer.

HR10 Persons with a family history of familial polyposis coli or cancer family syndrome.

HR11 Recent divorce, separation, unemployment, depression, alcohol or other drug abuse, serious medical illnesses, living alone, or recent bereavement.

HR12 Persons with children in the home or automobile.

HR13 Women at increased risk for osteoporosis (e.g., Caucasian, low bone mineral content, bilateral oophorectomy before menopause or early menopause, slender build) and who are without known contraindications (e.g., history of undiagnosed vaginal bleeding, active liver disease, thromboembolic disorders, hormone-dependent cancer).

HR14 Men who have risk factors for myocardial infarction (e.g., high blood cholesterol, smoking, diabetes mellitus, family history of early-onset CAD) and who lack a history of gastrointestinal or other bleeding problems, or other risk factors for bleeding or cerebral hemorrhage.

HR15 Persons with increased exposure to sunlight.

HR16 Homosexually active men, intravenous drug users, recipients of some blood products, or persons in health-related jobs with frequent exposure to blood or blood products.

Table 8.
Pregnant Women[1]

FIRST PRENATAL VISIT

SCREENING

History
Genetic and obstetric history
Dietary intake
Tobacco/alcohol/drug use
Risk factors for intrauterine
  growth retardation and
  low birthweight
Prior genital herpetic lesions

Laboratory/Diagnostic Procedures
Blood pressure
Hemoglobin and hematocrit
ABO/Rh typing
Rh(D) and other antibody
  screen
VDRL/RPR
Hepatitis B surface antigen
  (HBsAg)
Urinalysis for bacteriuria
Gonorrhea culture
HIGH-RISK GROUPS
  Hemoglobin electrophore-
    sis (HR1)
  Rubella antibodies (HR2)
  Chlamydial testing (HR3)
  Counseling and testing for
    HIV (HR4)

1. See also Tables 4–6 for other preventive services for women.
2. Women with access to counseling and follow-up services, skilled high-resolution ultrasound and amniocentesis capabilities, and reliable, standardized laboratories.

COUNSELING

Nutrition
Tobacco use
Alcohol and other drug use
Safety belts
HIGH-RISK GROUPS
  Discuss amniocentesis (HR5)
  Discuss risks of HIV infection (HR4)

Remain Alert For:
Signs of physical abuse

FOLLOW-UP VISITS

Schedule: See Footnote*

SCREENING

Blood pressure
Urinalysis for bacteriuria

Screening Tests at Specific Gestational Ages

14–16 Weeks:
  Maternal serum alpha-fetoprotein
    (MSAFP)[2]
  Ultrasound cephalometry (HR8)

24–28 Weeks:
  50 g oral glucose tolerance test
  Rh(D) antibody (HR9)
  Gonorrhea culture (HR10)
  VDRL/RPR (HR11)
  Hepatitis B surface antigen
    (HBsAg) (HR12)
  Counseling and testing for HIV
    (HR13)

36 Weeks:
  Ultrasound exam (HR14)

COUNSELING

Nutrition
Safety belts
Discuss meaning of upcom-
  ing tests
HIGH-RISK GROUPS
  Tobacco use (HR6)
  Alcohol and other drug
    use (HR7)

Remain Alert For:
Signs of physical abuse

This list of preventive services is not exhaustive. It reflects only those topics reviewed by the U.S. Preventive Services Task Force. Clinicians may wish to add other preventive services on a routine basis, and after considering the patient's medical history and other individual circumstances. Examples of target conditions not specifically examined by the Task Force include:
  Counseling on warning
    signs and symptoms
  Physical findings of ab-
    dominal and cervical
    examination
  Tay-Sachs disease
  Childbirth education
  Teratogenic and fetotoxic
    exposures

*Because of lack of data and differing patient risk profiles, the scheduling of visits and the frequency of the individual preventive services listed in this table are left to clinical discretion, except for those indicated at specific gestational ages.

Table 8.   Pregnant Women   High-Risk Categories

HR1   Black women.

HR2   Women lacking evidence of immunity (proof of vaccination after the first birthday or laboratory evidence of immunity.)

HR3   Women who attend clinics for sexually transmitted diseases, attend other high-risk health care facilities (e.g., adolescent and family planning clinics), or have other risk factors for chlamydial infection (e.g., multiple sexual partners or a sexual partner with multiple sexual contacts).

HR4   Women seeking treatment for sexually transmitted diseases; past or present intravenous (IV) drug users; women with a history of prostitution or multiple sexual partners; women whose past or present sexual partners were HIV-infected, bisexual, or IV drug users; women with long-term residence or birth in an area with high prevalence of HIV infection in women; or women with a history of transfusion between 1978 and 1985.

HR5   Women aged 35 and older.

HR6   Women who continue to smoke during pregnancy.

HR7   Women with excessive alcohol consumption during pregnancy.

HR8   Women with uncertain menstrual histories or risk factors for intrauterine growth retardation (e.g., hypertension, renal disease, short maternal stature, low prepregnancy weight, failure to gain weight during pregnancy, smoking, alcohol and other drug abuse, and history of a previous fetal death or growth-retarded baby).

HR9   Unsensitized Rh-negative women.

HR10   Women with multiple sexual partners or a sexual partner with multiple contacts, or sexual contacts of persons with culture-proven gonorrhea.

HR11   Women who engage in sex with multiple partners in areas in which syphilis is prevalent, or contacts of persons with active syphilis.

HR12   Women who engage in high-risk behavior (e.g., intravenous drug use) or in whom exposure to hepatitis B during pregnancy is suspected.

HR13   Women at high risk (see HR4) who have a nonreactive HIV test at the first prenatal visit.

HR14   Women with risk factors for intrauterine growth retardation (see HR8).

basis and do not apply to persons with special exposures to infected individuals. The reader is referred to Chapter 58 for detailed guidelines on immunization in such circumstances.

REFERENCES

1. American Cancer Society. Cancer statistics, 1989. CA 1989; 39:332.
2. National Center for Health Statistics. Advance report of final mortality statistics, 1986. Monthly Vital Statistics Report, vol. 37, no. 6. Hyattsville, Md.: Public Health Service, 1988. (Publication no. DHHS (PHS) 88–1120.)
3. Department of Transportation. Final regulatory impact assessment on amendments to Federal Motor Vehicle Safety Standard 208, Front Seat Occupant Protection. Washington, D.C.: Department of Transportation, 1984. (Publication no. DOT HS 806–572.)
4. Campbell BJ. Safety belt injury reduction related to crash severity and front seated position. J Trauma 1987; 27:733–9.
5. Baker SP, O'Neill B, Karpf R. The injury fact book. Lexington, Mass.: DC Heath and Company, 1984.
6. Waller JA. Injury control: a guide to causes and prevention of trauma. Lexington, Mass.: DC Heath and Company, 1985.
7. Centers for Disease Control. Summary of notifiable diseases, United States, 1987. MMWR 1988; 36:10.
8. Curran JW, Jaffe HW, Hardy AM, et al. Epidemiology of HIV infection and AIDS in the United States. Science 1988; 239:610–6.
9. American Academy of Pediatrics. Guidelines for health supervision. Elk Grove Village, Ill.: American Academy of Pediatrics, 1985.
10. *Idem*. Recommendations for preventive pediatric health care. Committee on Practice and Ambulatory Medicine. Elk Grove Village, Ill.: American Academy of Pediatrics, 1987.

iv.

Recommendations for Patient Education and Counseling

Empirical research and clinical experience yield certain principles that clinicians can use to induce behavior change among patients. Attention to these key concepts should enhance the effectiveness of physician counseling concerning all behavioral changes recommended in this report.

1. *Develop a therapeutic alliance.* See yourself as an expert consultant available to help patients who remain in control of their own health choices. This perspective facilitates development of a therapeutic alliance in which health is maintained or achieved through a provider-patient partnership.[1,2] Help motivate patients who smoke, abuse alcohol and other drugs, or do not exercise to change these behaviors. Assist them in acquiring the necessary attitudes and skills to succeed in their attempts.

2. *Counsel all patients.* Most patients are eager for health information and guidance and generally want more than physicians provide.[3] Whites tend to receive more information than blacks and Hispanics,[4,5] and middle class patients tend to receive more than working class patients.[6] Physicians tend to talk more with patients who pose more questions, but those who are quieter are often in greater need of education.[7] Make a concerted effort to respond to the educational needs of all your patients in ways appropriate to their age, race, sex, socioeconomic status, and interpersonal skills.

3. *Ensure that patients understand the relationship between behavior and health.* Inquire about what your patients already know or believe about the relationship between risk factors and health status. Do not assume that patients understand the health effects of smoking, lack of exercise, poor nutrition, and other lifestyle factors. Explain in simple terms the idea that certain factors can increase the risk of disease and that combinations of factors can sometimes work together to increase risk beyond the sum of their individual contributions. Respond to patients' questions, reinforce key points, and encourage patients to write down questions about risk factors for discussion at the next visit. Bear in mind that knowledge is a necessary, but not a sufficient, stimulus for behavior change.

4. *Work with patients to assess barriers to behavior change.* Anticipating obstacles to behavior change is fundamental to effective patient education since patients often do not follow physicians' advice concerning medication use or lifestyle changes.[8] According to one well-studied model, three areas of beliefs influence the adoption and maintenance of behavior change: (1) susceptibility to continuing problems if the advice is not followed; (2) severity of problems associated with not following the advice; and (3) the benefits of adopting the advice weighed against the potential risks, costs, side effects, and barriers.[9] Assess those areas and address those beliefs that are not conducive to healthful behaviors. In addition, try to determine other obstacles to change, including lack of skills, motivation,

resources, and social support, and help patients determine ways to overcome them.[10]

5. *Gain commitment from patients to change.* This is a critical step in patient education and counseling because patients typically come into the physician's office expecting to be treated for a condition. If patients do not agree that their behaviors are significantly related to health outcomes, attempts at patient education may be irrelevant.

6. *Involve patients in selecting risk factors to change.* Do not overwhelm patients by asking them to try to change all their unhealthful behaviors at the same time. Let patient need, patient preference, and your own assessment of relative importance to health dictate your recommendation of which risk factor to tackle first.[11] Patients who achieve success in one effort may attempt other changes, since many behavior patterns tend to be linked.[12] For example, quitting smoking may lead to renewed energy to begin exercising, which in turn may lead to better eating habits. There are situations, however, where it is advisable to address risk factors simultaneously, such as chemical dependence involving several substances.

7. *Use a combination of strategies.* Educational efforts that integrate individual counseling, group classes, audiovisual aids, written materials, and community resources are far more effective than those employing only one single technique.[13] Be flexible about tailoring programs to individual needs; for example, some patients will not attend group classes, and others may have inflexible work schedules. Ensure that printed materials are accurate, consistent with your views, and at a reading level appropriate to the patient population. Use written materials to strengthen the message, personalizing them by jotting pertinent comments in the margins; this will help to remind patients later of your suggestions. Be wary of excessive use of print materials as a substitute for verbal communication with patients. Multiple studies have demonstrated that clinicians' individual attention and feedback are more useful than media or other communication channels in changing patient knowledge and behavior.[14]

8. *Design a behavior modification plan.* Patient education should be oriented toward what patients should do, not merely what patients should know.[15] Ask patients if they have ever tried to change the specific behavior before and discuss the methods used, the barriers encountered, and the degree of success. If patients have tried and failed, ask them to identify what they have learned from the attempt. Agree on a specific, time-limited goal to be achieved and record the goal in the medical record.[16] Discuss the behaviors that need to be modified to achieve the goal, paying special attention to patient cultural beliefs and attitudes that might facilitate or impede success. Assist patients in writing action plans, review relevant instructional materials, and stress your willingness to be of continued assistance.[11] Remember, at best patients often recall only about 50% of what they are told by their physicians, and lifestyle recommendations are remembered less than are medication regimens.[17] Close your visit by summarizing your mutual expectations and expressing your confidence that the patient will make a good effort to modify his or her risk factors.

9. *Monitor progress through follow-up contact.* Once a strategy for behavior change has been developed, schedule a follow-up appointment or telephone call within the next few weeks to evaluate progress in achieving the goal. Reinforce successes through positive verbal feedback. If patients have not followed the plan, work with them to identify and overcome obstacles. Modify the plan if necessary to facilitate successful risk factor reduction. Strategies include referring patients to community agencies or self-help groups and eliciting support for the patient's prescribed regimen from family members or significant individuals in their social

networks.[8] Progressively transfer responsibility for self-care to patients by scheduling follow-up contacts with increasingly longer time intervals.[8] Evaluate your
office's capacity to monitor patient progress through computerized records or other
tracking systems, and make necessary improvements.

10. *Involve office staff.* Use the team approach to patient education. Share
responsibility for patients with nurses, health educators, dietitians, and other allied
health professionals, as appropriate. Ask your receptionist to encourage patients
to read materials that you have reviewed, approved, and placed in your reception
area. Ensure that team members and the office environment communicate consistent positive health messages.[18] Well-meaning comments such as "Well, you
know the doctor is a fanatic about exercise," or "I can't lose weight either" can
unintentionally sabotage patient education strategies.[19] If possible, form a patient
education committee to generate program ideas and promote staff commitment.[18]

Bear in mind that the physician's own health-promoting behavior should serve
as a role model for patients. It is difficult to assist patients to stop smoking, begin
exercising, change dietary patterns, reduce alcohol consumption, or manage stress
if you need to and do not make these changes in your own behavior. Rene Dubos
once said that "to ward off disease or recover from health, men as a rule find it
easier to depend on the healers than to attempt the more difficult task of living
wisely."[20] Physicians who both practice and preach prudent health behaviors should
be better able to foster health within themselves and their patients.[21]

REFERENCES

1. Rosenstock IM. Adoption and maintenance of lifestyle modifications. Am J Prev Med
   1988; 4:349–52.
2. Lipkin M. The medical interview and related skills. In Branch WT, ed. Office practice of
   medicine, 1st ed. Philadelphia: WB Saunders, 1987:1287–1306.
3. Woo B, Woo B, Cook F, et al. Screening procedures in the asymptomatic adult: comparisons of physicians' recommendations, patients' desires, published guidelines, and
   actual practice. JAMA 1985; 254:1480–4.
4. Hall JA, Roter DL, Katz NR. Meta-analysis of correlates of provider behavior in medical
   encounters. Med Care 1988; 26:657–75.
5. Roter DL, Hall JA, Katz NR. Patient-physician communication: a descriptive summary
   of the literature. Patient Educ Couns 1988; 12:99–119.
6. Waitzkin H. Information giving in medical care. J Health Soc Behav 1985; 26:81–101.
7. Roter DL. Patient participation in the patient-provider interaction. The effects of patient
   question asking on the quality of interaction, satisfaction, and compliance. Health Educ
   Monogr 1977; 5:281–315.
8. Green LW. How physicians can improve patients' participation and maintenance in self-
   care. West J Med 1987; 147:346–9.
9. Janz NK, Becker MH. The health belief model: a decade later. Health Educ Q 1984;
   11:1–47.
10. Ockene JK, Sorensen G, Kabat-Zinn J, et al. Benefits and costs of lifestyle change to
    reduce risk of chronic disease. Prev Med 1988; 17:224–34.
11. Fried RA, Iverson DC, Nagle JP. The clinician's health promotion handbook. Denver,
    Colo.: Mercy Medical Center, 1985:9–21.
12. Integration of risk factor interventions: two reports to the Office of Disease Prevention
    and Health Promotion. Washington, D.C.: Department of Health and Human Services,
    1986.
13. Kottke TE, Battista RN, DeFriese GH, et al. Attributes of successful smoking cessation
    interventions in clinical practice: a meta-analysis of 42 controlled trials. JAMA 1988;
    259:2882–9.
14. Mullen PD, Green LW, Persinger G. Clinical trials of patient education for chronic con-
    ditions: a comparative analysis of intervention types. Prev Med 1985; 14:753–81.

15. Bartlett EE. Introduction: eight principles from patient education research. Prev Med 1985; 14:667–9.
16. Simons-Morton BG, Pate RP, Simons-Morton DG. Prescribing physical activity to prevent disease. Postgrad Med 1988; 83:165–76.
17. Rost K, Roter D. Predictors of recall of medication regimens and recommendations for lifestyle change in elderly patients. Gerontologist 1987; 27:510–5.
18. Vogt HB, Kapp C. Patient education in primary care practice. Postgrad Med 1987; 81:273–8.
19. Richards JW, Blum A. Health promotion. In: Taylor RE, ed. Family medicine: principles and practice, 3rd ed. New York: Springer-Verlag, 1988:94–105.
20. Gutmann MC, Jackson TC. Facilitating behavior change. In: Sheridan DP, Winogrond IR, eds. The preventive approach to patient care. New York: Elsevier, 1987:49–68.
21. Shindell S, Sheridan DP. The healthy physician. In: Sheridan DP, Winogrond IR, eds. The preventive approach to patient care. New York: Elsevier, 1987:69–96.

I. Screening

1

Screening for Asymptomatic Coronary Artery Disease

Recommendation: Clinicians should emphasize the primary prevention of coronary artery disease (CAD) by periodically screening for high blood pressure (see Chapter 3) and high serum cholesterol (Chapter 2) and by routinely investigating behavioral risk factors for CAD such as tobacco use (Chapter 48), dietary fat and cholesterol intake (Chapter 50), and inadequate physical activity (Chapter 49). Secondary prevention of CAD (screening) by performing routine electrocardiography to screen asymptomatic persons is not recommended. It may be clinically prudent to perform screening electrocardiograms (ECGs) in certain high-risk groups (see *Clinical Intervention*). Routine resting or exercise ECG screening before entering athletic programs is not recommended for asymptomatic children, adolescents, or young adults.

Burden of Suffering

Coronary artery disease is the leading cause of death in the United States, accounting for about 1.5 million myocardial infarctions and 520,000 deaths each year.[1,2] Acute myocardial infarction is associated with high mortality despite recent advances in resuscitation and cardiac life support techniques; about 15% of patients who reach the hospital after acute myocardial infarction do not survive their hospitalization.[3] In addition, CAD is responsible for significant morbidity and disability among those suffering from angina pectoris and the complications of myocardial infarction. Medical care and lost productivity for cardiovascular diseases cost the United States nearly $80 billion in 1986.[2] Myocardial infarction and sudden death often occur without warning in persons without a history of angina pectoris or other clinical symptoms. The principal modifiable risk factors for CAD are cigarette smoking, hypertension, elevated serum cholesterol, and obesity. Age, sex, and family history are the principal nonmodifiable risk factors.

Efficacy of Screening Tests

There are two screening strategies to reduce morbidity and mortality from CAD. The first involves primary prevention by screening for cardiac risk factors, such as hypertension, elevated serum cholesterol, cigarette smoking, and physical inactivity. These topics are discussed in Chapters 2, 3, 48, and 49. The second strategy involves secondary prevention through early detection of coronary atherosclerotic disease. The principal tests considered for this form of screening include resting and exercise ECGs, which can provide evidence of previous silent myocardial infarctions. In addition, certain ECG findings may be useful in predicting the long-term risk of experiencing future coronary events. Prospective studies in asymptomatic persons suggest that Q-waves, ST-segment depression, T-wave inversion, left ventricular hypertrophy, and ventricular arrhythmias are associated with increased risk for coronary events and sudden death.[4-12] However, there are important limitations to the sensitivity and specificity of electrocardiography when used as a screening test. A normal ECG does not rule out coronary disease; ECG changes often do not become apparent until atherosclerotic narrowing has become great enough to significantly impede coronary blood flow.[13]

Conversely, an abnormal ECG cannot be relied on as conclusive evidence of underlying arterial disease. ST-segment changes, for example, occur commonly in the general population.[14] Thus, routine ECG testing in asymptomatic persons, in whom the probability of having CAD is relatively low, generates a large proportion of false-positive results.[15] Although precise data are lacking on the positive predictive value of the resting ECG, studies of exercise ECG (which has greater sensitivity and specificity than the resting ECG) indicate that most asymptomatic persons with abnormal results do not have underlying CAD. A series of reports have shown that angiographic evidence of significant stenosis (greater than 50% narrowing) is present in only 30–43% of middle-aged asymptomatic persons with abnormal exercise tests.[16-18] Abnormal resting ECG findings, although often associated with increased long-term risk of developing symptomatic disease, are of limited prognostic value. Prospective studies lasting between 5 and 30 years have found that CAD develops in only 3–15% of asymptomatic persons with resting ECG abnormalities.[4,5,9,12,19] An abnormal exercise test is of somewhat larger, but also limited, prognostic value in predicting CAD in asymptomatic persons.[20] Longitudinal studies lasting 3–13 years have shown that, depending on the population being studied and the end points used to define cardiac events, between 5% and 46% (or an average of about 25%) of persons with exercise-induced ST-segment depression developed symptomatic coronary disease such as angina pectoris or myocardial infarction.[21-30]

False-positive electrocardiography results are undesirable for several reasons. Persons with abnormal results often subsequently receive diagnostic procedures such as thallium scintigraphy and, if this is also positive, coronary angiography before it can be determined that the ECG is falsely positive. The initial abnormal ECG as well as the serial tests that follow may produce considerable anxiety among patients. Both the extent and precision of diagnostic testing can be modified to some extent by performing work-ups in accordance with a Bayesian model:[31] testing can be targeted to high-risk groups, such as men with a family history of premature CAD or those persons whose calculated pretest probability of developing CAD is greater than 10%. Nonetheless, even the initial abnormal ECG tracing may disqualify some patients from jobs, insurance eligibility, and other opportunities, although precise data on the magnitude of these problems are lacking.

Effectiveness of Early Detection

Although there is evidence from case-control and cohort studies that asymptomatic persons with selected ECG findings are at increased risk of cardiac death, myocardial infarction, and sudden death,[21,29,30,32-35] there is little evidence that the identification of these individuals through ECG screening and the treatment of their asymptomatic CAD can reduce the incidence of these outcomes. Studies have shown that antianginal drugs such as nitroglycerin, beta-adrenergic blockers, and calcium antagonists can reduce the frequency and the duration of silent ischemic episodes,[36-38] but there is no evidence that this treatment results in lowered incidence of cardiac events in persons with no history of angina or myocardial infarction. Other, more invasive treatment options such as coronary artery bypass grafting and angioplasty may be of benefit to asymptomatic persons with left main coronary or three-vessel disease.[39] For example, three-vessel disease accounts for about 25% of abnormal angiograms in asymptomatic middle-aged men.[40] However, it is unclear from current evidence that the detection of such individuals provides sufficient justification for routine screening of large asymptomatic populations.

Some argue that a screening ECG is valuable as a "baseline" to help interpret changes in subsequent ECGs.[41] Such ECG records are clinically useful on occasion, and changes in serial ECGs may help predict future coronary events,[11] but studies indicate that in actual practice, most baseline tracings are either unavailable or do not provide information that affects treatment decisions.[42] Even when important differences are noted between the baseline ECG and a subsequent tracing, it is often difficult to determine when during the interval the change occurred. Another argument for electrocardiography screening is that the early identification of persons at increased risk for CAD on the basis of ECG findings may help to modify other important cardiac risk factors such as cigarette smoking, hypertension, and high blood cholesterol.[41] While the efficacy of these behavioral changes is well established, these interventions are recommended independently of the ECG, and there is little evidence to suggest that patients who are aware of their ECG findings are more likely to change behavior or to experience a better outcome than those who do not obtain ECG results.

Periodic ECG screening has also been advocated for persons who might endanger public safety were they to experience myocardial infarction or sudden death at work (e.g., airline pilots, bus and truck drivers, railroad engineers).[43] Cardiac events in such individuals are more likely to affect the safety of a large number of persons, and clinical intervention, either through medical treatment or counseling to change job status, might prevent such catastrophes. There are no available data to confirm the efficacy of these measures, however.

Preliminary exercise ECG testing has been advocated for sedentary persons planning to begin vigorous exercise programs. There is evidence that strenuous exertion may increase the risk of sudden cardiac death,[44,45] usually as a result of underlying hypertrophic cardiomyopathy or congenital coronary anomalies in young persons[46] or CAD in older persons.[45] Cardiac events during exercise in persons without overt heart disease are relatively uncommon, however, and thus the number of cases that are preventable through preexercise testing of asymptomatic persons is limited. In addition, it has not been proved that restricted exertion in asymptomatic persons at risk for heart disease can prevent the occurrence of subsequent cardiac events. In populations at low risk for heart disease, such as healthy young persons engaged in athletic programs or recreational sports, the limited benefits of screening may be outweighed by the harmful effects of labeling and exercise restrictions for the large proportion of persons whose positive ECG results will be falsely positive.

Recommendations of Others

In 1977, a task force sponsored by the American College of Cardiology (ACC) recommended that all adults receive a baseline 12-lead ECG at an unspecified age, followed by periodic ECG testing every five years, or annually in high-risk persons.[47] The American Heart Association (AHA) recommends baseline electro-

cardiography at age 20 followed by repeated tracings at ages 40 and 60 in normotensive persons.[48] The Institute of Medicine has recommended obtaining a
baseline ECG at age 40 or 45.[49] Recommendations against routine electrocardiography have been issued by the Canadian Task Force[50] and a number of
reviewers.[51-53] The ACC and AHA recommend exercise electrocardiography testing of asymptomatic males over age 40 under the following circumstances: (a)
occupations affecting public safety (e.g., airline pilots, firemen, police officers, bus
or truck drivers, railroad engineers); (b) two or more cardiac risk factors (serum
cholesterol over 240 mg/dL [6.20 mmol/L], blood pressure greater than 160/90
mm Hg, cigarette smoking, diabetes mellitus, family history of CAD onset before
age 55); or (c) sedentary persons planning to begin a vigorous exercise program.[43]
The American College of Sports Medicine recommends preliminary exercise
ECG testing for all men and women over age 45 who plan to begin an exercise
program.[54]

Discussion

CAD is the leading cause of death in the United States, and thus even preventive
interventions of only modest benefit may have large public health implications.
The screening ECG has this potential due to its ability to detect previously unrecognized atherosclerotic heart disease and its prognostic value in predicting subsequent illness.

However, the ECG is an imperfect screening test. False-positive ECG results
are not uncommon in healthy persons, especially when screening is performed
routinely in low-risk asymptomatic populations. In these groups, the large majority
of persons with abnormal ECG results do not have CAD and are unlikely to develop
the disease in the near future. To minimize the physical, psychological, and economic effects of false-positive labeling, ECG screening should be targeted to
individuals at increased risk for CAD and to those whose sudden death or inca-
pacitation would endanger the safety of others.

There are major costs associated with the widespread performance of periodic
resting ECG on large numbers of asymptomatic persons. Exercise testing is an
even more expensive procedure. These expenses would be justified if the incidence of CAD could be significantly lowered in the process, but such evidence is
not yet available. Further research is necessary to demonstrate whether early
detection and treatment of asymptomatic CAD is effective in lowering morbidity
and mortality. In the meantime, the most effective proven means of preventing
CAD are the identification and control of major cardiac risk factors such as hypertension, elevated serum cholesterol, and cigarette smoking.

Clinical Intervention

Clinicians should emphasize primary prevention of CAD by periodically
screening for hypertension (see Chapter 3) and high serum cholesterol (Chapter
2) and by routinely investigating behavioral risk factors for CAD such as
tobacco use (Chapter 48), dietary fat and cholesterol intake (Chapter 50),
and inadequate physical activity (Chapter 49). Secondary prevention (screening) by performing routine electrocardiography in asymptomatic persons is
not recommended as an effective strategy to reduce the risk of CAD. It may
be clinically prudent to perform screening ECGs on asymptomatic males
over age 40 with two or more cardiac risk factors (hypercholesterolemia,
hypertension, cigarette smoking, diabetes mellitus, or family history of early-
onset CAD); on those who would endanger public safety were they to ex-

perience sudden cardiac events (e.g., commercial airline pilots); and as exercise tests for sedentary or high-risk males over age 40 who are planning to begin a vigorous exercise program. Due to the lack of data on the effectiveness of the screening ECG, the optimal interval for such testing is uncertain and is left to clinical discretion. The exercise ECG is a more sensitive and specific screening test than the resting ECG. Routine resting or exercise ECG screening to enter athletic programs is not recommended for children, adolescents, or young adults with no evidence of heart disease.

REFERENCES

1. National Center for Health Statistics. Advance report of final mortality statistics, 1986. Monthly Vital Statistics Report [Suppl], vol. 37, no. 6. Hyattsville, Md.: Public Health Service, 1988. (Publication no. DHHS (PHS) 88–1120.)
2. American Heart Association. 1989 heart facts. Dallas, Tex.: American Heart Association, 1988.
3. Furberg CD. Secondary prevention trials after acute myocardial infarction. Am J Cardiol 1987; 60:28A-32A.
4. Rose G, Baxter PJ, Reid DD, et al. Prevalence and prognosis of electrocardiographic findings in middle aged men. Br Heart J 1978; 40:636–43.
5. Knutsen R, Knutsen SF, Curb JD, et al. The predictive value of resting electrocardiograms for 12–year incidence of coronary heart disease in the Honolulu Heart Program. J Clin Epidemiol 1988; 41:293–302.
6. Cedres BL, Liu K, Stamler J, et al. Independent contribution of electrocardiographic abnormalities to risk of death from coronary heart disease, cardiovascular diseases and all causes: findings of three Chicago epidemiologic studies. Circulation 1982; 65:146–53.
7. Blackburn H, Taylor HL, Keys A. Coronary heart disease in seven countries. XVI. The electrocardiogram in prediction of five-year coronary heart disease incidence among men aged forty through fifty-nine. Circulation [Suppl 1] 1970; 41:154–61.
8. Cullen K, Stenhouse NS, Wearne KL, et al. Electrocardiograms and 13 year cardiovascular mortality in Busselton study. Br Heart J 1982; 47:209–12.
9. Higgins ITT, Kannel WB, Dawber TR. The electrocardiogram in epidemiological studies: reproducibility, validity, and international comparison. Br J Prev Soc Med 1965; 19:53–68.
10. Pooling Project Research Group. Relationship of blood pressure, serum cholesterol, smoking habit, relative weight and ECG abnormalities to incidence of major coronary events: final report of the Pooling Project. J Chron Dis 1978; 31:201–306.
11. Harlan WR, Cowie CC, Oberman A, et al. Prediction of subsequent ischemic heart disease using serial resting electrocardiograms. Am J Epidemiol 1984; 119:208–17.
12. Kannel WB, Anderson K, McGee DL, et al. Nonspecific electrocardiographic abnormality as a predictor of coronary heart disease: the Framingham Study. Am Heart J 1987; 113:370–6.
13. Detrano R, Froelicher V. A logical approach to screening for coronary artery disease. Ann Intern Med 1987; 106:846–52.
14. Kohli RS, Cashman PM, Lahiri A, et al. The ST segment of the ambulatory electrocardiogram in a normal population. Br Heart J 1988; 60:4–16.
15. Diamond GA, Forrester JS. Analysis of probability as an aid in the clinical diagnosis of coronary artery disease. N Engl J Med 1979; 300:1350–8.
16. Froelicher VF Jr, Yanowitz FG, Thompson AJ, et al. The correlation of coronary angiography and the electrocardiographic response to maximal treadmill testing in 76 asymptomatic men. Circulation 1973; 48:597–604.
17. Borer JS, Brensike JF, Redwood DR, et al. Limitations of the electrocardiographic response to exercise in predicting coronary-artery disease. N Engl J Med 1975; 293:367–71.

18. Froelicher VF Jr, Thompson AJ, Wolthuis R, et al. Angiographic findings in asymptomatic aircrewmen with electrocardiographic abnormalities. Am J Cardiol 1977; 39:32–8.
19. Multiple Risk Factor Intervention Trial Research Group. Baseline rest electrocardiographic abnormalities, antihypertensive treatment, and mortality in the Multiple Risk Factor Intervention Trial. Am J Cardiol 1985; 55:1–15.
20. Uhl GS, Froelicher V. Screening for asymptomatic coronary artery disease. J Am Coll Cardiol 1983; 1:946–55.
21. Bruce RA, DeRouen TA, Hossack KF. Value of maximal exercise tests in risk assessment of primary coronary heart disease events in healthy men: five years' experience of the Seattle Heart Watch Study. Am J Cardiol 1980; 46:371–8.
22. Aronow WS, Cassidy J. Five-year follow-up of double Master's test, maximal treadmill stress test, and resting and postexercise apex cardiogram in asymptomatic persons. Circulation 1975; 52:616–8.
23. Cumming GR, Samm J, Borysyk L, et al. Electrocardiographic changes during exercise in asymptomatic men: 3-year follow-up. Can Med Assoc J 1975; 112:578–81.
24. Froelicher VF Jr, Thomas MM, Pillow C, et al. Epidemiologic study of asymptomatic men screened by maximal treadmill testing for latent coronary artery disease. Am J Cardiol 1974; 34:770–6.
25. Allen WH, Aronow WS, Goodman P, et al. Five-year follow-up of maximal treadmill stress test in asymptomatic men and women. Circulation 1980; 62:522–7.
26. McHenry PL, O'Donnell J, Morris SN, et al. The abnormal exercise electrocardiogram in apparently healthy men: a predictor of angina pectoris as an initial coronary event during long-term follow-up. Circulation 1984; 70:547–51.
27. MacIntyre NR, Kunkler JR, Mitchell RE, et al. Eight-year follow-up of exercise electrocardiograms in healthy, middle-aged aviators. Aviat Space Environ Med 1981; 52:256–9.
28. Manca C, Dei Cas L, Albertini D, et al. Differential prognostic value of exercise electrocardiogram in men and women. Cardiology 1978; 63:312–9.
29. Giagnoni E, Secchi MB, Wu SC, et al. Prognostic value of exercise EKG testing in asymptomatic normotensive subjects: a prospective matched study. N Engl J Med 1983; 309:1085–9.
30. Gordon DJ, Ekelund LG, Karon JM, et al. Predictive value of the exercise tolerance test for mortality in North American men: the Lipid Research Clinics Mortality Follow-Up Study. Circulation 1986; 74:525–61.
31. Detrano R, Yiannikas J, Salcedo EE, et al. Bayesian probability analysis: a prospective demonstration of its clinical utility in diagnosing coronary disease. Circulation 1984; 69:541–7.
32. Erikssen J, Thaulow E. Follow-up of patients with asymptomatic myocardial ischemia. In: Rutishauser W, Roskamm H, eds. Silent myocardial ischemia. Berlin: Springer-Verlag, 1984:156–64.
33. Multiple Risk Factor Intervention Trial Research Group. Exercise electrocardiogram and coronary heart disease mortality in the Multiple Risk Factor Intervention Trial. Am J Cardiol 1985; 55:16–24.
34. Hickman JR Jr, Uhl GS, Cook RI, et al. A natural history study of asymptomatic coronary disease. Am J Cardiol 1980; 45:422.
35. Cohn PF. Silent myocardial ischemia. Ann Intern Med 1988; 109: 312–7.
36. Shell WE, Kivowitz CF, Rubins SB, et al. Mechanisms and therapy of silent myocardial ischemia: the effect of transdermal nitroglycerin. Am Heart J 1986; 112:222–9.
37. Frishman W, Teicher M. Antianginal drug therapy for silent myocardial ischemia. Am Heart J 1987; 114:140–7.
38. Pepine CJ, Hill JA, Imperi GA, et al. Beta-adrenergic blockers in silent myocardial ischemia. Am J Cardiol 1988; 61:18B-21B.
39. Epstein SE, Quyyumi AA, Bonow RO. Myocardial ischemia: silent or symptomatic. N Engl J Med 1988; 318:1038–43.
40. Erikssen J, Enge I, Forfang K, et al. False positive diagnostic tests and coronary angiographic findings in 105 presumably healthy males. Circulation 1978; 54:371–6.
41. Collen MF. The baseline screening electrocardiogram: is it worthwhile? An affirmative view. J Fam Pract 1987; 25:393–6.

42. Rubenstein L, Greenfield S. The baseline ECG in the evaluation of acute cardiac complaints. JAMA 1980; 224:2536–9.
43. American College of Cardiology. Guidelines for exercise testing: a report of the American College of Cardiology/American Heart Association Task Force on Assessment of Cardiovascular Procedures (Subcommittee on Exercise Testing). J Am Coll Cardiol 1986; 8:725–38.
44. Cobb LA, Weaver WD. Exercise: a risk for sudden death in patients with coronary artery disease. J Am Coll Cardiol 1986; 7:215–9.
45. Amsterdam EA, Laslett L, Holly R. Exercise and sudden death. Cardiol Clin 1987; 5: 337–43.
46. Epstein SE, Maron BJ. Sudden death and the competitive athlete: perspectives on preparticipation screening studies. J Am Coll Cardiol 1986; 7:220–30.
47. Resnekov L, Fox S, Selzer A, et al. Task Force IV: use of electrocardiograms in practice. Am J Cardiol 1978; 41:170–5.
48. American Heart Association. Cardiovascular and risk factor evaluation of healthy American adults: a statement for physicians by an ad hoc committee appointed by the steering committee, American Heart Association. Circulation 1987; 75:1340A-62A.
49. National Academy of Sciences, Institute of Medicine. Ad Hoc Advisory Group on Preventive Services. Preventive services for the well population. Washington, D.C.: National Academy of Sciences, 1978.
50. Canadian Task Force on the Periodic Health Examination. The periodic health examination: 1984 update. Can Med Assoc J 1984; 130:2–15.
51. Frame PS. A critical review of adult health maintenance. Part 1. prevention of atherosclerotic diseases. J Fam Pract 1986; 22:341–6.
52. Goldberger AL, O'Konski M. Utility of the routine electrocardiogram before surgery and on general hospital admission: critical review and new guidelines. Ann Intern Med 1986; 105:552–7.
53. Estes EH. Baseline screening electrocardiogram: an opposing view. J Fam Pract 1987; 25:395–6.
54. American College of Sports Medicine. Guidelines for exercise testing and prescription, 3rd ed. Philadelphia: Lea & Febiger, 1986.

2

Screening for High Blood Cholesterol

Recommendation: Periodic measurement of total serum cholesterol is most important for middle-aged men, and it may also be clinically prudent in young men, women, and the elderly (see *Clinical Intervention*). All patients should receive periodic counseling regarding dietary intake of fat (especially saturated fat) and cholesterol (see Chapter 50).

Burden of Suffering

High blood cholesterol, cigarette smoking, and hypertension are the principal modifiable risk factors for coronary artery disease (CAD), the leading cause of death in the United States.[1] About 1.5 million myocardial infarctions (MIs) and over 520,000 deaths from ischemic heart disease occur each year in the United States.[1,2] These cardiac events often occur without warning in persons with no previous history of angina pectoris or other clinical symptoms. The 30-day case-fatality rate for persons in whom MI is the initial manifestation of CAD is about 30%.[3] CAD is also associated with significant morbidity; the discomfort and exertional restrictions of angina pectoris and MI can limit productivity, functional independence, and quality of life. Cardiovascular diseases cost the United States about $80 billion each year.[2]

Efficacy of Screening Test

The principal screening test for high blood cholesterol is the measurement of total serum cholesterol in specimens obtained by either venipuncture or fingerstick. Due to biological variation and measurement error, such measurements may not always reflect the patient's true cholesterol level. Serum cholesterol levels normally undergo substantial physiologic fluctuations related to gender, stress, and season,[4] and therefore a single blood test may not always be representative. Repeated measurements on the same individual have a standard deviation of about 18 mg/dL (0.45 mmol/L), so that the 95% confidence interval for a typical adult whose blood cholesterol is 220 mg/dL (5.70 mmol/L) would be ±36 mg/dL (0.95 mmol/L), or 184–256 mg/dL (4.75–6.65 mmol/L).[5,6] Due to this variation, a single cholesterol measurement should not be relied on and the average of multiple tests should be used for therapeutic decisions.

In addition to biological variation, different laboratory instruments for measuring serum cholesterol are subject to systematic bias and random sources of error.[7] A number of instruments in routine use consistently overestimate (positive bias) or

underestimate (negative bias) the true cholesterol value by about 2–7%.[4,7-11] More extreme errors have also been reported. One study found that a serum cholesterol concentration of 250 mg/dL (6.45 mmol/L) was reported by one instrument as 285 mg/dL (7.35 mmol/L) (14% positive bias) and by another as 301 mg/dL (7.80 mmol/L) (20% positive bias).[4] Nearly half of all laboratory cholesterol results vary by 5% or more from the correct value.[12] Another potential source of error is poor precision (e.g., producing different results on the same specimen), although it is generally less of a problem than bias.[12] This accounts for about 3–4% of variation in the results of conventional clinical laboratory equipment[5,10] and desk-top office analyzers.[7,13-16] There is also significant variation between clinical laboratories (about 6%) and within individual laboratories (about 3.5%).[12]

Capillary sample measurements are often less accurate than analyses of venipuncture specimens. Inadequate training and the use of improper techniques in operating the equipment can introduce additional sources of error.[16] This is especially important in relation to desk-top chemical analyzers.[12] Further research is needed to fully evaluate these devices, and programs should be developed to assure acceptable performance standards before desk-top instruments are recommended for widespread screening.[12]

Since clinical decisions regarding treatment are affected by the report of a cholesterol level above a "desirable" level, there are potentially important clinical consequences resulting from laboratory underestimation or overestimation of the actual cholesterol level. Persons with high blood cholesterol requiring intervention may be advised incorrectly that their serum lipid levels are in the desirable range and thus not be retested for some time. Conversely, persons who receive falsely elevated test results may undergo the inconvenience and cost of follow-up testing. In some cases, erroneous cholesterol test results may generate unnecessary office visits to health care providers. Some patients may experience anxiety and the effects of labeling that have been observed in hypertension screening, such as absenteeism and psychological symptoms.[17] Finally, patients receiving inadequate follow-up testing may be exposed unnecessarily to treatment with cholesterol-lowering drugs.

To minimize the adverse effects of misclassification resulting from biological variance or laboratory error, an average of at least two blood test results is often recommended to provide a more accurate measure of the true concentration of total cholesterol; three tests are recommended if the difference between the first two tests is greater than 30 mg/dL [0.80 mmol/L].[18] In addition, rigorous standards for improving accuracy and precision in clinical laboratories are being developed and implemented by the College of American Pathologists, the Centers for Disease Control, and the National Cholesterol Coordinating Committee Laboratory Standardization Panel.[12,19] These groups have proposed the goal of improving standards for accuracy and precision in clinical laboratory measurement from the current range of ±5% to less than 3% by 1992.

Effectiveness of Early Detection

Early detection of high blood cholesterol in asymptomatic persons allows identification of an important modifiable risk factor for CAD. A large body of evidence gathered over several decades, including epidemiologic, pathologic, animal, genetic, and metabolic studies, supports the "lipid hypothesis," the causal relationship between serum cholesterol levels and the development of coronary atherosclerosis.[20-23]

The question of whether the lowering of serum cholesterol can achieve a significant reduction in the incidence of CAD in asymptomatic persons has been of

major clinical interest. Early efforts to answer this question involved controlled clinical trials in which asymptomatic middle-aged men with selected cardiac risk factors were given low-fat or modified-fat diets.[24-32] Such diets lowered serum cholesterol levels by about 10–15%, and in most trials, this was associated with a reduction in the incidence of cardiac events (e.g., myocardial infarction).[24,25,28-30,32] These early studies, however, suffered from a variety of design limitations, such as small sample size, selection bias in the recruitment of study groups and controls, confounding variables, inappropriate statistical analyses, and limited generalizability.[33,34] Probably due to inadequate sample size, most of these studies did not find a significant difference in either CAD or overall mortality between intervention and control groups.[24-27]

The ability of cholesterol-lowering drugs to reduce the incidence of CAD in asymptomatic persons has been demonstrated in three well-designed randomized controlled trials involving asymptomatic middle-aged men with high blood cholesterol. In the WHO Cooperative Trial, which involved over 15,000 men, subjects receiving clofibrate experienced a statistically significant 20% reduction in the overall rate of MI and 25% reduction in nonfatal MI when compared with controls receiving olive oil capsules.[35-37] The incidence of fatal MI was similar in both groups. The Lipid Research Clinics (LRC) Coronary Primary Prevention Trial, a multicenter study of cholestyramine involving 3806 men, reported an incidence of cardiac events of 7.0% in persons receiving cholestyramine and 8.6% in those receiving placebo.[38-42] This 19% reduction in the incidence of CAD was also statistically significant. Nonfatal MI and CAD mortality were 19% and 24% lower, respectively, in the group taking cholestyramine, and the incidence of angina, positive exercise tests, and coronary bypass surgery was also reduced. The Helsinki Heart Study, a trial involving 4081 asymptomatic men, reported a statistically significant 34% reduction in the incidence of cardiac events (nonfatal MI and cardiac death) in men receiving gemfibrozil.[43]

Taken together, these studies provide compelling evidence that the incidence of nonfatal MI and fatal cardiac disease can be reduced by lowering serum cholesterol. The randomized controlled trials that provide the strongest evidence, however, used drugs rather than diet to achieve this effect and involved a select population group, primarily white men aged 35–59 with serum cholesterol values above 255–265 mg/dL (6.60–6.85 mmol/L).[38,43] A current focus of interest is the extent to which this evidence is generalizable to other population groups (i.e., women, young men, the elderly, persons with less marked elevation of serum cholesterol) or to dietary measures.

Women, young men, and the elderly presumably benefit to some extent from lowering serum cholesterol. There are uncertainties, however, regarding the magnitude of benefit from screening these populations since elevated blood cholesterol is either a weaker risk factor or a less common abnormality in these groups.[34,44-47] Persons with borderline high cholesterol (200–240 mg/dL [5.15–6.20 mmol/L]), lacking the high blood cholesterol levels required of participants in the above trials, may benefit less by lowering cholesterol. A cohort study involving over 350,000 men[48,49] and 30-year longitudinal data from the Framingham Study[50] provide evidence that CAD risk increases in a continuous and graded fashion beginning with serum cholesterol levels as low as 180 mg/dL (4.65 mmol/L).[51] The risk rises sharply above 220–240 mg/dL (5.70–6.20 mmol/L), reaching a fourfold increase for levels above 260 mg/dL (6.70 mmol/L), which is the 90th percentile of middle-aged men. It follows that reductions in persons with borderline high cholesterol would be of less substantial benefit than for persons with severe elevations; a 50 mg/dL (1.30 mmol/L) reduction lowers absolute risk by about 50% in persons with a serum cholesterol of 300 mg/dL (7.75 mmol/L) but only by 25%

at a level of 250 mg/dL (6.45 mmol/L) and only 7.5% at 200 mg/dL (5.15 mmol/L).[22]

Cardiac risk factors other than high blood cholesterol are also important determinants of the benefits that can be expected from lowering blood cholesterol. Persons at increased risk for CAD because of a history of MI or angina, or asymptomatic persons with other cardiac risk factors, are thought to experience a greater reduction in risk for any given reduction in blood cholesterol than persons without these risk factors.[18,52] These risk factors include male sex, family history of premature CAD, cigarette smoking, hypertension, low high-density lipoprotein (HDL) cholesterol (less than 35 mg/dL [0.90 mmol/L]), diabetes mellitus, cerebrovascular or peripheral vascular disease, and severe obesity.

Another question concerns the magnitude of benefit associated with dietary measures. Animal studies, epidemiological data, and metabolic research support a beneficial effect from diets low in fat, primarily saturated fat. Clinical trials in which diet was the sole intervention have provided encouraging but not conclusive evidence of a significant reduction in the incidence of CAD.[21,22,44,53,54] The lack of conclusive evidence is due at least in part to design limitations (see above). It is reasonable to extrapolate from the drug trial findings that dietary restrictions, if successful in achieving significant reductions in serum cholesterol, can also lower the risk of CAD. Meta-analyses and other reviews of data pooled from dietary trials suggest that the dose-response relationship between dietary reduction of serum cholesterol and the risk of CAD is similar to that observed in data analyzed from drug trials.[55]

The ability of patients to achieve and maintain reductions in dietary fat is still under study. Low-fat diets that have been shown in experimental research to achieve significant reductions in serum cholesterol may not be adopted as readily by all members of the general population.[34,56] Thus, the more modest reductions in serum cholesterol level that result from ordinary fat-controlled diets may produce only modest reductions in CAD. Nonetheless, when compared with pharmacologic regimens to lower serum cholesterol, dietary measures are safer, less expensive, and may obviate the need for prescribing cholesterol-lowering drugs.

In summary, the magnitude of benefit of detecting high blood cholesterol may be reduced in women, young men, and the elderly; persons with borderline high cholesterol; and persons who use dietary measures that do not lower serum cholesterol significantly. Lowering serum cholesterol in low-risk populations may result in only minor changes in population-wide life expectancy.[47] On the other hand, low-risk individuals account for a large proportion of the population. It has been argued from a public health perspective that even modest benefits multiplied across large numbers of individuals can have significant public health implications.[57] Even a modest 5% reduction in the incidence of CAD would prevent about 75,000 MIs each year in the United States.[2]

It is also important to consider the potential health risks associated with lowering serum cholesterol. Long-term use of cholesterol-lowering drugs, such as nicotinic acid, clofibrate, and cholestyramine, is associated with a number of unpleasant and potentially serious side effects.[22,58,59] New classes of lipid-lowering drugs, such as lovastatin, also have adverse effects[60] and have not been in use for sufficient time to establish their long-term safety. The three major clinical trials involving lipid-lowering drugs each reported an increase in non-CAD deaths in intervention groups. An increase in violent deaths (accidents, suicide, homicide) reported in two of the three trials was not statistically significant and was attributed to chance by the investigators,[38,43] but the findings have raised concern among others.[61] The third trial reported a statistically significant 44% increase in all-cause mortality in men taking clofibrate.[35-37] Because clofibrate also causes gallstones,[35] its use for lowering cholesterol to prevent CAD is no longer recommended. Studies have reported associations between decreased levels of serum cholesterol and cancer[24,62-65] and gastrointestinal disease.[24,35,43] Evidence from a large longitudinal study, however, indicates that the association with cancer may represent an effect of preclinical cancer on blood cholesterol rather than an effect of low cholesterol on the development of the disease.[66] An increased incidence of cancer was also not apparent in the three drug trials discussed above.

Cholesterol screening during childhood has received increased attention in recent years. The detection of high blood cholesterol during childhood is of potential value in identifying those children who are at increased risk for developing CAD as adults and who might benefit from more intensive dietary interventions and follow-up than would be offered in the course of routine well-child care. Studies have shown that children with increased intake of dietary fat and cholesterol are at increased risk of having high blood cholesterol,[67] and children with high blood cholesterol are more likely than other children to have elevated cholesterol levels as adults.[68] Dietary habits learned in childhood may persist into adult life, and parents of children with high cholesterol levels are more likely to experience CAD.[69] High blood cholesterol may produce early atherosclerotic changes before adulthood; postmortem studies have demonstrated fatty streaks lining the aortas of children and adolescents with high blood cholesterol levels.[70] Autopsy studies have also noted evidence of CAD in adolescent and young adult war casualties.[71] It is unclear how strongly these pathologic changes are associated with subsequent CAD, however. A relationship between lowering cholesterol during childhood and decreased incidence of CAD during later life has yet to be demonstrated in controlled studies, in part due to the difficulty of performing such studies. This lack of evidence is of concern because it is currently unclear whether a policy of routine cholesterol screening of the 50–60 million children[72] in the United States would achieve sufficient clinical benefit in later years to justify the costs and potential adverse effects of widespread testing. Due to the low prevalence of high blood cholesterol in children, routine screening is likely to generate a large proportion of false positives. There is little information on the potential psychological effects on children of being "labeled" as having high blood cholesterol. Also, some pediatricians have expressed concern that dietary restrictions during childhood may affect the child's source of calories, calcium, and iron.[73] The issue is still under active study.

Recommendations of Others

The National Heart, Lung, and Blood Institute has issued recommendations on cholesterol screening in the clinical setting in the report of the Expert Panel on Detection, Evaluation, and Treatment of High Blood Cholesterol in Adults.[18] These recommendations were endorsed by the National Cholesterol Coordinating Committee, which includes representatives from the leading national medical organizations. The report recommends routine measurement of nonfasting serum cholesterol in all adults aged 20 and above at least once every five years and provides a detailed protocol to guide follow-up of test results. The protocol sets a lower treatment threshold for persons with CAD or who are at high risk for CAD and recommends averaging two to three separate measurements of total cholesterol and low-density lipoprotein (LDL) cholesterol to help guide drug treatment decisions. Specific recommendations to improve the effectiveness of public screening for high blood cholesterol have been issued through a workshop sponsored by the National Heart, Lung, and Blood Institute.[74] The American Academy of Pediatrics recommends regular elective testing for high blood cholesterol only for children over age 2 who have a family history of hyperlipidemia or early MI.[75] Others have recently recommended universal cholesterol screening for all children.[76] Recommendations on public screening outside the medical setting are currently being prepared by the National Cholesterol Coordinating Committee.

Discussion

Serum cholesterol testing of adults in the United States has the potential of achieving a significant reduction in the nationwide incidence of CAD. Care is, however, required for any program targeting more than 150 million people[72] for testing and follow-up to guard against unnecessary health care expenditures and adverse personal consequences. In particular, the use of inaccurate laboratory or desk-top instruments for screening can lead to large numbers of both false-negative and false-positive results. The former can delay needed clinical intervention and the latter can lead to considerable inconvenience, costs, and adverse psychological and medical consequences in persons not needing intervention. It is therefore important for clinicians to exercise discretion in selecting accurate and reliable methods of obtaining blood specimens in the clinical setting, to use clinical laboratories that adhere to accepted standards of quality control, and to properly design treatment strategies based on results confirmed by repeated tests.

Discretion is especially important in the use of cholesterol-lowering drugs. The efficacy of such drugs in preventing CAD has been demonstrated most convincingly in middle-aged men with serum cholesterol levels above 255–265 mg/dL (6.60–6.85 mmol/L).[38,43] The effect on CAD of using lipid-lowering drugs in young men, women, or elderly persons, or in those with only mild to moderate elevations in blood cholesterol, has not been studied in clinical trials of asymptomatic persons. It is therefore reasonable to limit the exposure of low- or moderate-risk individuals to the unpleasant side effects of lipid-lowering drugs, the inconvenience of daily, long-term administration, and the potential health risks of agents for which long-term safety has yet to be established. There are also economic implications to prescribing lipid-lowering drugs in light of their expense and the quantities required for long-term therapy. Some studies examining the economic benefits of preventing CAD have questioned the cost-effectiveness of routine drug therapy for elevations in blood cholesterol.[77-80]

It has been shown that a low level of HDL cholesterol is an independent predictor of CAD. Persons whose HDL cholesterol level is at the 20th percentile have two to four times the risk of developing CAD as persons whose level is at the 80th percentile.[81,82] Lipid-fractionation studies, which enable the calculation of HDL and LDL levels, can therefore provide more meaningful information on CAD risk and the effectiveness of therapy than can total cholesterol measurement. Concerns that total blood cholesterol measurements may fail to detect persons at increased risk due to low HDL cholesterol (despite a normal total cholesterol level) have led to recent recommendations to perform lipoprotein analysis routinely on all persons with borderline or high total blood cholesterol.[83]

There are substantial economic considerations in the performance of fractionation studies as a routine follow-up to finding elevated total cholesterol. For example, examining lipid profiles on all adults with high blood cholesterol (240 mg/dL [6.20 mmol/L] or greater) would require performing a $20–$40 test on nearly one-quarter of the 150 million adults in the United States.[72,84] Although it is likely that the information would be useful to clinicians, further research is necessary to determine the exact prevalence of low HDL cholesterol, the efficacy of measures to raise HDL cholesterol, and whether the added information provided by routine lipoprotein analysis results in an overall improvement in clinical outcome. Until this evidence becomes available, lipid fractionation studies may be best reserved for the smaller group of persons for whom the information is most important, such as those being considered for drug therapy and those being monitored for response to treatment with cholesterol-lowering drugs.

Clinical Intervention

All patients should receive periodic counseling regarding dietary intake of fat (especially saturated fat) and cholesterol (see Chapter 50). Periodic measurement of total serum cholesterol (nonfasting) is most important for middle-aged men, and it may also be clinically prudent in young men, women, and the elderly. The optimal frequency for cholesterol measurement in asymptomatic persons has not been determined on the basis of scientific evidence and is left to clinical discretion; an interval of every five years (and more frequently for persons with previous evidence of elevated cholesterol) has been recommended on the basis of expert opinion.[18] Cholesterol tests should be performed on venous blood samples analyzed by an accredited laboratory that meets current standards of accuracy and reliability. Abnormal results should be confirmed by a second measurement of nonfasting total cholesterol, and the mean of both results should be used for subsequent therapeutic decisionmaking.

All adults with high blood cholesterol (at or above 240 mg/dL [6.20 mmol/ L]) and those persons with borderline high cholesterol (200–239 mg/dL [5.15–6.15 mmol/L]) who have known CAD or two or more cardiac risk factors should receive information about the meaning of results, intensive dietary counseling, and follow-up evaluation. The most important cardiac risk factors to be considered include male gender, premature CAD in a first-degree relative, smoking, hypertension, serum HDL cholesterol less than 35 mg/dL (0.90 mmol/L) (when this information is available), diabetes mellitus, previous stroke or peripheral vascular disease, and severe obesity. The recommended two-step dietary program to lower serum cholesterol has been described in detail elsewhere.[18] The primary objective of the Step-One diet is to reduce all dietary fat intake to less than 30% of total calories (with saturated fat contributing less than 10% of total calories) and to reduce dietary cholesterol intake to less than 300 mg/day. The Step-Two diet, which is recommended if the goals of therapy are not achieved after three months, differs from the first by further restricting intake of saturated fats (to 7% of total calories) and dietary cholesterol (200 mg/day).

Cholesterol-lowering drugs should be considered in middle-aged men in whom blood cholesterol remains significantly elevated after a thorough six-month trial of dietary intervention. A suggested threshold for drug treatment is 240 mg/dL (6.20 mmol/L) or greater in persons with CAD or at least two cardiac risk factors and 265 mg/dL (6.85 mmol/L) or greater in persons without risk factors. The patient should receive information on the potential benefits and risks of long-term therapy before beginning treatment on cholesterol-lowering drugs. It is clinically prudent to perform lipid fractionation studies on persons being considered for drug treatment and those being monitored for response to drug therapy over time.

REFERENCES

1. National Center for Health Statistics. Advance report of final mortality statistics, 1986. Monthly Vital Statistics Report [Suppl], vol. 37, no. 6. Hyattsville, Md.: Public Health Service, 1988. (Publication no. DHHS (PHS) 88–1120.)

2. American Heart Association. 1989 heart facts. Dallas, Tex.: American Heart Association, 1988.

3. Elveback LR, Connolly DC, Melton LJ III. Coronary heart disease in residents of Rochester, Minnesota. Incidence, 1950 through 1982. Mayo Clin Proc 1986; 61:896–900.

4. Blank DW, Hoeg JM, Kroll MH, et al. The method of determination must be considered in interpreting blood cholesterol levels. JAMA 1986; 256:2767–70.

5. Jacobs DR, Barrett-Connor E. Retest reliability of plasma cholesterol and triglyceride: the Lipid Research Clinics Prevalence Study. Am J Epidemiol 1982; 116:878–85.

6. Wyngaarden JB. Variability in individual cholesterol level clouds risk assessment. JAMA 1988; 260:759.

7. Burke JJ II, Fischer PM. A clinician's guide to the office measurement of cholesterol. JAMA 1988; 259:3444–8.

8. Koch TR, Mehta U, Lee H, et al. Bias and precision of cholesterol analysis by physician's office analyzers. Clin Chem 1987; 33:2262–7.

9. Kroll MH, Lindsey H, Greene J, et al. Bias between enzymatic methods and the reference method for cholesterol. Clin Chem 1988; 34:131–5.

10. Rastam L, Admire JB, Frantz ID, et al. Measurement of blood cholesterol with the Reflotron analyzer evaluated. Clin Chem 1988; 34:426.

11. Lasater TM, Lefebvre RC, Assaf AR, et al. Rapid measurement of blood cholesterol: evaluation of a new instrument. Am J Prev Med 1987; 3:311–6.

12. Laboratory Standardization Panel of the National Cholesterol Education Program. Current status of blood cholesterol measurement in clinical laboratories in the United States. Clin Chem 1988; 34:193–201.

13. Hicks JM, Iosefsohn M. Another physician's office analyzer: the Abbott "Vision" evaluated. Clin Chem 1987; 33:817–9.

14. Nanji AA, Sincennes F, Poon R, et al. Evaluation of the Boehringer Mannheim "Reflotron" analyzer. Clin Chem 1987; 33:1254–5.

15. von Schenck H, Treichl L, Tilling B, et al. Laboratory and field evaluation of three desktop instruments for assay of cholesterol and triglyceride. Clin Chem 1987; 33:1230–2.

16. Belsey R, Vandenbark M, Goitein RK, et al. Evaluation of a laboratory system intended for use in physicians' offices. II. Reliability of results produced by health care workers without formal or professional training. JAMA 1987; 258:357–61.

17. Lefebvre RC, Hursey KG, Carleton RA. Labeling of participants in high blood pressure screening programs: implications for blood cholesterol screenings. Arch Intern Med 1988; 148:1993–7.

18. Report of the National Cholesterol Education Program Expert Panel on Detection, Evaluation, and Treatment of High Blood Cholesterol in Adults. Arch Intern Med 1988; 148:36–69.

19. Cotton P. CAP moves to improve lipid tests. Medical World News, June 1988:55.

20. Stamler J. Lifestyles, major risk factors, proof and public policy. Circulation 1978; 58: 3–19.

21. Stallones RA. Ischemic heart disease and lipids in blood and diet. Ann Rev Nutr 1983; 3:155–85.

22. Grundy SM. Cholesterol and coronary heart disease: a new era. JAMA 1986; 256: 2849–58.

23. National Institutes of Health. Lowering blood cholesterol to prevent heart disease. JAMA 1985; 253:2080–6.

24. Dayton S, Pearce ML, Hashimoto S, et al. A controlled clinical trial of a diet high in unsaturated fat in preventing complications of atherosclerosis. Circulation [Suppl II] 1969; 40:II-1–63.

25. Hjermann I, Velve Byre K, Holme I, et al. Effect of diet and smoking intervention on the incidence of coronary heart disease. Report from the Oslo Study Group of a randomized trial in healthy men. Lancet 1981; 2:1303–10.

26. Multiple Risk Factor Intervention Trial Research Group. Multiple risk factor intervention trial: risk factor changes and mortality results. JAMA 1982; 248:1465–77.

27. World Health Organization European Collaborative Group. European collaborative trial

of multifactorial prevention of coronary heart disease: final report on the 6–year results. Lancet 1986; 1:869–72.

28. Pinnlar O. Primary prevention of coronary heart disease by diet. Bull NY Acad Med 1968; 44:936–49.

29. Turpeinen O, Karvonen MJ, Pekkarinen M, et al. Dietary prevention of coronary heart disease: the Finnish Mental Hospital Study. Int J Epidemiol 1979; 8:99–118.

30. Miettinen M, Turpeinen O, Karvonen MJ, et al. Effect of cholesterol-lowering diet on mortality from coronary heart disease and other causes. Lancet 1972; 2:835–8.

31. Stamler J. Acute myocardial infarction, progress in primary prevention. Br Heart J 1971; 33:145–64.

32. Frantz ID, Dawson EA, Kuba K. The Minnesota Coronary Survey: effect of diet on cardiovascular events and deaths. Circulation [Suppl II] 1975; 52:II-4.

33. Borhani NO. Primary prevention of coronary heart disease: a critique. Am J Card 1977; 40:251–9.

34. Ahrens EH. The diet-heart question in 1985; has it really been settled? Lancet 1985; 1:1085–7.

35. Report from the Committee of Principal Investigators. A cooperative trial in the primary prevention of ischaemic heart disease using clofibrate. Br Heart J 1978; 40:1069–118.

36. Report of the Committee of Principal Investigators. W.H.O. cooperative trial on primary prevention of ischaemic heart disease using clofibrate to lower serum cholesterol: mortality follow-up. Lancet 1980; 2:379–85.

37. Idem. W.H.O. cooperative trial on primary prevention of ischaemic heart disease with clofibrate to lower serum cholesterol: final mortality follow-up. Lancet 1984; 2:600–4.

38. The Lipid Research Clinics Coronary Primary Prevention Trial Results. I. Reduction in incidence of coronary heart disease. JAMA 1984; 251:351–64.

39. The Lipid Research Clinics Coronary Primary Provention Trial Results. II. The relationship of reduction in incidence of coronary heart disease to cholesterol lowering. JAMA 1984; 251:365–74.

40. The Lipid Research Clinics Program. The coronary primary prevention trial: design and implementation. J Chron Dis 1979; 32:609–31.

41. Idem. Pre-entry characteristics of participants in the Lipid Research Clinics Coronary Primary Prevention Trial. J Chron Dis 1983; 36:467–79.

42. Idem. Participant recruitment to the Coronary Primary Prevention Trial. J Chron Dis 1983; 36:451–65.

43. Frick MH, Elo O, Haapa K, et al. Helsinki Heart Study: primary prevention trial with gemfibrozil in middle-aged men with dyslipidemia. Safety of treatment, changes in risk factors, and incidence of coronary heart disease. N Engl J Med 1987; 317:1237–45.

44. Kronmal RA. Commentary on the published results of the Lipid Research Clinics Coronary Primary Prevention Trial. JAMA 1985; 253:2091–3.

45. Rahimtoola SH. Some unexpected lessons from large multicenter randomized clinical trials. Circulation 1985; 72:449–55.

46. Borhani NO. Prevention of coronary heart disease in practice: implications of the results of recent clinical trials. JAMA 1985; 254:257–62.

47. Taylor WC, Pass TM, Shepard D, et al. Cholesterol reduction and life expectancy: a model incorporating multiple risk factors. Ann Intern Med 1987; 106:605–14.

48. Stamler J, Wentworth D, Neaton JD. Is relationship between serum cholesterol and risk of premature death from coronary heart disease continuous and graded? JAMA 1986; 256:2823–8.

49. Martin MJ, Hulley SB, Browner WS, et al. Serum cholesterol, blood pressure, and mortality: implications from a cohort of 361,662 men. Lancet 1986; 2:933–6.

50. Anderson KM, Castelli WP, Levy D. Cholesterol and mortality: 30 years of follow-up from the Framingham Study. JAMA 1987; 257:2176–80.

51. Neaton JD, Kuller LH, Wentworth D, et al. Total and cardiovascular mortality in relation to cigarette smoking, serum cholesterol concentration, and diastolic blood pressure among black and white males followed up for five years. Am Heart J 1984; 108: 759–70.

52. Siegel D, Grady D, Browner WS, et al. Risk factor modification after myocardial infarction. Ann Intern Med 1988; 109:213–8.
53. Rahimtoola SH. Cholesterol and coronary heart disease: a perspective. JAMA 1985; 253:2094–5.
54. Kaplan RM. Behavioral epidemiology, health promotion, and health services. Med Care 1985; 23:564–83.
55. Tyroler HA. Review of lipid-lowering clinical trials in relation to observational epidemiologic studies. Circulation 1987; 76:515–22.
56. Hulley SB, Lo B. Choice and use of blood lipid tests: an epidemiologic perspective. Arch Intern Med 1983; 143:667–73.
57. Blackburn H. Public policy and dietary recommendations to reduce population level of blood cholesterol. Am J Prev Med 1985; 1:3–11.
58. Oliver MF. Risks of correcting the risks of coronary disease and stroke with drugs. N Engl J Med 1982; 306:297–8.
59. Knodel LC, Talbert RL. Adverse effects of hypolipidaemic drugs. Med Toxicol 1987; 2:10–32.
60. Lovastatin for hypercholesterolemia. Medical Letter 1987; 29:99–101.
61. Kolata G. Heart panel's conclusions questioned. Science 1985; 227:40–1.
62. Rose G, Shipley MJ. Plasma lipids and mortality: a source of error. Lancet 1980; 1: 523–6.
63. Neugut AI, Johnsen CM, Fink DJ. Serum cholesterol levels in adenomatous polyps and cancer of the colon: a case-control study. JAMA 1986; 255:365–7.
64. International Collaborative Group. Circulating cholesterol level and risk of death from cancer in men aged 40 to 69 years. JAMA 1982; 248:2853–9.
65. Williams RR, Sorlie PD, Feinleib M, et al. Cancer incidence by levels of cholesterol. JAMA 1981; 245:247–52.
66. Sherwin RW, Wentworth DN, Cutler JA, et al. Serum cholesterol levels and cancer mortality in 361,662 men screened for the Multiple Risk Factor Intervention Trial. JAMA 1987; 257:943–8.
67. Nicklas TA, Farris RP, Smoak CG, et al. Dietary factors relate to cardiovascular risk factors in early life. Arteriosclerosis 1988; 8:193–9.
68. Lauer RM, Lee J, Clarke WR. Factors affecting the relationship between childhood and adult cholesterol levels: the Muscatine Study. Pediatrics 1988; 82:309–18.
69. Croft JB, Cresanta JL, Webber LS, et al. Cardiovascular risk in parents of children with extreme lipoprotein cholesterol levels: the Bogalusa Heart Study. South Med J 1988; 81:341–9.
70. Berenson GS, Srinivasan SR, Nicklas TA, et al. Cardiovascular risk factors in children and early prevention of heart disease. Clin Chem 1988; 34:B115–22.
71. Enos WF, Holmes RH, Beyer J. Coronary disease among United States soldiers killed in action in Korea. JAMA 1953; 152:1090–3.
72. National Center for Health Statistics. Health, United States, 1988. Washington D.C.: Government Printing Office, 1989:41. (Publication no. DHHS (PHS) 89–1232.)
73. American Academy of Pediatrics. Prudent lifestyle for children: dietary fat and cholesterol. Pediatrics 1986; 78:521–5.
74. National Heart, Lung, and Blood Institute. Recommendations regarding public screening for measuring blood cholesterol: summary of a National Heart, Lung, and Blood Institute workshop. Bethesda, Md.: National Heart, Lung, and Blood Institute, 1988.
75. American Academy of Pediatrics. Indications for cholesterol testing in children. Pediatrics 1989; 83:141–2.
76. Merz B. New studies fuel controversy over universal cholesterol screening during childhood. JAMA 1989; 261:814.
77. Oster G, Epstein AM. Cost-effectiveness of antihyperlipemic therapy in the prevention of coronary heart disease: the case of cholestyramine. JAMA 1987; 258:2381–7.
78. Kinosian BP, Eisenberg JM. Cutting into cholesterol: cost-effective alternatives for treating hypercholesterolemia. JAMA 1988; 259:2249–54.
79. Weinstein MC, Stason WB. Cost effectiveness of interventions to prevent or treat coronary heart disease. Ann Rev Public Health 1985; 6:41–63.

80. Himmelstein DU, Woolhandler S. Costs and effects: the lipid research trial and the Rand experiment. N Engl J Med 1985; 311:1512–3.
81. Castelli WP, Garrison RJ, Wilson PW, et al. Incidence of coronary heart disease and lipoprotein cholesterol levels: the Framingham Study. JAMA 1986; 256:2835–8.
82. Wilson PW, Abbott RD, Castelli WP. High density lipoprotein cholesterol and mortality: the Framingham Heart Study. Arteriosclerosis 1988; 8:737–41.
83. Merz B. Is it time to include lipoprotein analysis in cholesterol screening? JAMA 1989; 261:497–8.
84. Herman M, Health Care Financing Administration. Personal communication, February 1989.

3

Screening for Hypertension

Recommendation: Blood pressure should be measured regularly in all persons aged 3 and above (see *Clinical Intervention*).

Burden of Suffering

Hypertension may occur in as many as 58 million Americans.[1] It is a leading risk factor for coronary artery disease, congestive heart failure, stroke, renal disease, and retinopathy. These complications of hypertension are among the most common and serious diseases in the United States, and successful efforts to lower blood pressure could thus have substantial impact on population morbidity and mortality. Heart disease is the leading cause of death in the United States, accounting for over 765,000 deaths each year, and cerebrovascular disease, the third leading cause of death, accounts for 150,000 deaths each year.[2] Hypertension is more common in blacks and the elderly.[1]

Efficacy of Screening Tests

The most accurate devices for measuring blood pressure (e.g., intraarterial catheters) are not appropriate for routine screening because of their invasiveness, technical limitations, and cost. Office sphygmomanometry (the blood pressure cuff) remains the most appropriate screening test for hypertension in the asymptomatic population. Although this test is highly accurate when performed correctly, false-positive and false-negative results (i.e., recording a blood pressure that is not representative of the patient's mean blood pressure) do occur in clinical practice.[3] A recent study found that 21% of persons diagnosed as mildly hypertensive based on office sphygmomanometry had no evidence of hypertension when 24-hour ambulatory recordings were obtained.[4]

Errors in measuring blood pressure may result from instrument, observer, and/or patient factors.[5] Examples of instrument error include manometer dysfunction, pressure leaks, stethoscope defects, and bladders of incorrect width and length for the patient's arm size. The observer can introduce errors due to sensory impairment (difficulty hearing Korotkoff sounds or reading the manometer), inattention, inconsistency in recording Korotkoff sounds (e.g., Phase IV vs. Phase V), and subconscious bias (e.g., "digit preference" for numbers ending with zero or preconceived notions of "normal" pressures). The patient can be the source of misleading readings due to posture and biological factors. Posture (i.e., lying, standing, sitting) and arm position in relation to the heart can affect results by as much as 10 mm Hg.[5] Biological factors include anxiety, meals, tobacco, temperature changes, exertion, and pain. Due to these limitations in the test-retest reliability of blood pressure measurement, it is commonly recommended that hypertension be diagnosed only after more than one elevated reading is obtained on each of three separate visits.[1]

Additional factors affect accuracy when performing sphygmomanometry on children; these difficulties are especially common when testing infants and toddlers under age 3.[6] First, there is increased variation in arm circumference, requiring greater care in the selection of cuff sizes. Second, the examination is more frequently complicated by the anxiety and restlessness of the patient. Third, the disappearance of Korotkoff sounds (Phase V) is often difficult to hear in children and Phase IV values are often substituted. Fourth, erroneous Korotkoff sounds can be produced inadvertently by the pressure of the stethoscope diaphragm against the antecubital fossa. Finally, the definition of pediatric hypertension has itself been uncertain because of confusion over normal values during childhood. Previous criteria using population data to define the 95th percentile at different ages were erroneously high.[7] Revised criteria for pediatric hypertension, based on data from over 70,000 children, have recently been published[6] (see *Clinical Intervention*).

Effectiveness of Early Detection

There is a direct relationship between the magnitude of blood pressure elevation and the benefit of lowering pressure. In persons with malignant hypertension, the benefits of intervention are most dramatic; treatment increases five-year survival from near zero (data from historical controls) to 75%.[8] The efficacy of treating moderate hypertension (diastolic blood pressure above 104 mm Hg) is also clear, as demonstrated in the Veterans Administration Cooperative Study on Antihypertensive Agents.[9-11] In this randomized double-blind controlled trial, middle-aged men with diastolic blood pressure above 104 mm Hg experienced a significant reduction in cardiovascular events after treatment with antihypertensive medication.

Persons with mild hypertension (diastolic blood pressure of 90–104 mm Hg) also benefit from treatment. This was confirmed in the Hypertension Detection and Follow-Up Program, a randomized controlled trial involving nearly 11,000 hypertensives.[12] The intervention group received standardized pharmacologic treatment ("stepped care") while the control group was referred for community medical care. There was a statistically significant 17% reduction in five-year all-cause mortality in the group receiving standardized drug therapy; the subset with mild hypertension experienced a 20% reduction in mortality.[12] Deaths due to cerebrovascular disease, ischemic heart disease, and other causes were also significantly reduced in the stepped care group.[13] Similar results have been reported in other studies, such as the Australian National Blood Pressure Study[14] and the Medical Research Council trial.[15] Although treatment of hypertension is associated with multiple benefits, the greatest effect appears to be in the prevention of cerebrovascular disease.[16] Improved treatment of high blood pressure has been credited with the greater than 50% reduction in age-adjusted stroke mortality that has been observed since 1972.[1,17]

Although the efficacy of antihypertensive treatment has been well established in clinical research, certain factors may influence the magnitude of benefit achieved in actual practice. First, the benefits of treatment may be less significant or less well proven in certain population groups, such as children. Second, nonpharmacologic first-line therapy (e.g., weight reduction, exercise, sodium restriction, decreased alcohol intake) may be less effective than drug therapy in achieving significant and consistent blood pressure reductions. Although it is known that weight reduction and sodium restriction can lower blood pressure,[18,19] the magnitude and duration of reduction in actual practice may be limited by biological factors (o.g., hypertensives who are not "salt-sensitive") and the difficulties of maintaining behavioral changes (e.g., weight loss). Finally, compliance with drug therapy may be limited by the inconvenience, side effects, and cost of these agents.[20,21]

Recommendations of Others

Revised recommendations for adults from the National Heart, Lung, and Blood Institute were issued recently by the Joint National Committee on Detection, Evaluation, and Treatment of High Blood Pressure,[1] and similar recommendations have been issued by the American Heart Association.[22] These call for routine blood pressure measurement at least once every two years for persons with a diastolic blood pressure below 85 mm Hg and a systolic pressure below 140 mm Hg. Measurements are recommended annually for persons with a diastolic blood pressure of 85–89 mm Hg. Persons with higher blood pressures require more frequent measurements. The Canadian Task Force recommends that all persons aged 25 and over receive a blood pressure measurement during any visit to a physician.[23] The American Academy of Pediatrics and the National Heart, Lung, and Blood Institute recommend that children and adolescents receive annual blood pressure measurements from ages 3–20.[6]

Discussion

It is clear from several large clinical trials that lowering blood pressure is beneficial and that the population incidence of several leading causes of death can be reduced through the detection and treatment of high blood pressure. An average diastolic blood pressure reduction of 6–8 mm Hg across the population could reduce the incidence of coronary artery disease by 25% and the incidence of strokes by 50%.[24] At the same time, it is important for clinicians to minimize the potential harmful effects of detection and treatment. For example, if performed incorrectly, sphygmomanometry can produce misleading results. Some hypertensive patients thereby escape detection (false negatives) and some normotensive persons receive inappropriate labeling (false positives), which may have certain psychological, behavioral, and even financial consequences.[25] Treatment of hypertension can also be harmful as a result of medical complications, especially related to drugs. Clinicians can minimize these effects by using proper technique when performing sphygmomanometry, making appropriate use of nonpharmacologic methods, and prescribing antihypertensive drugs with careful adherence to current guidelines.

Clinical Intervention

Blood pressure should be measured regularly in all persons aged 3 and above. The optimal interval for blood pressure screening has not been determined and is left to clinical discretion. Current expert opinion is that persons thought to be normotensive should receive blood pressure measurements at least once every two years if their last diastolic and systolic blood pressure readings were below 85 mm Hg and 140 mm Hg, respectively, and annually if the last diastolic blood pressure was 85–89 mm Hg.[1] Sphygmomanometry should be performed in accordance with recommended tech-

nique.*[1] **Hypertension should not be diagnosed on the basis of a single measurement; elevated readings** should be confirmed on more than one reading at each of three separate visits.** Once confirmed, patients should **receive counseling regarding exercise (see Chapter 49), weight reduction, dietary sodium intake (Chapter 50), and alcohol consumption (Chapter 47).**[1] **Other cardiovascular risk factors, such as smoking and elevated serum cholesterol, should also be discussed (Chapters 2 and 48).** Antihypertensive drugs should be prescribed in accordance with recent guidelines[1] and with attention to current techniques for improving compliance.**[20,21]

REFERENCES

1. 1988 Joint National Committee. The 1988 report of the Joint National Committee on Detection, Evaluation, and Treatment of High Blood Pressure. Arch Intern Med 1988; 148:1023–38.
2. National Center for Health Statistics. Advance report of final mortality statistics, 1986. Monthly Vital Statistics Report [Suppl], vol. 37, no. 6. Hyattsville, Md.: Public Health Service, 1988. (Publication no. DHHS (PHS) 88–1120.)
3. Tifft CP. Are the days of the sphygmomanometer past? Arch Intern Med 1988; 148:518–9.
4. Pickering TG, James GD, Boddie C, et al. How common is white coat hypertension? JAMA 1988; 259:225–8.
5. Kirkendall WM, Feinleib M, Freis ED, et al. Recommendations for human blood pressure determination by sphygmomanometers. Subcommittee of the AHA Postgraduate Education Committee. Circulation 1980; 62:1146A-55A.
6. Task Force on Blood Pressure Control in Children. Report of the Second Task Force on Blood Pressure Control in Children—1987. Pediatrics 1987; 79:1–25.
7. Mehta SK. Pediatric hypertension: a challenge for pediatricians. Am J Dis Child 1987; 141:893–4.

---

*Guidelines for Sphygmomanometry
• Patient should be seated with arm bared, supported, and positioned at heart level.
• Patient should have refrained from smoking or ingesting caffeine within 30 minutes before measurement.
• Measurement should begin after five minutes of quiet rest.
• An appropriate cuff size (child, adult, large adult) should be selected; the rubber bladder should encircle at least two thirds of the arm.
• Measurements should be taken with a mercury sphygmomanometer, a recently calibrated aneroid manometer, or a validated electronic device.
• Both systolic and diastolic pressures should be recorded; the disappearance of sound (Phase V) indicates the diastolic pressure.
• Two or more readings should be averaged; if the first two differ by more than 5 mm Hg, additional readings should be obtained.

**In adults, current blood pressure criteria for the diagnosis are a diastolic pressure of 90 mm Hg or greater or a systolic pressure of 140 mm Hg or greater.[1] In children, the criteria vary with age:[6]

	Pediatric Blood Pressure	
Age (Yrs)	Diastolic (mm Hg)	Systolic (mm Hg)
0–2	74	112
3–5	76	116
6–9	78	122
10–12	82	126
13–15	86	136

8. Hansson L. Current and future strategies in the treatment of hypertension. Am J Cardiol 1988; 61:2C-7C.
9. Veterans Administration Cooperative Study Group on Antihypertensive Agents. Effects of treatment on morbidity in hypertension. III. Influence of age, diastolic pressure, and prior cardiovascular disease: further analysis of side effects. Circulation 1972; 45:991–1004.
10. *Idem*. Effects of treatment on morbidity in hypertension: results in patients with diastolic pressures averaging 115 through 129 mm Hg. JAMA 1967; 202:1028–34.
11. *Idem*. Effects of treatment on morbidity in hypertension. II. Results in patients with diastolic pressures averaging 90 through 114 mm Hg. JAMA 1970; 213:1143–52.
12. Hypertension Detection and Follow-Up Program Cooperative Group. Five-year findings of the Hypertension Detection and Follow-Up Program. I. Reduction in mortality of persons with high blood pressure, including mild hypertension. JAMA 1979; 242: 2562–72.
13. *Idem*. Persistence of reduction in blood pressure and mortality of participants in the Hypertension Detection and Follow-Up Program. JAMA 1988; 259:2113–22.
14. Management Committee of the Australian National Blood Pressure Study. The Australian therapeutic trial in mild hypertension. Lancet 1980; 1:1261–7.
15. Medical Research Council Working Party. MRC trial of treatment of mild hypertension: principal results. Br Med J 1985; 291:97–104.
16. MacMahon SW, Cutler JA, Furberg CD, et al. The effects of drug treatment for hypertension on morbidity and mortality from cardiovascular disease: a review of randomized, controlled trials. Prog Cardiovasc Dis [Suppl] 1986; 29:99–118. and the declining incidence of stroke. JAMA 1987; 258:214–7.
17. Garraway WM, Whisnant JP. The changing pattern of hypertension and the declining incidence of stroke. JAMA 1987; 258:214–7.
18. Nonpharmacological approaches to the control of high blood pressure. Final report of the Subcommittee on Nonpharmacological Therapy of the 1984 Joint National Committee on Detection, Evaluation, and Treatment of High Blood Pressure. Hypertension 1986; 8:444–67.
19. Stamler J, Stamler R. Intervention for the prevention and control of hypertension and atherosclerotic diseases: United States and international experience. Am J Med 1984, 76:13–36.
20. McClellan WM, Hall WD, Brogan D, et al. Continuity of care in hypertension: an important correlate of blood pressure control among aware hypertensives. Arch Intern Med 1988; 148:525–8.
21. National Institutes of Health. The physician's guide: improving adherence among hypertensive patients. Working Group on Health Education and High Blood Pressure Control. Bethesda, Md.: Department of Health and Human Services, 1987.
22. Grundy SM, Greenland P, Herd A, et al. Cardiovascular and risk factor evaluation of healthy American adults. A statement for physicians by an ad hoc committee appointed by the Steering Committee, American Heart Association. Circulation 1987; 75:1340A-62A.
23. Canadian Task Force on the Periodic Health Examination. 1984 update. Can Med Assoc J 1984; 130:2–15.
24. Blackburn H. Public policy and dietary recommendations to reduce the population level of blood cholesterol. Am J Prev Med 1985; 1:3–11.
25. MacDonald LA, Sackett DL, Haynes RB, et al. Labelling in hypertension: a review of the behavioral and psychological consequences. J Chron Dis 1984; 37:933–42.

4

Screening for
Cerebrovascular Disease

Recommendation: There is currently insufficient evidence to recommend for or against auscultation for carotid bruits or noninvasive testing for carotid stenosis as effective screening strategies to prevent cerebrovascular disease in asymptomatic persons. It may be clinically prudent to include cervical auscultation in the physical examination of patients with established risk factors for cerebrovascular or cardiovascular disease (see *Clinical Intervention*). All patients should be screened for hypertension (see Chapter 3), and some persons should be tested for high blood cholesterol (Chapter 2). Clinicians should also provide counseling about smoking (Chapter 48), exercise (Chapter 49), and dietary fat consumption (Chapter 50).

Burden of Suffering

Cerebrovascular disease is the third leading cause of death in the United States, accounting for nearly 150,000 deaths in 1986.[1] Strokes can result in substantial neurologic deficits as well as serious medical and psychological complications. This illness places an enormous burden on family members and caretakers, and it often necessitates skilled care in an institutional setting. The cost of stroke care in the United States has been estimated at $5 billion per year.[2] The principal risk factors for ischemic stroke are increased age, hypertension, smoking, coronary artery disease, atrial fibrillation, and diabetes.[3-5] Of these, the most important modifiable risk factor is hypertension. Improved treatment of high blood pressure has been credited with the greater than 50% reduction in age-adjusted stroke mortality that has been observed since 1972.[6,7]

Efficacy of Screening Tests

Population-based cohort studies have established that persons with carotid artery stenosis are at substantially increased risk for subsequent stroke, myocardial infarction, and death.[8,9] The risk is greater for persons with neurologic symptoms such as transient ischemic attacks. Even in asymptomatic persons, however, it has been proposed that stroke can be prevented by identifying individuals with carotid stenosis and performing endarterectomy on these vessels. Two methods are used to detect carotid artery stenosis: clinical auscultation for carotid bruits and noninvasive studies of the artery. Neck auscultation is an inadequate screening test for carotid stenosis. There is considerable interobserver variation among clinicians in the interpretation of the key auditory characteristics—intensity, pitch, and duration—of importance in predicting stenosis.[10] In addition, a cervical bruit can be heard in 4% of the population over age 40, but the finding is not specific for significant carotid artery stenosis. Between 40% and 75% of arteries with asymptomatic bruits do not have significant compromise in blood flow;[11] similar sounds can also be produced by anatomic variation and tortuosity, venous hum, goiter, and transmitted cardiac murmur.[10,12-14] Finally, hemodynamically significant stenotic lesions may exist in the absence of an audible bruit.[10,12,15]

Persons with cervical bruits can be further evaluated with greater accuracy by noninvasive study of the carotid arteries. Techniques include the evaluation of auditory or visual features (spectral analysis phonoangiography, continuous-wave or pulsed Doppler ultrasound, B-mode real-time ultrasound, and duplex scanning combining the latter two) and tests of blood flow in ophthalmic and cranial tributaries of the carotid arteries (oculoplethysmography, ophthalmodynamometry, periorbital directional Doppler ultrasound, and thermography).[12,16] Several of these tests compare favorably with conventional angiography, the reference standard for confirming carotid artery disease.[12] Continuous-wave Doppler ultrasound, for example, has a sensitivity of 87% and a specificity of 91% when angiography is used as the reference criterion.[17] Duplex scanning is also reported to have good agreement with angiographic results.[18]

Effectiveness of Early Detection

The rationale for testing for carotid artery stenosis is that persons with asymptomatic bruits are at increased risk for cerebrovascular disease and myocardial infarction;[8,9,19] thus, information about the degree of stenosis may facilitate interventions to help prevent subsequent stroke. An awareness of the diagnosis may motivate patients to modify other risk factors (e.g., high blood pressure, smoking, hypercholesterolemia, physical inactivity) and to notify clinicians when they first become aware of symptoms of transient ischemic attack. Moreover, performing carotid endarterectomy in some individuals may prevent subsequent cerebral infarction distal to the obstruction.

Rigorous evidence that these interventions improve outcome in asymptomatic persons is lacking. It has not been proved, for example, that asymptomatic persons with stenoses detected through screening have a better outcome than do those who first present with symptoms. The proportion of persons with asymptomatic bruits who will experience stroke is relatively small; the annual incidence of stroke (unheralded by transient ischemic attacks) in this population is only 1–3%.[8,9,13,19-21] In those persons who will suffer a stroke, it is unclear from current evidence whether the degree of carotid stenosis provides meaningful information on the risk of infarction[13,19,22] or its location.[8,9] Carotid artery lesions may be less a predictor of thromboembolic strokes than of generalized atherosclerotic disease; persons with carotid artery disease are considerably more likely to die from ischemic heart disease than from a cerebrovascular event.[8,9] Finally, no controlled studies have examined changes in the behavior of patients on learning the results of carotid artery examinations.

Nonetheless, the performance of carotid endarterectomy for lesions detected through screening may provide an important means of preventing subsequent stroke. Reliable data about the benefits and risks of performing this procedure on asymptomatic persons are lacking. Two studies reporting improved outcomes after endarterectomy suffered from selection biases and inconsistent measurement criteria.[14,23] Other trials often involved persons with neurologic symptoms (e.g., transient ischemic attacks) and do not provide compelling evidence of substantial benefit [24-26] In response to the need for more reliable data, four large multicenter trials are currently under way.[21,20] They are expected to provide results in coming years on the efficacy of endarterectomy in both asymptomatic and symptomatic persons.

In the meantime, data from a number of studies have generated some concern that the risks associated with carotid endarterectomy, especially when performed at centers with high complication rates, may exceed potential benefits in asymptomatic persons with bruits, who have a relatively low risk of subsequent stroke even without treatment (see above). A number of studies have reported a perioperative mortality of about 3%,[29-31] and a perioperative stroke rate ranging between 2% and 24%, depending on the surgical expertise of the center.[11,30-35] However, these studies suffer from important methodologic problems, and definitive data on the risk-benefit ratio await the completion of the trials in progress. Until this information becomes available, it remains uncertain whether the detection of asymptomatic carotid artery stenoses through screening results in improved outcome.

Recommendations of Others

Although auscultation of the carotid arteries is widely considered a routine component of the physical examination, the Canadian Task Force[36] and other reviewers[15,37] have argued against routine screening for carotid bruits in asymptomatic persons. A consensus panel has recently recommended a baseline noninvasive study of the carotid arteries in persons considered at high risk for extracranial carotid arterial disease.[38]

Discussion

The most effective interventions to prevent stroke are recommended even in the absence of cerebrovascular disease: the identification and treatment of hypertension, smoking cessation, and lowering of serum cholesterol.[32] By comparison, the relative effectiveness of screening for carotid artery disease is less certain. Although the auscultation of bruits can detect some cases of carotid artery stenosis and noninvasive testing can confirm the presence of significant obstructive lesions, the detection of these lesions may be of limited clinical value if the diagnosis cannot be followed by an intervention that prevents subsequent stroke. Until evidence regarding carotid endarterectomy becomes available from ongoing clinical trials, the effectiveness of screening for carotid artery disease remains in question. Nonetheless, there is little evidence of harm from cervical auscultation, a procedure widely considered a routine component of the physical examination, and the auscultatory findings may provide especially useful risk assessment information for patients with other risk factors for cerebrovascular and cardiovascular disease. This is especially important for persons with a history of transient ischemic attacks. In the absence of careful questioning by the clinician about previous neurologic symptoms, elderly patients are often presumed erroneously to be "asymptomatic."

Although noninvasive testing can provide more accurate information on the degree of stenosis, economic considerations preclude routine noninvasive testing of the general population. About 1 million Americans have carotid bruits, and it is estimated that it would cost as much as $200 million to perform noninvasive testing on all of them.[15] The costs of carotid endarterectomy are also an important consideration. Over 100,000 carotid endarterectomies were performed in 1985,[39] making it the third most common operation in the United States.[40] In light of the substantial costs associated with the treatment and support of stroke victims, the expense of diagnostic testing and surgery are justified if these procedures prove to be effective in preventing stroke, but evidence of this awaits the results of ongoing research.

As an alternative to screening, antiplatelet therapy with aspirin offers a possible method of reducing the risk of stroke in asymptomatic persons. Most clinical trials to date, however, have examined the role of aspirin only as a secondary prevention strategy (i.e., in persons with previous transient ischemic attacks or strokes) and have often failed to demonstrate a statistically significant effect on subsequent strokes.[41-44] A recent meta-analysis of 25 trials of antiplatelet therapy concluded that antiplatelet treatment of low-risk persons may be of some benefit in preventing subsequent disease, but only if the risk of serious side effects (e.g., cerebral hemorrhage) remains quite low.[45] A stronger body of evidence exists for the role of aspirin in the primary prevention of coronary artery disease (see Chapter 60).

Clinical Intervention

There is currently insufficient evidence to recommend for or against auscultation for carotid bruits and noninvasive testing for carotid stenosis as an effective screening strategy to prevent cerebrovascular disease in asymptomatic persons. It may be clinically prudent to include cervical auscultation in the physical examination of asymptomatic patients with established risk factors for cerebrovascular or cardiovascular disease (e.g., increased age, hypertension, smoking, coronary artery disease, atrial fibrillation, diabetes) and in all patients with neurologic symptoms (e.g., transient ischemic attacks) or a previous history of cerebrovascular disease. Elderly patients should be asked whether they have experienced previously the symptoms of transient ischemic attack or other neurologic illnesses. All patients should receive routine screening for hypertension (see Chapter 3), and some persons should be tested for high blood cholesterol (Chapter 2). Clinicians should provide counseling to stop smoking (Chapter 48), to engage in regular exercise (Chapter 49), and to decrease intake of dietary fat (Chapter 50).

REFERENCES

1. National Center for Health Statistics. Advance report of final mortality statistics, 1986. Monthly Vital Statistics Report, vol. 37, no. 6. Hyattsville, Md.: Public Health Service, 1988. (Publication no. DHHS (PHS) 88–1120.)
2. Hodgson TA, Kopstein AN. Health care expenditures for major diseases in 1980. Health Care Fin Rev 1984; 5:1–12.
3. Schoenberg BS. Epidemiology of cerebrovascular disease. South Med J 1979; 72: 331–6.
4. Davis PH, Dambrosia JM, Schoenberg DG, et al. Risk factors for ischemic stroke: a prospective study in Rochester, Minnesota. Ann Neurol 1987; 22:319–27.
5. Wolf PA, D'Agostino RB, Kannel WB, et al. Cigarette smoking as a risk factor for stroke: the Framingham Study. JAMA 1988; 259:1025–9.
6. 1988 Joint National Committee. The 1988 Report of the Joint National Committee on Detection, Evaluation, and Treatment of High Blood Pressure. Arch Intern Med 1988; 148:1023–38.
7. Garraway WM, Whisnant JP. The changing pattern of hypertension and the declining incidence of stroke. JAMA 1987; 258:214–7.
8. Heyman A, Wilkinson WE, Heyden S, et al. Risk of stroke in asymptomatic persons with cervical arterial bruits: a population study in Evans County, Georgia. N Engl J Med 1980; 302:838–41.

9. Wolf PA, Kannel WB, Sorlie P, et al. Asymptomatic carotid bruit and risk of stroke: the Framingham study. JAMA 1981, 245.1442–5.
10. Chambers BR, Norris JW. Clinical significance of asymptomatic neck bruits. Neurology 1985; 35:742–5.
11. Quinones-Baldrich WJ, Moore WS. Asymptomatic carotid stenosis: rationale for management. Arch Neurol 1985; 42:378–82.
12. Caplan LR. Carotid-artery disease. N Engl J Med 1986; 315:886–8.
13. Chambers BR, Norris JW. Outcome in patients with asymptomatic neck bruits. N Engl J Med 1986; 315:860–5.
14. Thompson JE, Patman RD, Talkington CM. Asymptomatic carotid bruit: long-term outcome of patients having endarterectomy compared with unoperated controls. Ann Surg 1978; 188:308–16.
15. Kuller LH, Sutton KC. Carotid artery bruit: is it safe and effective to auscultate the neck? Stroke 1984; 15:944–7.
16. Solomon S. Recent developments in the diagnosis and management of stroke. Bull NY Acad Med 1986; 62:250–61.
17. D'Alton JG, Norris JW. Carotid Doppler evaluation in cerebrovascular disease. Can Med Assoc J 1983; 129:1184–9.
18. Stavenow L, Bjerre P, Lindgarde F. Experiences of duplex ultrasonography of carotid arteries performed by clinicians: correlation to angiography. Acta Med Scand 1987; 222:31–6.
19. Bogousslavsky J, Despland PA, Regli F. Asymptomatic tight stenosis of the internal carotid artery: long-term prognosis. Neurology 1986; 36:861–3.
20. Meissner I, Wiebers DO, Whisnant JP, et al. The natural history of asymptomatic carotid artery lesions. JAMA 1987; 258:2704–7.
21. Hennerici M, Hulsbomer HB, Hefter H, et al. Natural history of asymptomatic extracranial arterial disease: results of a long-term prospective study. Brain 1987; 110:777–91.
22. Yatsu FM, Fields WS. Asymptomatic carotid bruit: stenosis or ulceration, a conservative approach. Arch Neurol 1985; 42:383–5.
23. Busuttil RW, Baker JD, Davidson RK, et al. Carotid artery stenosis: hemodynamic significance and clinical course. JAMA 1981; 245:1438–41.
24. Fields WS, Maslenikov V, Meyer JS, et al. Joint study of extracranial arterial occlusion. V. Progress report of prognosis following surgery or nonsurgical treatment for transient cerebral ischemic attacks and cervical carotid artery lesions. JAMA 1970; 211:1993–2003.
25. Bauer RB, Meyer JS, Gotham JE, et al. A controlled study of surgical treatment of cerebrovascular disease: forty-two months' experience with 183 cases. In: Millikan CH, Siekert RG, Whisnant JP, eds. Cerebral vascular diseases. New York: Grune and Stratton, 1966.
26. Shaw DA, Venables GS, Cartlidge NEP, et al. Carotid endarterectomy in patients with transient cerebral ischemia. J Neurol Sci 1984; 64:45–53.
27. Walker MD, National Institute of Neurological and Communicative Disorders and Stroke. Personal communication, February 1988.
28. Callow AD, Caplan LR, Correll JW, et al. Carotid endarterectomy: what is its current status? Am J Med 1988; 85:835–8.
29. Dyken ML, Pokras R. The performance of endarterectomy for disease of the extracranial arteries of the head. Stroke 1984; 15:948–50.
30. Brott T, Labutta RJ, Kempozinski RF. Changing patterns in the practice of carotid endarterectomy in a large metropolitan area. JAMA 1986; 255:2609–12.
31. Slavish LG, Nicholas GG, Gee W. Review of a community hospital experience with carotid endarterectomy. Stroke 1984; 15:956–9.
32. Grotta JC. Current medical and surgical therapy for cerebrovascular disease. N Engl J Med 1987; 317:1505–16.
33. Warlow C. Carotid endarterectomy: does it work? Stroke 1984; 15:1068–76.
34. Rubin JR, Pitluk HC, King TA, et al. Carotid endarterectomy in a metropolitan community: the early results after 8535 operations. J Vasc Surg 1988; 7:256–60.
35. Zurbruegg HR, Seiler RW, Grolimund P, et al. Morbidity and mortality of carotid endar-

terectomy: a literature review of the results in the last 10 years. Acta Neurochir (Wien) 1987; 84:3–12.

36. Canadian Task Force on the Periodic Health Examination. 1984 update. Can Med Assoc J 1984; 130:1–16.

37. Frame PS. A critical review of adult health maintenance. Part 1. Prevention of atherosclerotic diseases. J Fam Pract 1986; 22:341–6.

38. Toole JF, Adams H Jr, Dyken M, et al. Evaluation for asymptomatic carotid artery atherosclerosis: a multidisciplinary consensus statement. South Med J 1988; 81: 1549–52.

39. Winslow CM, Solomon DH, Chassin MR, et al. The appropriateness of carotid endarterectomy. N Engl J Med 1988; 318:721–7.

40. Barnett HJM, Plum F, Walton JN. Carotid endarterectomy: an expression of concern. Stroke 1984; 15:941–3.

41. Fields WS, Lemak NA, Frankowski RF, et al. Controlled trial of aspirin in cerebral ischemia. Circulation 1980; 62:V90–6.

42. Canadian Cooperative Study Group. A randomized trial of aspirin and sulfinpyrazone in threatened stroke. N Engl J Med 1978; 299:53–9.

43. Bousser MG, Eschwege E, Haguenau M, et al. "AICLA" controlled trial of aspirin and dipyrimadole in the secondary prevention of atherothrombotic cerebral ischemia. Stroke 1983; 14:5–14.

44. UK-TIA Study Group. United Kingdom transient ischemic attack (UK-TIA) aspirin trial: interim results. Br Med J 1988; 296:316–20.

45. Antiplatelet Trialists' Collaboration. Secondary prevention of vascular disease by prolonged antiplatelet treatment. Br Med J 1988; 296:320–31.

5

Screening for Peripheral Arterial Disease

Recommendation: Routine screening for peripheral arterial disease in asymptomatic persons is not recommended. Clinicians should be alert to signs of peripheral arterial disease in persons at increased risk (see *Clinical Intervention*) and should thoroughly evaluate those patients with clinical evidence of vascular disease.

Burden of Suffering

Peripheral arterial disease (PAD) becomes increasingly common with age; it is estimated that 12–15% of the population over age 50 have this disease.[1-3] Increased mortality has been documented in patients with PAD, a disease that is strongly associated with coronary artery disease and that shares many of the same risk factors.[1,2,4-7] Although only a small proportion of individuals with PAD and intermittent claudication develop skin breakdown or limb loss, pain and associated disability often restrict ambulation and the overall quality of life.[1,4,7] Persons at increased risk for PAD include cigarette smokers and persons with diabetes mellitus or hypertension.[1,4,7] Diabetic PAD is responsible for about one-half of all amputations.[1]

Efficacy of Screening Tests

There is evidence that a history of intermittent claudication and the palpation of peripheral pulses are unreliable techniques for the detection of PAD.[1,3,6,8] In one study, a battery of noninvasive tests for PAD were administered to 624 hyperlipidemic subjects aged 38–82.[5] In this population, the positive predictive value and sensitivity of a classic history of claudication were only 54.5% and 9.2%, respectively, when compared with the results of formal noninvasive testing. The sensitivity of an abnormal posterior tibial pulse was 71.2%, the positive predictive value was 48.7%, and the specificity was 91.3%. An abnormal dorsalis pedis pulse had a sensitivity of only 50%; this artery is congenitally absent in 10–15% of the population.[8] The authors concluded that symptoms and abnormal pulses are not pathognomonic for PAD.[5] Greater accuracy has been achieved with noninvasive testing using Doppler ankle-arm pressure ratios, measurement of reactive hyperemia after exercise, pulse reappearance time, ultrasound duplex scanning, and plethysmography.[1,9,10] At present, however, additional data on sensitivity, specificity, and positive predictive value in asymptomatic populations are needed before noninvasive testing can be considered for routine screening.

Effectiveness of Early Detection

The rationale for the early detection of PAD is that risk factor modification following detection might lower subsequent morbidity and mortality from PAD and systemic atherosclerotic disease. By virtue of its strong association with coronary atherosclerosis, the early diagnosis of PAD might also lead to the detection of asymptomatic coronary artery disease. Firm evidence of these benefits is lacking, however; there has been little research to examine whether asymptomatic persons with PAD have lower morbidity or mortality with treatment than do symptomatic patients. It is clear that certain interventions are beneficial in symptomatic persons. There is evidence, for example, that patients who stop smoking have marked improvement in PAD symptoms and reduced overall cardiovascular mortality.[1,7,11] Certain antithrombotic drugs may also be of benefit.[12] These and other measures used in the treatment of PAD symptoms may also be effective preventive interventions in asymptomatic persons, but the evidence is less rigorous.[1,4] Examples include walking programs, control of weight and blood pressure, correction of elevated serum lipids and glucose, proper foot care, and certain drugs.

Recommendations of Others

There are no official recommendations for physicians to screen asymptomatic persons for PAD, although inspection of the skin and palpation of peripheral pulses are often included in the physical examination of the extremities.

Discussion

There is insufficient evidence that routine screening for PAD in asymptomatic persons is effective in reducing morbidity or mortality from this disease. However, many of the behavioral interventions that are prescribed after detecting PAD—smoking cessation (see Chapter 48), blood pressure control (Chapter 3), and exercise (Chapter 49)—can be recommended even in the absence of screening and are of proven value in the prevention of other atherosclerotic conditions, such as coronary artery and cerebrovascular disease.

Clinical Intervention

Routine screening for peripheral arterial disease in asymptomatic persons is not recommended. Clinicians should be alert to signs of PAD in persons at increased risk (persons over age 50, smokers, diabetics) and should thoroughly evaluate those patients with clinical evidence of vascular disease. Clinicians should screen for hypertension (see Chapter 3) and hypercholesterolemia (Chapter 2), and they should provide appropriate counseling regarding the use of tobacco products (Chapter 48), exercise (Chapter 49), and nutritional risk factors for atherosclerotic disease (Chapter 50).

REFERENCES

1. Strandness DE, Didisheim P, Clowes AW, et al, eds. Vascular diseases: current research and clinical applications. Orlando, Fla.: Grune and Stratton, Inc., 1987.
2. Criqui MH, Fronek A, Barrett-Connor E, et al. The prevalence of peripheral arterial disease in a defined population. Circulation 1985; 71:510–5.
3. Lombardi G, Polotti R, Polizzi N, et al. Prevalence of asymptomatic peripheral vascular disease in a group of patients older than 50. J Am Geriatr Soc 1986; 34:551–2.

4. Kannel WB, McGee DL. Update on some epidemiologic features of intermittent claudication: the Framingham study. J Am Geriatr Soc 1985; 33:13-8

5. Criqui MH, Fronek A, Klauber MR, et al. The sensitivity, specificity, and predictive value of traditional clinical evaluation of peripheral arterial disease: results from noninvasive testing in a defined population. Circulation 1985; 71:516-22.

6. Criqui MH, Coughlin SS, Fronek A. Noninvasively diagnosed peripheral arterial disease as a predictor of mortality: results from a prospective study. Circulation 1985; 72: 768-73.

7. Rutherford RB, ed. Vascular surgery, 2nd ed. Philadelphia: WB Saunders Company, 1984:553.

8. Kappert A, Winsor T. Diagnosis of peripheral vascular diseases. Philadelphia: FA Davis Company, 1972:26.

9. Barnes RW. Noninvasive diagnostic techniques in peripheral vascular disease. Am Heart J 1979; 97:241-4.

10. Moneta GL, Strandness DE. Peripheral arterial duplex scanning. J Clin Ultrasound 1987; 15:645-51.

11. Jonason T, Bergstrom R. Cessation of smoking in patients with intermittent claudication: effects of the risk of peripheral vascular complications, myocardial infarction and mortality. Acta Med Scand 1987; 221:253-60.

12. Arcan JC, Blanchard J, Boissel JP, et al. Multicenter double-blind study of ticlopidine in the treatment of intermittent claudication and the prevention of its complications. Angiology 1988; 39:802-11.

6

Screening for Breast Cancer

Recommendation: All women over age 40 should receive an annual clinical breast examination. Mammography every one to two years is recommended for all women beginning at age 50 and concluding at approximately age 75 unless pathology has been detected. It may be prudent to begin mammography at an earlier age for women at high risk for breast cancer (see *Clinical Intervention*). Although the teaching of breast self-examination is not specifically recommended at this time, there is insufficient evidence to recommend any change in current breast self-examination practices.

Burden of Suffering

In the United States in 1989, an estimated 142,000 new cases of breast cancer will occur in women, and 43,000 women will die of this disease.[1] Breast cancer accounts for 28% of all newly diagnosed cancers in women and 18% of female cancer deaths.[1] The age-adjusted mortality rate from breast cancer has been almost unchanged over the past 10 years. Breast cancer is the leading contributor to premature cancer mortality in women.[2] Because women of the "baby boom" generation are now reaching age 40, the number of breast cancer cases and deaths will increase substantially over the next 40 years unless age-specific incidence and mortality rates decline.

Important risk factors for breast cancer include sex, geographic location, and age. Breast cancer is much more common in women than men,[1] and the highest rates of breast cancer exist in North America and northern Europe. In American women, the annual incidence of breast cancer increases rapidly with age, from approximately 20 per 100,000 at age 30 to 180 per 100,000 at age 60.[3] The risk for women with a family history of premenopausally diagnosed breast cancer in a first-degree relative is about two to three times that of the average woman of the same age in the general population.[3-5] Women with previous breast cancer are at increased risk, as are women with a history of benign breast disease.[3,4,6] Other factors with some clinical or statistical association with breast cancer include first pregnancy after age 30, menarche before age 12, menopause after age 50, obesity, high socioeconomic status, and a history of ovarian or endometrial cancer.[3,4,7]

Efficacy of Screening Tests

The three screening tests usually considered for breast cancer are clinical examination of the breast, x-ray mammography, and breast self-examination (BSE).

The sensitivity and specificity of clinical examination of the breast varies with the skill and experience of the examiner and with the characteristics of the individual breast being examined. Over the five years of the Breast Cancer Detection Demonstration Project (BCDDP), the estimated sensitivity of clinical examination alone was 45%.[8] Data from studies using manufactured breast models show that mean sensitivity among registered nurses was 65% compared with 55% for untrained women.[8,9] Detection by physicians was 87% for lumps 1.0 cm in diameter, a size comparable to that used in the studies involving nurses and women.[8,10]

Estimates of the sensitivity of mammography depend on a number of factors, including the size of the lesion, the age of the patient, and the extent of follow-up to determine the proportion of "negative" masses that are later found to be malignant (i.e., false negatives). The average sensitivity of the combined clinical examination and mammography in the five years of the BCDDP was 75%. The estimated sensitivity for mammography alone was 71%.[8] A recent report from a multicenter trial estimated the sensitivity of an initial mammographic examination to be about 75%.[11] In a study of 499 women, mammography had an overall sensitivity of 78%, but it was reduced to 70% when only lesions under 1.0 cm in diameter were considered.[12] Sensitivity for all breast cancers in women over 50 was 87%, while sensitivity in women under 51 was 56%. In the 10-year follow-up of a Dutch study, the sensitivity of mammography was 80% for women aged 50 and above and 60% for those under 50.[13]

The specificity of mammography is about 94–99%.[11,13] Even with this excellent specificity, however, false positives can occur frequently if the test is performed routinely in populations with a low prevalence of breast cancer. Thus, most abnormal results of mammograms performed on young women without known risk factors for breast cancer are likely to be false positives. BCDDP data show that only 10% of women with positive (mammography and clinical examination) screening results were found to have cancer,[14] and a recent multicenter trial reported a positive predictive value of only 7% for initial mammographic examinations.[11] There is no study that shows that the sensitivity or specificity of mammography is increased when "baseline" mammograms are available for comparison.

Studies of mammography have shown large variations in observer (radiologist interpreter) performance.[15-17] In a study using 100 xeroradiographic mammograms, including 10 of women with proven cancers, the number of lesions identified as "suspicious for cancer" by 9 radiologists ranged from 10 to 45.[15] In a large breast cancer screening study in Canada, agreement was poor between radiologists at five screening centers and a single reference radiologist.[16]

Because exposure to ionizing radiation can be carcinogenic, widespread testing by mammography has the potential of producing some cases of radiation-induced cancer. However, radiation exposure from mammography has decreased dramatically with the development of dedicated mammography equipment and low-dose techniques.[18,19] Radiation exposure varies with breast size as well as with the specific equipment and technique used.[17-19] Thus, it is important for operators to use low-dose equipment and proper technique to limit unnecessary exposure to ionizing radiation during mammography.

Self-examination of the breast appears to be a less sensitive form of screening than clinical examination, and its specificity remains uncertain. Using reasonable assumptions applied to data from the BCDDP, the estimated overall sensitivity of BSE alone was found to be 26% in women also screened by mammography and physical examination.[8] Estimated BSE sensitivity in the BCDDP varied by age group; it was most sensitive for women 35–39 years of age (41%) and least sensitive for women aged 60–74 (21%).[8] Among participants in a breast cancer registry, BSE was reported to detect 34% of cancers.[8,20]

In a study of women's ability to detect breast lumps, untrained volunteers were able to detect 25% of lumps ranging in size from 0.25 to 3.0 cm in diameter.[0,21] The study showed that the sensitivity of BSE can be improved by training. A 30-minute training session increased the mean lump detection rate to 50%.[21] Although training sessions have increased detection rates, they also increase false-positive rates. False-positive BSE may result in unnecessary physician visits, heightened anxiety levels in women, and increased radiographic and surgical procedures. No study yet reported has directly compared the sensitivity or specificity of self-examination with that of clinical examination and mammography, in part due to the methodologic difficulties with properly designing such a study.

Effectiveness of Early Detection

The results of several large studies have convincingly demonstrated the effectiveness of clinical examination and mammographic screening for breast cancer in women aged 50 and older. The Health Insurance Plan of Greater New York (HIP) in 1963 began a randomized prospective study of clinical examination and mammography in 62,000 women.[22] The follow-up of this group now exceeds 18 years. In women who were over age 50 at the time of entry into the study, mortality from breast cancer in the screened group was more than 50% lower than in the unscreened group at five years. This effect has gradually decreased to about 21% after 18 years.

In the Swedish "two county study," a randomized controlled trial was begun in 1977 using single-view mammograms to screen about 78,000 women every 20 to 36 months.[23] After six years of follow-up, the group of women who were over age 50 at the time of entry showed a significant decrease in breast cancer mortality. A recently reported randomized controlled trial in Malmo, Sweden, found that in 8.8 years of follow-up women aged 55 and older who received periodic mammographic screening had a significant reduction in mortality from breast cancer.[24] In the Netherlands, a screening program of single-view mammography every two years for women over age 35 was introduced in 1975.[25] After seven years, this case-control study showed that mammography significantly reduced the risk of mortality from breast cancer in women 50 and over. A case-control study in Italy also reported a strong inverse relationship between mortality from breast cancer and mammographic screening in women aged 50 and older.[26]

More than 280,000 women in the United States were screened with a combination of clinical examination and mammography during the Breast Cancer Detection Demonstration Project.[27] This demonstration project was not designed as a research study, however, and lacked a control group. Effectiveness was inferred by comparing the outcome among BCDDP participants with that observed in national cancer surveillance programs. These comparisons showed that BCDDP participants had higher survival rates than those of breast cancer cases in national sample groups.[27] The finding of increased five-year survival was confirmed in a recent analysis of the BCDDP data, which also demonstrated that cumulative mortality from breast cancer was 80% of that expected of BCDDP participants without diagnosed breast cancer at the start of the study.[28] Due to the absence of internal controls in the original design of this study, however, it is unclear to what extent these differences were due to selection bias, lead-time bias, and other sources of bias.[29]

Although most authorities agree on the benefits of screening women aged 50 and over for breast cancer, there has been some uncertainty about the effectiveness of mammographic screening in women between the ages of 40 and 49.[29-31] Mammography for women under 50 has not been shown to be effective in reducing breast cancer mortality in the Swedish "two county" trial[23] or the Dutch study,[25] although the follow-up period may not have been of sufficient duration to detect an effect on mortality. The Malmo, Sweden, trial also reported no benefit for women under age 55, but the mean follow-up period was less than 9 years; moreover, 24% of women in the control group are thought to have received mammography outside of the screening program and as many as 26% of women in the intervention program did not attend screening.[24]

Follow-up data from the HIP study suggest that women aged 40–49 who receive periodic mammography and clinical examination may experience a reduction of about 25% in breast cancer mortality, but the investigators and others have not found this difference to be statistically significant.[22,32] Interpretations of statistical significance when analyzing these data are influenced by a number of factors, some of which include the definition of the 40–49 age group (i.e., age at entry into study vs. age at diagnosis), the length of follow-up, and the denominator chosen to calculate mortality (women entering the study vs. cases of breast cancer). The difference in mortality is statistically significant when cases of breast cancer are used as the denominator and age at entry defines the age group.[33] Statistical significance may, however, be less a consideration than clinical significance. Although nearly 28,000 women aged 40–49 entered the HIP trial, after over 18 years there were only 16 fewer breast cancer deaths among screened women (61 deaths) than in the control group (77 deaths), a difference of about 12 in 10,000 women screened.[33,34]

There are few data regarding the optimal frequency of mammography or the age at which to discontinue screening in the asymptomatic elderly. Although an annual interval is widely recommended, a recent analysis of data from the Swedish "two county" study found little evidence that an annual interval conferred greater benefit than screening every two years.[35] Although there are no reliable data on the optimal age to conclude mammographic screening, there are uncertainties regarding the effectiveness of screening beyond age 75 in asymptomatic women with consistently normal results on previous examinations. The incidence of new disease in this population may be relatively low and thus the effectiveness of screening may be limited, but reliable data are lacking.

Although no large study has quantitated the effectiveness of breast cancer screening for women in high-risk groups, it is apparent that these women have a greater probability of developing the disease.[30] If screening can reduce the risk of mortality from breast cancer, there may be a greater effect from screening those in high-risk groups, but studies confirming this effect are lacking. Further, established risk factors are present in less than one-quarter of women with breast cancer, so that a screening program restricted to high-risk groups is likely to miss the majority of cases.

Retrospective studies of the effectiveness of BSE have produced mixed results, and BSE has not been studied in a prospective controlled trial with mortality as an outcome.[8] A recent meta-analysis of pooled data from 12 studies found that women who practiced BSE before their illness were less likely to have a tumor of 2.0 cm or more in diameter or to have evidence of extension to lymph nodes.[36] The studies from which these data were obtained, however, suffer from important design limitations and provide little information on clinical outcome (e.g., breast cancer mortality).

Recommendations of Others

The American Cancer Society[37] and the National Cancer Institute[38] recommend monthly BSE and regular clinical examination of the breast for all women; baseline mammography between ages 35 and 40, followed by annual or biennial mammograms from ages 40–49, and annual mammograms beginning at age 50. These recommendations have been supported by other groups such as the American Medical Association,[39] the American College of Obstetricians and Gynecologists,[40] and the American College of Radiology.[41] A joint statement on screening for breast cancer involving many of these organizations is currently being developed under the organization of the American College of Radiology.[42]

In contrast, the Canadian Task Force,[43] American College of Physicians,[44] and other authorities[45,46] support annual clinical breast examinations for all women starting at age 40 but do not recommend beginning yearly mammography until age 50.

The World Health Organization states that there is insufficient evidence that BSE is effective in reducing mortality from breast cancer.[47] Thus, it does not recommend BSE screening programs as public health policy, although it finds equally insufficient evidence to change such programs where they already exist.

Discussion

At this time, there is little doubt that breast cancer screening by clinical examination and mammography has the potential of reducing mortality from breast cancer for women aged 50 and above. Most studies have not shown a clear benefit from mammography in women aged 40–49. Studies that will provide important information on this topic are in progress.[48] In the meantime, it is unclear whether the effects on breast cancer mortality achieved by screening women aged 40–49 are of sufficient magnitude to justify the costs and potential adverse effects from false-positive results that may occur as a result of widespread screening.[34] Until more definitive data become available, it is reasonable to concentrate the large effort and expense associated with mammography on women in the age group for which benefit has been most clearly demonstrated: those aged 50 and above. Annual clinical breast examination is a prudent recommendation for women aged 40–49.

Conclusions about the cost-effectiveness of mammography have not been universally accepted. Charges vary greatly in the United States, but in 1984 they averaged about $80–$100 per procedure.[30] For screening mammography to be widely used, it is likely that this charge would have to be reduced to $50 or less.[49] Even if only $50 were charged per mammogram, surveying all of the women in the United States over 40 years of age would cost more than $2 billion a year.[50] Others have drawn attention to the additional costs of biopsies performed on the basis of false-positive mammography results.[30] There are also concerns about the availability of the large numbers of trained radiologists needed to interpret additional screening examinations.[50,51]

Wide variation is found in the quality and consistency of mammography, as well as in the accuracy of interpretation, radiation exposure, and cost.[15-18,30] Radiation exposure during routine mammography is frequently much higher than the optimal doses or the minimal achievable doses usually quoted.[17-19] All of the above caveats about mammography argue for caution in the recommendation of mammographic screening, as well as for the selection of mammographers who maintain only the highest standards of quality.

The accuracy of BSE as currently practiced appears to be considerably inferior to that of the combination of clinical breast examination and mammography. False-positive BSE, especially among younger women in whom breast cancer is uncommon, can lead to needless anxiety and expense. With the present state of knowledge, it is difficult to make a recommendation about the inclusion or exclusion of teaching BSE during the periodic health examination. The WHO policy, neither recommending new BSE teaching programs nor changing existing ones, appears to be a prudent interim approach pending new data.[47]

Clinical Intervention

Annual clinical breast examination is recommended for all women aged 40 and above. Mammography every one to two years is recommended for all women beginning at age 50 and concluding at approximately age 75 unless pathology is detected. Obtaining "baseline" mammograms before age 50 is not recommended. For the special category of women at high risk because of a family history of premenopausally diagnosed breast cancer in first-degree relatives, it may be prudent to begin regular clinical breast examination and mammography at an earlier age (e.g., age 35). Clinicians should refer patients to mammographers who use low-dose equipment and adhere to high standards of quality control. Although teaching BSE is not specifically recommended at this time, there is insufficient evidence to recommend any change in current BSE practices.

Note: See Appendix A for the U.S. Preventive Services Task Force Table of Ratings for this topic. See also the relevant Task Force background paper: O'Malley MS, Fletcher SW. U.S. Preventive Services Task Force: screening for breast cancer with breast self-examination: a critical review. JAMA 1987; 257:2196–203.

REFERENCES

1. American Cancer Society. Cancer statistics, 1989. CA 1989; 39:3–20.
2. Leads from MMWR. Premature mortality due to breast cancer—United States, 1984. JAMA 1987; 3:229–31.
3. McLellan GL. Screening and early diagnosis of breast cancer. J Fam Pract 1988; 26: 561–8.
4. Kelsey JL, Hildreth NG, Thompson WD. Epidemiological aspects of breast cancer. Radiol Clin North Am 1983; 21:3–12.
5. Kelsey JL. A review of the epidemiology of human breast cancer. Epidemiol Rev 1979; 1:74–109.
6. Dupont WD, Page DL. Risk factors for breast cancer in women with proliferative breast disease. N Engl J Med 1985; 312:146–51.
7. Seidman H, Stellman SD, Mushinski MH. A different perspective on breast cancer risk factors: some implications of nonattributable risk. CA 1982; 32:301–13.
8. O'Malley MS, Fletcher SW. Screeening for breast cancer with breast self examination. JAMA 1987; 257:2197–293.
9. Haughey BP, Marshall JR, Mettlin C, et al. Nurses' ability to detect nodules in silicone breast models. Oncol Nurs Forum 1984; 1:37–42.
10. Fletcher SW, O'Malley MS, Bunce LA. Physicians' abilities to detect lumps in silicone breast models. JAMA 1985; 253:2224–8.
11. Baines CJ, McFarlane DV, Miller AB. Sensitivity and specificity of first screen mammography in 15 NBSS centres. Can Assoc Radiol J 1988; 39:273–6.
12. Eideiken S. Mammography and palpable cancer of the breast. Cancer 1988; 61: 263–5.
13. Peeters PH, Verbeck AL, Hendricks JH, et al. The predictive value of positive test results in screening for breast cancer by mammography in the Nijmegen programme. Br J Cancer 1987; 56:667–71.
14. Wright CJ. Breast cancer screening: a different look at the evidence. Surgery 1986; 100:594–8.

15. Boyd NF, Wolfson C, Moskowitz M, et al. Observer variation in the interpretation of xeromammograms. JNCI 1982; 68:357–63.
16. Baines CJ, McFarlane DV, Wall C. Audit procedures in the national breast screening study: mammography interpretation. J Can Assoc Radiol 1986; 37:256–60.
17. Gadkin BM, Feig SA, Muir HD. The technical quality of mammography in centers participating in a regional breast cancer awareness program. Radiographics 1988; 8: 133–45.
18. Kimme-Smith C, Bassett LW, Gold RH. Evaluation of radiation dose, focal spot, and automatic exposure of newer film-screen mammography units. AJR 1987; 149:913–7.
19. Prado KL, Rakowski JT, Barragan F, et al. Breast radiation dose in film/screen mammography. Health Physics 1988; 55:81–3.
20. Gould-Martin K, Paganini-Hill A, Cassagrande C, et al. Behavioral and biological determinants of surgical stage of breast cancer. Prev Med 1982; 11:441–53.
21. Hall DC, Adams CK, Stein GH, et al. Improved detection of human breast lesions following experimental training. Cancer 1980; 46:408–11.
22. Shapiro S, Venet W, Strax P, et al., eds. Periodic screening for breast cancer. Baltimore, Md.: Johns Hopkins Press, 1988.
23. Tabar L, Fagerberg CJG, Gad A, et al. Reduction in mortality from breast cancer after mass screening with mammography: randomised trial from the Breast Cancer Screening Working Group of the Swedish National Board of Health and Welfare. Lancet 1985; 1:829–32.
24. Andersson I, Aspegren K, Janzon L, et al. Mammographic screening and mortality from breast cancer: the Malmo Mammographic Screening Trial. Br Med J 1988; 297:943–8.
25. Verbeek ALM, Hendricks JHCL, Hollan PR, et al. Reduction of breast cancer mortality through mass screeening with modern mammography: first results of the Nijmegen Project, 1975–1981. Lancet 1984; 1:1222–4.
26. Palli D, Del Turco MR, Buiatti E, et al. A case-control study of the efficacy of a non-randomized breast cancer screening program in Florence (Italy). Int J Cancer 1986; 38:501–4.
27. Seidman H, Gelb SK, Silverberg E, et al. Survival experience in the breast cancer detection demonstration project. CA 1987; 37:258–90.
28. Morrison AS, Brisson J, Khalid N. Breast cancer incidence and mortality in the Breast Cancer Detection Demonstration Project. JNCI 1988; 80:1540–7.
29. Bailar JC. Mammography before age 50 years? An editorial. JAMA 1988; 259:1548–9.
30. Eddy DM, Hasselblad V, McGivney W, et al. The value of mammography screening in women under age 50 years. JAMA 1988; 259:1512–9.
31. Dodd GD, Taplin S. Is screening mammography routinely indicated for women between 40 and 50 years of age? J Fam Pract 1988; 27:313–20.
32. Day NE, Baines CJ, Chamberlain J, et al. UICC project on screening for cancer: report of the workshop on screening for breast cancer. Int J Cancer 1986; 38:303–8.
33. Chu KC, Smart CR, Tarone RE. Analysis of breast cancer mortality and stage distribution by age for the Health Insurance Plan clinical trial. JNCI 1988; 80:1125–32.
34. Eddy DM. Breast cancer screening (letter). JNCI 1989; 81:234–5.
35. Tabar L, Faberberg G, Day NE, et al. What is the optimum interval between mammographic screening examinations? An analysis based on the latest results of the Swedish two-county breast cancer screening trial. Int J Cancer 1987; 55:547–51.
36. Hill D, White V, Jolley D, et al. Self examination of the breast: is it beneficial? Meta-analysis of studies investigating breast self examination and extent of disease in patients with breast cancer. Br Med J 1988; 297:271–5.
37. American Cancer Society. Summary of current guidelines for the cancer-related checkup: recommendations. New York: American Cancer Society, 1988.
38. National Cancer Institute. Working guidelines for early detection: rationale and supporting evidence to decrease mortality. Bethesda, Md.: National Cancer Institute, 1987.
39. American Medical Association. Mammography screening in asymptomatic women 40 years and older (Resolution 93, I-87). Report of the Council on Scientific Affairs, Report F (A-88). Chicago, Ill.: American Medical Association, 1988.
40. American College of Obstetricians and Gynecologists. Standards for obstetric-gyne-

cologic services, 6th ed. Washington, D.C.: American College of Obstetricians and Gynecologists, 1985.
41. American College of Radiology. Policy statement: guidelines for mammography. Reston, Va.: American College of Radiology, 1982.
42. Dodd GD, American College of Radiology. Personal communication, February 1989.
43. Canadian Task Force on the Periodic Health Examination. The periodic health examination: 2. 1985 update. Can Med Assoc J 1986; 134:724–9.
44. American College of Physicians. The use of diagnostic tests for screening and evaluating breast lesions. Ann Intern Med 1985; 103:147–51.
45. Baines CJ. Breast-cancer screening: current evidence on mammography and implications for practice. Can Fam Physician 1987; 33:915–22.
46. Frame PS. A critical review of adult health maintenance. Part 3. Prevention of cancer. J Fam Pract 1986; 22:511–20.
47. World Health Organization. Self-examination in the early detection of breast cancer. Bull WHO 1984; 62:861–9.
48. Miller AB. Screening for breast cancer. Breast Cancer Res Treat 1983; 3:143–56.
49. Sickles EA, Weber WN, Galvin HB, et al. Mammographic screening: how to operate successfully at low cost. Radiology 1986; 160:95–7.
50. Dodd GD. The history and present status of radiographic screening for breast carcinoma. Cancer [Suppl 7] 1987; 1:1671–4.
51. Bassett LW, Diamond JJ, Gold RH, et al. Survey of mammography practices. AJR 1987; 149:1149–52.

7

Screening for Colorectal Cancer

Recommendation: There is insufficient evidence to recommend for or against fecal occult blood testing or sigmoidoscopy as effective screening tests for colorectal cancer in asymptomatic persons. There are also inadequate grounds for discontinuing this form of screening where it is currently practiced or for withholding it from persons who request it. It may be clinically prudent to offer screening to persons aged 50 and older with known risk factors for colorectal cancer (see *Clinical Intervention*).

Burden of Suffering

Colorectal cancer is the second most common form of cancer in the United States and has the second highest mortality rate, accounting for over 150,000 new cases and 61,000 deaths each year.[1] On average, clinically diagnosed colorectal cancer deprives its victims of about six to seven years of life.[2] Estimated 10-year survival is 74% in persons with localized disease, 36% in persons with regional metastases, and only 5% in those with disseminated disease.[3] In addition to the mortality associated with colorectal cancer, this disease and its treatment can produce significant morbidity; surgical resection, colostomies, chemotherapy, and radiotherapy can cause considerable discomfort and disruption of lifestyle. Principal risk factors for colorectal cancer include a family history of colorectal cancer, familial polyposis coli, or cancer family syndrome; a personal history of endometrial, ovarian, or breast cancer; and a history of longstanding ulcerative colitis, adenomatous polyps, or previous colorectal cancer.

Efficacy of Screening Tests

The principal screening tests for detecting colorectal cancer in asymptomatic persons are the digital rectal examination, fecal occult blood testing, and sigmoidoscopy. The digital rectal examination is of limited value as a screening test for colorectal cancer. The examining finger, which is only 7–8 cm long, has limited access even to the rectal mucosa, which is 11 cm in length.[4] It is estimated that less than 10% of colorectal cancers can be palpated by digital rectal examination.[4]

A second screening maneuver is fecal occult blood testing. Positive reactions on guaiac-impregnated cards, the most common form of testing, can signal the presence of bleeding from premalignant adenomas and early-stage colorectal cancers. The guaiac test can also produce false-positive results, however. The ingestion of foods containing peroxidases,[5] iron compounds,[6] and gastric irritants such as salicylates and other anti-inflammatory agents[7,8] can produce false-positive test results for neoplasia. Gastrointestinal bleeding can be caused by conditions other than colorectal adenomas or cancer, such as hemorrhoids, diverticulosis, and peptic ulcers. As a result, when occult blood testing is performed on asymptomatic persons, the majority of positive reactions are falsely positive for neoplasia. When fecal occult blood testing is performed in groups of asymptomatic persons over age 50, the positive predictive value is only about 5–10% for carcinoma and 30% for adenomas.[9-14] This large proportion of false-positive results is an important concern because of the discomfort, cost, and occasional complications associated with follow-up diagnostic tests, such as barium enema and colonoscopy.[15]

Fecal occult blood testing can also miss cases, especially small adenomas and colorectal malignancies that do not bleed or bleed only intermittently.[16,17] About 20 mL of daily blood loss is necessary to produce consistently positive results on guaiac cards.[18-20] Other causes of false-negative results include nonuniform distribution of blood in feces,[21] antioxidants such as ascorbic acid that interfere with test reagents,[22] and extended delays in testing stool samples.[18] Rehydration of stored slides can improve sensitivity, but this also increases the number of false-positive reactions.[23] The exact sensitivity of fecal occult blood testing in asymptomatic persons is not known; reported sensitivities of 50–92% are based on studies of persons with known colorectal malignancies[16,24-27] and are not applicable to the general population. The reported sensitivity in asymptomatic persons ranges from 20–25% in some studies (which were not properly designed to measure sensitivity)[14,28] to about 75% in preliminary data from ongoing clinical trials.[29,30]

HemoQuant (SmithKline Diagnostics, Sunnyvale, CA), a test for quantitative measurement of hemoglobin in the stool, has been suggested as a more sensitive and specific screening test for occult blood loss.[31-33] In addition to providing quantitative information, the test may be less influenced by dietary peroxidases, specimen storage, hydration, ascorbic acid, and upper gastrointestinal bleeding. The increased sensitivity and specificity for blood, however, may come at the expense of decreased specificity for neoplasia.[34] Also, the test is considerably more expensive than conventional guaiac cards.[34,35] Since specific cut-point criteria for defining a positive test have yet to be developed, the HemoQuant test is not ready for widespread clinical use.

The third screening test for colorectal cancer is sigmoidoscopy. Sigmoidoscopic screening in asymptomatic persons detects approximately 1–4 cancers per 1000 examinations.[36,37] However, the sensitivity and diagnostic yield of this form of screening varies with the type of instrument: the rigid (25 cm) sigmoidoscope, the short (35 cm) flexible fiberoptic sigmoidoscope, and the long (60 cm or 65 cm) flexible fiberoptic sigmoidoscope. Since only 30% of colorectal cancers occur in the distal 20 cm of bowel, and only 50–60% occur in or distal to the sigmoid colon,[38-41] the length of the sigmoidoscope has a direct effect on case detection.[42-46] The rigid sigmoidoscope, which has an average depth of insertion of about 20 cm[42-48] and allows examination to just above the rectosigmoid junction,[49] can detect only about 25–30% of colorectal cancers. The 35 cm flexible sigmoidoscope, however, can visualize about 50–75% of the sigmoid colon. Longer 60 cm and 65 cm instruments can reach the proximal end of the sigmoid in 80% of examinations[50,51] and thus can detect 50–60% of colorectal cancers. Researchers have recently examined the feasibility of introducing the 105 cm flexible sigmoidoscope into the family practice setting,[52] but it is as yet unclear whether the added length substantially increases the rate of detection of premalignant or malignant lesions.

Sigmoidoscopy can also produce "false-positive" results, primarily by detecting polyps that are unlikely to become malignant during the patient's lifetime. Autopsy studies have shown that as many as 10–33% of older adults have colonic polyps at death,[63] but only 2–3% have colorectal cancer.[54-56] Depending on the type of adenomatous polyp, an estimated 5–40% eventually become malignant,[57] a process that takes an average of 10–15 years.[58,59] It follows that the majority of asymptomatic persons with colonic polyps discovered on routine sigmoidoscopic examination will not develop clinically significant malignancy during their lifetime. For these persons, interventions that typically follow such a discovery (i.e., biopsy, polypectomy, frequent colonoscopy), procedures that are costly, anxiety provoking, and potentially harmful, are unlikely to be of significant clinical benefit.

Effectiveness of Early Detection

Persons with early-stage colorectal cancer on diagnosis appear to have longer survival than persons with advanced disease. The estimated 10–year survival is 74% for localized lesions (Dukes' A or B), 36% for tumors with regional invasion (Dukes' C) and 5% for disseminated disease (Dukes' D).[3] There is little information, however, on the extent to which lead-time and length biases account for these differences, or whether asymptomatic persons detected through screening have lower mortality than cases detected without screening. Two controlled trials in the United States[9-12] and three additional clinical trials under way in Europe[29,30,60] are expected to provide this information, primarily for fecal occult blood testing, but final results will not be available for several years.

A randomized controlled trial of multiphasic health examinations has often been cited as evidence that sigmoidoscopic screening can lower mortality from colon cancer.[61-63] Study group participants were urged annually to schedule a multiphasic checkup; controls received no such urging. Among the many interventions in the multiphasic checkup, persons aged 40 and older were encouraged to receive a rigid sigmoidoscopic examination. After 16 years of follow-up, the investigators found that the study group had significantly lower mortality from colorectal cancer, one-half the incidence of cancer of the distal bowel, a greater proportion of localized tumors, and a lower case-fatality rate.[64] The investigators have urged that these results be interpreted cautiously, however, since the trial was not designed specifically to examine the effect of sigmoidoscopy, but rather the multiphasic checkup as a whole. In addition, the role of sigmoidoscopy has been questioned by the investigators after a recent data analysis revealed little difference between study and control groups in the proportion of subjects receiving sigmoidoscopy or in the rate of detection or removal of polyps.[64]

The results of two large screening programs have also been cited in support of sigmoidoscopic screening.[65-67] Both studies found that persons receiving periodic rigid sigmoidoscopic examinations had less advanced disease and better survival from colon cancer than was typical of the general population. One program, which performed 21,150 initial examinations and 92,650 subsequent sigmoidoscopies, reported an incidence of colorectal cancer that was 85% less than that of the general population within the state.[65,66] The participants in both studies, however, were recruited in a nonrandomized fashion and may not have been entirely comparable to the general population in terms of risk for colorectal cancer. Since neither study included internal controls, it is difficult to conclude with certainty that the favorable outcomes observed in the studies were due to sigmoidoscopic screening rather than to other characteristics of the screening program or participants. Other methodologic concerns relating to the designs of these investigations have been outlined in recent reviews.[64,68]

An important consideration in assessing the effectiveness of sigmoidoscopic screening is the potential iatrogenic risk associated with the procedure. Complications from sigmoidoscopy are relatively rare in asymptomatic persons but can be potentially serious. Perforations occur in approximately 1 out of 5000–7000 rigid sigmoidoscopic examinations.[36,69] Although there are fewer data available on flexible sigmoidoscopy, the complication rate appears to be less than or equal to that observed for rigid sigmoidoscopy.

Even if screening is effective in reducing colorectal cancer mortality, there is little information on the optimal age to begin screening or the frequency with which it should be performed. Theoretically, the potential yield from screening increases beyond age 50 since the incidence of colorectal cancer after this age doubles every seven years.[3] In the absence of direct evidence from clinical studies, some have attempted to evaluate the effectiveness of different screening schedules through mathematical modeling. One such study suggested that delaying the onset of screening from age 40 to age 50 would reduce effectiveness by about 5–10% in persons with a family history of colon cancer.[2] The same study estimated that a screening interval of three to five years would preserve 70–90% of the effectiveness of annual screening in persons with a family history of colon cancer.[2] Another modeling study found that an interval of two to four years would allow detection of 95% of all polypoid lesions greater than 13 mm in diameter.[70]

Recommendations of Others

The American Cancer Society recommends annual digital rectal examination for all adults beginning at age 40 and annual stool occult blood testing beginning at age 50. Sigmoidoscopy every three to five years is recommended beginning at age 50.[71] Similar recommendations have been issued by the National Cancer Institute,[72] the American Gastroenterological Association,[73] the American Society for Gastrointestinal Endoscopy,[73] and other groups. The Canadian Task Force makes no mention of sigmoidoscopy but recommends annual stool occult blood testing for high-risk persons over age 45.[74] Other experts on the periodic health examination have advised against routine sigmoidoscopy but advocate fecal occult blood testing every two years between ages 40 and 50 and annually thereafter.[37,75]

Discussion

An important limitation to the effectiveness of screening for colorectal cancer is the ability of patients and clinicians to comply with testing. Patients may not comply with fecal occult blood testing for a variety of reasons,[60,76] but compliance rates are generally higher than for sigmoidoscopy. Although the introduction of flexible fiberoptic instruments has made sigmoidoscopy more acceptable to patients,[77] the procedure remains uncomfortable, embarrassing, and expensive, and therefore many patients may be reluctant to agree to this test. A recent survey of patients over age 50 found that only 13% indicated a desire to receive sigmoidoscopy after being informed of recommendations that they should receive the test every three to five years;[71] the most common reasons cited by the patients for declining the test were cost (31%), discomfort (12%), and fear (9%).[78] In a study in which sigmoidoscopy was repeatedly recommended, only 31% of participants consented to the procedure,[61-63] but this study was performed during years when the rigid sigmoidoscope was typically used for the procedure. Compliance rates as low as 6–12% have been reported.[37] Physicians may also be reluctant to perform screening sigmoidoscopy on asymptomatic persons. It has been estimated that a typical family physician with 3000 active patients (one-third aged 50 or older) would have to perform five sigmoidoscopies daily to initially screen the population and two daily procedures for subsequent screening.[37] In addition, examinations using the more effective long (60 cm or 65 cm) flexible sigmoidoscopes are more time-consuming[39-43] and require more extensive training[79-81] than do those using shorter instruments.

Another limitation to screening is cost. Although a formal cost-effectiveness analysis of screening for colorectal cancer is beyond the scope of this chapter, it should be noted that the economic implications associated with the widespread performance of fecal occult blood testing and sigmoidoscopy are not insignificant. A single flexible sigmoidoscopic examination costs between $100 and $200.[2,15,82] A policy of routine occult blood and sigmoidoscopic screening of all persons in the United States over age 50 (about 62 million persons) would be expected to cost over $1 billion per year in direct charges.[82] Others have calculated that Hemoccult (SmithKline Diagnostics, Sunnyvale, CA) screening alone could cost the United States and Canada between $500 million and $1 billion each year.[83] The costs of performing screening tests on a large proportion of the U.S. population may be justified if morbidity and mortality from colorectal cancer can be prevented through screening, but firm evidence to this effect is not yet available.

In summary, whether screening asymptomatic persons will significantly reduce mortality from colorectal cancer remains uncertain and awaits the results of ongoing clinical trials. In the absence of such evidence, widespread screening of asymptomatic persons for colonic polyps or colorectal cancer appears to be premature. The logistical difficulties of performing fecal occult blood tests and sigmoidoscopy on a large proportion of the U.S. population are not insignificant, due to the limited acceptability of the tests and the expense of performing screening and follow-up on a large proportion of the population. Moreover, the tests have potential adverse effects that must be considered, such as false-positive results that lead to expensive and potentially harmful diagnostic procedures. Screening of persons at increased risk for colorectal cancer may be justified on the basis of clinical prudence, but direct evidence that screening of this population is effective is also lacking.

Clinical Intervention

There is insufficient evidence to recommend for or against fecal occult blood testing or sigmoidoscopy as effective screening tests for colorectal cancer in asymptomatic persons. There are also inadequate grounds for discontinuing this form of screening where it is currently practiced or for withholding it from persons who request it. It may be clinically prudent to offer screening to persons aged 50 and older who have first-degree relatives with colorectal cancer; a personal history of endometrial, ovarian, or breast cancer; or a previous diagnosis of inflammatory bowel disease, adenomatous polyps, or colorectal cancer. These patients should receive current information regarding the benefits, risks, and uncertainties of both occult blood tests and sigmoidoscopy. Fecal occult blood testing should adhere to current guidelines for dietary preparation, sample collection, and storage.[84] Sigmoidoscopy should be performed by a trained examiner. The instrument should be selected on the basis of examiner expertise and patient comfort. The optimal interval for colorectal cancer screening is uncertain and is left to clinical discretion. Periodic colonoscopy is recommended for all persons with a family history of familial polyposis coli or cancer family syndrome.

Note: See Appendix A for the U.S. Preventive Services Task Force Table of Ratings for this topic. See also the relevant Task Force background papers: Knight KK, Fielding JE, Battista RN. Occult blood screening for colorectal cancer. JAMA 1989; 261:587–93; and

Selby JV, Friedman GD. Sigmoidoscopy in the periodic health examination of asymptomatic adults. JAMA 1989; 261:595–601.

REFERENCES

1. American Cancer Society. Cancer statistics, 1989. CA 1989; 39:3–20.
2. Eddy DM, Nugent FW, Eddy JF, et al. Screening for colorectal cancer in a high-risk population: results of a mathematical model. Gastroenterology 1987; 92:682–92.
3. National Cancer Institute. Surveillance, epidemiology and end-results: incidence and mortality data, 1973–77. National Cancer Institute Monograph No. 57. Bethesda, Md.: National Cancer Institute, 1981.
4. Schottenfeld D, Winawer SJ. Large intestine. In: Schottenfeld D, Sherlock P, eds. Colorectal cancer: prevention, epidemiology, and screening. New York: Raven Press, 1980:175–80.
5. Illingworth DG. Influence of diet on occult blood tests. Gut 1965; 6:595–8.
6. Lifton LJ, Kreiser J. False-positive stool occult blood tests caused by iron preparations: a controlled study and review of the literature. Gastroenterology 1982; 83:860–3.
7. Grossman MI, Matsumoto KK, Lichter RJ. Fecal blood loss produced by oral and intravenous administration of salicylates. Gastroenterology 1961; 40:383–8.
8. Rees WD, Turnberg LA. Reappraisal of the effects of aspirin on the stomach. Lancet 1980; 2:410–3.
9. Winawer SJ, Andrews M, Flehinger B, et al. Progress report on controlled trial of fecal occult blood testing for the detection of colorectal neoplasia. Cancer 1980; 45: 2959–64.
10. Gilbertsen VA, Church TR, Grewe FJ. The design of a study to assess occult-blood screening for colon cancer. J Chron Dis 1980; 33:107–14. 11. Gilbertsen VA, McHugh RB, Schuman LM, et al. The earlier detection of colorectal cancers: a preliminary report of the results of the occult blood study. Cancer 1980; 45:2899–901.
12. Gilbertsen V. Colon cancer screening: the Minnesota experience. Gastrointest Endosc 1980; 26:31S-2S.
13. Windeler J, Kobberling J. Colorectal cancer and Haemoccult. A study of its value in mass screening using meta-analysis. Int J Color Dis 1987; 2:223–8.
14. Bang KM, Tillett S, Hoar SK, et al. Sensitivity of fecal Hemoccult testing and flexible sigmoidoscopy for colorectal cancer screening. J Occup Med 1986; 28:709–13.
15. Brandeau ML, Eddy DM. The workup of the asymptomatic patient with a positive fecal occult blood test. Med Decis Making 1987; 7:32–46.
16. Crowley ML, Freeman LD, Mottet MD, et al. Sensitivity of guaiac-impregnated cards for the detection of colorectal neoplasia. J Clin Gastroenterology 1983; 5:127–30.
17. Griffith CDM, Turner DJ, Saunders JH. False-negative results of Hemoccult test in colorectal cancer. Br Med J 1981; 283:472.
18. Morris DW, Hansell JR, Ostrow D, et al. Reliability of chemical tests for fecal occult blood in hospitalized patients. Dig Dis 1976; 21:845–52.
19. Heinrich HC, Icagic F. Comparative studies on the "in vivo" sensitivity of four commercial pseudoperoxidase-based faecal occult blood tests in relation to actual blood losses as calculated from measured whole body 59Fe-elimination rates. Klin Wochenschr 1980; 58:1283–97.
20. Stroehlein JR, Fairbanks VF, McGill DB, et al. Hemoccult detection of fecal occult blood quantitated by radioassay. Dig Dis 1976; 21:841–4.
21. Rosenfield RE, Kochwa S, Kaczera Z, et al. Nonuniform distribution of occult blood in feces. Am J Clin Pathol 1979; 71:204–9.
22. Jaffe RM, Kasten B, Young DS, et al. False-negative stool occult blood tests caused by ingestion of ascorbic acid (vitamin C). Ann Intern Med 1975; 83:824–6.
23. Wells HJ, Pagano JF. "Hemoccult" (TM) test-reversal of false-negative results due to storage. Gastroenterology 1977; 72:1148.
24. Doran J, Hardcastle JD. Bleeding patterns in colorectal cancer: the effect of aspirin and the implications for faecal occult blood testing. Br J Surg 1982; 69:711–3.
25. Macrae FA, St John DJB. Relationship between patterns of bleeding and Hemoccult

sensitivity in patients with colorectal cancers or adenomas. Gastroenterology 1982; 82:091–0.

26. Ribet A, Frexinos J, Escourrou J, et al. Occult blood tests and colorectal tumours. Lancet 1980; 1:417.

27. Applegate WB, Spector MH. Colorectal cancer screening. J Commun Health 1981; 7:138–51.

28. Rozen P, Ron E, Fireman Z, et al. The relative value of fecal occult blood tests and flexible sigmoidoscopy in screening for large bowel neoplasia. Cancer 1987; 60: 2553–8.

29. Kewenter J, Bjork S, Haglind E, et al. Screening and rescreening for colorectal cancer: a controlled trial of fecal occult blood testing in 27,700 subjects. Cancer 1988; 62: 645–51.

30. Hardcastle JD, Armitage NC, Chamberlain J, et al. Fecal occult blood screening for colorectal cancer in the general population: results of a controlled trial. Cancer 1986; 58:397–403.

31. Schwartz S, Dahl J, Ellefson M, et al. The "HemoQuant" test: a specific and quantitative determination of heme (hemoglobin) in feces and other materials. Clin Chem 1983; 29:2061–7.

32. Ahlquist DA, McGill DB, Schwartz S, et al. HemoQuant, a new quantitative assay for fecal hemoglobin: comparison with Hemoccult. Ann Intern Med 1984; 101:297–302.

33. *Idem*. Fecal blood levels in health and disease: a study using HemoQuant. N Engl J Med 1985; 312:1422–8.

34. Joseph AM, Crowson TW, Rich EC. Cost effectiveness of HemoQuant versus Hemoccult for colorectal cancer screening. J Gen Intern Med 1988; 3:132–8.

35. Peterson WL, Fordtran JS. Quantitating the occult. N Engl J Med 1985; 312:1448–9.

36. Bolt RJ. Sigmoidoooopy in detection and diagnosis in the asymptomatic individual. Cancer 1971; 28:121–2.

37. Frame PS. Screening flexible sigmoidoscopy: is it worthwhile? An opposing view. J Fam Pract 1987; 25:604–7.

38. Cady N, Persson AV, Monson DO, et al. Changing patterns of colorectal carcinoma. Cancer 1974; 33:422–6.

39. Rhodes JB, Holmes FF, Clark GM. Changing distribution of primary cancers in the large bowel. JAMA 1977; 238:1641–3.

40. Abrams JS, Reines HD. Increasing incidence of right-sided lesions in colorectal cancer. Am J Surg 1979; 137:522–6.

41. Greene FL. Distribution of colorectal neoplasms. A left-to-right shift of polyps and cancer. Am J Surg 1983; 49:62–5.

42. Winnan G, Berci G, Panish J, et al. Superiority of the flexible to the rigid sigmoidoscope in routine proctosigmoidoscopy. N Engl J Med 1980; 302:1011–2.

43. Bohlman TW, Katon RM, Lipshutz GR, et al. Fiberoptic pansigmoidoscopy: an evaluation and comparison with rigid sigmoidoscopy. Gastroenterology 1977; 72:644–9.

44. Winawer SJ, Leidner SD, Boyle C, et al. Comparison of flexible sigmoidoscopy with other diagnostic techniques in the diagnosis of rectocolon neoplasia. Dig Dis Sci 1979; 24:277–81.

45. Marks G, Boggs HW, Castro AF, et al. Sigmoidoscopic examinations with rigid and flexible fiberoptic sigmoidoscopes in the surgeon's office. Dis Col Rect 1979; 22: 162–9.

46. Protell RL, Buenger N, Gilbert DA, et al. The short colonoscope: preliminary analysis of a comparison with rigid sigmoidoscopy and Hemoccult testing. Gastrointest Endosc 1978; 24:208.

47. Nivatvongs S, Fryd DS. How far does the proctosigmoidoscope reach? N Engl J Med 1980; 303:380–2.

48. Nicholls RJ, Dube S. The extent of examination by rigid sigmoidoscopy. Br J Surg 1982; 69:438.

49. Shatz BA, Freitas EL. Area of colon visualized through the sigmoidoscope. JAMA 1954; 156:717–9.

50. Gillespie PE, Chambers TJ, Chan KW, et al. Colonic adenomas: a colonoscopic survey. Gut 1979; 20:240–5.
51. Lehman GA, Buchner DM, Lappas JC. Anatomical extent of fiberoptic sigmoidoscopy. Gastroenterology 1983; 84:803–8.
52. Dervin JV. Feasibility of 105–cm flexible sigmoidoscopy in family practice. J Fam Pract 1986; 23:341–4.
53. Correa P, Strong JP, Reif A, et al. The epidemiology of colorectal polyps: prevalence in New Orleans and international comparisons. Cancer 1977; 39:2258–64.
54. Hughes LE. The incidence of benign and malignant neoplasms of the colon and rectum: a post mortem study. NZ J Surg 1968; 38:30–5.
55. Rickert RR, Auerback O, Garfinke L, et al. Adenomatous lesions of the large bowel: an autopsy survey. Cancer 1979; 43:1847–57.
56. Williams AR, Balasooriy BAW, Day DW. Polyps and cancer of the large bowel: a necropsy study in Liverpool. Gut 1982; 23:835–42.
57. Muto T, Bussey HJR, Morson BC. The evolution of cancer of the colon and rectum. Cancer 1975; 36:2251–70.
58. Morson BC. Evolution of cancer of the colon and rectum. Cancer 1974; 34:845–9.
59. Idem. The evolution of colorectal carcinoma. Clin Radiol 1984; 35:425–31.
60. Kronborg O, Fenger C, Sndergaard O, et al. Initial mass screening for colorectal cancer with fecal occult blood test. A prospective randomized study at Funen in Denmark. Scan J Gastroenterol 1987; 22:677–86.
61. Cutler JL, Ramcharan S, Feldman R, et al. Multiphasic checkup evaluation study. 1. Methods and population. Prev Med 1973; 2:197–206.
62. Dales LG, Friedman GD, Collen MF. Evaluating periodic multiphasic health checkups: a controlled trial. J Chronic Dis 1979; 32:385–404.
63. Friedman GD, Collen MF, Fireman BH. Multiphasic health checkup evaluation: a 16–year follow-up. J Chronic Dis 1986; 39:453–63.
64. Selby JV, Friedman GD, Collen MF. Sigmoidoscopy and mortality from colorectal cancer: the Kaiser Permanente Multiphasic Evaluation Study. J Clin Epidemiol 1988; 41:427–34.
65. Gilbertsen VA. Proctosigmoidoscopy and polypectomy in reducing the incidence of rectal cancer. Cancer 1974; 34:936–9.
66. Gilbertsen VA, Nelms JM. The prevention of invasive cancer of the rectum. Cancer 1978; 41:1137–9.
67. Hertz REL, Deddish MR, Day E. Value of periodic examinations in detecting cancer of the colon and rectum. Postgrad Med 1960; 27:290–4.
68. Morrison A. Screening in chronic disease. New York: Oxford University Press, 1985.
69. Nelson RL, Abcarian H, Prasad ML. Iatrogenic perforation of the colon and rectum. Dis Colon Rectum 1982; 25:305–8.
70. Carroll RLA, Klein M. How often should patients be sigmoidoscoped? A mathematical perspective. Prev Med 1980; 9:741–6.
71. American Cancer Society. Guidelines for the cancer-related checkup: guidelines and rationale. CA 1980; 30:194–240.
72. National Cancer Institute. Working guidelines for early cancer detection: rationale and supporting evidence to decrease mortality. Bethesda, Md.: National Cancer Institute, 1987.
73. Fleischer DE, Goldberg SB, Browning TH, et al. Detection and surveillance of colorectal cancer. JAMA 1989; 261:580–5.
74. Canadian Task Force on the Periodic Health Examination. The periodic health examination. Can Med Assoc J 1979; 1193–1254.
75. Frame PS. A critical review of adult health maintenance. Part 3. Prevention of cancer. J Fam Pract 1986; 22:511–20.
76. Blalock SJ, DeVellis BM, Sandler RS. Participation in fecal occult blood screening: a critical review. Prev Med 1987; 16:9–18.
77. Winawer SJ, Miller C, Lightdale C, et al. Patient response to sigmoidoscopy: a randomized, controlled trial of rigid and flexible sigmoidoscopy. Cancer 1987; 60:1905–8.

78. Petravage J, Swedberg J. Patient response to sigmoidoscopy recommendations via mailed reminders. J Fam Pract 1988; 27:387–9.
79. Shapiro M. Flexible fiberoptic sigmoidoscopy: the long and the short of it. Gastrointest Endosc 1984; 30:114–6.
80. Griffin JW. Flexible fiberoptic sigmoidoscopy: longer may not be better for the "nonendoscopist." Gastrointest Endosc 1985; 31:347–8.
81. Weissman GS, Winawer SJ, Baldwin MP, et al. Multicenter evaluation of training of nonendoscopists in flexible sigmoidoscopy. CA 1987; 37:26–30.
82. Clayman CB. Mass screening for colorectal cancer: are we ready? JAMA 1989; 261:609.
83. Frank JW. Occult-blood screening for colorectal carcinoma: the yield and the costs. Am J Prev Med 1985; 1:18–24.
84. Gnauck R, Macrae FA, Fleisher M. How to perform the fecal occult blood test. CA 1984; 34:134–7.

8

Screening for Cervical Cancer

Recommendation: Regular Papanicolaou (Pap) testing is recommended for all women who are or have been sexually active (see *Clinical Intervention*). Pap smears should begin with the onset of sexual activity and should be repeated every one to three years at the physician's discretion. They may be discontinued at age 65 if previous smears have been consistently normal.

Burden of Suffering

Approximately 13,000 new cases of cervical cancer are diagnosed each year, and about 7000 women die from this disease annually.[1] Although the five-year survival rate is about 90% for persons with localized cervical cancer, it is considerably lower (about 40%) for persons with advanced disease.[1] The incidence of invasive cervical cancer has decreased significantly over the last 40 years, due in large part to organized early detection programs.[2] Although all sexually active women are at risk for cervical cancer, the disease is more common among women of low socioeconomic status and those with a history of multiple sexual partners or early onset of sexual intercourse.[3-5]

Efficacy of Screening Test

The principal screening test for cervical cancer is the Pap smear. Precise data on the sensitivity and specificity of this test are lacking due to methodologic problems. Depending on study design, false-negative rates of 1–80% have been reported;[6,7] a range of 20–45% has been most frequently quoted, primarily in studies comparing normal test results with subsequent smears.[8-12] Although reliable data are lacking, specificity is probably greater than 90%[7] and may be as high as 99%.[12] The test-retest reliability of Pap smears is also influenced by variations in the expertise and procedures of different cytopathology laboratories. A significant proportion of diagnostic errors may be attributable to laboratory error. In one study of over 300 laboratories given slides with known cytologic diagnoses, false-negative diagnoses were made in 7.5% of smears with moderate dysplasia or frank malignancy, and false-positive diagnoses were made in 8.9% of smears with no more than benign atypia.[6]

There are important potential adverse effects associated with errors in the interpretation of Pap smears. False-negative results are of significance because carcinoma in situ or more invasive lesions may escape detection and progress to more advanced disease during the period between tests. The potential adverse effects of false-positive results include patient anxiety regarding the risk of cervical cancer, as well as the unnecessary inconvenience, discomfort, and expense of follow-up diagnostic procedures.

Effectiveness of Early Detection

Early detection of cervical neoplasia provides an opportunity to prevent or delay progression to invasive cancer by performing clinical interventions such as colposcopy, conization, localized excision, and, when necessary, hysterectomy.[13] There is evidence that early detection through routine Pap testing and treatment of precursor cervical intraepithelial neoplasia can lower mortality from cervical cancer. Correlational studies in the United States, Canada, and several European countries comparing cervical cancer data over time have shown dramatic reductions in the incidence of invasive disease following the implementation of cervical screening programs.[14-19] Case-control studies have shown a strong negative association between screening and invasive disease, also suggesting that screening is protective.[20-23] These observational studies do not constitute direct evidence that screening was responsible for the findings,[24] and randomized controlled trials to provide such evidence have not been performed. Nonetheless, the large body of supportive evidence accumulated to date has prompted the adoption of routine cervical cancer screening in many countries and makes performance of a controlled trial of Pap smears unlikely for ethical reasons.

The effectiveness of cervical cancer screening increases when Pap testing is performed more frequently.[2,21] Aggressive dysplastic and premalignant lesions are less likely to escape detection when the interval between smears is short. There are, however, diminishing returns as frequency is increased.[2,20,25] Although studies have shown that reducing the interval between Pap smears from 10 years to 5 years is likely to achieve a significant reduction in the risk of invasive cervical cancer, case-control studies and mathematical modeling have demonstrated that increasing to a 2- to 3-year interval offers only slight added benefit.[2,5,20] There is little evidence that women who receive annual screening are at significantly lower risk for invasive cervical cancer than are women who are tested every three to five years. These findings were confirmed in a major study of eight cervical cancer screening programs in Europe and Canada involving over 1.8 million women.[26] According to this report, the cumulative incidence of invasive cervical cancer was reduced 64.1% when the interval between Pap tests was 10 years, 83.6% at 5 years, 90.8% at 3 years, 92.5% at 2 years, and 93.5% at 1 year. These estimates were for women aged 35–64 who had at least one screen before age 35, and they are based on the assumption of 100% compliance.

Recommendations of Others

Although inconsistent guidelines on Pap testing have been issued in the past, a consensus recommendation was adopted recently by the American Cancer Society, the National Cancer Institute, the American College of Obstetricians and Gynecologists, the American Medical Association, the American Nurses Association, the American Academy of Family Physicians, and the American Medical Women's Association.[27] It recommends annual Pap smears for all women who are or have been sexually active or have reached age 18. The recommendation permits Pap testing less frequently once three or more annual smears have been normal and if recommended by the physician. The organizations did not recommend an age to discontinue Pap testing.

The 1980 National Institutes of Health Consensus Conference on Cervical

Cancer Screening[3] and the 1982 Canadian Task Force on Cervical Cancer Screening Programs[28] recommended that Pap testing begin when a woman becomes sexually active or reaches age 18, and that it be discontinued at age 60 if previous screening has been adequate and Pap smears have been consistently negative. The consensus conference recommended an interval of one to three years after two normal annual smears. The Canadian Task Force recommended annual Pap testing until age 35 followed by rescreening every five years.

Discussion

There are important economic considerations to performing Pap tests every year, rather than every two to three years, since this policy could double or triple the total number of smears taken on over 77 million American women at risk.[29] Although there is at least some epidemiologic data to support Pap testing as frequently as every two to three years,[5,20] annual testing appears to be of only limited added benefit in lowering mortality.[26] It has been estimated that screening women aged 20–64 every three years reduces cumulative incidence of invasive cervical cancer by 91%, requires about 15 tests per woman, and yields 96 cases for every 100,000 Pap smears. Annual screening reduces incidence by 93%, but requires 45 tests and yields only 33 cases for every 100,000 tests.[26]

Annual testing, however, is common. A survey of recently trained gynecologists found that 97% recommend a Pap test at least once a year.[30] The preference of many clinicians for performing annual Pap smears is based on concerns that less frequent testing may result in more harm than good, but reliable scientific data to support these opinions are lacking. Specifically, advocates of annual testing have expressed concerns that data demonstrating little added value to annual testing are based on retrospective studies and mathematical models that are subject to biases and invalid assumptions; that an interval longer than one year may permit aggressive, rapidly growing cancers to escape early detection; that the public may obtain Pap smears at a lower frequency than that publicized in recommendations; that a longer interval might affect compliance among high-risk women, a group with poor coverage even with an annual testing policy; that repeated testing may offset the false-negative rate of the Pap smear; that the test is inexpensive and safe; and that a large proportion of women believe it is important to have an annual Pap test and, while visiting the clinician, may receive other preventive interventions.[31] Definitive evidence to support these concerns is lacking.

Women who do not engage in sexual intercourse are not at risk for cervical cancer and therefore do not require screening.[3,4,28] In addition, screening of women who have only recently become sexually active (e.g., adolescents) is likely to have low yield. The incidence of invasive cancer in women under age 25 is only about 1–3 per 100,000, a rate that is much lower than that of older age groups.[12] One study found that most women with cervical intraepithelial neoplasia who had become sexually active at age 18 were not diagnosed with severe dysplasia or carcinoma in situ until age 30.[4]

Although invasive cervical cancer is uncommon at young ages, a number of authorities advocate starting screening with the onset of sexual activity.[3,27,28] This policy is based in part on the concern that a proportion of young women with cervical intraepithelial neoplasia may have an aggressive cell type that can progress rapidly and undetected if screening is delayed to a later age. The exact incidence and natural history of aggressive disease in young women remains uncertain, however. Another reason given for early screening is the concern that the incidence of cervical dysplasia occurring in young women appears to be on the rise, coincident with the increasing sexual activity of adolescents. On these grounds, testing should begin by age 18, since about 60% of American teenagers are sexually active by this age.[32] Screening in the absence of a history of sexual intercourse may be justified if the credibility of the sexual history is in question.

When screening is initiated, it is frequently recommended that the first two to three smears be obtained one year apart as a means of detecting aggressive tumors at a young age. There is little evidence to suggest, however, that young women whose first two tests are separated by two or three years, rather than one, have a greater mortality or person-years life lost.[2] Recommendations to perform these first tests annually are based primarily on expert opinion.

Elderly women do not appear to benefit from Pap testing if repeated cervical smears have consistently been normal.[2,4,28] Many older women have had inadequate screening, however; nearly half of women over age 65 have never received a Pap test and 75% have not received regular screening.[33,34] Further screening in this group of older women is important[2,34] and has been shown to be cost-effective.[35]

The effectiveness of cervical cancer screening is more likely to be improved by extending testing to women who are not currently being screened and by improving the accuracy of Pap smears than by efforts to increase the frequency of testing. Studies suggest that those at greatest risk for cervical cancer are the very women least likely to have access to testing.[33,36] Inadequate Pap testing is most common among blacks, the poor, uninsured persons, the elderly, and persons living in rural areas. In addition, many women who are tested receive inaccurate results due to interpretative or reporting errors by cytopathology laboratories or specimen collection errors by clinicians.[37] The failure of some physicians to provide adequate follow-up for abnormal Pap smears is another source of delay in the management of cervical dysplasia.[37]

Clinical Intervention

Regular Papanicolaou tests are recommended for all women who are or have been sexually active. Testing should begin at the age when the woman first engages in sexual intercourse. Adolescents whose sexual history is thought to be unreliable should be presumed to be sexually active at age 18. Pap tests are appropriately performed at an interval of one to three years, to be recommended by the physician based on the presence of risk factors (e.g., early onset of sexual intercourse, history of multiple sexual partners, low socioeconomic status). Pap smears may be discontinued at age 65, but only if the physician can document previous Pap screening in which smears have been consistently normal. Physicians should submit specimens to laboratories having adequate quality control measures to ensure optimal accuracy in the interpretation and reporting of results. Thorough follow-up of test results should also be ensured.

REFERENCES

1. American Cancer Society. Cancer statistics, 1989. CA 1989; 39:3–20.
2. Yu S, Miller AB, Sherman GJ. Optimising the age, number of tests, and test interval for cervical screening in Canada. J Epidemiol Community Health 1982; 36:1–10.
3. Cervical cancer screening: summary of an NIH consensus statement. Br Med J 1980; 281:1264–6.
4. Wright VC, Riopelle MA. Age at time of intercourse v. chronologic age as a basis for Pap smear screening. Can Med Assoc J 1982; 127:127–31.
5. Brinton LA, Tashima KT, Lehman HF, et al. Epidemiology of cervical cancer by cell type. Cancer Res 1987; 47:1706–11.

6. Yobs AR, Swanson RA, Lamotte LC. Laboratory reliability of the Papanicolaou smear. Obstet Gynecol 1985, 65.235–43.

7. I awa R, Forsythe A, Cove JR, et al. A comparison of the Papanicolaou smear and the cervigram: sensitivity, specificity, and cost analysis. Obstet Gynecol 1988; 71:229–35.

8. Foltz AM, Kelsey JL. The annual Pap test: a dubious policy success. Milbank Mem Fund Q 1978; 56:426–62.

9. Coppleson LW, Brown B. Estimation of the screening error rate from the observed detection rates in repeated cervical cytology. Am J Obstet Gynecol 1974; 119:953–8.

10. Benoit AG, Krepart GV, Lotocki RJ. Results of prior cytologic screening in patients with a diagnosis of Stage I carcinoma of the cervix. Am J Obstet Gynecol 1984; 148: 690–4.

11. Jones DE, Creasman WT, Dombroski RA, et al. Evaluation of the atypical Pap smear. Am J Obstet Gynecol 1987; 157:544–9.

12. Boyes DA, Morrison B, Knox EG, et al. A cohort study of cervical cancer screening in British Columbia. Clin Invest Med 1982; 5:1–29.

13. American College of Obstetricians and Gynecologists. Cervical cytology: evaluation and management of abnormalities. ACOG Technical Bulletin No. 81. Washington, D.C.: American College of Obstetricians and Gynecologists, 1984.

14. Cramer DW. The role of cervical cytology in the declining morbidity and mortality of cervical cancer. Cancer 1974; 34:2018–27.

15. Miller AB, Lindsay J, Hill GB. Mortality from cancer of the uterus in Canada and its relationship to screening for cancer of the cervix. Int J Cancer 1976; 17:602–12.

16. Anderson GH, Boyes DA, Benedet JL, et al. Organisation and results of the cervical cytology screening programme in British Columbia, 1955–85. Br Med J 1988; 296: 975–8.

17. Johanneson G, Geirsson G, Day N. The effect of mass screening in Iceland, 1965–1974, on the incidence and mortality of cervical carcinoma. Int J Cancer 1978; 21: 418–25.

18. Hakama M. Mass screening for cervical cancer in Finland. In: Miller AB, ed. Screening in cancer: a report of a UICC workshop in Toronto. UICC Technical Report Series Vol. 40. Geneva: UICC, 1978.

19. Laara E, Day NE, Hakama M. Trends in mortality from cervical cancer in the Nordic countries: association with organized screening programmes. Lancet 1987; 1:1247–9.

20. La Vecchia C, Decarli A, Gentile A, et al. Pap smear and the risk of cervical neoplasia: quantitative estimates from a case-control study. Lancet 1984; 2:779–82.

21. Clarke EA, Anderson TW. Does screening by Pap smears help prevent cervical cancer? A case-control study. Lancet 1979; 2:1–4.

22. Aristizabal N, Cuello C, Correa P, et al. The impact of vaginal cytology on cervical cancer risks in Cali, Colombia. Int J Cancer 1984; 34:5–9.

23. Berrino F, Gatta G, d'Alto M, et al. Efficacy of screening in preventing invasive cervical cancer: a case-control study in Milan, Italy. IARC Sci Publ 1986; 76:111–23.

24. Skrabanek P. Cervical cancer screening. Lancet 1987; 1:1432–3.

25. Miller AB, Visentin T, Howe GR. The effect of hysterectomies and screening on mortality from cancer of the uterus in Canada. Int J Cancer 1981; 27:651–7.

26. International Agency for Research on Cancer Working Group on Evaluation of Cervical Cancer Screening Programmes. Screening for squamous cervical cancer: duration of low risk after negative results of cervical cytology and its implication for screening policies. Br Med J 1986; 293:659–64.

27. Fink DJ. Change in American Cancer Society checkup guidelines for detection of cervical cancer. CA 1988; 38:127–8.

28. Canadian Task Force on Cervical Cancer Screening Programs. Cervical cancer screening programs: summary of the 1982 Canadian task force report. Can Med Assoc J 1982; 127:581–9.

29. National Center for Health Statistics. Health United States 1986. Washington, D.C.: Department of Health and Human Services, 1986:72. (Publication no. DHHS (PHS) 87–1232.)

30. Weisman CS, Celentano DD, Hill MN, et al. Pap testing: opinion and practice among young obstetricians-gynecologists. Prev Med 1986; 15:342–51.
31. American College of Obstetricians and Gynecologists. Periodic cancer screening for women: statement of the Task Force on Periodic Cancer Screening for Women. Washington, D.C.: American College of Obstetricians and Gynecologists, 1980.
32. *Idem*. The adolescent obstetric-gynecologic patient. ACOG Technical Bulletin No. 94. Washington, D.C.: American College of Obstetricians and Gynecologists, 1986.
33. Kleinman JC, Kopstein A. Who is being screened for cervical cancer? Am J Public Health 1981; 71:73–5.
34. Mandelblatt J, Gopaul I, Wistreich M. Gynecologic care of elderly women: another look at Papanicolaou smear testing. JAMA 1986; 256:367–71.
35. Mandelblatt JS, Fahs MC. The cost-effectiveness of cervical cancer screening for low-income elderly women. JAMA 1988; 259:2409–13.
36. Hayward RA, Shapiro MF, Freeman HE, et al. Who gets screened for cervical and breast cancer? Results from a new national survey. Arch Intern Med 1988; 148:1177–81.
37. Koss LG. The Papanicolaou test for cervical cancer detection: a triumph and a tragedy. JAMA 1989; 261:737–43.

9

Screening for Prostate Cancer

Recommendation: There is insufficient evidence to recommend for or against routine digital rectal examinations as an effective screening test for prostate cancer in asymptomatic men. Transrectal ultrasound and serum tumor markers are not recommended for routine screening in asymptomatic men.

Burden of Suffering

Prostate cancer is the most common cancer in American men and has the third highest cancer mortality rate.[1] It has the second highest cancer mortality rate in men over age 75.[1] Prostate cancer will account for an estimated 103,000 new cases and 28,500 deaths in the United States in 1989.[1] There has been no improvement in the age-adjusted death rate from this disease since 1949.[2] Risk increases with age, beginning at ages 55–60. After age 80, the incidence is as high as 1000 cases per 100,000 men.[3] Because local extension beyond the capsule of the prostate rarely produces symptoms, between 35% and 75% of patients already have metastases to the bones or lymph nodes at the time of diagnosis.[4,5] Survival is substantially decreased at this stage.[4]

Efficacy of Screening Tests

The principal screening tests for detecting prostate cancer in asymptomatic men are the digital rectal examination, transrectal ultrasound, and serum tumor markers. The digital rectal examination is limited in sensitivity because the examining finger can palpate only the posterior and lateral aspects of the gland. Studies have shown that tumors often occur in portions of the prostate not accessible to the examining finger.[5-7] In addition, Stage A tumors by definition are nonpalpable. The digital rectal examination also has limited specificity, producing a large proportion of false-positive results. Several studies involving largely asymptomatic populations have shown that only 26–34% of men with suspicious findings on digital rectal examination have histological evidence of prostate cancer on needle biopsy.[8-10] The exact sensitivity and specificity of digital palpation are, however, unknown because biopsies are rarely performed on persons with normal rectal examinations. Studies in which a battery of other diagnostic tests were performed along with the rectal examination found the examination to have a sensitivity of 69–73% and a specificity of 77–89%, but these data were obtained in men with urinary obstructive symptoms and presumably are not generalizable to asymptomatic men.[11,12] A study in asymptomatic men found a digital rectal examination to have a sensitivity of only 33%.[13] It has recently been suggested that the actual sensitivity of the digital rectal examination may be as low as 2–9% in detecting cancer.[14]

Transrectal ultrasonography is a second means of identifying prostate cancer, but there are as yet few data on the performance characteristics of this test in asymptomatic persons. Most sensitivity and specificity data for transrectal ultrasound derive from studies involving patients with suspected or confirmed prostate cancer, in which ultrasound is generally performed on a selected group of patients.[15-17] In one study, for example, transrectal ultrasound was performed on men with abnormal digital rectal examinations; the sonographers correctly identified cancer in 19 out of 28 (68%) men with biopsy-proven cancers and correctly ruled out cancer in 26 of 60 (43%) patients without histologic evidence of cancer.[15] In a recent prospective study, digital rectal examination and transrectal ultrasound were performed on nearly 800 community volunteers; biopsies were taken if either test was positive.[10] The positive predictive value of ultrasound in this study was 31%. The large proportion of false positives is due in part to the similarity in sonographic appearance between prostatic carcinoma and benign inflammatory conditions such as prostatitis and prostatic infarction.[18]

Serum tumor markers such as prostatic acid phosphatase (PAP) and prostate-specific antigen (PSA) are often elevated in persons with prostate cancer, but they do not appear to be useful screening tests for the detection of preclinical disease. The reported sensitivity of PAP is between 20% and 45%.[11,19] PSA is highly sensitive but lacks specificity (about 38–56%), in part because of difficulties in distinguishing between cancer and benign prostatic inflammation.[19,20]

Effectiveness of Early Detection

There is little direct evidence that early detection of prostate cancer improves outcome. Survival appears to be longer for persons with early disease; five-year survival is 85% for Stage A tumors, 77% for Stage B, 65% for Stage C, and 29% for Stage D.[21] It is not known, however, to what extent lead-time and length biases account for these differences. Autopsy studies indicate that prostate cancer is present in nearly half of older men, suggesting that a large proportion of occult cancers detected through screening would not manifest themselves during the patient's lifetime. In these persons, the detection of slow-growing malignancies through screening, followed by potentially unpleasant or harmful therapeutic interventions, might offer little clinical benefit.

It is estimated that only 1 in 380 men with histologic evidence of prostate cancer die from the disease.[9] Even in these individuals there is little evidence that treatment can significantly alter the course of the disease. Stage C and Stage D disease are generally resistant to intervention, and the efficacy of treatment for Stage B prostatic cancer remains in question. The major randomized controlled trial comparing treatment of prostate cancer with no treatment found that radical prostatectomy was no better than placebo in altering five-year survival.[22] Finally, the morbidity associated with complications from invasive diagnostic/staging procedures (e.g., needle biopsy, lymphadenectomy) and treatment (e.g., radical prostatectomy) must also be considered in assessing the overall benefits of clinical intervention.

Prospective studies are needed to provide evidence that persons with prostate cancer detected through screening have a better outcome than those who are not screened. A multicenter trial, the National Prostatic Cancer Ultrasound Detection Project, is currently under way to compare the effectiveness of different screening protocols, but this study does not include a control group in which screening is not offered.[23] Published evidence to date on the benefits of screening are largely descriptive uncontrolled studies that lack conclusive evidence of clinical benefit. In a frequently cited screening program, for example, annual digital rectal examinations were performed on nearly 6000 men over the course of 21 years, resulting in the detection of 75 cases of prostate cancer.[24] Five-year survival for these patients was 77%, and the investigators noted that the subgroup receiving total prostatectomies experienced a higher five-year survival rate (91%) than men of the same age in the general population (83%). Other centers have reported that screened cohorts are more likely to have localized (Stage A and B) disease on diagnosis, but there is no direct evidence of improved clinical outcome.[8,9,25] There is also reason to question the accuracy of the clinical staging of these Stage A and Stage B cancers; several studies have shown that two-thirds of patients classified clinically as Stage A or Stage B are subsequently found to have Stage C or Stage D disease when staging lymphadenectomy is performed.[8,9,25] Mathematical modeling studies have suggested modest benefit from screening by digital rectal examination, but these findings are sensitive to certain assumptions about the natural history of the disease and the efficacy of treatment.[26]

Recommendations of Others

The American Cancer Society[27] and the National Cancer Institute[28] recommend an annual digital rectal examination for both prostate and colorectal cancer beginning at age 40. The Canadian Task Force[29] and other experts[30] on the periodic health examination have advised against routine screening for prostate cancer. A technology assessment panel convened by the American Medical Association recently concluded that the role of transrectal ultrasound in screening for prostate cancer is investigational.[31] Similar recommendations have been issued by other experts.[32,33]

Clinical Intervention

There is insufficient evidence to recommend for or against routine digital rectal examination as an effective screening test for prostate cancer in asymptomatic men. Transrectal ultrasound and serum tumor markers are not recommended for routine screening in asymptomatic men.

REFERENCES

1. American Cancer Society. Cancer statistics, 1989. CA 1989; 39:3–20.
2. *Idem*. Cancer facts and figures. New York: American Cancer Society, 1985.
3. Young JL Jr, Percy CL, Asire AJ (eds). SEER Program: incidence and mortality, 1973–77. National Cancer Institute Monograph 57. Washington, D.C.: Government Printing Office, 1981.
4. Chodak GW, Schoenberg HW. Early detection of prostate cancer by routine screening. JAMA 1984; 252:3261–4.
5. Resnick MI. Background for screening: epidemiology and cost effectiveness. Prog Clin Biol Res 1988; 269:111–20.
6. Spigelman SS, McNeal JE, Freiha FS, et al. Rectal examination in volume determination of carcinoma of the prostate: clinical and anatomical correlations. J Urol 1986; 136: 1228–30.
7. McNeal JE, Price HM, Redwine EA, et al. Stage A versus Stage B adenocarcinoma of the prostate: morphological comparison and biological significance. J Urol 1988; 139: 61–5.
8. Thompson IM, Ernst JJ, Gangai MP, et al. Adenocarcinoma of the prostate: results of routine urological screening. J Urol 1984; 132:690–2.

9. Chodak GW, Keller P, Schoenberg H. Routine screening for prostate cancer using the digital rectal examination. Prog Clin Biol Res 1988; 269:87–98.
10. Lee F, Littrup PJ, Torp-Pedersen ST, et al. Prostate cancer: comparison of transrectal US and digital rectal examination for screening. Radiology 1988; 168:389–94.
11. Guinan P, Bush I, Ray V, et al. The accuracy of the rectal examination in the diagnosis of prostatic carcinoma. N Engl J Med 1980; 303:499–503.
12. Guinan P, Ray P, Bhatti R, et al. An evaluation of five tests to diagnose prostate cancer. Prog Clin Biol Res 1987; 243A:551–8.
13. Vihko P, Kontturi O, Ervast J, et al. Screening for carcinoma of the prostate: rectal examination and enzymatic radioimmunologic measurements of serum acid phosphatase compared. Cancer 1985; 56:173–7.
14. Stamey TA. Cancer of the prostate. Monographs Urol 1983; 4:65–132.
15. Chodak GW, Wald V, Parmer E, et al. Comparison of digital examination and transrectal ultrasonography for the diagnosis of prostatic cancer. J Urology 1986; 135:951–4.
16. Clements R, Griffiths GJ, Peeling WB, et al. How accurate is the index finger? A comparison of digital and ultrasound examination of the prostatic nodule. Clin Radiol 1988; 39:87–9.
17. Brooman PJC, Peeling WB, Griffiths GJ, et al. A comparison between digital examination and per-rectal ultrasound in the evaluation of the prostate. Br J Urol 1981; 53:617–20.
18. Kadmon D. Methods of detecting prostatic tumors. In: Ratliff TL, Catalona WJ, eds. Genitourinary cancer. Boston, Mass.: Martinus Nijhoff, 1987:77–93.
19. Stamey TA, Yan N, Hay AR, et al. Prostate-specific antigen as a serum marker for adenocarcinoma of the prostate. N Engl J Med 1987; 317:909–16.
20. Huber PR, Schnell Y, Hering F, et al. Prostate-specific antigen: experimental and clinical observations. Scand J Urol Nephrol 1987; 104:33–9.
21. Mettlin C, Natarajan N. End results for urologic cancers: trends and interhospital differences. Cancer 1987; 60:474–9.
22. Byar DK, Corle DK. VACURG randomized trial of radical prostatectomy for Stages I and II prostate cancer. Veterans Administration Cooperative Urological Research Group. Urol [Suppl] 1981; 17:7–11.
23. Murphy GP. Screening for prostatic carcinoma: useful or not? Prog Clin Biol Res 1988; 269:131–7.
24. Gilbertsen VA. Cancer of the prostate gland: results of early diagnosis and therapy undertaken for cure of the disease. JAMA 1971; 215:81–4.
25. Thompson IM, Rounder JB, Teague JL, et al. Impact of routine screening for adenocarcinoma of the prostate on stage distribution. J Urol 1987; 137:424–6.
26. Love RR, Fryback DG, Kimbrough SR. A cost-effectiveness analysis of screening for carcinoma of the prostate by digital examination. Med Decis Making 1985; 5:263–78.
27. American Cancer Society. Guidelines for the cancer-related checkup: recommendations and rationale. CA 1980; 30:4.
28. National Cancer Institute. Working guidelines for early cancer detection: rationale and supporting evidence to decrease mortality. Bethesda, Md.: National Cancer Institute, 1987.
29. Canadian Task Force on the Periodic Health Examination. The periodic health examination. Can Med Assoc J 1979; 121:1194–254.
30. Frame PS. A critical review of adult health maintenance. Part 3. Prevention of cancer. J Fam Pract 1986; 22:511–20.
31. Diagnostic and Therapeutic Technology Assessment (DATTA). Transrectal ultrasonography in prostatic cancer. JAMA 1988; 259:2757–9.
32. McClellan BL. Transrectal US of the prostate: is the technology leading the science? Radiology 1988; 168:571–5.
33. Chodak GW. Transrectal ultrasonography: is it ready for routine use? JAMA 1988; 259:2744–5.

10

Screening for Lung Cancer

Recommendation: Screening asymptomatic persons for lung cancer by performing routine chest radiography or sputum cytology is not recommended.

Burden of Suffering

Cancer of the lung is the leading cause of deaths from cancer in the United States.[1] It is responsible for over 140,000 deaths annually; 155,000 new cases will be diagnosed in 1989.[1] The five-year survival rate is only 13%, representing the poorest prognosis for any cancer site other than the pancreas, liver, and esophagus.[1] Important risk factors for lung cancer include the use of tobacco and occupational exposure to certain carcinogens.[2] Tobacco alone is responsible for over 90% of all cases of cancer of the lung, trachea, and bronchus.[2]

Efficacy of Screening Tests

Although the chest radiograph and the sputum cytological examination are capable of detecting lung cancer in its early stages, they lack sufficient accuracy to be used as routine screening tests in asymptomatic persons. The accuracy of the chest radiograph is limited by the capabilities of the technology and observer variation among radiologists. Suboptimal technique, insufficient exposure, and poor positioning and cooperation of the patient can obscure pulmonary nodules or introduce artifacts into the film.[3] Once the x-ray is taken, there can be significant inconsistencies in the interpretations made by different radiologists. The extent of this problem is difficult to measure in terms of sensitivity and specificity because of the absence of a "gold standard" to confirm the accuracy of the radiologist's report.[3] Studies do indicate, however, that radiologists frequently disagree on the interpretation of chest radiographs and that over 40% of these are significant or potentially significant.[4] Most errors are false-negative interpretations, and about 10–20% are incorrect radiologic diagnoses and "indeterminate" results that require follow-up testing for clarification.[4] Interpretation of chest x-rays by primary care physicians may be less accurate than those of radiologists.[5]

Furthermore, the yield of screening chest radiography to detect cancer is low, largely due to the low prevalence of lung cancer in the general population and even among asymptomatic smokers. Of the initial 31,360 screening radiographs performed on asymptomatic smokers in the National Cancer Institute Cooperative Early Lung Cancer Detection Program, only 256 (0.82%) were interpreted as "suspicious for cancer," and only 121 of these patients (0.39% of the screened population) were ultimately diagnosed as having lung cancer.[6] Other studies have confirmed the low yield of performing chest radiographs on asymptomatic persons.[7,8]

Data from the same studies suggest that sputum cytology is a less effective screening test than chest radiography. The investigators found that, of the 160 lung cancers detected by administering both tests, 123 (77%) would have been detected by x-ray alone and 67 (42%) would have been detected by cytological examination alone.[6] In addition, the majority of incident cases detected in subsequent screenings were detected by x-ray.[9]

Effectiveness of Early Detection

Lung cancers first detected when symptomatic usually present at an advanced stage for which the treatment outcome is poor. Overall five-year survival for lung cancer is less than 13%.[1] If therapy is initiated early, while the tumor is still localized (Stage I), five-year survival is about 27–33%,[1] and under optimal conditions Stage I cases can have a five-year survival of 60–75%.[9-11] Once tumors have metastasized, however, the benefits of resection are limited.[10] Early detection of Stage I tumors through screening might therefore provide an opportunity to improve survival. However, there is little convincing evidence that screening programs using radiography or cytology, either alone or in combination, actually succeed in reducing lung cancer mortality.

The efficacy of chest x-ray screening for lung cancer was first investigated in the 1960s. A controlled prospective study involving over 55,000 persons found that those receiving chest radiographs every six months had a larger proportion of resectable tumors but the same mortality from lung cancer when compared with controls who received x-rays at the beginning and end of the trial.[12] Similar findings were reported in the Philadelphia Pulmonary Neoplasm Research Project[13] and, more recently, in a case-control study.[14] In addition, the results of one of the three centers participating in the National Cancer Institute Cooperative Early Lung Cancer Detection Program (see below) provide indirect evidence of the limited efficacy of x-ray screening. In this study, persons receiving chest radiography and sputum cytology every four months had the same outcome (lung cancer mortality) as persons receiving advice to obtain annual testing.[15] However, no study to date has compared chest x-ray screening for lung cancer with no screening in a prospective design with adequate follow-up time. Thus, although the efficacy of chest x-ray screening can be questioned on the basis of the preceding studies, conclusive evidence that chest radiography screening does not lower lung cancer mortality is not available.

Three large clinical trials published by the National Cancer Institute Cooperative Early Lung Cancer Detection Program have examined the efficacy of dual screening (chest x-ray and sputum cytology) in over 30,000 male smokers.[6,9,16-21] Two trials comparing annual dual screening with annual radiographic screening tested the incremental benefit of adding sputum cytology to x-ray screening.[17,18] The third trial, which compared dual screening every four months with advice to receive the same tests annually, examined the benefit of frequent dual screening compared with usual medical care.[19] In each study, lung cancer mortality did not differ between experimental groups and control groups. Although early-stage, resectable tumors were more common and five-year survival significantly higher in groups receiving regular dual screening, lead-time and length biases may have been responsible for these findings. A recent randomized prospective trial of dual screening in Czechoslovakia produced similar results; the investigators found no substantial difference in the number or causes of death between groups.[22]

Recommendations of Others

There is a consensus that current evidence is insufficient to support routine screening for lung cancer among asymptomatic persons. This is the official policy of the American Cancer Society,[23] the National Cancer Institute,[24] the Food and Drug Administration,[25] the American College of Radiology,[26] the Royal College of Radiologists,[27] and the World Health Organization.[28] Recent reviews of the evidence by the Canadian Task Force[29] and others[3,30] have reached the same conclusion. Some experts defend screening smokers even in the face of the limited evidence because of the poor prognosis of lung cancer patients who present with symptoms.[31] There are no official recommendations to screen nonsmokers. All authorities strongly endorse the value of smoking cessation in the prevention of lung cancer.

Discussion

Although lung cancer is the leading cause of cancer deaths and early detection might improve survival, there is little rigorous evidence that screening programs can lower mortality from this disease. To the weakness of the evidence for screening must be added the substantial cost of routine population testing. It is estimated that $1.5 billion is spent annually for screening chest radiographs,[8] and it is known that false-positive results from these films lead to unnecessary expense and morbidity in follow-up procedures.[32] Primary prevention may be a more effective strategy than screening to reduce the morbidity and mortality of lung cancer. Cigarette smoking is responsible for over 90% of all lung cancers[2] and should therefore serve as the principal focus of clinical efforts to help prevent this disease.

Clinical Intervention

Screening asymptomatic persons for lung cancer by performing routine chest radiography or sputum cytology is not recommended. All persons should be counseled about the use of tobacco products (see Chapter 48).

REFERENCES

1. American Cancer Society. Cancer statistics, 1989. CA 1989; 39:3–20.
2. Department of Health and Human Services. Reducing the health consequences of smoking: 25 years of progress. A report of the Surgeon General. Rockville, Md.: Department of Health and Human Services, 1989. (Publication no. DHHS (PHS) 89–8411.)
3. Tape TG, Mushlin AI. The utility of routine chest radiographs. Ann Intern Med 1986; 104:663–70.
4. Herman PG, Gerson DE, Hessel SJ, et al. Disagreements in chest roentgen interpretation. Chest 1975; 68:278–82.
5. Kuritzky L, Haddy RI, Curry RW Sr. Interpretation of chest roentgenograms by primary care physicians. South Med J 1987; 80:1347–51.
6. The National Cancer Institute Cooperative Early Lung Cancer Detection Program. Summary and conclusions. Am Rev Resp Dis 1984; 130:565–7.
7. Rucker L, Frye EB, Staten MA. Usefulness of screening chest roentgenograms in preoperative patients. JAMA 1983; 250:3209–11.
8. Hubbel FA, Greenfield S, Tyler JL, et al. The impact of routine admission chest x-ray films on patient care. N Engl J Med 1985; 312:209–13.
9. Melamed MR, Flehinger BJ, Zaman MB, et al. Screening for early lung cancer: results of the Memorial Sloan-Kettering study in New York. Chest 1984; 86:44–53.
10. Wright JL, Coppin C, Mullen BJ, et al. Surgical treatment of lung cancer: promise and problems of early diagnosis. Can J Surg 1986; 29:205–8.

11. Moores DW, McKneally MF. Treatment of Stage I lung cancer (T1N0M0, T2N0M0). Surg Clin North Am 1987; 67:937–43.
12. Brett GZ. The value of lung cancer detection by six-monthly chest radiographs. Thorax 1968; 23:414–20.
13. Weiss W. Survivorship among men with bronchogenic carcinoma: three studies in populations screened every six months. Arch Environ Health 1971; 22:168–73.
14. Ebeling K, Nischan P. Screening for lung cancer: results from a case-control study. Int J Cancer 1987; 40:141–4.
15. Sanderson DR. Lung cancer screening: the Mayo study. Chest 1986; 89:324S.
16. Berlin NI, Buncher CR, Fontana RS, et al. The National Cancer Institute Cooperative Early Lung Cancer Detection Program: results of the initial screen (prevalence): introduction. Am Rev Resp Dis 1984; 130:545–9.
17. Flehinger BJ, Melamed MR, Zaman MB, et al. Early lung cancer detection: results of the initial (prevalence) radiologic and cytologic screening in the Memorial Sloan-Kettering study. Am Rev Resp Dis 1984; 130:555–60.
18. Frost JK, Ball WC Jr, Levin ML, et al. Early lung cancer detection: results of the initial (prevalence) radiologic and cytologic screening in the Johns Hopkins study. Am Rev Resp Dis 1984; 130:549–54.
19. Fontana RS, Sanderson DR, Taylor WF, et al. Early lung cancer detection: results of the initial (prevalence) radiologic and cytologic screening in the Mayo Clinic study. Am Rev Resp Dis 1984; 130:561–5.
20. Fontana RS. Screening for lung cancer: recent experience in the United States. In: Hansen HH, ed. Lung cancer. Boston, Mass.: Martinus Nijhoff, 1986:91–111.
21. Tockman MS, Frost JK, Stitik FP, et al. Screening and detection of lung cancer. In: Aisner J, ed. Lung cancer. New York: Churchill Livingston, 1985:25–40.
22. Kubik A, Polak J. Lung cancer detection: results of a randomized prospective study in Czechoslovakia. Cancer 1986; 57:2427–37.
23. American Cancer Society. Guidelines for the cancer-related check-up. CA 1980; 30:199–207.
24. National Cancer Institute. Cancer control objectives for the nation: 1985–2000. Washington, D.C.: Public Health Service, 1986. (Publication no. DHHS (NIH) 86–2880.)
25. National Center for Devices and Radiologic Health. The selection of patients for x-ray examinations: chest x-ray screening examinations. Rockville, Md.: Food and Drug Administration, 1983. (Publication no. DHHS (FDA) 83–8204.)
26. American College of Radiology. Policy statement: referral criteria for chest x-ray examinations. Chicago, Ill.: American College of Radiology, 1982.
27. Royal College of Radiologists Working Party on the Effective Use of Diagnostic Radiology. Preoperative chest radiology: national study by the Royal College of Radiologists. Lancet 1979; 2:83–6.
28. WHO Scientific Group on the Indications for and Limitations of Major X-Ray Diagnostic Investigations. A rational approach to radiodiagnostic investigations. WHO Technical Report Series No. 689. Geneva: World Health Organization, 1983:7–28.
29. Morrison B. Lung cancer: report for the Canadian Task Force on the Periodic Health Examination. Can Med Assoc J (in press).
30. Frame PS. A critical review of adult health maintenance. Part 3. Prevention of cancer. J Fam Pract 1986; 22:511–20.
31. Melamed MR, Flehinger BJ. Screening for lung cancer. Chest 1984; 86:2–3.
32. Bailar JC. Screening for lung cancer: where are we now? Am Rev Resp Dis 1984; 130:541–2.

11

Screening for Skin Cancer

Recommendation: Routine screening for skin cancer is recommended for persons at high risk (see *Clinical Intervention*). Clinicians should advise all patients with increased outdoor exposure to use sunscreen preparations and other measures to protect their skin from ultraviolet rays. Currently there is no evidence for or against counseling patients to perform skin self-examination.

Burden of Suffering

Over 500,000 new cases of skin cancer are diagnosed each year.[1] Most of these are basal cell and squamous cell carcinomas, which are highly treatable and rarely metastasize. These tumors can, however, be disfiguring if they are not detected early, and they account for over 2000 deaths each year.[2] The most serious form of skin cancer is malignant melanoma, which accounts for 74% of all skin cancer deaths.[3] An estimated 27,000 new cases of malignant melanoma will occur in the United States in 1989, and 6000 persons will die of this disease.[2] An increasing number of new cases and deaths from malignant melanoma are being reported in the United States.[3] Malignant melanoma usually presents in persons over age 40 and is uncommon in young persons.[3] The principal risk factors are precursor lesions (e.g., dysplastic nevi, certain congenital nevi) and a family history of malignant melanoma.[3,4] A number of other risk factors for malignant melanoma have also been identified.[5]

Efficacy of Screening Tests

The principal screening test for skin cancer is physical examination of the skin. Detection of a suspicious lesion constitutes a positive screening test, which then should be confirmed by skin biopsy. There are few studies evaluating the accuracy of the skin examination, however, and most suffer from important design flaws. Estimates of sensitivity and specificity (33–98% and 45–95%, respectively) vary with the type of skin cancer being sought.[6-9] A randomized community study found that the positive predictive value of a suspicious skin lesion is limited; biopsy-proven carcinoma was present in only 38–59% of lesions identified as suspicious for skin cancer by expert dermatologists.[7] Primary care physicians and others lacking specialized training in dermatology would be expected to have greater difficulty in evaluating skin lesions.[10-12] In one study, in which skin photographs were shown to dermatologists and nondermatologists, five of the six photographs of malignant melanoma were correctly identified by 69% of the dermatologists but only by 12% of the nondermatologists.[10] Both of the two photographs of dysplastic nevi were recognized by most of the dermatologists, but only 31% of the nondermatologists were able to identify one.[10]

Other factors affecting the yield of screening for skin cancer are the proportion of the body surface examined and the frequency of the examination. Only 20% of malignant melanomas occur on normally exposed body surfaces (in contrast to 85–90% of basal cell and squamous cell carcinomas); many melanomas occur on the back and legs.[13] Dermatologists estimate the detection of malignant melanoma is over six times as likely with a total-body skin examination.[13] A second factor affecting yield is the frequency of the examination. If the interval between examinations is too long, new cancers may not be detected before they have progressed to an advanced stage. There are no data, however, with which to determine the optimal frequency of examination, and therefore annual or biennial intervals have been recommended on the basis of clinical judgment.

Patient self-examination would be expected to be less accurate than physician examination in evaluating skin lesions. There are no data, however, on the accuracy of skin self-examination, the efficacy of self-examination instructions in reducing errors, or the proportion of lesions brought to medical attention that would be benign (false positives). It is known that persons who detect malignant lesions often delay seeking medical care until the lesion becomes symptomatic. In one study, patients with malignant melanoma reported seeking medical attention 11–18 months after the melanoma was first detected.[14] Symptomatic lesions were seen by clinicians within 2–6 months but were more advanced on presentation.[14]

Effectiveness of Early Detection

Although there is little proven reduction in mortality associated with the early diagnosis of basal and squamous cell cancers, early treatment may reduce morbidity and disfigurement. In the case of malignant melanoma, there is stronger evidence that survival is directly related to the stage of the disease. Five-year survival for Stage I melanoma is greater than 80–90%, but it is only 27–57% with Stage II disease.[15] In more advanced cases of disseminated metastatic melanoma, for which there is no effective treatment,[4] the median survival time is about 5–9 months.[16] The likelihood of recurrence after resection is also related to the thickness of the melanoma. A lesion thickness less than 0.76 mm is associated with a 10-year disease-free survival rate in excess of 99%.[3,17] The rate is only 48% for lesions greater than 3 mm in thickness.[3] Although it is possible that lead-time and length biases account for some of these differences, the data suggest that persons in whom malignant melanoma is detected early may experience a better outcome than those detected with more advanced disease.

Recommendations of Others

The American Academy of Dermatology[18] and others[3] recommend annual, complete skin examination by a physician, to be supplemented by monthly self-examinations of the skin. The American Cancer Society[19] and the National Cancer Institute[20] recommend including a complete skin examination as part of the routine periodic health examination. The Canadian Task Force advises against routine screening but recommends skin examinations for those in high-risk groups, such as persons with dysplastic nevi and their relatives, outdoor workers, and persons exposed to chemical skin carcinogens.[21] Others have advised physicians not to screen for skin cancer but to instruct patients to perform self-examinations.[22] Most dermatologists recommend examining the entire body; some recommend performing complete skin examinations only on those patients with a history of actinic lesions, skin cancer, and extensive or obscure dermatologic disorders.[10] The American Academy of Dermatology also recommends advising patients to limit sun exposure and to use sunscreens and protective clothing when exposed to sunlight.[18] Others emphasize the importance of counseling parents to use sunscreens and other measures to prevent skin damage in children.[24]

Discussion

Although screening for skin cancer is of some value in detecting basal cell and squamous cell carcinoma, its principal benefit lies in discovering and treating early-stage malignant melanoma. This disease is, however, relatively uncommon in the general population (lifetime risk of 0.7%).[3] Since over 99% of patients who would be examined under routine screening would never have malignant melanoma, it is important to consider the potential adverse effects of routine skin examinations. Medical expenses, for example, might be increased; physician office visits would be lengthened by performing a thorough skin examination and teaching self-examination.[23] A total-body examination may be embarrassing for some patients;[23] skin biopsy may be uncomfortable and may increase physician charges ($36–$125 or more per procedure);[25] and patient anxiety may be generated by lesions that ultimately prove to be benign (false positives). In light of these concerns, a more prudent approach might be to limit screening by total-body examination to population groups at increased risk for skin cancer.

As an alternative to early detection, many authorities have advocated primary prevention of skin cancer by limiting exposure to sunlight and by applying sunscreen preparations rated 15 SPF (Sun-Protective Factor) or more. These maneuvers are more clearly relevant to preventing nonmelanomatous skin cancers (e.g., basal cell and squamous cell carcinoma) for which ultraviolet rays are an established risk factor. Malignant melanoma may be linked to certain patterns of sunlight exposure, such as sunburns or exposure at young ages, but the association remains uncertain.[26-29] There have been few studies examining the effectiveness of counseling patients to protect themselves from sunlight in reducing the incidence of skin cancer. It is known that sunscreen agents can block carcinogenic ultraviolet rays[30] and can reduce the incidence of skin tumors in laboratory animals.[31,32] There is also some evidence that public education can increase knowledge about the health risks of sunlight.[33] At the same time, it is not certain that patients act on this information, perhaps due to the perceived personal benefits of sunbathing or obtaining a suntan.[34] A recent survey found that although 54% of adults and 37% of adolescents are aware of the risks of sun exposure, 30% of adults and 50% of adolescents continue to engage in suntanning. Fully 23% of adults and 33% of adolescents failed to use protective measures while engaged in suntanning.[35]

Clinical Intervention

Routine screening by complete skin examination is recommended for persons with a family or personal history of skin cancer, clinical evidence of precursor lesions (e.g., dysplastic nevi, certain congenital nevi), and those with increased occupational or recreational exposure to sunlight. The optimal frequency of such examinations has not been determined and is left to clinical discretion. Although routine screening for skin cancer is not recommended for the general population, clinicians should be alert to skin lesions with malignant features when examining patients for other reasons.

When examining pigmented lesions, a malignant appearance should be judged by established dermatologic criteria (i.e., asymmetry, border irregularity, color variability, diameter greater than 6 mm). Appropriate biopsy specimens should be taken of suspicious lesions. Clinicians should advise patients with increased occupational or recreational exposure to sunlight to use sunscreen preparations, protective clothing, and other measures to limit exposure to ultraviolet rays. Currently, there is no evidence for or against counseling patients to perform periodic self-examination of the skin.

REFERENCES

1. American Cancer Society. Cancer facts and figures—1987. New York: American Cancer Society, 1987.
2. American Cancer Society. Cancer statistics, 1989. CA 1989; 39:3–20.
3. Friedman RJ, Rigel DS, Kopf AW. Early detection of malignant melanoma: the role of physician examination and self-examination of the skin. CA 1985; 35:130–51.
4. Fitzpatrick TB, Rhodes AR, Sober AJ. Prevention of malignant melanoma by recognition of its precursors. N Engl J Med 1985; 312:115–6.
5. Evans RD, Kopf AW, Lew RA, et al. Risk factors for the development of malignant melanoma. I. Review of case-control studies. J Dermatol Surg Oncol 1988; 14:393–408.
6. Lightstone AC, Kopf AW, Garfinkel L. Diagnostic accuracy: a new approach to its evaluation. Arch Dermatol 1965; 91:497–502.
7. Green A, Leslie D, Weedon D. Diagnosis of skin cancer in the general population: clinical accuracy in the Nambour survey. Med J Aust 1988; 148:447–50.
8. Kopf AW, Mintzis M, Bart RS. Diagnostic accuracy in malignant melanoma. Arch Dermatol 1975; 111:1291–2.
9. Presser SE, Taylor JR. Clinical diagnostic accuracy of basal cell carcinoma. J Am Acad Dermatol 1987; 16:988–90.
10. Cassileth BR, Clark WH, Lusk EJ. How well do physicians recognize melanoma and other problem lesions? J Am Acad Dermatol 1986; 14:555–60.
11. Ramsey DL, Fox AB. The ability of primary care physicians to recognize the common dermatoses. Arch Dermatol 1981; 117:620–2.
12. Wanger RF, Wagner D, Tomich JM, et al. Diagnoses of skin diseases: dermatologists vs. nondermatologists. J Dermatol Surg Oncol 1985; 11:476–9.
13. Rigel DS, Friedman RJ, Kopf AW, et al. Importance of complete cutaneous examination for the detection of malignant melanoma. J Am Acad Dermatol 1986; 14:857–60.
14. Cassileth BR, Lusk EJ, Guerry D, et al. "Catalyst" symptoms in malignant melanoma. J Gen Intern Med 1987; 2:1–4.
15. Hartley JW, Fletcher WS. Improved survival of patients with Stage II melanoma of the extremity using hyperthermic isolation perfusion with 1–phenylalanine mustard. J Surg Oncol 1987; 36:170–4.
16. Hena MA, Emrich LJ, Nambisan RN, et al. Effect of surgical treatment on Stage IV melanoma. Am J Surg 1987; 153:270–5.
17. Veronesi U, Cascinelli N, Adamus J, et al. Thin Stage I primary cutaneous malignant melanoma: comparison of excision with margins of 1 or 3 cm. N Engl J Med 1988; 318:1159–62.
18. Martin G, American Academy of Dermatology. Personal communication, January 1989.
19. American Cancer Society. Guidelines for the cancer-related checkup: recommendations and rationale. New York: American Cancer Society, 1980.
20. National Cancer Institute. Working guidelines for early cancer detection: rationale and supporting evidence to decrease mortality. Bethesda, Md.: National Cancer Institute, 1987.
21. Canadian Task Force on the Periodic Health Examination. The periodic health examination: 2. 1984 update. Can Med Assoc J 1984; 130:2–16.

22. Frame PS. A critical review of adult health maintenance. Part 3. Prevention of cancer. J Fam Pract 1986; 22:511–20.

23. Epstein E. Crucial importance of the complote skin examination (letter). J Am Acad Dermatol 1985; 13:151–3.

24. Stern RS, Weinstein MC, Baker SG. Risk reduction for nonmelanoma skin cancer with childhood sunscreen use. Arch Dermatol 1986; 122:537–45.

25. Fewkes JL, Sober AJ. Skin biopsy: the four types and how best to do them. Primary Care and Cancer 1988; March:11–6.

26. Lew RA, Sober AJ, Cook N, et al. Sun exposure habits in patients with cutaneous malignant melanoma: a case control study. J Dermatol Surg Oncol 1983; 9:981–6.

27. Holman CD, Armstrong BK, Heenan PJ. Relationship of cutaneous malignant melanoma to individual sunlight-exposure habits. JNCI 1986; 76:403–14.

28. MacKie RM. The role of sunlight in the etiology of cutaneous malignant melanoma. Clin Exp Dermatol 1981; 6:407–10.

29. MacKie RM, Aitchison T. Severe sunburn and subsequent risk of primary cutaneous malignant melanoma in Scotland. Br J Cancer 1982; 46:955–60.

30. Pathak MA. Sunscreens and their use in the preventive treatment of sunlight-induced skin damage. J Dermatol Surg Oncol 1987; 13:739–50.

31. Wulf HC, Poulsen T, Brodthagen H, et al. Sunscreens for delay of ultraviolet induction of skin tumors. J Am Acad Dermatol 1982; 7:194–202.

32. Kligman LH, Akin FJ, Kligman AM. Sunscreens prevent ultraviolet photocarcinogenesis. J Am Acad Dermatol 1980; 3:30–5.

33. Putnam GL, Yanagisako KL. Skin cancer comic book: evaluation of a public educational vehicle. Cancer Det Prev 1982; 5:349–56.

34. Keesling B, Friedman HS. Psychosocial factors in sunbathing and sunscreen use. Health Psychol 1987; 6:477–93.

35. Public awareness of the effects of sun on skin. A survey conducted for the American Academy of Dermatology. Princeton, N.J.: Opinion Research Corporation, 1987.

12

Screening for Testicular Cancer

Recommendation: Periodic screening for testicular cancer by testicular examination is recommended for men with a history of cryptorchidism, orchiopexy, or testicular atrophy. There is insufficient evidence of clinical benefit or harm to recommend for or against routine screening of other asymptomatic men for testicular cancer. Clinicians should advise adolescent and young adult males to seek prompt medical attention for testicular symptoms such as pain, swelling, or heaviness. Currently, there is insufficient evidence for or against counseling patients to perform periodic self-examination of the testicles (see *Clinical Intervention*).

Burden of Suffering

Testicular cancer is the most common form of cancer in young men.[1] It will account for an estimated 5700 new cases and 350 deaths in the United States in 1989.[2] Diagnostic techniques and therapeutic interventions, while successful in reducing the previously high mortality of this disease, nonetheless produce considerable morbidity. Orchiectomy, for example, is frequently required for diagnostic purposes; lymph node dissection often results in ejaculatory dysfunction; and effective chemotherapeutic agents, such as cis-platin and bleomycin, are associated with a variety of serious side effects.[3] Testicular cancer is most common in white adolescents and young adults, in whom the annual incidence is about 1 per 10,000.[4] Leading risk factors for testicular cancer are a history of cryptorchidism, orchiopexy, or testicular atrophy.[5]

Efficacy of Screening Tests

The principal screening test for testicular cancer is palpation of the testes by an examiner. Detection of a suspicious testicular mass constitutes a positive test, and accuracy is confirmed by pathological examination of tissue. There is little information on the sensitivity, specificity, or positive predictive value of the testicular examination in asymptomatic persons. Sensitivity, which depends in large part on the palpability of the mass, would be expected to be poor in detecting small testicular tumors or when an improper examination technique is used.[6,7] Even when the physician is aware of a testicular mass or symptoms, however, sensitivity may be poor in recognizing cancer because of the variety of other causes of symptomatic testicular masses. There is evidence that between 26% and 56% of patients presenting initially to their physician with testicular cancer are first diagnosed as having epididymitis, testicular trauma, hydrocele, or other benign disorders,[8-10] and they often receive treatment for these conditions before the cancer is diagnosed.[6,9,11] An alternative means of screening for testicular cancer is instructing patients to periodically examine themselves for testicular masses. Reliable information on the accuracy of testicular self-examination is not available. There have been few studies of whether counseling men to perform self-examination motivates them to adopt this practice or to perform it correctly. Research to date has demonstrated only that education about testicular cancer and self-examination may enhance knowledge and self-reported claims of performing testicular examination.[12,13] One study found that men who reviewed an educational checklist on how to perform self-examination were able to demonstrate greater skill when self-examination was performed moments later, and they were able to recall the contents of the checklist in a telephone survey months later.[14] Few studies, however, have examined whether education or self-examination instructions actually increase the performance of self-examination. It is also unclear whether persons who detect testicular abnormalities seek medical attention promptly. Patients with testicular symptoms may wait as long as several months before contacting a physician.[8] Finally, no studies have proved that persons who perform testicular self-examination are more likely to detect early-stage tumors or have improved survival than those who do not practice self-examination.[15] Rather, published evidence that self-examination can detect testicular cancer in asymptomatic persons is limited to a small number of anecdotal reports.[16]

Effectiveness of Early Detection

The outcome of treatment is considerably better in patients with Stage I testicular cancer than in those with more advanced disease. The current five-year survival for Stage I seminoma treated with radiotherapy is 91–99%.[3] Stage I nonseminomatous cancers (e.g., teratomas, embryonal carcinoma) treated with radical retroperitoneal lymph node dissection have a reported 3–5-year survival approaching 90%.[3] With the advent of cisplatin-based chemotherapeutic regimens, a 3-year survival of 90–100% has been reported.[3] Reported survival in patients with disseminated testicular cancer, however, is lower (about 60–75%), and these persons require intensive treatment with chemotherapeutic agents that produce a variety of systemic side effects.[17,18]

Although lead-time and length biases may account for part of the improved survival observed for persons with early-stage testicular cancer, it is likely that the prognosis is, in fact, better for persons with less advanced disease. There is, however, no evidence that screening (i.e., detection of testicular cancer in asymptomatic persons) is effective in improving the detection of Stage I testicular cancer or its outcome. Even without screening, 60–80% of seminomas present as Stage I disease.[3] There is evidence that once testicular symptoms have appeared, diagnostic delays are associated with more advanced disease and lower survival.[8,9,19] But there is no evidence to date that diagnosis before symptoms appear (i.e., through screening) is of benefit in improving outcome.

Recommendations of Others

The American Cancer Society[20] and the National Cancer Institute[21] recommend that testicular examination be included as part of the periodic health examination of men. The Canadian Task Force, however, recommends that screening should be performed only on patients with a history of cryptorchidism, testicular atrophy, or ambiguous sex.[22] Recommendations differ on whether patients should be counseled to perform testicular self-examination. The American Cancer Society[23] and the National Cancer Institute[24] recommend that all postpubertal males should perform monthly testicular self-examination. Physicians have been advised to instruct male patients on how to perform this examination,[25] and some authorities believe the technique should be reviewed at every periodic health visit beginning with puberty and continuing throughout life.[26] Others, citing the lack of evidence that self-examination is effective, have advised physicians against routinely devoting time to discussing testicular self-examination.[15,27]

Discussion

Although screening for testicular cancer may be beneficial, conclusive evidence of benefit is lacking. It is also clear from the rarity of this disease that a program of routine screening of all asymptomatic males would have low yield. Testicular cancer accounts for less than 1% of all male neoplasms, and the lifetime probability of a white male (the race at greatest risk for the disease) developing this disease is 0.2%.[18] Thus, the vast majority of men would have normal examinations; of those with suspicious masses, most would have benign disease (false positives). Many of these cases, however, would require referral to urologists, radiographic studies, or invasive procedures (e.g., orchiectomy, inguinal exploration) before malignancy could be ruled out.[3] Similarly, routine performance of self-examination by all males would detect some malignancies, but the vast majority of findings would be benign. The discovery by patients of testicular masses might generate anxiety and increased physician office visits, but data supporting such adverse effects are lacking. Finally, some authors have expressed concern about the cost of physician time to teach self-examination.[15]

Clinical Intervention

Periodic screening for testicular cancer by testicular examination is recommended for men with a history of cryptorchidism, orchiopexy, or testicular atrophy. The optimal frequency of such examinations has not been determined and is left to clinical discretion. There is insufficient evidence of clinical benefit or harm to recommend for or against routine screening of other asymptomatic men for testicular cancer. Clinicians should advise adolescent and young adult males to seek prompt medical attention for testicular symptoms such as pain, swelling, or heaviness. Currently, there is insufficient evidence for or against counseling patients to perform periodic self-examination of the testicles.

REFERENCES

1. Davies JM. Testicular cancer in England and Wales: some epidemiological aspects. Lancet 1981; 1:928–32.
2. American Cancer Society. Cancer statistics, 1989. CA 1989; 39:3–20.
3. Fung CY, Garnick MB. Clinical stage I carcinoma of the testis: a review. J Clin Oncol 1988; 6:734–50.
4. Edson M. Testis cancer: the pendulum swings. Experience in 430 patients. J Urol 1979; 122:763–5.
5. Henderson BE, Benton B, Jing J, et al. Risk factors for cancer of the testes in young men. Cancer 1979; 23:598–602.
6. Prout GR, Griffin PP. Testicular tumors: delay in diagnosis and influence on survival. Am Fam Physician 1984; 29:205–9.

7. Peterson LJ, Catalona WJ, Koehler RE. Ultrasonic localization of a non-palpable testis tumor. J Urol 1979; 122:843–4.
8. Bosl GJ, Vogelzang NJ, Goldman A, et al. Impact of delay in diagnosis on clinical stage of testicular cancer. Lancet 1981; 2:970–2.
9. Field TE. Common errors occurring in the diagnosis of testicular neoplasms and the effect of these errors on prognosis. J R Army Med Corps 1964; 110:152–5.
10. Patton JF, Hewitt CB, Mallis N. Diagnosis and treatment of tumors of the testis. JAMA 1959; 171:2194–8.
11. Earlier diagnosis of testicular tumors (editorial). Br Med J 1980; 280:961.
12. Marty PJ, McDermott RJ. Three strategies for encouraging testicular self-examination among college-aged males. J Am Coll Health 1986; 34:253–8.
13. Ostwald SK, Rothenberger J. Development of a testicular self-examination program for college men. J Am Coll Health 1985; 33:234–9.
14. Friman PC, Finney JW, Glasscock SG, et al. Testicular self-examination: validation of a training strategy for early cancer detection. J Appl Behav Anal 1986; 19:87–92.
15. Westlake SJ, Frank JW. Testicular self-examination: an argument against routine teaching. Fam Pract 1987; 4:143–8.
16. Garnick MB, Mayer RJ, Richie JP. Testicular self-examination (letter). N Engl J Med 1980; 302:297.
17. Einhorn LH, Williams SD. Chemotherapy of disseminated testicular cancer. Cancer 1980; 46:1339–44.
18. Paulson DF. Testicular carcinoma. Curr Prob Cancer 1982; 6:1–44.
19. Post GJ, Belis JA. Delayed presentation of testicular tumors. South Med J 1980; 73: 33–5.
20. American Cancer Society. Guidelines for the cancer-related checkup: recommendations and rationale. New York: American Cancer Society, 1980.
21. National Cancer Institute. Working guidelines for early cancer detection: rationale and supporting evidence to decrease mortality. Bethesda, Md.: National Cancer Institute, 1987.
22. Canadian Task Force on the Periodic Health Examination. The periodic health examination, 1984 update. Can Med Assoc J 1984; 130:2–16.
23. American Cancer Society. For men only—testicular cancer and how to do testicular self examination. New York: American Cancer Society, 1984.
24. National Cancer Institute. Testicular self-examination. Washington, D.C.: Government Printing Office, 1986. (Publication no. DHHS (NIH) 87–2636.)
25. Frame PS. A critical review of adult health maintenance. Part 3. Prevention of cancer. J Fam Pract 1986; 22:511–20.
26. Goldenring JM. Equal time for men: teaching testicular self-examination. J Adol Health Care 1986; 7:273–4.
27. Goldbloom RB. Self-examination by adolescents. Pediatrics 1985; 76:126–8.

13

Screening for Ovarian Cancer

Recommendation: Screening of asymptomatic women for ovarian cancer is not recommended. It is prudent to examine the uterine adnexa when performing gynecologic examinations for other reasons.

Burden of Suffering

Ovarian cancer is the fifth leading cause of cancer deaths among U.S. women[1] and has the highest mortality of any of the gynecologic cancers.[2] It will account for about 20,000 new cases and 12,000 deaths in 1989.[1] It is estimated that 1 in every 70–100 American women is destined to die from this disease.[3,4] The overall five-year survival rate is about 30–35%[3,5] and decreases to 4% in women diagnosed with advanced disease.[5] Symptoms usually do not become apparent until the tumor compresses or invades adjacent structures, ascites develops, or metastases become clinically evident.[2] As a result, two-thirds of women with ovarian cancer have advanced (Stage III or IV) disease at the time of diagnosis.[5,6] Carcinoma of the ovary is most common in women over age 60.[7] Other important risk factors include increased ovulatory activity (nulliparity, late first pregnancy, late menopause) and a family history of ovarian cancer.[8,9]

Efficacy of Screening Tests

Potential screening tests for ovarian cancer include the bimanual pelvic examination, the Papanicolaou (Pap) smear, cytologic examination of peritoneal lavage, tumor markers, and ultrasound imaging. The pelvic examination, which can detect a variety of gynecologic disorders, is of unknown sensitivity and specificity in detecting ovarian cancer. However, small, early-stage ovarian tumors are often not detected by palpation, due to the deep anatomic location of the ovary. Thus, ovarian cancers detected by pelvic examination are generally advanced[7,8,10,11] and associated with poor survival.[8] The pelvic examination may also produce false positives when benign adnexal masses (e.g., functional cysts) are found.[4,8]

The Pap smear may occasionally reveal malignant ovarian cells,[12] but it is not considered a reliable screening test for ovarian carcinoma.[3,8,10,11,13] Studies indicate that the Pap smear has a sensitivity of only 40% in detecting ovarian cancer,[12] and some authors report even lower values (10–30%).[8] Another potential test for ovarian cancer, cytologic examination of peritoneal lavage obtained by culdocentesis, is also considered inappropriate for routine screening. This procedure is impractical in primary care, technically difficult, uncomfortable for patients, and has poor sensitivity in detecting early-stage disease.[4,8,13,14] In one study,[15] only

36% of patients with Stage Ia ovarian cancer had positive cytology when culdocentesis was performed prior to diagnostic laparotomy. This study also demonstrated the poor positive predictive value of the test: only 5.4% of women with positive cytology were subsequently shown to have ovarian cancer.

Serum tumor markers are often elevated in women with ovarian cancer. Examples of these markers include carcinoembryonic antigen, ovarian cystadenocarcinoma antigen, and CA-125 tumor-associated antigen. CA-125 is elevated in 82% of women with advanced (Stage III or IV) ovarian cancer,[16] and it is also elevated, although less frequently, in women with earlier stage disease.[17] Measurements taken prior to diagnostic laparoscopy indicate that CA-125 is elevated in one-half of women with Stage I tumors;[18-20] preoperative elevations are more common in women with nonmucinous tumors.[20] These cases are not representative of asymptomatic women in the general population, however. It is not known whether tumor markers become elevated early enough in the natural history of occult ovarian cancer to provide adequate sensitivity for screening. A recent study found that elevated CA-125 levels (greater than 30 U/mL) were present in 24% of blood specimens obtained from women five or more years before ovarian cancer was diagnosed.[17] However, further research is needed to provide more reliable data on the sensitivity of this and other tumor markers in detecting early-stage ovarian cancer in asymptomatic women.

Tumor markers may have limited specificity. It has been reported that CA-125 is elevated in 1% of healthy women, 6–40% of women with benign masses (e.g., uterine fibroids, endometriosis, pancreatic pseudocyst, pulmonary hamartoma), and 29% of women with nongynecologic cancers (e.g., pancreas, stomach, colon, breast).[16,21] It may be possible to improve the specificity of CA-125 measurement by selective screening of postmenopausal women,[22] through modifications in the assay technique,[23] or by combining CA-125 measurement with ultrasound (see below). However, prospective studies involving asymptomatic women are needed to provide definitive data on the performance characteristics of these techniques when used as screening tests.

Ultrasound imaging has also been evaluated as a screening test for ovarian cancer, since it is able to accurately estimate ovarian size, detect masses as small as 1 cm, and distinguish solid lesions from cysts.[10,24] Studies have shown, however, that routine ultrasound testing of asymptomatic women has a low yield in detecting ovarian cancer and generates a large proportion of false-positive results that often require diagnostic laparotomy or laparoscopy. In one study, ultrasound screening of 805 high-risk women led to 39 laparotomies, which revealed one ovarian carcinoma, two borderline tumors, one cancer of the cecum, and five cystadenomas.[25] In a larger study, ultrasound was performed routinely on 5678 asymptomatic female volunteers over age 45 or with a history of previous breast or gynecologic cancer.[14] Two Stage I ovarian cancers were detected in a total of 6920 scans performed over two years. A recent preliminary report from the same center indicated that 14,356 ultrasound examinations performed over three years on 5489 asymptomatic women over age 45 detected five ovarian cancers.[26] Although the sensitivity and specificity of the test were excellent (100% and 94.6%, respectively), the positive predictive value in this low-risk study population was only 2.6%. It has been calculated from these results and other data that ultrasound screening of 100,000 women over age 45 would detect 40 cases of ovarian cancer, but at a cost of 5398 false positives and over 160 complications from diagnostic laparoscopy.[27]

It may be possible to improve accuracy by combining ultrasound with other screening tests, such as the measurement of CA-125. This approach has been shown to be a useful method of discriminating between benign and malignant adnexal masses in preoperative patients.[28] Further research is needed, however, to determine the sensitivity, specificity, and positive predictive value of performing these tests in combination to screen asymptomatic women. One prospective study[29] screened 1010 asymptomatic postmenopausal women over age 45 with pelvic examination and CA-125 measurement; those with abnormal results received an ultrasound examination. Although one ovarian cancer was detected (all three screening tests were positive in this woman), the study demonstrated poor positive predictive value with each of the three screening tests. No abnormality was discovered in 28 of the 31 women with elevated CA-125. Fibroids and benign cysts were responsible for over half of the 28 abnormal pelvic examinations. There were 13 abnormal ultrasound examinations; 12 of these women consented to laparotomy, which revealed six benign ovarian cysts, two fimbrial cysts, two women with no surgical findings, one woman with adhesions, and the ovarian cancer.

Effectiveness of Early Detection

There is no direct evidence from prospective studies that women with early-stage ovarian cancer detected through screening have lower mortality from ovarian cancer than do women with more advanced disease. A large body of indirect evidence, however, suggests that this is the case. Although lead-time and length biases may be responsible, it is known that survival from ovarian cancer is related to stage at diagnosis. The five-year survival rate is 66.4% at Stage I, 45% at Stage II, 13.3% at Stage III, and only 4.1% at Stage IV.[5] Studies have shown that the most important prognostic factor in patients with advanced ovarian cancer is the size of residual tumor after treatment.[2,6] Surgical debulking, abdominal radiotherapy, and chemotherapy for ovarian cancer appear to be more effective in reducing the size of residual tumor when ovarian cancer is detected early.[2] Although these observations provide suggestive evidence that early detection may be beneficial, conclusive proof will require properly conducted prospective studies comparing long-term mortality from ovarian cancer between screened and non-screened cohorts.

Recommendations of Others

Although some authors have advocated selective screening for ovarian cancer by ultrasound,[10,30] and even by culdocentesis in certain high-risk groups,[4,8] there are no official recommendations to screen for ovarian cancer in asymptomatic women. The pelvic examination is, however, mentioned in a recent consensus recommendation on Pap testing issued by the American Cancer Society, National Cancer Institute, American College of Obstetricians and Gynecologists, American Medical Association, American Nurses Association, American Academy of Family Physicians, and the American Medical Women's Association.[31] Specifically, the pelvic examination (and Pap smear) are recommended annually for all women who are or have been sexually active or have reached age 18. Although Pap testing may be performed less frequently once three annual smears have been normal, the organizations did not specifically recommend reducing the frequency of pelvic examinations. An annual pelvic examination has been advocated in the past by the American College of Obstetricians and Gynecologists[32] and the American Cancer Society.[3] The pelvic examination is considered by the National Cancer Institute[33] and others[8,11] to be a necessary component of the complete physical examination. Recently, however, a number of authors have advised against performing periodic pelvic examinations to detect ovarian cancer.[34,35] There are no recommendations to perform routine ultrasound examinations to detect ovarian cancer.

Clinical Intervention

Screening of asymptomatic women for ovarian cancer is not recommended. It is clinically prudent to examine the uterine adnexa when performing gynecologic examinations for other reasons.

REFERENCES

1. American Cancer Society. Cancer statistics, 1989. CA 1989; 39:3–20.
2. Slotman BJ, Rao BR. Ovarian cancer: etiology, diagnosis, prognosis, surgery, radiotherapy, chemotherapy and endocrine therapy. Anticancer Res 1988; 8:417–34.
3. American Cancer Society. Cancer facts and figures, 1987. New York: American Cancer Society, 1987.
4. Griffiths CT. Carcinoma of the ovary and fallopian tube. In: Holland JF, Frei E, eds. Cancer medicine. Philadelphia: Lea and Febiger, 1982:1958–69.
5. Richardson GS, Scully RE, Nikrui N, et al. Common epithelial cancer of the ovary. N Engl J Med 1985; 312:415–24.
6. Young RC. Ovarian cancer treatment: progress or paralysis. Semin Oncol 1984; 11: 327–9.
7. Young JL, Percy CL, Asire AJ, eds. SEER Program: incidence and mortality, 1973–1977. National Cancer Institute, Monograph 57. Washington, D.C.: Government Printing Office, 1981:75.
8. Smith LH, Oi RH. Detection of malignant ovarian neoplasm: a review of the literature. 1. Detection of the patient at risk; clinical, radiological and cytological detection. Obstet Gynecol Surv 1984; 39:313–28.
9. Hildreth NG, Kelsey JL, LiVolsi VA, et al. An epidemiological study of epithelial carcinoma of the ovary. Am J Epidemiol 1981; 114:398–405.
10. Lynch HT, Albano WA, Lynch JF, et al. Surveillance and management of patients at high genetic risk for ovarian carcinoma. Obstet Gynecol 1982; 59:589–96.
11. Hall DJ, Hurt WG. The adnexal mass. J Fam Pract 1982; 14:135–40.
12. Graham JB, Graham RM, Schueller EF. Preclinical detection of ovarian cancer. Cancer 1964; 17:1414.
13. Rubin P, Bennett JM. Ovarian cancer. In: Bakeman RP, ed. Clinical oncology for medical students and physicians: a multidisciplinary approach, 5th ed. New York: American Cancer Society, 1978:114–20.
14. Goswamy RK, Campbell S. Screening for ovarian cancer. IARC Sci Publ 1986; 76: 305–9.
15. Keettel WC, Pixley EE, Buckshaum HJ. Experience with peritoneal cytology in management of gynecologic malignancies. Am J Obstet Gynecol 1974; 120:174.
16. Bast RC, Klug TL, St John E, et al. A radioimmunoassay using a monoclonal antibody to monitor the course of epithelial ovarian carcinoma. N Engl J Med 1983; 309:883–7.
17. Zurawski VR Jr, Orjaseter H, Andersen A, et al. Elevated serum CA 125 levels prior to diagnosis of ovarian cancer neoplasia: relevance for early detection of ovarian cancer. Int J Cancer 1988; 42:677–80.
18. Jacobs I. Screening for ovarian cancer by CA-125 measurement. Lancet 1988; 1:889.
19. Mann WJ, Patsner B, Cohen H, et al. Preoperative serum CA-125 levels in patients with surgical stage I invasive ovarian adenocarcinoma. JNCI 1988; 80:208–9.
20. Zurawski VR Jr, Knapp RC, Einhorn N, et al. An initial analysis of preoperative serum CA 125 levels in patients with early stage ovarian carcinoma. Gynecol Oncol 1988; 30:7–14.
21. Di-Xia C, Schwartz P, Xinguo L, et al. Evaluation of CA 125 levels in differentiating malignant from benign tumors in patients with pelvic masses. Obstet Gynecol 1988; 72:23–7.
22. Zurawski VR Jr, Broderick SF, Pickens P, et al. Serum CA 125 levels in a group of nonhospitalized women: relevance for the early detection of ovarian cancer. Obstet Gynecol 1987; 69:606–11.
23. Klug TL, Green PJ, Zurawski VR Jr, et al. Confirmation of a false-positive result in CA

125 immunoradiometric assay caused by human anti-idiotypic immunoglobulin. Clin Chem 1988; 34:1071–6.
24. Campbell S, Goessens I, Goswamy R, et al. Real time ultrasound for determination of ovarian morphology and volume: a possible early screening test for ovarian cancer? Lancet 1982; 1:425–6.
25. Andolf E, Svalenius E, Astedt B. Ultrasonography for early detection of ovarian carcinoma. Br J Obstet Gynecol 1986; 93:1286–9.
26. Campbell S, Bhan V, Royston J, et al. Screening for early ovarian cancer. Lancet 1988; 1:710–1.
27. Jacobs I. Screening for early ovarian cancer. Lancet 1988; 2:171–2.
28. Finkler NJ, Benacerraf B, Lavin PT, et al. Comparison of serum CA 125, clinical impression, and ultrasound in the preoperative evaluation of ovarian masses. Obstet Gynecol 1988; 72:659–64.
29. Jacobs I, Stabile I, Bridges J, et al. Multimodal approach to screening for ovarian cancer. Lancet 1988; 1:268–71.
30. Ferrucci JT Jr. Screening for ovarian cancer. JAMA 1986; 255:3169.
31. Fink DJ. Change in American Cancer Society checkup guidelines for detection of cervical cancer. CA 1988; 38:127–8.
32. American College of Obstetricians and Gynecologists. Standards for obstetric-gynecologic services, 6th ed. Washington, D.C.: American College of Obstetricians and Gynecologists, 1985:53–5.
33. National Cancer Institute, Division of Cancer Prevention and Control. Working guidelines for early detection: rationale and supporting evidence to decrease mortality. Bethesda, Md.: National Cancer Institute, 1987.
34. Frame PS. A critical review of adult health maintenance. Part 3. Prevention of cancer. J Fam Pract 1986; 22:511–20.
35. Qaniats TQ. Screening for ovarian cancer. JAMA 1986; 256:1892.

(reference list — illegible)

14

Screening for Pancreatic Cancer

Recommendation: Routine screening for pancreatic cancer in asymptomatic persons is not recommended.

Burden of Suffering

Pancreatic cancer is the fifth leading cause of cancer deaths in the United States, accounting for 25,000 deaths in 1989.[1] The age-adjusted incidence and mortality of pancreatic cancer have been increasing since the 1930s.[2,3] Since initial symptoms are usually nonspecific and are frequently disregarded, about 85% of symptomatic patients have regional and distant metastases by the time they are diagnosed.[4] At this stage, the disease is usually inoperable.[5] Only 4% of the 26,000 new cases of pancreatic cancer diagnosed annually live more than three years after diagnosis.[6] Pancreatic cancer is more common in older persons (80% of cases occur between ages 60 and 80), blacks, and cigarette smokers.[2,3,6]

Efficacy of Screening Tests

There are no reliable screening tests for detecting pancreatic cancer in asymptomatic persons. The deep anatomic location of the pancreas makes detection of small localized tumors unlikely during the routine abdominal examination. Even in patients with confirmed pancreatic cancer, an epigastric mass is palpable in only 12–20% of cases.[5,7] The most accurate tests for pancreatic cancer, such as computerized axial tomography and endoscopic retrograde cholangio-pancreatography, are inappropriate for routine screening due to their cost and invasiveness. A noninvasive screening test, ultrasonography, can detect some tumors in the head of the pancreas, where cancers are more resectable.[8] Although ultrasound has a reported sensitivity of 79% and a specificity of 94%,[9] data from most ultrasound studies are based on examinations of symptomatic patients with suspected disease. They thus provide little information on the efficacy of abdominal ultrasound as a screening test in asymptomatic persons.

Persons with pancreatic cancer often have elevated levels of certain serologic markers. These include carcinoembryonic antigen, carbohydrate antigen 19–9, pancreatic oncofetal antigen, tissue polypeptide antigen, inhibited leukocyte adherence, galactosyl transferase isoenzyme II, and a number of other peptides and hormones. Although studies suggest that serologic markers are elevated in most patients with pancreatic cancer,[8-13] no single marker has achieved acceptance as a suitable screening test for asymptomatic persons. This is because most tests have only been studied in high-risk populations, such as symptomatic patients with suspected or confirmed pancreatic cancer. Many of these tests lack adequate sensitivity and specificity, and some serologic markers are elevated only after the tumor has progressed to an advanced stage. Also, routine testing for serologic markers in asymptomatic persons would generate a large proportion of false-positive results, due to the low prevalence of pancreatic cancer in the general population.[10] Studies indicate that 15–50% of elevations of various serologic markers are due to benign gastrointestinal diseases or malignancies other than pancreatic cancer.[8-13]

Effectiveness of Early Detection

There is little conclusive evidence that early detection can lower morbidity or mortality from pancreatic cancer. The current five-year survival for localized disease is 5%, only slightly higher than five-year survival with regional (4%) and distant (1%) metastases.[6] There is some evidence to suggest that surgically treated patients with resectable tumors survive longer than those with more advanced disease,[14,15] but the designs of most studies of surgical outcome suffer from lead-time, length, and selection biases.[15] Surgery is performed in less than 10% of patients with pancreatic cancer,[15] and it is not without risk; estimates of perioperative mortality range between 3% and 20%.[16]

Recommendations of Others

There are no official recommendations to perform routine screening for pancreatic cancer in asymptomatic persons, and some authors[15] have specifically advised against the practice.

Discussion

Primary prevention of pancreatic cancer may be possible through clinical efforts directed at the use of tobacco products. Studies suggest that cigarette smoking is an important risk factor for this disease.[2] Although the causal relationship between smoking and pancreatic cancer requires further study, counseling patients to discontinue smoking (see Chapter 48) is easily justified by its established efficacy in preventing other malignancies (e.g., lung cancer), coronary artery disease, and other serious disorders.

Clinical Intervention

Routine screening for pancreatic cancer in asymptomatic persons is not recommended. All patients should be counseled regarding the use of tobacco products (see Chapter 48).

REFERENCES

1. American Cancer Society. Cancer statistics, 1988. CA 1989; 39:3–20.
2. Gordis L, Gold EB. Epidemiology of pancreatic cancer. World J Surg 1984; 8:808–21.
3. Levin DL, Connelly RR, Devesa SS. Demographic characteristics of cancer of the pancreas: mortality, incidence, survival. Cancer 1981; 47:1456–68.
4. Go VLW, Taylor WF, DiMagno EP. Efforts at early diagnosis of pancreatic cancer: the Mayo Clinic experience. Cancer 1981; 47:1698–703.
5. Macdonald JS, Widerlite L, Schein PS. Current diagnosis and management of pancreatic carcinoma. JNCI 1976; 56:1093–9.
6. American Cancer Society. Cancer facts and figures, 1987. New York: American Cancer Society, 1987.

7. Gudjonsson B, Livstone EM, Spiro HM. Cancer of the pancreas: diagnostic accuracy and survival statistics. Cancer 1978; 42:2494–506.
8. Moossa AR, Levin B. The diagnosis of "early" pancreatic cancer: the University of Chicago experience. Cancer 1981; 47:1688–97.
9. Wang TH, Lin JT, Chen DS, et al. Noninvasive diagnosis of advanced pancreatic cancer by real-time ultrasonography, carcinoembryonic antigen, and carbohydrate antigen 19–9. Pancreas 1986; 1:219–23.
10. Podolsky DK. Serologic markers in the diagnosis and management of pancreatic carcinoma. World J Surg 1984; 8:822–30.
11. Evaluation of CA 19–9 as a serum tumour marker in pancreatic cancer. Br J Cancer 1986; 53:197–202.
12. Basso D, Fabris C, Del Favero G, et al. Combined determination of serum CA 19–9 and tissue polypeptide antigen: why not improvement in pancreatic cancer diagnosis? Oncology 1988; 45:24–9.
13. Podolsky DK, McPhee MS, Alpert E, et al. Galactosyltransferase isoenzyme II in the detection of pancreatic cancer: comparison with radiologic, endoscopic, and serologic tests. N Engl J Med 1981; 304:1313–8.
14. Cancer of the Pancreas Task Force. Staging of cancer of the pancreas. Cancer 1981; 47:1631–7.
15. Early diagnosis and screening for pancreatic cancer. Lancet 1986; 2:785–6.
16. Trede M. The surgical treatment of pancreatic carcinoma. Surgery 1985; 97:28–35.

Screening for Oral Cancer

Recommendation: Routine screening of asymptomatic persons for oral cancer by primary care clinicians is not recommended. It may be prudent for clinicians to perform careful examinations for cancerous lesions of the oral cavity in patients who use tobacco or excessive amounts of alcohol, as well as in those with suspicious symptoms or lesions detected through self-examination. All patients should be counseled to receive regular dental examinations (see Chapter 55), to discontinue the use of all forms of tobacco (Chapter 48), and to limit consumption of alcohol (Chapter 47). Persons with increased exposure to sunlight should be advised to take protective measures to protect their lips and skin from the harmful effects of ultraviolet rays (Chapter 11).

Burden of Suffering

Oral cancer will account for over 30,000 new cases and about 8600 deaths in the United States in 1989.[1] Since over half of these cancers have metastasized or become invasive at the time of diagnosis,[2,3] overall five-year survival from this form of cancer is poor (30–50%).[1,4] Carcinoma of the tongue, the most frequent site of oral cancer (excluding the lip), has an overall five-year survival of less than 15%.[2] About half of all oropharyngeal cancers and the majority of deaths from this disease occur in persons over age 65.[5] In addition to age, other major risk factors include the use of tobacco (smoking of cigarettes, pipes, or cigars; smokeless tobacco, i.e., chewing tobacco or snuff) and the excessive consumption of alcohol.[5]

Efficacy of Screening Tests

The principal screening test for oropharyngeal cancer in asymptomatic persons is inspection and palpation of the oral cavity. Studies indicate that many oral cancers occur on the floor of the mouth, the ventral and lateral regions of the tongue, and the soft palate, anatomic sites that may be inaccessible to routine visual inspection.[3,5] The recommended examination technique involves a careful exploration of the oral cavity with a gloved hand and a gauze pad, retraction of the tongue to expose ventral and posterolateral surfaces and the floor of the mouth, and bidigital palpation for masses.[2,6] There is little information, however, on the sensitivity of this procedure in detecting oral cancer or on the frequency of false-positive results when a lesion is found. In addition, it may be impractical for physicians to perform a complete examination in this manner on all patients. The abbreviated oral inspection that is more typical of the routine physical examination is also of unknown accuracy and predictive value. Some studies suggest that dentists are more effective than physicians in routinely performing a complete mouth examination and detecting early-stage oral cancer.[7] Unfortunately, older Americans, the population at greatest risk for oral cancer, visit the dentist infrequently (an average of less than once every five years); physician visits are six times as common at this age.[2]

Alternative screening tests for oral cancer have been proposed, such as tolonium chloride rinses to stain suspicious lesions,[8] but further research is needed to evaluate the accuracy and acceptability of these techniques before routine use in the general population can be considered.

Effectiveness of Early Detection

There is evidence that persons with early-stage oral cancer have a better prognosis than those diagnosed with more advanced disease. In one study, overall five-year survival was 63% for persons with localized disease, 30% for those with regional extension, and 17% for persons with cancers with distant metastases.[7] Similar findings have been published in other series. However, the role of lead-time bias, length bias, and other factors in the interpretation of these data has not been fully considered; some authors have questioned the effectiveness of early detection in improving prognosis.[9] Further research is needed to demonstrate in a prospective fashion that the outcome of oral cancer is improved when lesions are detected in asymptomatic persons.

Recommendations of Others

The Canadian Task Force recommends that an annual visual inspection of the mouth include an examination for oral cancer in males and in all smokers.[10] Similarly, the National Cancer Institute[11] and the American Cancer Society[12] recommend that a complete oral examination for cancer be included in the periodic health examination.

Discussion

Available screening tests for oral cancer are limited to the physical examination of the mouth, a test of undetermined sensitivity, specificity, and positive predictive value. The primary care physician faces logistical difficulties in performing a thorough mouth examination on every patient. There is also inadequate evidence that early detection of oral cancer necessarily improves outcome. Although direct evidence of benefit is lacking, examinations for oral cancer in asymptomatic persons may be clinically prudent in persons at significantly increased risk for the disease (i.e., persons with a smoking or alcohol history, or those with suspicious lesions). It is also appropriate to refer patients for regular visits to the dentist, for whom complete examination of the oral cavity is often more feasible (see Chapter 55).

Primary prevention strategies, such as counseling patients regarding the use of tobacco and alcohol, may have a greater impact on the morbidity and mortality associated with oral cancer than measures aimed at early detection. There is good evidence that smoking and excessive consumption of alcohol are both independent and synergistic risk factors for oral cancer.[5] Over 90% of oropharyngeal cancer deaths are associated with smoking.[13] In addition to smoking and alcohol, oral cancer is also associated with the use of snuff and chewing tobacco.[14,15] Smokeless tobacco is used by over 10 million Americans[14,16] and a growing number of young persons under the age of 21 (currently estimated at 3 million).[18] Between 8% and 36% of male high school and college students are regular users of smokeless tobacco, and there is evidence that young children (aged 8–13) may also have significant exposure in some geographic areas.[15] Young people who use smokeless tobacco may be more likely to switch to cigarette smoking as they grow older.[17] Efforts by patients to reduce or eliminate exposure to these substances will have benefits that extend beyond the prevention of oral cancer. Smoking is a leading risk factor for lung cancer, atherosclerosis, and a number of other serious diseases (see Chapter 48), and alcohol abuse is associated with addictive behavior, medical disorders, and increased risk of injuries (Chapter 47). Finally, measures to reduce outdoor exposure to sunlight may reduce the risk of lip cancer, along with other forms of skin cancer (Chapter 11).

Clinical Intervention

Routine screening examinations for oral cancer by primary care clinicians are not recommended for all asymptomatic persons. It may be clinically prudent to include an examination for cancerous and precancerous lesions of the oral cavity in the periodic health examination of persons with exposure to tobacco and excessive amounts of alcohol, as well as in persons with suspicious symptoms or lesions detected through self-examination. All patients, especially those over age 65, should be advised to receive a complete dental examination on a regular basis (see Chapter 55). All adolescent and adult patients should be asked to describe their use of tobacco (Chapter 48) and alcohol (Chapter 47). Appropriate counseling should be offered to those persons who smoke cigarettes, pipes, or cigars, those who use chewing tobacco or snuff, and those who have evidence of alcohol abuse. Persons with increased exposure to sunlight should be advised to take protective measures when outdoors to protect their lips and skin from the harmful effects of ultraviolet rays (Chapter 11).

Note: See Appendix A for the U.S. Preventive Services Task Force Table of Ratings for this topic. See also the relevant Task Force background paper: Greene JC. Preventive dentistry. In: Goldbloom RB, Lawrence RS, eds. Preventing disease: beyond the rhetoric. New York: Springer-Verlag (in press).

REFERENCES

1. American Cancer Society. Cancer statistics, 1989. CA 1989; 39:3–20.
2. Chiodo GT, Eigner T, Rosenstein DI. Oral cancer detection: the importance of routine screening for prolongation of survival. Postgrad Med 1986; 80:231–6.
3. Mashberg A, Meyers H. Anatomical site and size of 222 early asymptomatic oral squamous carcinomas. Cancer 1976; 37:2149–57.
4. Orlian AI. Cancer of the soft tissues of the oral cavity. NY State Dent J 1983; 49:704–9.
5. Baden E. Prevention of cancer of the oral cavity and pharynx. CA 1987; 37:49–62.
6. Hahn W. Clinical signs for the early recognition of cancer of the oral cavity. Int Dent J 1977; 27:165–71.
7. Elwood JM, Gallagher RP. Factors influencing early diagnosis of cancer of the oral cavity. Can Med Assoc J 1985; 133:651–6.
8. Mashberg A. Final evaluation of tolonium chloride rinse for screening of high-risk patients with asymptomatic squamous carcinoma. J Am Dent Assoc 1983; 106:319–23.

9. William RG. The early diagnosis of carcinoma of the mouth. Ann R Coll Surg Engl 1981; 63:423–5.
10. Canadian Task Force on the Periodic Health Examination. The periodic health examination. Can Med Assoc J 1979; 121:1–45.
11. National Cancer Institute. Working guidelines for early cancer detection: rationale and supporting evidence to decrease mortality. Bethesda, Md.: National Cancer Institute, 1987.
12. American Cancer Society. Guidelines for the cancer-related checkup: recommendations and rationale. CA 1980; 30:4–50.
13. Department of Health and Human Services. Reducing the health consequences of smoking: 25 years of progress. A report of the Surgeon General. Rockville, Md.: Department of Health and Human Services, 1989. (Publication no. DHHS (PHS) 89–8411.)
14. Idem. The health consequences of smokeless tobacco: a report of the advisory committee to the Surgeon General. Washington, D.C.: Government Printing Office, 1986. (Publication no. DHHS (PHS) 86–2874.)
15. Connoly GN, Winn DM, Hecht SS, et al. The reemergence of smokeless tobacco. N Engl J Med 1986; 314:1020–7.
16. National Institutes of Health. Consensus development conference statement: health implications of smokeless tobacco use. Bethesda, Md.: National Institutes of Health, 1986.
17. Glover ED, Laflin M, Edwards SW. Age of initiation and switching patterns between smokeless tobacco and cigarettes among college students in the United States. Am J Public Health 1989; 79:207–8.

16

Screening for Diabetes Mellitus

Recommendation: An oral glucose tolerance test for gestational diabetes mellitus is recommended for all pregnant women between 24 and 28 weeks of gestation. Routine screening for diabetes in asymptomatic nonpregnant adult patients, using plasma glucose measurement or urinalysis, is not recommended for the general population, but it may be appropriate in selected high-risk groups (see *Clinical Intervention*).

Burden of Suffering

Approximately 11 million persons in the United States have diabetes mellitus, and about 5 million of them have not been diagnosed.[1,2] Diabetes can cause life-threatening metabolic complications, and it is an important risk factor for other leading causes of death, such as coronary artery disease, congestive heart failure, and cerebrovascular disease. Diabetes is the seventh leading cause of death in the United States, accounting for over 130,000 deaths each year.[3,4] It is an important contributor to deaths from other causes as well.[4] Diabetes is a leading cause of neuropathy, which develops in at least 50% of patients within 25 years of diagnosis.[5] Diabetic peripheral vascular disease accounts for about 50,000 amputations each year.[6] Diabetic microvascular disease can lead to renal failure and blindness. Diabetic nephropathy, a complication in about 10% of cases, accounts for one-quarter of all new dialysis patients.[1] Diabetes is the leading cause of blindness in adults, with about 5800 people each year losing their sight as a result of this disease.[7] Infants born of diabetic women are at increased risk of prematurity, perinatal mortality, macrosomia, congenital malformations, and metabolic derangements.[8,9] Direct and indirect costs of diabetes in the United States total at least $14 billion per year.[10]

About 90% of all cases of diabetes are Type II, or noninsulin-dependent diabetes mellitus (NIDDM).[2] This form of diabetes generally occurs in adults and is increasingly common after age 40. About 2 million older Americans have diabetes.[11] NIDDM is more common in blacks, Hispanics, and Native Americans. About 1 million black Americans have diabetes.[12] Other important risk factors for NIDDM include family history, obesity, and a history of gestational diabetes. Type I diabetes, or insulin-dependent diabetes mellitus (IDDM), accounts for about 10% of all cases of diabetes and characteristically has an acute onset during childhood or adolescence.

Gestational diabetes, the development of impaired glucose tolerance during pregnancy in nondiabetic women, occurs in about 3% of pregnancies. This condition is a risk factor for fetal macrosomia and may also be associated with other maternal and neonatal complications. Although macrosomia by itself is not a morbid condition, it is associated with increased risk of birth trauma from skull and clavicular fracture, shoulder dystocia, and peripheral nerve injury.[13-16] As mentioned, a history of gestational diabetes is also a maternal risk factor for the development of NIDDM, and it may be an indicator of long-standing impaired glucose tolerance.[17]

Efficacy of Screening Tests

Although a number of techniques are available to test for diabetes (e.g., hemoglobin A_1c), the principal screening test for asymptomatic persons is blood glucose measurement. Glucose can be measured at random, after the patient has fasted, following a meal (postprandial), or at specified intervals after the administration of a known oral dose of glucose (oral glucose tolerance test [GTT]). These tests are used to detect impaired glucose tolerance, a condition that is present in diabetes but that can also occur before diabetes develops. To be classified as having diabetes rather than impaired glucose tolerance alone, an individual must have a fasting plasma glucose of 140 mg/dL (7.8 mmol/L) or greater, an elevated plasma glucose following a 75 g oral glucose tolerance test (200 mg/dL [11.1 mmol/L] or greater at both the 2-hour test and between 0 and 2 hours), or the presence of classic symptoms such as polyuria, polydypsia, and ketonuria.[18] (A higher, 100 g dose and different threshold criteria have been used since the 1960s for the detection of gestational diabetes in pregnant women.[19]) An individual is thought to have impaired glucose tolerance in the absence of diabetes if plasma glucose is between 140 mg/dL (7.8 mmol/ L) and 200 mg/dL (11.1 mmol/L) two hours after a 75 g challenge and the plasma glucose prior to two hours equals or exceeds 200 mg/dL (11.1 mmol/L).[18]

The need for such complex criteria is due in part to the difficulty of using a single glucose value as a basis for screening for diabetes. No specific glucose level discriminates completely between persons with impaired glucose tolerance or diabetes and the normal population. There is a wide overlap in the range of blood glucose concentrations within such populations. Even within individuals, there is considerable temporal variation in blood glucose in relation to meals. Thus, adopting a low threshold criteria for defining hyperglycemia will result in high sensitivity but poor specificity for impaired glucose tolerance and diabetes. Conversely, a blood glucose above 200 mg/dL (11.1 mmol/L) is considered an unequivocal sign of impaired glucose tolerance,[20] but many cases would be overlooked if this high threshold value were adopted for screening.

There are advantages and disadvantages to the various glucose screening tests. Fasting glucose measurement is less practical for routine screening than random measurement because the patient must not eat for 8 to 10 hours before the test, but it is generally more accurate. Nonetheless, its sensitivity as a screening test is limited; in one survey, only 25% of persons with undiagnosed diabetes had fasting glucose levels greater than 140 mg/dL (7.8 mmol/L).[21] Postprandial testing (levels above 200 mg/dL [11.1 mmol/L] 90–120 minutes after a meal) may be more convenient for patients and more sensitive in detecting impaired glucose tolerance, but it is not ideal for screening purposes due to the time constraints. The 75 g oral GTT provides the greatest accuracy, but the test is not suited for routine screening due to the inconvenience and cost associated with glucose administration and multiple venipunctures over a period of several hours. Rather than being used as a routine screening test, the GTT is often used as a confirmatory test once diabetes is suspected.

A shorter (one hour) and lower dose (50 g) GTT is now used as a routine screening test for gestational diabetes. A level of 140 mg/dL (7.8 mmol/L) or greater one hour after the 50 g glucose challenge has a reported sensitivity of 83% and a specificity of 87% when compared with the 100 g GTT.[22] Assuming a prevalence of 3% for gestational diabetes, routine use of the 50 g test in pregnant women would generate five false positives for every case of gestational diabetes detected. The test may also have limited reproducibility; up to 75% of patients with a positive GTT have been found to be negative on subsequent testing.[23,24] The high false-positive rate is of significance because mislabeled patients may experience anxiety and inconvenience from follow-up diagnostic testing. Dietary restrictions and unnecessary fetal monitoring and operative deliveries may also result if the error is not disclosed in subsequent testing. There are, however, few reliable data regarding the magnitude of these problems.

Urine testing for glucosuria is considered a poor screening test for diabetes, primarily because the concentration of glucose in urine is variable and because glucosuria may occur at normal blood glucose levels in persons with a low renal threshold for glucose.[25] Urine glucose measurement has been reported to have a sensitivity of less than 30%.[26] In addition, urinalysis is subject to inaccuracies caused by improper specimen collection and testing. Even in persons with known diabetes, urinalysis is being replaced by self-monitoring of blood glucose as a more effective technique for daily assessment of glycemic control.[27,28]

Effectiveness of Early Detection

The detection of impaired glucose tolerance or diabetes in asymptomatic persons provides an opportunity to attempt to prevent or delay the complications of diabetes through dietary and pharmacologic measures to achieve euglycemia. The presumed benefits of early detection are based on evidence that many of the complications of diabetes are directly related to the duration and severity of hyperglycemia.[29-32] There is little direct evidence that asymptomatic persons benefit from the detection and treatment of impaired glucose tolerance in the absence of overt diabetes.[33,34] Most asymptomatic persons with impaired glucose tolerance do not develop diabetes even in the absence of treatment; longitudinal data suggest that only 15–30% of such cases progress to frank diabetes.[35-37] Among persons with impaired glucose tolerance who are destined to develop diabetes, there is conflicting evidence regarding the ability of early hypoglycemic therapy to prevent the progression of the disease. One prospective trial found that dietary and pharmacologic treatment did reduce progression to diabetes,[35] but other prospective studies have reported no beneficial effect.[36-38] Thus, although impaired glucose tolerance is an important risk factor for diabetes, it is not by itself an established indication for treatment.

It is also unclear whether treatment reduces the risk of long-term complications after diabetes (IDDM or NIDDM) has developed. Aggressive clinical maneuvers to maintain euglycemia ("tight control") are efficacious in achieving normal plasma glucose levels and reducing the risk of metabolic derangements. Longitudinal studies demonstrate a correlation between the level of glucose control and the incidence of microvascular complications (e.g., diabetic nephropathy and retinopathy).[39-42] However, the benefits of tightened control have been difficult to demonstrate with certainty under controlled experimental conditions. Two controlled trials that examined the efficacy of continuous subcutaneous insulin infusion in reducing progression of microvascular disease in IDDM were unable to demonstrate significant slowing of retinal deterioration within the first year of treatment. In fact, tightened control produced an early acceleration in retinal deterioration.[43,44] Follow-up data from both research groups suggest that reduced progression of retinopathy may become more apparent two years after treatment, but the data are inconclusive due to limitations in study design.[45,46] Both groups also reported that renal function, as measured by urinary albumin excretion, was improved in those who received continuous insulin treatment.[45,47] Another controlled trial, which found that progression of retinopathy and neuropathy was reduced after two years of treatment with continuous insulin infusion, suffered from small sample size and other design limitations.[48]

Macrovascular benefits from treatment, such as reduced cardiovascular disease, have also been presumed but not proved convincingly in clinical trials. Although a large trial reported that glucose control in patients with NIDDM did not appear to lower the rate of vascular complications or deaths in over 12 years of observation, there is substantial controversy regarding the design of this study.[49,50] A clear association between glucose control and overall mortality has also been difficult to demonstrate in longitudinal studies.[51] A multicenter randomized trial is currently under way to provide further data on the health benefits of maintaining euglycemia in patients with IDDM.[52]

In women with IDDM who become pregnant, glycemic control may have a direct effect on maternal and neonatal outcome. A temporal relationship between metabolic control during certain periods of pregnancy and the incidence of maternal and fetal complications has been demonstrated in a number of studies.[53] Women with IDDM who are enrolled in intensive programs to maintain euglycemia during pregnancy appear to have better outcomes than matched controls, although selection biases in these studies may contribute to some of these differences.[54] Historical data demonstrate a dramatic decline in the rate of maternal deaths and neonatal complications (e.g., perinatal death, macrosomia, congenital malformations, postpartum metabolic derangements) in the years following the introduction of insulin.[55,56] Factors other than strict glycemic control, such as closer monitoring of both mother and fetus and vigorous management of the infant after delivery, may have also contributed significantly to this trend.

In addition to instituting hypoglycemic therapy, another possible argument for routine screening is the identification of candidates for laser photocoagulation therapy, which can slow the progression of diabetic retinopathy.[57] However, retinopathy requiring treatment is rare early in the course of the disease,[58,59] and therefore it is unlikely that screening would result in increased benefit from the procedure. Since diabetes is often associated with other serious diseases (e.g., coronary artery disease, peripheral vascular disease), the discovery of diabetes might lead to early detection and treatment of these other conditions. There are, however, few data regarding the accuracy and efficiency of using diabetes screening as a means of detecting other diseases. In addition, more sensitive and specific screening tests are available for most of the conditions associated with diabetes (see Chapters 1–5).

Pregnant women with an abnormal oral GTT are at significantly increased risk of macrosomia, preeclampsia, and other complications.[60] The early detection and treatment of gestational diabetes to achieve euglycemia has been associated in observational studies with significantly lower neonatal mortality and morbidity (macrosomia, birth trauma, operative delivery).[61-66] However, the designs of these studies, which are often nonrandomized and lack proper controls, do not permit the conclusion that the treatment of gestational diabetes (rather than other components of prenatal care) was by itself responsible for the improved outcome. Two controlled trials have provided stronger evidence of treatment efficacy.[67,68] In both studies, diet and insulin treatment of gestational diabetes were associated with a significant decrease in the incidence of macrosomia; no differences were reported in neonatal mortality or other outcome measures. In a more recent randomized controlled trial, there were no differences in outcome between women treated with diet and insulin and those treated with diet alone.[69]

Thus, the principal benefit of screening for gestational diabetes that has been proved under controlled experimental conditions is the prevention of macrosomia, a condition associated with increased risk of birth trauma and operative delivery.[13-16] The majority of macrosomic infants are born to women without gestational or insulin-dependent diabetes;[70] other factors such as maternal obesity may be more important. In a study of 574 macrosomic infants, gestational diabetes was present in only 5% of the mothers, whereas 45% were overweight (greater than 90 kg).[71] It is therefore unclear whether the overall incidence of macrosomia in the population will be affected significantly by early detection of gestational diabetes or whether the effect will be of sufficient magnitude and clinical value to justify routine screening of all pregnant women.

Recommendations of Others

Recommendations against routine screening for diabetes in nonpregnant adults have been issued by the Canadian Task Force[72] and other experts on the periodic health examination.[73] The American Diabetes Association (ADA) recommends screening high-risk groups by performing fasting or random blood glucose measurements.[74] The Canadian Task Force recommends screening pregnant women for gestational diabetes by assessing risk factors and by repeated urine glucose testing.[72] In 1985, the Second International Workshop-Conference on Gestational Diabetes Mellitus recommended that all pregnant women receive a 50 g oral glucose tolerance test between 24 and 28 weeks of gestation; women with a one-hour plasma glucose level of 140 mg/dL (7.8 mmol/L) or greater should then receive the 100 g oral glucose tolerance test.[75] This is also the official recommendation of the ADA.[76] The American College of Obstetricians and Gynecologists recommends screening for gestational diabetes in all pregnant women over age 30 and in those with glucosuria, hypertension, or a risk factor for gestational diabetes.[77] The ADA and the American College of Physicians are currently preparing revised recommendations on screening for diabetes.[78]

Discussion

Screening for diabetes in the clinical setting suffers from two important limitations: the lack of a screening test that combines accuracy with practicality, and the absence of adequate evidence that early detection and treatment improve outcome in asymptomatic persons. The uncertainties regarding the benefits of early treatment of asymptomatic persons must be weighed against the potential adverse effects of screening (e.g., false-positive labeling) and treatment (e.g., dietary restrictions, insulin injections). In high-risk groups (see *Clinical Intervention*), in which the prevalence of diabetes is increased, the frequency of false-positive results from screening is likely to be lower. Proponents of screening emphasize that the implications of false-positive labeling can be minimized through subsequent diagnostic testing; moreover, the principal forms of treatment, dietary modification and exercise, are of low cost and of considerable health benefit for numerous target conditions.[78]

A stronger scientific rationale exists for screening pregnant women for gestational diabetes, but there are important limitations to this evidence as well. It has not been demonstrated in properly conducted controlled trials (as opposed to observational studies) that treatment can prevent most of the health risks associated with gestational diabetes (perinatal mortality, neonatal metabolic derangements, congenital anomalies). The ability to prevent macrosomia has been proved, but it is uncertain to what extent screening would reduce the overall incidence of birth trauma and operative delivery. Nonetheless, since treatment is unlikely to result in significant maternal or fetal harm, routine screening for gestational diabetes may be a reasonable measure.

In persons who are not pregnant, primary prevention rather than screening may be an important means of preventing diabetes and its complications. Among the many benefits of exercise and weight reduction, for example, are improved glucose tolerance and reduced obesity, important risk factors for diabetes as well as for other serious chronic diseases (see Chapter 18). A number of dietary interventions (e.g., increased dietary fiber) have also been examined in the prevention and treatment of NIDDM.[79] Since these healthy behaviors are widely recommended even in the absence of diabetes, patients should be encouraged to adopt these behaviors independently of diabetes screening (see Chapters 49 and 50).

Clinical Intervention

A 50 g oral glucose tolerance test for gestational diabetes is recommended for all pregnant women between 24 and 28 weeks of gestation. Women with a one-hour plasma glucose level of 140 mg/dL (7.8 mmol/L) or greater should receive a confirmatory three-hour 100 g oral glucose tolerance test. Routine screening for diabetes in asymptomatic nonpregnant adults, using plasma glucose measurement or urinalysis, is not recommended. Periodic fasting plasma glucose measurements may be appropriate in persons at high risk for diabetes mellitus, such as the markedly obese, persons with a family history of diabetes, or women with a history of gestational diabetes.

Note: See Appendix A for the U.S. Preventive Services Task Force Table of Ratings for this topic. See also the relevant Task Force background paper: Singer DE, Samet JH, Coley CM, et al. Screening for diabetes mellitus. In: Goldbloom RB, Lawrence RS, eds. Preventing disease: beyond the rhetoric. New York: Springer-Verlag (in press).

REFERENCES

1. American Diabetes Association. Diabetes facts and figures. Alexandria, Va.: American Diabetes Association, 1986.
2. Harris MI. Prevalence of non-insulin-dependent diabetes and impaired glucose tolerance. In: National Diabetes Data Group. Diabetes in America: diabetes data compiled 1984. Washington, D.C.: Department of Health and Human Services, 1985:VI-1 to VI-31. (Publication no. DHHS (NIH) 85–1468.)
3. Kovar MG, Harris MI. The scope of diabetes in the United States population. Am J Public Health 1987; 77:1549–50.
4. Centers for Disease Control. Trends in diabetes mellitus mortality. MMWR 1988; 37: 769–73.
5. Harati Y. Diabetic peripheral neuropathies. Ann Intern Med 1987; 107:546–59.
6. Bild D, Selby JV, Sinnock P, et al. Lower extremity amputation in persons with diabetes: epidemiology and prevention. Diabetes Care 1989; 12:24–31.
7. The Carter Center. Closing the gap: the problem of diabetes mellitus in the United States. Diabetes Care 1985; 8:391–406.
8. Miodonovik M, Mimouni F, Dignan PSJ, et al. Major malformations in infants of IDDM women: vasculopathy and early-trimester poor glycemic control. Diabetes Care 1988; 11:713–8.
9. Mimouni F, Miodonovik M, Siddiqi TA, et al. High spontaneous premature labor rate in

insulin-dependent diabetic pregnant women: an association with poor glycemic control and urogenital infection. Obstet Gynecol 1988; 72:175–00.

10. Entmacher PS, Sinnock P, Bostic E, et al. Economic impact of diabetes. In. National Diabetes Data Group. Diabetes in America: diabetes data compiled 1984. Washington, D.C.: Department of Health and Human Services, 1985:XXXII-1 to XXXII-13. (Publication no. DHHS (NIH) 85–1468.)

11. Bennett PH. Diabetes in the elderly: diagnosis and epidemiology. Geriatrics 1984; 39: 37–41.

12. National Center for Health Statistics. Prevalence of known diabetes among black Americans. Advance Data from Vital and Health Statistics, no. 130. Hyattsville, Md.: Public Health Service, 1987. (Publication no. DHHS (PHS) 87–1250.)

13. Sandmire HF, O'Halloin TJ. Shoulder dystocia: its incidence and associated risk factors. Int J Gynaecol Obstet 1988; 26:65–73.

14. Gross TL, Sokol RJ, Williams T, et al. Shoulder dystocia: a fetal-physician risk. Am J Obstet Gynecol 1987; 156:1408–18.

15. McFarland LV, Raskin M, Daling JR, et al. Erb/Duchenne's palsy: a consequence of fetal macrosomia and method of delivery. Obstet Gynecol 1986; 68:784–8.

16. Modanlou HD, Dorchester WL, Thorosian A, et al. Macrosomia—maternal, fetal, and neonatal complications. Obstet Gynecol 1980; 55:420–4.

17. Harris MI. Gestational diabetes may represent discovery of preexisting glucose intolerance. Diabetes Care 1988; 11:402–11.

18. National Diabetes Data Group. Classification and diagnosis of diabetes mellitus and other categories of glucose tolerance. Diabetes 1979; 28:1039–57.

19. O'Sullivan JB, Mahan CM. Criteria for the oral glucose tolerance test in pregnancy. Diabetes 1964; 13:278–85.

20. World Health Organization. Expert Committee on Diabetes Mellitus. WHO Technical Report Series 646. Geneva: World Health Organization, 1980:1–80.

21. Harris MI, Hadden WC, Knowler WC, et al. Prevalence of diabetes and impaired glucose tolerance and plasma glucose levels in U.S. population aged 20–74 yr. Diabetes 1987; 36:523–34.

22. Carpenter MW, Coustan DR. Criteria for screening tests for gestational diabetes. Am J Obstet Gynocol 1982; 144:708–73.

23. Abell DA, Beischer NA. Evaluation of the three hour oral glucose tolerance test in detection of significant hyperglycemia in pregnancy. Diabetes 1975; 24:874–80.

24. McDonald GW, Fisher GF, Burnham C. Reproducibility of the oral glucose tolerance test. Diabetes 1965; 14:473–80.

25. Lind T. Antenatal screening using random blood glucose values. Diabetes [Suppl 2] 1985; 34:17–20.

26. Bitzen PO, Schersten B. Assessment of laboratory methods for detection of unsuspected diabetes in primary health care. Scand J Prim Health Care 1986; 4:85–95.

27. McCall AL, Mullin CJ. Home monitoring of diabetes mellitus—a quiet revolution. Clin Lab Med 1986; 6:215–39.

28. Consensus statement on self-monitoring of blood glucose. Diabetes Care 1987; 10: 95–9.

29. Burditt AGF, Caird FI, Draper GJ. The natural history of diabetic retinopathy. Q J Med 1968; 37:303–17.

30. Nathan DM, Singer DE, Godine JE, et al. Retinopathy in older type II diabetics: association with glucose control. Diabetes 1986; 35:797–801.

31. Davidson MB. The case for control in diabetes mellitus. West J Med 1978; 129:193–200.

32. West KM, Erdreich LJ, Stober JA. A detailed study of risk factors for retinopathy and nephropathy in diabetes. Diabetes 1980; 29:501–8.

33. Genuth SM, Houser HB, Carter JR Jr, et al. Observations on the value of mass indiscriminate screening for diabetes mellitus based on a five-year follow-up. Diabetes 1978; 27:377–83.

34. Bennett PH, Knowler WC. Early detection and intervention in diabetes mellitus: is it effective? J Chronic Dis 1984; 37:653–6.

35. Sartor G, Schersten B, Carlstrom S, et al. Ten-year follow-up of subjects with impaired glucose tolerance: prevention of diabetes by tolbutamide and diet regulation. Diabetes 1980; 29:41–9.

36. Keen H, Jarrett RJ, McCartney P. The ten-year follow-up of the Bedford survey (1962–1972): glucose tolerance and diabetes. Diabetologia 1982; 22:73–8.

37. Jarrett RJ, Keen H, McCartney P. The Whitehall Study: ten year follow-up report on men with impaired glucose tolerance with reference to worsening of diabetes and predictors of death. Diabetic Med 1984; 1:279–83.

38. Jarrett RJ, Keen H, Fuller JH, et al. Treatment of borderline diabetes: controlled trial using carbohydrate restriction and phenformin. Br Med J 1977; 2:861–5.

39. Chase HP, Jackson WE, Hoops SL, et al. Glucose control and the renal and retinal complications of insulin-dependent diabetes. JAMA 1989; 261:1155–60.

40. Pirart J. Diabetes mellitus and its degenerative complications: a prospective study of 4,400 patients observed between 1947 and 1973. Diabetes Care 1978; 1:168–88, 252–63.

41. Miki E, Fukuda M, Kuzuya T, et al. Relation of the course of retinopathy to control of diabetes, age, and therapeutic agents in diabetic Japanese patients. Diabetes 1969; 18:773–80.

42. Takazakura E, Nakamoto Y, Hayakawa H, et al. Onset and progression of diabetic glomerulosclerosis: a prospective study based on serial renal biopsies. Diabetes 1975; 24:1–9.

43. Kroc Collaborative Study Group. Blood glucose control and the evolution of diabetic retinopathy and albuminuria: a preliminary multicenter trial. N Engl J Med 1984; 311: 365–72.

44. Lauritzen T, Frost-Larsen K, Larsen HW, et al. Effect of 1 year of near-normal blood glucose levels on retinopathy in insulin-dependent diabetics. Lancet 1983; 1:200–4.

45. Kroc Collaborative Study Group. Diabetic retinopathy after two years of intensified insulin treatment: follow-up of the Kroc Collaborative Study. JAMA 1988; 260:37–41.

46. Lauritzen T, Frost-Larsen K, Larsen HW, et al. The Steno Study Group: two-year experience with continuous subcutaneous insulin infusion in relation to retinopathy and neuropathy. Diabetes [Suppl 3] 1985; 34:74–9.

47. Feldt-Rasmussen B, Mathiesen ER, Deckert T. Effect of two years of strict metabolic control on progression of incipient nephropathy in insulin-dependent diabetes. Lancet 1986; 2:1300–4.

48. Dahl-Jorgensen K, Brinchmann-Hansen O, Hanssen KF, et al. Effect of near normoglycaemia for two years on progression of early diabetic retinopathy, nephropathy, and neuropathy: the Oslo Study. Br Med J 1986; 293:1195–9.

49. Knatterud GL, Klimt CR, Levin ME, et al. Effects of hypoglycemic agents on vascular complications in patients with adult-onset diabetes. VII: Mortality and selected nonfatal events with insulin treatment. JAMA 1978; 240:37–42.

50. University Group Diabetes Program. Effects of hypoglycemic agents on vascular complications in patients with adult-onset diabetes. VIII. Evaluation of insulin therapy: final report. Diabetes [Suppl 5] 1982; 31:1–81.

51. Hadden DR, Blair AR, Wilson EA, et al. Natural history of diabetes presenting age 40–69 years: a prospective study of the influence of intensive dietary therapy. Q J Med 1986; 59:579–98.

52. The DCCT Research Group. Diabetes Control and Complications Trial (DCCT): results of feasibility study. Diabetes Care 1987; 10:1–19.

53. Mimouni F, Tsang RC. Pregnancy outcome in insulin-dependent diabetes: temporal relationships with metabolic control during specific pregnancy periods. Am J Perinatol 1988; 5:334–8.

54. Jovanovic L, Druzin M, Peterson CM. Effect of euglycemia on the outcome of pregnancy in insulin-dependent diabetic women as compared with normal control subjects. Am J Med 1981; 71:921–7.

55. O'Sullivan JB, Harris MI, Mills JL. Maternal diabetes in pregnancy. In: National Diabetes Data Group. Diabetes in America: diabetes data compiled 1984. Washington, D.C.: Department of Health and Human Services, 1985:XX-1 to XX-17. (Publication no. DHHS (NIH) 85–1468.)

56. Mills JL, O'Sullivan JB. The infant of the diabetic mother. In: National Diabetes Data Group. Diabetes in America: diabetes data compiled 1984. Washington, D.C.: Department of Health and Human Services, 1985:XXI-1 to XXI-19. (Publication no. DHHS (NIH) 85–1468.)

57. Diabetic Retinopathy Research Group. Preliminary report on effects of photocoagulation therapy. Am J Ophthalmol 1976; 81:383–96.

58. Dorf A, Ballantine EJ, Bennett PH, et al. Retinopathy in Pima Indians: relationship to glucose level, duration of diabetes, age at diagnosis of diabetes, and age at examination in a population with a high prevalence of diabetes mellitus. Diabetes 1976; 25:554–60.

59. Dwyer MS, Melton LJ III, Ballard DJ, et al. Incidence of diabetic retinopathy and blindness: a population-based study in Rochester, Minnesota. Diabetes Care 1985; 8:316–22.

60. Lindsay MK, Graves W, Klein L. The relationship of one abnormal glucose tolerance test value and pregnancy complications. Obstet Gynecol 1989; 73:103–6.

61. Gyves MT, Rodman HM, Little AB, et al. A modern approach to management of pregnant diabetics: a two-year analysis of perinatal outcomes. Am J Obstet Gynecol 1977; 128: 606–16.

62. Roversi GD, Gargiulo M, Nicolini U, et al. A new approach to the treatment of diabetic women: report of 479 cases seen from 1963 to 1975. Am J Obstet Gynecol 1979; 135:567–76.

63. Adashi EY, Pinto H, Tyson JE. Impact of maternal euglycemia on fetal outcome in diabetic pregnancy. Am J Obstet Gynecol 1979; 133:268–74.

64. Coustan DR, Imarah J. Prophylactic insulin treatment of gestational diabetes reduces the incidence of macrosomia, operative delivery, and birth trauma. Am J Obstet Gynecol 1984; 150:836–42.

65. Karlsson K, Kjellmer I. The outcome of diabetic pregnancies in relation to the mother's blood sugar level. Am J Obstet Gynecol 1972; 112:213–20.

66. Gabbe SG, Mestman JH, Freeman RK, et al. Management and outcome of class A diabetes mellitus. Am J Obstet Gynecol 1977; 127:475–9.

67. O'Sullivan JB, Gellis SS, Dandrow RV, et al. The potential diabetic and her treatment in pregnancy. Obstet Gynecol 1966; 27:683–9.

68. Coustan DR, Lewis SB. Insulin therapy for gestational diabetes. Obstet Gynecol 1978; 51:306–10.

69. Persson B, Stangenberg M, Hansson U, et al. Gestational diabetes mellitus (GDM): comparative evaluation of two treatment regimens, diet versus insulin and diet. Diabetes [Suppl 2] 1985; 34:101–5.

70. Braveman P, Showstack J, Browner W, et al. Evaluating outcomes of pregnancy in diabetic women: epidemiologic considerations and recommended indicators. Diabetes Care 1988; 11:281–7.

71. Spellacy WN, Miller S, Winegar A, et al. Macrosomia—maternal characteristics and infant complications. Obstet Gynecol 1985; 66:158–61.

72. Canadian Task Force on the Periodic Health Examination. The periodic health examination. Can Med Assoc J 1979; 121:1193–254.

73. Frame PS. A critical review of adult health maintenance. Part 4. Prevention of metabolic, behavioral, and miscellaneous conditions. J Fam Pract 1986; 23:29–39.

74. American Diabetes Association. Physician's guide to non-insulin dependent (type II) diabetes. Diagnosis and Treatment. Alexandria, Va.: American Diabetes Association, 1988.

75. Summary and Recommendations of the Second International Workshop-Conference on Gestational Diabetes Mellitus. Diabetes 1985; 34:123–6.

76. American Diabetes Association. Gestational diabetes mellitus. Ann Intern Med 1986; 105:461.

77. American College of Obstetricians and Gynecologists. Management of diabetes mellitus in pregnancy. ACOG Technical Bulletin No. 92. Washington, D.C.: American College of Obstetricians and Gynecologists, 1986.

78. Stolar MH, American Diabetes Association. Personal communication, March 1989.

79. National Institutes of Health Consensus Development Conference. Diet and exercise in noninsulin-dependent diabetes mellitus. Bethesda, Md.: National Institutes of Health, 1986.

17

Screening for Thyroid Disease

Recommendation: Screening for congenital hypothyroidism is recommended for all neonates during the first week of life (see *Clinical Intervention*). Routine screening for thyroid disorders is otherwise not warranted in asymptomatic adults or children. Persons with a history of upper-body irradiation may benefit from regular physical examination of the thyroid.

Burden of Suffering

The thyroid disorders for which screening is most often considered, hyperthyroidism, hypothyroidism, and thyroid cancer, account for significant morbidity and mortality in the United States. About 2–3% of the U.S. population have either hypothyroidism or hyperthyroidism, conditions that are especially common in women and the elderly.[1] The diverse symptoms that are characteristic of these diseases can have significant impact on the health and behavior of victims. Hyperthyroidism, for example, can cause restlessness, emotional lability, insomnia, heat intolerance, dyspnea, palpitations, ophthalmopathy, diarrhea, muscle atrophy, weakness, tremors, and tachycardia. Hypothyroidism can produce lethargy, confusion, poor memory, cold intolerance, weight gain, constipation, alopecia, dyspnea, myalgias, and paresthesias. Thyroid dysfunction may even lead to death; examples include thyroid storm in hyperthyroidism and myxedema coma in hypothyroidism. The nonspecific nature of many thyroid symptoms introduces added difficulties for patients, especially for those with hypothyroidism, because many thyroid symptoms are easily confused with those of other medical and psychiatric conditions. The patient may receive an incorrect diagnosis or none at all, and this may delay the initiation of appropriate treatment.

Congenital hypothyroidism occurs each year in about 1 out of every 3500–4000 newborns.[2] Most children who do not receive prompt treatment for this condition develop irreversible mental retardation and a variety of neuropsychological deficits comprising the syndrome of cretinism.[2] These complications have become less common in recent years following the introduction of routine neonatal screening and early treatment with l-thyroxine.

Thyroid cancer will account for an estimated 11,300 new cases and 1000 deaths in the United States in 1989.[3] Current five-year survival with treatment is over 90%.[3] Persons at increased risk for thyroid cancer, in addition to those with characteristic symptoms (e.g., neck mass, hoarseness), include women, persons with a family history of multiple endocrine neoplasia syndrome II, and the estimated 1 million Americans who have received low-dose upper-body irradiation during infancy, childhood, or adolescence. It has been calculated that at least 90,000 of these persons have irradiation-related cancers.[4,5]

Efficacy of Screening Tests

Many different thyroid function tests can provide useful information in the evaluation of persons with symptoms of thyroid disease, but the yield is considerably less when these tests are performed routinely for screening purposes in asymptomatic individuals or those with nonspecific symptoms. This has been apparent when thyroid function tests are included as a routine component of the periodic health examination. When this was done in one study, total T_4 or free T_4 levels were abnormal in 5–6% of persons, and over two-thirds of these persons were found to be euthyroid on further testing.[6] The positive predictive value of an abnormal total T_4, total T_3, or free T_4 was between 15% and 26%.[6] In another study, only 1.5% of the population had an abnormal free T_4 index and nearly a third of these were false positives.[7] Similar results have been reported in other studies.[8] In a study of hospitalized patients, where 9.4% had an abnormal serum T_4 screening test, only 0.6% were found to have newly discovered thyroid disease after further testing.[9]

This is, in part, because the serum levels of thyroid hormones that are characteristic of hypothyroidism and hyperthyroidism are not uniform and are often influenced by a variety of biological and diagnostic factors. Thus, although T_4 is usually elevated in hyperthyroidism, sole reliance on this hormone to detect the disease may produce false-negative results because 15–25% of cases have normal levels of T_4 but an elevated T_3 (T_3 toxicosis).[10] Conversely, false-positive elevations in T_4 and T_3 can be produced by increased levels of serum thyroid hormone-binding proteins, certain drugs, and pregnancy.[10] The presence of nonthyroidal illness can produce spuriously low levels of T_3 and T_4 ("euthyroid sick syndrome") or may raise thyroid-stimulating hormone (TSH) and T_4 levels.[10-12] Also, psychiatric diseases may produce transient increases in thyroid hormones that later revert to normal during recovery.[10] For these reasons, estimates of the sensitivity and specificity of thyroid function tests vary with the type of test and the type of thyroid dysfunction being sought. For thyroid tests commonly recommended for screening purposes (total T_4, free T_4, and free T_4 index), specificity is in excess of 90% but sensitivity ranges between 32% and 100%.[6,7,13,14]

A new method of measuring TSH offers promise as a more accurate first-line screening test for thyroid disease. For many years viewed as an important means of evaluating hypothyroidism, TSH is now of potential value in detecting hyperthyroidism as well because of recent advances in immunoradiometric assays that permit measurement of low serum levels of TSH. Its use as a first-line test of thyroid function has been widely investigated.[15-19] One group of investigators, reporting a sensitivity and specificity for this technique in excess of 90% in detecting thyroid disease, has recommended that this test be used for routine screening.[20] Other researchers, however, have raised concerns about its predictive value when used as a first-line test in the general population.[21]

Screening for congenital hypothyroidism in neonates involves the radioimmunoassay of T_4 and/or TSH from heel-prick specimens applied to filter paper. These tests have been used routinely for many years throughout the United States and other countries.[22] In the United States, T_4 is measured initially on all specimens and TSH is then measured if the T_4 level is low; in Europe and elsewhere, TSH is measured first. Currently in the United States, only 1 out of 120 neonates with congenital hypothyroidism escapes detection, usually as a result of biological factors or screening errors.[23] False-positive results are not uncommon, occurring at a ratio of 24–44 for every proven case, but they are easily corrected with follow-up testing.[22] Nonetheless, some investigators have called attention to the evidence that families receiving false-positive results from thyroid function tests may suffer increased anxiety and long-term effects years after the error is corrected.[24]

Screening tests for the detection of thyroid cancer include palpation to detect nodules and diagnostic procedures such as scintigraphy, ultrasonography, and thin-needle aspiration with cytology. With the exception of neck palpation, these tests are generally reserved for persons with evidence of nodular disease or goiter, and they are not recommended as screening tests for asymptomatic persons. There is little information on the accuracy of neck palpation in detecting thyroid disease. Accuracy varies with the technique of the examiner and the size of the mass. Other factors affect the sensitivity and specificity of the examination; for example, autopsy studies have shown that most thyroid nodules are not palpable and those that are palpable are usually benign.[25] Scintigraphy, as mentioned, is generally not performed on asymptomatic individuals without evidence of nodular or diffuse disease, but this test has been recommended to screen asymptomatic persons with a history of upper-body irradiation during childhood. In programs combining scintigraphy with a complete physical examination, nodular disease (benign and malignant) is discovered in as many as 30% of these high-risk participants.[26]

Effectiveness of Early Detection

The early detection of thyroid disease with thyroid function tests and the prompt initiation of treatment is thought to be of value in preventing the steady progression of symptoms that is typical of thyroid dysfunction. The results of thyroid screening tests may also benefit the patient by providing an explanation for nonspecific and insidious symptoms attributed mistakenly to other medical or psychiatric causes.[13] This is especially important in older persons, a population in which the classic clinical presentation of hypothyroidism and hyperthyroidism is often masked. Although the elderly are at increased risk for hypothyroidism, less than a third display the typical signs and symptoms.[27] Many older persons with hyperthyroidism experience "apathetic hyperthyroidism,"[10] lacking the goiter, ophthalmopathy, and signs of sympathetic nervous system overactivity that are typically seen in younger age groups.[28]

It has not been proved, however, that adults with thyroid dysfunction who are identified early and receive treatment prior to the appearance of symptoms have a better outcome than those who receive treatment after symptoms become apparent.[8] Although it is known that treatment of hypothyroid persons with l-thyroxine can improve thyroid function test results and certain indices of cardiac function,[29] there is limited evidence that these alterations result in meaningful health benefits for persons with subclinical hypothyroidism.[30,31] Evidence supporting early treatment comes primarily from a randomized placebo-controlled trial of 33 persons with subclinical hypothyroidism.[29] When compared with controls, those persons treated with l-thyroxine had milder symptoms and improved myocardial contractility; there were no differences in other outcome measures such as basal metabolic rate, pulse, body weight, and skin texture.[29] Although persons with subclinical hypothyroidism are known to have higher levels of serum cholesterol,[32] there was no significant decrease in serum lipids with treatment.[29] Similar questions exist about the efficacy of treating subclinical hyperthyroidism. These uncertainties about treatment benefits are important because of the costs and potential health effects of antithyroid medications, radioactive iodine ablation, and subtotal thyroidectomy.[30]

In contrast, there is good evidence that early treatment of congenital hypothyroidism is effective. It has been known for many years that delay of treatment for this disorder beyond the first few months of life is likely to result in irreversible mental retardation.[2,33] With the advent of early detection and treatment, longitudinal studies have shown that children who receive treatment within the first weeks of life have normal or near-normal intellectual performance when tested at ages 4 to 7.[33-36] These children may have lower IQ scores than their siblings, and many continue to manifest subtle deficits in language, perception, and fine motor skills;[35,37,38] however, the reduced incidence of severe neuropsychological effects observed with early treatment has prompted most Western governments to require routine screening for all neonates.

The benefits of early detection of thyroid cancer are not well defined. Five-year survival is currently over 90%,[3] but it has not been determined whether asymptomatic persons receiving treatment have a better outcome than those who present with symptoms or physical findings. In addition, there is reason to believe that many cancers detected through screening are not destined to manifest themselves clinically during the life of the patient.[4] Autopsy studies[39,40] indicate that 3–36% of the population have occult thyroid carcinoma, but the incidence of overt disease is only about 11,000 cases per year.[3] One group more likely to benefit from early detection of thyroid cancer are those persons with a history of upper-body irradiation during infancy, childhood, or adolescence, since 12% of this population does develop palpable thyroid disease.[4]

Recommendations of Others

Newborn screening for congenital hypothyroidism is mandatory in all states[41] and is recommended by most authorities, including the Canadian Task Force[42] and the American Academy of Pediatrics and American Thyroid Association.[43] There is disagreement about the role of thyroid function tests in screening asymptomatic adults. In its 1979 report, the Canadian Task Force found little scientific evidence to screen for hyperthyroidism but recommended clinical examination of postmenopausal women for hypothyroidism.[42] Others have recommended routine thyroid screening of the elderly,[30] and some authors have advocated routine screening of all asymptomatic persons.[7] Recommendations against any form of screening for thyroid disease in adults have also been made.[44] Routine screening for thyroid cancer has not been recommended for the general population, but annual examinations for thyroid nodules have been advocated for persons with a history of upper-body irradiation during infancy, childhood, or adolescence.[4,26]

Clinical Intervention

Screening for congenital hypothyroidism is recommended for all neonates during the first week of life. Heel-prick specimens for T_4 and TSH should be obtained, preferably between days 3 and 6. Testing procedures and follow-up treatment for abnormal results should follow current guidelines.[43] Routine thyroid function testing is otherwise not recommended for asymptomatic children or adults. Thyroid screening in the absence of symptoms, however, may be clinically prudent for populations at increased risk, such as older persons, especially women. The specific tests most frequently recommended as first-line screening tests are the serum T_4 or the free T_4 index (FTI);[7,9,11,14,45,46] further investigation is needed into the role of new, sensitive thyroid-stimulating hormone assays as a first-line test. It may be prudent to

perform regular physical examinations of the thyroid in persons with a history of upper-body irradiation

REFERENCES

1. Tunbridge WMG, Evered DC, Hall R, et al. The spectrum of thyroid disease in a community: the Whickham survey. Clin Endocrinol 1977; 7:481–93.
2. Postellon DC, Abdallah A. Congenital hypothyroidism: diagnosis, treatment, and prognosis. Compr Ther 1986; 12:67–71.
3. American Cancer Society. Cancer statistics, 1989. CA 1989; 39:3–20.
4. Stockwell RM, Barry M, Davidoff F. Managing thyroid abnormalities in adults exposed to upper body irradiation in childhood: a decision analysis. Should patients without palpable nodules be scanned and those with scan defects be subjected to subtotal thyroidectomy? J Clin Endocrinol Metab 1984; 58:804–12.
5. Krenning EP, Ausema L, Bruining HA, et al. Clinical and radiodiagnostic aspects in the evaluation of thyroid nodules with respect to thyroid cancer. Eur J Cancer Clin Oncol 1988; 24:299–304.
6. Fukazawa H, Sakurada T, Yoshida K, et al. Free thyroxine estimation for the screening of hyper- and hypothyroidism in an adult population. Tohoku J Exp Med 1966; 148:411–20.
7. dos Remedios LV, Weber PM, Feldman R, et al. Detecting unsuspected thyroid dysfunction by the free thyroxine index. Arch Intern Med 1980; 140:1045–9.
8. White GH, Walmsley RN. Can the initial assessment of thyroid function be improved? Lancet 1978; 2:933–5.
9. Nolan JP, Tarsa NJ, DiBenedetto G. Case-finding for unsuspected thyroid disease: costs and health benefits. Am J Clin Pathol 1985; 83:346–55.
10. Gavin LA. The diagnostic dilemmas of hyperthyroxinemia and hypothyroxinemia. Adv Intern Med 1988; 33:185–204.
11. Wong ET, Steffes MW. A fundamental approach to the diagnosis of diseases of the thyroid gland. Clin Lab Med 1984; 4:655–70.
12. Wilke TJ. Estimation of free thyroid hormone concentrations in the clinical laboratory. Clin Chem 1986; 32:585–92.
13. Ericsson UB, Thorell JI. A prospective critical evaluation of in vitro thyroid function tests. Acta Med Scand 1986; 220:47–56.
14. Wilke TJ, Eastment HT. Discriminative ability of tests for free and total thyroid hormones in diagnosing thyroid disease. Clin Chem 1986; 32:1746–50.
15. Klee GG, Hay ID. Sensitive thyrotropin assays: analytic and clinical performance criteria. Mayo Clin Proc 1988; 63:1123–32.
16. Ross DS. New sensitive immunoradiometric assays for thyrotropin. Ann Intern Med 1986; 104:718–21.
17. Alexander WD, Kerr DJ, Ferguson MM. First-line test of thyroid function. Lancet 1984; 2:647.
18. Roddis MJ, Burrin JM, Johannssen A, et al. Serum thyrotropin: a first-line discriminatory test of thyroid function. Lancet 1985; 1:277–8.
19. Hershman JM, Pekary AE, Smith VP, et al. Evaluation of five high-sensitivity thyrotropin assays. Mayo Clin Proc 1988; 63:1133–9.
20. Caldwell G, Kellett HA, Gow SM, et al. A new strategy for thyroid function testing. Lancet 1985; 1:1117–9.
21. Ericsson UB, Fernlund P, JI Thorell. Evaluation of the usefulness of a sensitive immunoradiometric assay for thyroid stimulating hormone as a first-line thyroid function test in an unselected patient population. Scan J Clin Lab Invest 1987; 47:215–21.
22. Fisher DA. Effectiveness of newborn screening programs for congenital hypothyroidism: prevalence of missed cases. Pediatr Clin North Am 1987; 34:881–90.
23. Holtzman C, Slazyk WE, Cordero JF, et al. Descriptive epidemiology of missed cases of phenylketonuria and congenital hypothyroidism. Pediatrics 1986; 78:553–8.
24. Fyro K, Bodegard G. Four-year follow-up of psychological reactions to false positive screening tests for congenital hypothyroidism. Acta Paediatr Scand 1987; 76:107–14.

25. Mortensen JB, Woolner LB, Bennett WA. Gross and microscopic findings in clinically normal thyroid glands. J Clin Endocrinol Metab 1955; 15:1270–80.
26. Shimaoka K, Bakri K, Sciascia M, et al. Thyroid screening program: follow-up evaluation. NY State J Med 1982; 82:1184–7.
27. Bahemuka M, Hodkinson HM. Screening for hypothyroidism in elderly inpatients. Br Med J 1975; 2:601–3.
28. Feit H. Thyroid function in the elderly. Clin Ger Med 1988; 4:151–61.
29. Cooper DS, Halpern R, Wood LC, et al. L-thyroxine therapy in subclinical hypothyroidism: a double-blind, placebo-controlled trial. Ann Intern Med 1984; 101:18–24.
30. Screening for thyroid disease (editorial). Lancet 1981; 2:128–30.
31. Fraser WD, Biggart EM, O'Reilly DJ, et al. Are biochemical tests of thyroid function of any value in monitoring patients receiving thyroxine replacement? Br Med J 1986; 293: 808–10.
32. Althaus BU, Staub JJ, Ryff-De Leche A, et al. LDL/HDL changes in subclinical hypothyroidism: possible risk factors for coronary heart disease. Clin Endocrinol 1988; 28: 157–63.
33. Glorieux J, Dussault JH, Letarte J, et al. Preliminary results on the mental development of hypothyroid infants detected by the Quebec Screening Program. J Pediatr 1983; 102:19–22.
34. New England Congenital Hypothyroidism Collaborative. Effects of neonatal screening for hypothyroidism: prevention of mental retardation by treatment before clinical manifestations. Lancet 1981; 2:1095–8.
35. Glorieux J, Dussault JH, Morisette J, et al. Follow-up at ages 5 and 7 years on mental development in children with hypothyroidism detected by Quebec Screening Program. J Pediatr 1985; 107:913–5.
36. Ilicki A, Larsson A. Psychomotor development of children with congenital hypothyroidism diagnosed by neonatal screening. Acta Paediatr Scan 1988; 77:142–7.
37. Rovet JF. A prospective investigation of children with congenital hypothyroidism identified by neonatal thyroid screening in Ontario. Can J Public Health [Suppl 1] 1986; 77:164–73.
38. Murphy G, Hulse JA, Jackson D, et al. Early treated hypothyroidism: development at 3 years. Arch Dis Child 1986; 61:761–5.
39. Holm LE, Lowhagen T, Silfversward C. The reliability of malignant thyroid tumor diagnosis in the Swedish cancer registry. Acta Pathol Microbiol Scand A 1980; 88:251–4.
40. Franssila KO, Harach R. Occult papillary carcinoma of the thyroid in children and young adults. Cancer 1986; 58:715–9.
41. Stevens MB, Rigilano JC, Wilson CC. State screening for metabolic disorders in newborns. Am Fam Physician 1988; 37:223–8.
42. Canadian Task Force on the Periodic Health Examination. The periodic health examination. Can Med Assoc J 1979; 121:1–45.
43. American Academy of Pediatrics, American Thyroid Association. Newborn screening for congenital hypothyroidism: recommended guidelines. Pediatrics 1987; 80:745–9.
44. Frame PS. A critical review of adult health maintenance. Part 4. Prevention of metabolic, behavioral, and miscellaneous conditions. J Fam Pract 1986; 23:29–39.
45. Schultz AL. Thyroid function tests: selective use for cost containment. Postgrad Med 1986; 80:219–28.
46. Penney MD, O'Sullivan DJ. Total or free thyroxin as a primary test of thyroid function. Clin Chem 1987; 33:170–1.

18

Screening for Obesity

Recommendation: All children and adults should receive periodic height and weight measurements (see *Clinical Intervention*).

Burden of Suffering

Obesity has been defined as being 20% or more above desirable body weight.[1] Increasingly, body mass index (body weight in kilograms divided by the square of height in meters) and other parameters are replacing crude weight measurements in the definition of obesity. About 32 million American adults (aged 25–74) are obese.[2] The prevalence of obesity among children is uncertain, but it is estimated to be between 5% and 25%.[3] There are reports that the prevalence of childhood obesity is increasing.[4] There is also evidence that childhood obesity may be a significant risk factor for adult obesity and that this risk becomes greater when obesity occurs among older children and adolescents.[1,5]

Increased mortality in adults has been clearly documented as a result of morbid obesity, weight that is at least twice (or 100 pounds over) the desirable weight.[1,6] In the case of moderate obesity, however, experts differ on whether the observed decrease in longevity is due to the effect of obesity alone or to the effect of closely related variables such as smoking, concurrent diseases, physical inactivity, socioeconomic status, or diet.[7-12] It is known, however, that the overweight are more likely to have diabetes, hypertension, and risk factors for other diseases.[1] The prevalence of diabetes and hypertension is three times higher in overweight persons[13] than in those of normal weight. Research has established a clear association between obesity and hypercholesterolemia and a possible independent relationship between obesity and coronary artery disease.[1,3,9,10,13,14] Obesity may influence the risk of cancer of the colon, rectum, prostate, gallbladder, biliary tract, breast, cervix, endometrium, and ovary.[1] Finally, obesity affects the quality of life through social discrimination and by limiting mobility, physical endurance, and other functional measures.[1]

Efficacy of Screening Tests

Extremely overweight individuals can be identified easily in the clinical setting by their physical appearance. More precise methods are often necessary, however, to evaluate persons who are mildly or moderately overweight. The complications of obesity occur among those with elevated body fat composition, which is most accurately measured by underwater (hydrostatic) weighing, isotopic dilution measures, and other sophisticated techniques that are not suited to clinical practice. Body fat distribution, which may be an independent predictor of the complications of obesity, can be measured in the clinical setting by comparing the circumference or skinfold thickness of the trunk and limbs. For example, a waist/hip circumference ratio greater than 1.0 in men and 0.8 in women may be a reliable predictor of complications from obesity, and studies have shown that such anthropometric measurements compare favorably with estimates obtained from hydrostatic weighing.[15] Further research is needed, however, to develop standardized diagnostic criteria for these tests and to minimize interobserver variation due to differences in anthropometric measurement techniques among clinicians.[16,17]

The most common clinical method for detecting obesity, the evaluation of body weight and height based on tables of average weights, only approximates the extent of overweight. The criteria for desirable body weight are a matter of controversy among experts and vary considerably as presented in different weight-for-height tables.[18]

Effectiveness of Early Detection

The purpose of screening for obesity is to convince the individual to lose weight and thereby prevent the complications of obesity. Interventions reserved for persons at high risk for coronary artery disease may also be implemented as a result of the diagnosis. The identification of individuals at increased risk of becoming obese (e.g., children) because of family history or other risk factors may also help in the primary prevention of obesity. Although there is little evidence from prospective studies that losing weight improves longevity,[19] there is evidence that obesity increases mortality[12] and that weight loss reduces important risk factors such as hypertension, elevated serum cholesterol, and impaired glucose tolerance.[1] To benefit from the detection of obesity, however, patients must be motivated by nutritional and exercise counseling to lose weight, must have access to an efficacious method of reducing body weight, and must maintain the resulting weight loss.

Although a variety of weight-reducing regimens are available, many have only short-term efficacy and fail to achieve long-term weight loss.[3,6,20-23] The lowest failure rates have been reported for conservative weight-loss regimens such as behavior therapy, nutrition education, and exercise programs, primarily involving persons with mild to moderate obesity.[23] One study reported that only 27% of patients on behavior therapy had regained their weight one year after treatment had ended.[23] More intensive approaches, such as very-low-calorie diets, are appropriate only for highly selected individuals.[22,24] Surgery is indicated for an even smaller group of patients,[25] and pharmacotherapy is effective only when used for an indefinite period of time.[26] Recent evidence suggests that some intensive weight-loss measures, such as the insertion of a gastric balloon,[27] may not be effective. Weight loss during childhood and adolescence may reduce growth velocity and produce other complications.[28,29]

Recommendations of Others

The Institute of Medicine recommends height and weight measurement at five age intervals during adulthood (18–24, 25–39, 40–59, 60–74, over 75).[30] The American Heart Association recommends a body weight measurement every five years.[31] Others have suggested a periodicity of four years[20] and two to three years.[32] The American Academy of Pediatrics recommends height and weight measurements for children throughout infancy, annually from ages 1–6, and every two years thereafter.[33] The Canadian Task Force recommends measurement of height, weight, and head circumference throughout infancy, at ages 18 months,

2–3 years, 4 years, 5–6 years, 10–11 years, and at the clinician's discretion during adolescence and adulthood.[34]

Discussion

Evidence that screening for obesity and weight-reducing strategies are effective in reducing long-term morbidity and mortality is unlikely to improve in the near future due to the difficulty of conducting controlled trials of weight loss with these outcome measures and of separating the effect of obesity from that of other risk factors. It is clear, however, that weight loss reduces an individual's risk for major chronic diseases such as diabetes, hypertension, and coronary artery disease. Periodic height and weight measurements, although not proven to be effective, are inexpensive, rapid, and acceptable to patients. They may also be useful for the detection of medical conditions causing unintended weight loss and weight gain, such as cancer or thyroid disorders. The intervention is especially prudent in children to detect growth abnormalities and obesity in early childhood.[35] The reliability of other methods of detecting obesity, such as the measurement of skinfold thickness and limb circumference, requires further study before these techniques are deemed suitable for widespread implementation in the clinical setting. There are inadequate data to determine the optimal frequency of obesity screening, and this is best left to clinical discretion.

Clinical Intervention

The height and weight of all adults should be routinely measured and evaluated, using a table of desirable weights (e.g., Metropolitan Life Insurance Company Table)[36] or a body mass index (body weight in kilograms divided by the square of height in meters) above 27.8 in men or 27.3 in women as a basis for further intervention.[1] The height and weight of children should be measured regularly and plotted on a growth chart throughout infancy and childhood. The optimal frequency for measuring height and weight in adults is a matter of clinical discretion. Those individuals who are 20% or more above desirable weight should receive appropriate nutritional (Chapter 50) and exercise (Chapter 49) counseling.

REFERENCES

1. Foster WR, Burton BT, eds. National Institutes of Health consensus conference: health implications of obesity. Ann Intern Med 1985; 103:977–1077.
2. Department of Health and Human Services, Department of Agriculture. Nutrition monitoring in the United States. Washington, D.C.: Government Printing Office, 1986:2,54, 59–62.
3. Dietz WH. Childhood obesity: susceptibility, cause, and management. J Pediatr 1983; 103:676–86.
4. Gortmaker SL, Dietz WH, Sobol AM, et al. Increasing pediatric obesity in the United States. Am J Dis Child 1987; 141:535–40.
5. Epstein LH, Wing RR, Valoski A, et al. Childhood obesity. Pediatr Clin North Am 1985; 32:363–79.
6. Van Itallie TB, Kral JG. The dilemma of morbid obesity. JAMA 1981; 246:999–1003.
7. Manson JE, Stampfer MJ, Hennekens CH, et al. Body weight and longevity: a reassessment. JAMA 1987; 257:353–8.
8. Ernsberger P. Body weight and longevity (letter). JAMA 1987; 257:1895–6.
9. Keys A. Overweight, obesity, coronary heart disease and mortality. Nutr Rev 1980; 38:297–307.

10. Simopoulos AP, Van Itallie TB. Body weight, health, longevity. Ann Intern Med 1984; 100:285–95.
11. Stallones RA. Epidemiologic studies of obesity. Ann Intern Med 1985; 103:1003–5.
12. Harris T, Cook EF, Garrison R, et al. Body mass index and mortality among nonsmoking older persons: the Framingham Heart Study. JAMA 1988; 259:1520–4.
13. Van Itallie TB. Health implications of overweight and obesity in the United States. Ann Intern Med 1985; 103:983–8.
14. Hubert HB, Feinleib M, McNamara PM, et al. Obesity as an independent risk factor for cardiovascular disease: a 26–year follow-up of participants in the Framingham Heart Study. Circulation 1983; 67:968–77.
15. Latin RW, Johnson SC, Ruhling RO. An anthropometric estimation of body composition of older men. J Gerontol 1987; 42:24–8.
16. Kispert CP, Merrifield HH. Interrater reliability of skinfold fat measurements. Phys Ther 1987; 67:917–20.
17. Jung E, Kaufman JJM, Narins DC, et al. Skinfold measurements in children: a comparison of Lange and McGaw calipers. Clin Pediatr 1984; 23:25–8.
18. Schulz LO. Obese, overweight, desirable, ideal: where to draw the line in 1986? J Am Diet Assoc 1986; 86:1702–4.
19. Kannel WB. Weight loss as a homeostatic stress (letter). JAMA 1986; 256:2881.
20. Frame PS. A critical review of adult health maintenance. Part 4. Prevention of metabolic, behavioral, and miscellaneous conditions. J Fam Pract 1986; 23:29–39.
21. Currey H, Malcolm R, Riddle E, et al. Behavioral treatment of obesity: limitations and results with the chronically obese. JAMA 1977; 237:2829–31.
22. Wadden TA, Stunkard AJ, Brownell KD. Very low calorie diets: their efficacy, safety, and future. Ann Intern Med 1983; 99:675–84.
23. Stunkard AJ. Conservative treatments for obesity. Am J Clin Nutr 1987; 45:1142–54.
24. Wadden TA, Stunkard AJ. Controlled trial of very-low-calorie diet, behavior therapy and their combination in the treatment of obesity. J Consult Clin Psychol 1986; 54:482–8.
25. Mason EE. Surgical treatment of obesity. Philadelphia: WB Saunders, 1981.
26. Stunkard AJ. Anorectic agents lower a body weight set point. Life Sciences 1982; 30:2043–55.
27. Kramer FM, Stunkard AJ, Spiegel TA, et al. Limited weight losses with a gastric balloon. Arch Intern Med 1989; 149:411–3.
28. Dietz WH, Hartung R. Changes in height velocity of obese preadolescents during weight reduction. Am J Dis Child 1985; 139:705–7.
29. Mallick MJ. Health hazards of obesity and weight control in children: a review of the literature. Am J Public Health 1983; 73:78–82.
30. National Academy of Sciences, Institute of Medicine. Ad Hoc Advisory Group on Preventive Services. Preventive services for the well population. Washington, D.C.: National Academy of Sciences, 1978.
31. Grundy SM, Greenland P, Herd A, et al. Cardiovascular and risk factor evaluation of healthy American adults. Circulation 1987; 75:1340A-62A.
32. Breslow L, Somers AR. The lifetime health-monitoring program. N Engl J Med 1977; 296:601–8.
33. American Academy of Pediatrics, Committee on Practice and Ambulatory Medicine. Guidelines for health supervision. Elk Grove, Ill.: American Academy of Pediatrics, 1987.
34. Canadian Task Force on the Periodic Health Examination. The periodic health examination. Can Med Assoc J 1979; 121:1194–254.
35. Peckham C, Stark O, Moynihan C. Obesity in school children: is there a case for screening? Public Health (London) 1985; 99:3–9.
36. 1983 Metropolitan height and weight tables. Stat Bull Metrop Insur Co 1983; 64:3.

19

Screening for
Phenylketonuria

Recommendation: Screening for phenylketonuria (PKU) is recommended for all newborns prior to discharge from the nursery. Infants who are tested before 24 hours of age should receive a repeat screening test before the third week of life. Routine prenatal screening for maternal PKU is not recommended.

Burden of Suffering

Phenylketonuria occurs once in every 15,000 births.[1-3] In the absence of treatment during infancy, most persons with this disorder develop severe, irreversible mental retardation. Many experience neurobehavioral symptoms such as seizures, tremors, gait disorders, athetoid movements, and psychotic episodes with autism.[4] These clinical manifestations of PKU have rarely developed in children born after the mid-1960s, when routine screening was legislated and early treatment for PKU became common. A cohort of healthy phenylketonuric females have now entered childbearing age, however, thus increasing the incidence of *maternal* PKU (estimated at 1 per 30,000–40,000 pregnancies).[5] These women are at increased risk of giving birth to a child with mental retardation, microcephaly, congenital heart disease, and low birthweight.[6] It has been estimated that, if treatment is not made available to protect offspring from the teratogenic effects of maternal phenylalanine, the incidence of PKU-related mental retardation could return to previous levels after only one generation.[7]

Efficacy of Screening Tests

Automated blood phenylalanine determinations, such as the Guthrie test, have been the principal screening tests for phenylketonuria for over two decades.[8] Although well-designed evaluations of the sensitivity and specificity of the Guthrie test have never been performed,[1] international experience with its use in millions of newborns suggests that missed cases are very uncommon; most appear to be due to administrative or laboratory errors. Fluorometric assays are an alternative form of testing that offers excellent sensitivity.[1] False-positive results can occur in PKU screening. In certain situations and population conditions, the ratio of false positives to true positives could be as high as 32 to 1.[1] Although false positives have been viewed for many years as less important than false-negative results because they can be corrected easily by repeating the test, it should be noted that recalling patients for a second PKU test does generate significant parental anxiety.[9,10]

The sensitivity of the Guthrie test is influenced by the age of the newborn when the sample is obtained. The current trend toward early discharge from the nursery (resulting in PKU screening being performed as early as 1 to 2 days of age) has raised concerns that test results obtained during this early period may be inaccurate. This is because the blood level of phenylalanine is typically normal in affected neonates immediately after birth and increases progressively during the first days of life. Using the conventional cutoff of 4 mg/dL, diagnostic levels of phenylalanine may not be present in some phenylketonuric newborns for several days. Early data on the frequency of this problem were inconsistent: one group found that all cases could be detected within the first 48 hours of life,[11] but others reported that the false-negative rate during the first 24 hours might be 2–6%[1] or as high as 15–16%.[12,13] The error rate in these studies decreased to 0.6–2% on the second day and to 0.3% by the third day.[1,12,13] Current rates may be lower as a result of recent improvements in laboratory standardization. Moreover, fluorometric assays have been reported to have higher sensitivity than the Guthrie test.[1] Two additional solutions to improve sensitivity, repeat testing of all newborns after early discharge and lowering the cutoff value to reduce the false-negative rate, have encountered criticism for several reasons. Repeat testing would have low yield and cost-effectiveness;[13,14] it has been estimated that detecting even one case of PKU in this manner would require performing from 600,000 to perhaps 6 million tests.[1,14] Lowering the cutoff value, on the other hand, would improve sensitivity at the expense of specificity, thereby increasing the ratio of false positives to true positives.[1] Nonetheless, many screening programs now use a cutoff level of 2 mg/dL.

Routine screening of pregnant women for *maternal* PKU has been recommended as a means of preventing fetal complications.[5,15,16] This disorder is rare in the general population, however, and many women with PKU are already aware of the diagnosis. Thus, the yield from screening all pregnant women would be very low. One program that has provided this form of prenatal screening reports performing 260,000 tests to detect 9 cases of previously unknown hyperphenylalaninemia.[17] Of the 11 resulting pregnancies, 5 were in women with benign hyperphenylalaninemia and 4 of their offspring were normal (the fifth pregnancy was terminated by abortion). In Massachusetts, routine screening of cord blood for 10 years detected only 22 mothers with previously undiagnosed hyperphenylalaninemia.[16,18]

Effectiveness of Early Detection

Before treatment with dietary phenylalanine restriction became common in the early 1960s, severe mental retardation was a common outcome in children with PKU. A review in 1953 reported that 85% of patients had an intelligence quotient (IQ) less than 40, and 37% had IQ scores below 10; less than 1% had scores above 70.[4] The majority of proven cases of the disease resided in mental institutions.[4] Since dietary phenylalanine restriction was introduced, however, over 95% of children with PKU have developed normal or near-normal intelligence.[19-22] A large longitudinal study reports a mean IQ of 100 in children who have been followed to age 8,[23] and other reports show adolescent and young adult patients are functioning well in society.[24] The efficacy of dietary treatment has never been proved in a properly designed controlled trial,[25] and the performance of such a study in the future is unlikely for ethical reasons. Nonetheless, the compelling contrast in outcome between children receiving treatment and historical controls prompted most Western governments to require routine neonatal screening as early as the late 1960s.

Nevertheless, there are limitations to the effectiveness of dietary treatment. It is essential that phenylalanine restrictions be instituted in early infancy to prevent the irreversible effects of PKU.[19,21,23,26] Adherence to the diet must continue for at least four to eight years,[19,21,23,26,27] and there are now data suggesting that continuation of the diet through adolescence and perhaps into the adult years may be advisable.[23,26] Finally, even if these precautions are taken, dietary treatment may not offer full protection from subtle effects of PKU. Intelligence scores in treated persons with PKU, although often in the normal range for the general population, may be significantly lower than those of siblings and parents,[19] and mild psychological deficits, such as perceptual motor dysfunction and academic difficulties, have also been reported.[28-30] Early detection of *maternal* PKU in pregnant women may also be beneficial. The incidence of maternal PKU is increasing with the growing number of healthy phenylketonuric females now entering childbearing age. Maternal hyperphenylalaninemia can produce teratogenic effects, even on normal fetuses who have not inherited PKU. If the mother does not follow a low phenylalanine diet during pregnancy, there is an overwhelming risk of birth of an abnormal child: over 90% of these children will have mental retardation, 75% microcephaly, 40–50% intrauterine growth retardation, and 10–25% other birth defects.[5,6] Uncertainties exist, however, as to whether these outcomes can be prevented by instituting treatment with dietary phenylalanine restriction.[6,31] Although some pregnant women under treatment have given birth to normal children, a number of investigators[6,31-33] have found that dietary intervention fails to prevent fetal damage. Many believe restrictions must be instituted prior to conception to achieve efficacy.[6,16,17,33,34] There are also concerns that the low-phenylalanine diet may produce deficiencies in calories, protein, and other nutrients that are needed for proper fetal growth.[5,31] A number of studies examining the health effects of such diets during pregnancy are currently under way.[35]

Recommendations of Others

Routine screening of all newborns for PKU is required in every state.[36] The American Academy of Pediatrics recommends that a heel blood specimen be obtained before leaving the nursery and as close as possible to discharge.[37] Premature infants and those being treated for illness should be tested on or near the seventh day. The Academy recommends that infants who are tested before 24 hours of age receive a repeat screening test before the third week of life. Routine prenatal screening for maternal PKU has been advocated by some authors,[15] but most groups have not recommended this approach due to concerns about cost-effectiveness.[5]

Clinical Intervention

A heel-prick test for blood phenylalanine level is recommended for all newborns before discharge from the nursery, preferably after 3 days of age. Infants who are tested in the first 24 hours of age should receive a repeat screening test before the third week of life. Premature infants and those with illnesses should be tested at or near 7 days of age. All parents should receive adequate information regarding the proper interpretation of PKU test results, including the probability of false positives. Routine prenatal screening for maternal PKU is not recommended.

REFERENCES

1. Kirkman HN, Carroll CL, Moore EG, et al. Fifteen-year experience with screening for phenylketonuria with an automated fluorometric method. Am J Hum Genet 1982; 34: 743–52.
2. Walker V, Clayton BE, Ersser RS, et al. Hyperphenylalaninaemia of various types among three-quarters of a million neonates tested in a screening programme. Arch Dis Child 1981; 56:759–64.
3. Somens DG, Favreau L. Newborn screening for phenylketonuria: incidence and screening procedures in North America. Can J Public Health 1982; 73:206–7.
4. Jervis GA. Phenylpyruvic oligophrenia (phenylketonuria). Res Publ Assoc Res Nerv Ment Dis 1953; 33:259–82.
5. Hanley WB, Clarke JTR, Schoonheyt W. Maternal phenylketonuria (PKU): a review. Clin Biochem 1987; 20:149–56.
6. Lenke RR, Levy HL. Maternal phenylketonuria and hyperphenylalaninemia: an international survey of the outcome of untreated and treated pregnancies. N Engl J Med 1980; 303:1202–8.
7. Kirkman HN. Projections of mental retardation from PKU. Pediatr Res 1979; 13:414.
8. Guthrie R, Susi A. A simple phenylalanine method for detecting phenylketonuria in large populations of newborn infants. Pediatrics 1963; 32:338–43.
9. Rothenberg MB, Sills EM. Iatrogenesis: the PKU anxiety syndrome. J Am Acad Child Psychiatry 1968; 7:689–92.
10. Sorenson JR, Levy HL, Mangione TW, et al. Parental response to repeat testing of infants with "false-positive" results in a newborn screening program. Pediatrics 1984; 73:183–7.
11. Meryash DL, Levy HL, Guthrie R, et al. Prospective study of early neonatal screening for phenylketonuria. N Engl J Med 1981; 304:294–6.
12. Holtzman NA, McCabe ERB, Cunningham GC, et al. Screening for phenylketonuria. N Engl J Med 1981; 304:1300.
13. Schneider AJ. Newborn phenylalanine/tyrosine metabolism: implications for screening for phenylketonuria. Am J Dis Child 1983; 137:427–32.
14. Sepe SJ, Levy HL, Mount FW. An evaluation of routine follow-up blood screening of infants for phenylketonuria. N Engl J Med 1979; 300:606.
15. MacCready RA, Levy HL. The problem of maternal phenylketonuria. Am J Obstet Gynecol 1972; 123:121–8.
16. Waisbren SE, Doherty LB, Bailey IV, et al. The New England Maternal PKU Project: identification of at-risk women. Am J Public Health 1988; 78:789–92.
17. Buist NRM, Lis EW, Tuerck JM, et al. Maternal phenylketonuria. Lancet 1979; 2:589.
18. Levy HL, Waisbren SE. Effects of untreated maternal phenylketonuria and hyperphenylalaninemia in the fetus. N Engl J Med 1983; 309:1269–74.
19. Berman PW, Waisman HA, Graham FK. Intelligence in treated phenylketonuric children: a developmental study. Child Develop 1966; 37:731–47.
20. Hudson FP, Mordaunt VL, Leahy I. Evaluation of treatment begun in first three months of life in 184 cases of phenylketonuria. Arch Dis Child 1970; 45:5–12.
21. Williamson ML, Koch R, Azen C, et al. Correlates of intelligence test results in treated phenylketonuric children. Pediatrics 1981; 68:161–7.
22. Hsia DY. Phenylketonuria 1967. Dev Med Child Neurol 1967; 9:531–40.
23. Holtzman NA, Kronmal RA, van Doorninck W, et al. Effect of age at loss of dietary control on intellectual performance and behavior of children with phenylketonuria. N Engl J Med 1986; 314:593–8.
24. Koch R, Yusin M, Fishler K. Successful adjustment to society by adults with phenylketonuria. J Inherited Metab Dis 1985; 8:209–11.
25. Birch HG, Tizard J. The dietary treatment of phenylketonuria: not proven? Dev Med Child Neurol 1967; 9:9–12.
26. Waisbren SE, Mahon BE, Schnell RR, et al. Predictors of intelligence quotient and intelligence quotient change in persons treated for phenylketonuria early in life. Pediatrics 1987; 79:351–5.

27. Hackney IM, Hanley WB, Davidson W, et al. Phenylketonuria: mental development behavior and termination of low phenylalanine diet. J Pediatr 1968; 72:646–55.
28. Pennington BF, van Doorninck WJ, McCabe LL, et al. Neuropsychological deficits in early treated phenylketonuric children. Am J Ment Defic 1985; 5:467–74.
29. Smith I, Beasley MG, Wolff OH, et al. Behavior disturbance in 8–year-old children with early treated phenylketonuria. Report from the MRC/DHHS Phenylketonuria Register. J Pediatr 1988; 112:403–8.
30. Faust D, Libon D, Pueschel S. Neuropsychological functioning in treated phenylketonuria. Int J Psych Med 1986–87; 16:169–77.
31. Lenke RR, Levy HL. Maternal phenylketonuria: results of dietary therapy. Am J Obstet Gynecol 1982; 142:548–53.
32. Murphy D, Saul I, Kirby M. Maternal PKU and phenylalanine-restricted diet: studies of seven pregnancies and of offspring produced. Ir J Med Sci 1985; 154:66–70.
33. Scott TM, Fyfe WM, Hart DM. Maternal phenylketonuria: abnormal baby despite low phenylalanine diet during pregnancy. Arch Dis Child 1980; 55:634–7.
34. Rohn FJ, Doherty LB, Waisborn SE, et al. The New England Maternal PKU Project: prospective study of untreated and treated pregnancies and their outcomes. J Pediatr 1987; 110:391–8.
35. de la Cruz F, National Institute of Child Health and Human Development. Personal communication, September 1988.
36. Stevens MB, Rigilano JC, Wilson CC. State screening for metabolic disorders in newborns. Am Fam Physicisn 1988; 37:223–8.
37. Committee on Genetics. New issues in newborn screening for phenylketonuria and congenital hypothyroidism. Pediatrics 1982; 69:104–6.

20

Screening for Hepatitis B

Recommendation: All pregnant women should be tested for hepatitis B surface antigen at their first prenatal visit. The test may be repeated in the third trimester in women at increased risk of exposure during pregnancy (see *Clinical Intervention*). See Chapter 57 for recommendations on vaccination against hepatitis B in high-risk groups and Chapter 58 for information about immunization of persons with possible exposure to infected individuals or blood products.

Burden of Suffering

Each year in the United States, over 300,000 persons become infected with hepatitis B virus (HBV) and more than 10,000 require hospitalization.[1] Although most infections resolve with time, 6–10% of patients develop an asymptomatic chronic carrier state that places them at risk for developing chronic active hepatitis, cirrhosis, and primary hepatocellular carcinoma.[2] The United States has an estimated pool of 500,000 to 1 million chronic carriers of HBV.[2] An estimated 4000 hepatitis B-related deaths occur each year as a result of cirrhosis, and more than 1000 occur as a result of liver cancer.[2] An estimated 16,500 births occur to HBV-infected women each year in the United States.[3] Infants whose mothers are positive for hepatitis B "e" antigen have a 70–90% chance of becoming infected perinatally, and virtually all (85–90%) infants who do become infected develop chronic HBV carrier status.[4,5] It has been estimated that more than 25% of chronic HBV carriers die from primary hepatocellular carcinoma or cirrhosis of the liver, with the median age of death in the fifth decade of life.[6-8] The principal risk factors for HBV infection in the United States are intravenous drug abuse; heterosexual contact with HBV-infected persons, HBV chronic carriers, or multiple partners; and male homosexual activity.[9] Certain population groups, such as immigrants from Asia and Africa, may also be at increased risk.[2] In recent years, a growing number of intravenous drug abusers have become infected; currently, between 60% and 80% of persons who use illicit parenteral drugs have serologic evidence of HBV infection.[2] This population now accounts for the largest proportion of HBV cases in the United States.[9]

Efficacy of Screening Tests

The principal screening test for detecting current HBV infection or carrier state in asymptomatic persons is the identification of hepatitis B surface antigen (HBsAg). The immunoassay for detecting HBsAg has a reported sensitivity of 97.5% and a specificity of 98%.[10] Spontaneous clearance of HBsAg occurs each year in 1–2% of carriers.

Effectiveness of Early Detection

The most important benefit of detecting HBV infection or carrier state in asymptomatic persons is the prevention of transmission of the virus to others. There is little evidence that early detection reduces the risk of developing chronic liver disease or its complications. Theoretically, the results of screening tests coupled with counseling have the potential to influence high-risk behaviors (e.g., sexual intercourse, sharing needles among drug abusers, donating blood products) in infected persons, and thereby prevent transmission. Sexual contacts and persons with possible percutaneous exposure may be identified in the process and offered vaccination (see Chapter 58). However, the effectiveness of routine screening of asymptomatic persons in the clinical setting as a means of reducing HBV transmission requires further study. Counseling on preventive behaviors to reduce the risk of infection and transmission currently appears to be a more effective strategy (see Chapter 53).

There is evidence that early detection of HBsAg in pregnant women can help prevent infection in the newborn. Studies have shown that treatment beginning 2–12 hours after birth with hepatitis B immune globulin and hepatitis B vaccine is 85–95% effective in preventing the development of the HBV chronic carrier state during childhood.[5,11-13] Based on this evidence, prenatal testing for HBsAg has been recommended for pregnant women at high risk of having acquired hepatitis B.[14] Recent studies have shown, however, that only 35–65% of HBsAg-positive mothers are identified when testing is restricted to high-risk groups.[15-19] It is thought that many women at risk are not tested because their sexual and drug-related histories are not discussed with clinicians or because their clinicians are unfamiliar with perinatal transmission of HBV and recommended preventive measures.[3] In addition, many women who are carriers may not have known risk factors even after a careful history is taken.

For these reasons, routine HBsAg testing of all pregnant women may be a more effective strategy. It has been calculated that screening all of the 3.5 million pregnant women per year in the United States would detect about 16,500 HBsAg-positive mothers. Treatment of their newborns would prevent the development of HBV carrier status in an estimated 3500 neonates each year.[3] At $12–$20 per test,[20] the HBsAg assay is an expensive screening test to be performed on large numbers of women. Several studies have demonstrated, however, that the long-term benefits of preventing chronic liver disease make routine prenatal HBsAg testing as cost-effective as other widely implemented prenatal and blood-donor screening practices.[19-21] In certain populations in the United States in which HBV infection is endemic (e.g., Alaskan Natives, Pacific Islanders), universal vaccination of newborns with HBV vaccine may be a more practical strategy than prenatal screening.[3]

Recommendations of Others

Routine testing of asymptomatic persons for HBV infection is recommended primarily as a means of identifying persons in high-risk groups who require vaccination (see Chapter 57). Screening of pregnant women is, however, widely recommended. The Immunization Practices Advisory Committee of the Centers for Disease Control, in consultation with the American College of Obstetricians and Gynecologists and the American Academy of Pediatrics, has recently recommended that all pregnant women be tested for HBsAg during an early prenatal visit.[3] The test may be repeated in the third trimester if acute hepatitis is suspected, an exposure to hepatitis has occurred, or the woman practices a high-risk behavior such as intravenous drug abuse.

Clinical Intervention

All pregnant women should be tested for HBsAg at their first prenatal visit. The test may be repeated in the third trimester if the mother engages in high-risk behavior such as intravenous drug abuse or if exposure to hepatitis B during pregnancy is suspected. Infants born to HBsAg-positive mothers should receive hepatitis B immune globulin (0.5 mL) intramuscularly within 12 hours of birth. Hepatitis B vaccine, either plasma-derived (10 mcg per dose) or recombinant (5 mcg per dose), should be administered intramuscularly concurrently with immune globulin (at a different injection site) or within seven days. The second and third doses should be given one and six months after the first dose. Persons with sexual or percutaneous exposure to the mother should be tested to determine susceptibility to HBV and vaccinated if susceptible. See Chapter 57 for further recommendations on HBV vaccination in high-risk groups and Chapter 58 for information about passive and active immunization of persons with possible exposure to HBV-infected individuals or blood products.

Note: See Appendix A for the U.S. Preventive Services Task Force Table of Ratings for this topic. See also the relevant Task Force background paper: LaForce FM. Immunizations, immunoprophylaxis, and chemoprophylaxis to prevent selected infections. JAMA 1987; 257:2464–70.

REFERENCES

1. Immunization Practices Advisory Committee. Update on hepatitis B prevention. MMWR 1987; 36:353–60,366.
2. *Idem*. Recommendations for protection against viral hepatitis. MMWR 1985; 34:313–24, 329–35.
3. *Idem*. Prevention of perinatal transmission of hepatitis B virus: prenatal screening of all pregnant women for hepatitis B surface antigen. MMWR 1988; 37:341–6, 351.
4. Stevens CE, Beasley RP, Tsui J, et al. Vertical transmission of hepatitis B antigen in Taiwan. N Engl J Med 1975; 292:771–4.
5. Stevens CE, Toy PT, Tong MJ, et al. Perinatal hepatitis B virus transmission in the United States: prevention by passive-active immunization. JAMA 1985; 253:1740–5.
6. Beasley RP, Hwang LY. Epidemiology of hepatocellular carcinoma. In: Vyas GN, Dienstag JL, Hoofnagle JH, eds. Viral hepatitis and liver disease. Orlando, Fla.: Grune and Stratton, 1984:209–24.
7. Beasley RP. Hepatitis B virus as the etiologic agent in hepatocellular carcinoma: epidemiologic considerations. Hepatology 1982; 2:21S-6S.
8. Beasley RP, Hwang LY, Lin CC, et al. Hepatocellular carcinoma and HBV: a prospective study of 22,707 men in Taiwan. Lancet 1981; 2:1129–33.
9. Centers for Disease Control. Changing patterns of groups at high risk for hepatitis B in the United States. MMWR 1988; 37:429–32,437.
10. Holland P. Hepatitis B surface antigen and antibody (HBsAg/anti HBs). In: Gerety RJ, ed. Hepatitis B. Orlando, Fla.: Academy Press, 1985.
11. Beasley RP, Hwang LY, Lee GCY, et al. Prevention of perinatally transmitted hepatitis B virus infections with hepatitis B immune globulin and hepatitis B vaccine. Lancet 1983; 2:1099–102.
12. Wong VCW, Ip HMH, Reesink HW, et al. Prevention of the HBsAg carrier state in newborn

infants of mothers who are chronic carriers of HBsAg and HBeAg by administration of hepatitis-B vaccine and hepatitis-B immunoglobulin: double-blind randomised placebo controlled study. Lancet 1984; 1:921–6.

13. Stevens CE, Taylor PE, Tong MJ, et al. Yeast-recombinant hepatitis B vaccine: efficacy with hepatitis B immune globulin in prevention of perinatal hepatitis B virus transmission. JAMA 1987; 257:2612–6.

14. Immunization Practices Advisory Committee. Postexposure prophylaxis of hepatitis B. MMWR 1984; 33:285–90.

15. Kumar ML, Dawson NV, McCullough AJ, et al. Should all pregnant women be screened for hepatitis B? Ann Intern Med 1987; 107:273–7.

16. Jonas MM, Schiff ER, O'Sullivan MJ, et al. Failure of Centers for Disease Control criteria to identify hepatitis B infection in a large municipal obstetrical population. Ann Intern Med 1987; 107:335–7.

17. Summers PR, Biswas MK, Pastorek JG II, et al. The pregnant hepatitis B carrier: evidence favoring comprehensive antepartum screening. Obstet Gynecol 1987; 69: 701–4.

18. Wetzel AM, Kirz DS. Routine hepatitis screening in adolescent pregnancies: is it cost effective? Am J Obstet Gynecol 1987; 156:166–9.

19. Delage G, Montplaisir S, Remy-Prince S, et al. Hepatitis B Virus Transmission Study Group. Prevalence of hepatitis B virus infection in pregnant women in the Montreal area. Can Med Assoc J 1986; 134:897–901.

20. Arevalo JA, Washington AE. Cost-effectiveness of prenatal screening and immunization for hepatitis B virus [Published erratum appears in JAMA 1988; 260:478]. JAMA 1988; 259:365–9.

21. Kane MA, Hadler SC, Margolis HS, et al. Routine prenatal screening for hepatitis B surface antigen. JAMA 1988; 259:408–9.

21

Screening for Tuberculosis

Recommendation: Tuberculin skin testing of asymptomatic persons should be performed on those at high risk of acquiring tuberculosis (see *Clinical Intervention*). The indications for bacille Calmette-Guerin (BCG) vaccination are discussed in Chapter 58.

Burden of Suffering

Over 22,000 reported cases of tuberculosis (TB) occurred in the United States in 1987.[1] This disease is associated with considerable morbidity from pulmonary and extrapulmonary symptoms. Pulmonary symptoms are progressive and include cough, hemoptysis, dyspnea, and pleuritis. Extrapulmonary TB can involve the bones, joints, pericardium, and lymphatics, and it can cause spinal cord compression from Pott's disease. Death is more common in older patients, with estimated case-fatality rates ranging from 0.8–2.1% in adolescents to 16.5% in the elderly.[2] The incidence of TB is greatest in Asians, Pacific Islanders, blacks, American Indians, Alaska Natives, and Hispanics.[3] About one-third of all reported cases in the United States occur in blacks,[4] 14% occur in Hispanics,[5] 11% occur in Asians and Pacific Islanders,[6] and 2% occur in American Indians and Alaska Natives.[7] TB is 150–300 times as common in the homeless as in the general population; the prevalence in homeless persons is 2–7% for clinically active TB and 22–50% for asymptomatic infection.[8] The incidence of TB has recently increased after experiencing a steady decline from 1963 to 1985.[3] A disproportionately large number of new cases are occurring among black and Hispanic persons.[3] There is also evidence that compromised immunity due to infection with human immunodeficiency virus (HIV) is contributing to the rise in incidence.[9]

Efficacy of Screening Tests

Tuberculin skin testing is the principal means of detecting TB infection in asymptomatic persons. Although some authors continue to recommend chest radiography as a first-line test in high-risk populations,[10] roentgenography is generally considered to be inappropriate as the initial screening test for detecting TB in asymptomatic persons. It is important, however, as a follow-up test to identify active pulmonary TB in infected persons identified through tuberculin testing. The most accurate tuberculin skin test is the Mantoux test, in which 5 units (5 TU) of tuberculin purified protein derivative (PPD) are injected intradermally to detect delayed hypersensitivity; induration of 10 mm or more in diameter is generally considered a positive test.

The frequency of false-positive and false-negative tuberculin skin tests depends on a number of variables, including immunologic status, the size of the hypersensitivity reaction and the prevalence of atypical mycobacteria.[11,12] In certain geographic areas, cross-reacting atypical mycobacteria (as well as previous BCG vaccination) can produce intermediate size reactions, thereby limiting the specificity of the test.[11-14] False-positive results can also be produced by improper technique (e.g., measuring erythema rather than induration), hypersensitivity to PPD constituents, an Arthus reaction, and cellulitis.[11-14] False-negative reactions, which are estimated to occur in about 5–10% of patients, can be observed early in infection before hypersensitivity develops, in anergic individuals and those with severe illnesses (including active TB), and as a result of improper technique in handling the PPD solution, administering the intradermal injection, and interpreting the results.[11-15] Other limitations of the Mantoux test include the time and skill required for proper administration and variability among clinicians in interpreting results.[16] In recent years, multiple puncture tests (e.g., tine, Heaf, Mono-Vacc) have become available that are less expensive and easier to administer than the Mantoux test. Studies evaluating the accuracy of these devices, however, have produced inconsistent results. In general, the evidence suggests that multiple puncture tests have poor specificity and may have inadequate sensitivity when compared with the Mantoux test.[11,15,17,18] Patient compliance can also affect the effectiveness of tuberculin skin testing because patients must either return to the clinician or telephone results 48–72 hours after the injection. Studies in pediatric patients report noncompliance rates of 28–82%.[19-21]

Persons who are tuberculin test negative may need repeat testing, but there are inadequate data from which to determine the optimal frequency of PPD screening. In the absence of such data, clinical decisions regarding the need for repeat testing and its frequency should be based on the likelihood of further exposure to TB and the clinician's level of confidence in the accuracy of the test results.

Effectiveness of Early Detection

The early detection of tuberculin reactivity is of potential benefit because chemoprophylaxis with isoniazid (INH) is an effective means of preventing the subsequent development of active TB.[22] A review of 14 controlled trials found that efficacy ranges between 25% and 88% among persons assigned to a one-year course of INH.[22] Among compliant individuals, efficacy is greater than 90%.[23,24] This intervention is also of potential public health value in preventing transmission of the organism to household members and other close contacts. A number of factors limit the effectiveness of INH chemoprophylaxis, however. Some organisms are resistant to INH and other agents.[25-28] Patient compliance with a one-year regimen is often difficult, especially in certain populations.[26] The most important limitation of INH is its potential hepatotoxicity. INH-induced hepatitis occurs in about 0.3– 2.3% of patients,[2] the frequency increasing with age. The condition can be fatal, but the exact frequency of this complication of INH-induced hepatitis is uncertain. Mortality was reported to be as high as 4–7% in one major study.[29] These data may overestimate the actual mortality from INH-induced hepatitis because the local incidence of cirrhosis-related deaths was increased in one of the communities participating in the study.[30] In persons who develop complications from INH, the resulting interruption of INH therapy before completion of the one-year course may also lower the effectiveness of TB prevention.[24]

Although the benefits of INH probably outweigh its side effects in persons at high risk for TB (see *Clinical Intervention*), it is uncertain from available data whether low-risk, asymptomatic persons with a reactive tuberculin skin test are at sufficient risk of developing TB to justify the risks of INH-induced hepatitis. The annual incidence of TB in a low-risk population is less than 0.1%,[31,32] and the calculated lifetime probability of developing active TB ranges from 1.2% at age 20 to 0.37% at age 80.[33] Depending on the risk of INH-induced hepatitis, it is possible for complications from INH treatment to be more likely than the development of TB. In the absence of definitive clinical studies to clarify this issue, investigators have used decision analysis techniques to compare the benefits and risks of INH in tuberculin skin reactors of different ages. The results of these analyses have been inconsistent. One group concluded that benefits outweigh risks until the patient exceeds age 45;[34] another found that treatment was beneficial at all ages;[2] and another analysis concluded that INH should be withheld at all ages in the absence of other risk factors.[33] A decision analysis in young persons concluded that treatment was not beneficial in this age group.[31] An analysis for elderly tuberculin skin reactors concluded that INH would neither improve nor worsen five-year survival but would decrease the risk of developing active disease.[32]

Recommendations of Others

The Centers for Disease Control (CDC) recommends routine tuberculin skin testing of persons at increased risk of developing TB, such as immigrants or refugees from Asia or the Pacific Islands,[6] American Indians, and Alaska Natives.[7] The CDC also recommends testing homeless persons if there is a commitment to complete the diagnostic evaluation and the prescribed therapy.[8] Staff members and volunteers working at homeless shelters should be screened upon employment and every 6–12 months thereafter.[8] The American Thoracic Society (ATS) and the CDC recommend offering a 6- to 12-month course of isoniazid to all persons under 35 years of age who have positive tuberculin skin reactions and to those over 35 with one of the following risk factors: household members or other close contacts of potentially infectious TB cases; history of previous, nonprogressing, inadequately treated TB; abnormal chest x-ray consistent with inactive TB; or other illnesses (e.g., silicosis, diabetes mellitus, steroid therapy, acquired immunodeficiency syndrome).[35] The ATS and CDC also recommend chest radiography for every person with a large reaction to a tuberculin skin test.[35] The CDC screening recommendations are currently undergoing revision by the Advisory Committee for Elimination of Tuberculosis.[36]

Clinical Intervention

The Mantoux skin test for tuberculosis infection should be performed on all persons at increased risk of developing tuberculosis. Asymptomatic persons at increased risk include household members of persons with TB and others at risk for close contact with tuberculosis (e.g., staff members of tuberculosis clinics, shelters for the homeless, nursing homes, substance abuse treatment facilities, dialysis units, correctional institutions); recent immigrants or refugees from countries in which tuberculosis is common (e.g., Asia, Africa, Central and South America, the Pacific Islands, Caribbean); migrant workers; residents of nursing homes, correctional institutions, and homeless shelters; and persons with certain underlying medical disorders (e.g., HIV infection). The Mantoux test involves the intradermal injection of 5 units of tuberculin purified protein derivative and the subsequent examination of the injection site 48–72 hours later; induration greater than 10 mm in diameter is considered positive. The frequency of tuberculin skin testing is a matter of clinical discretion.

Persons with a positive PPD test should receive a chest x-ray and clinical evaluation for tuberculosis. Those lacking evidence of active infection should receive INH prophylaxis in accordance with established guidelines.[35] **Vaccination with BCG is discussed in Chapter 58.**

Note: See Appendix A for the U.S. Preventive Services Task Force Table of Ratings for this topic. See also the relevant Task Force background paper: LaForce FM. Immunizations, immunoprophylaxis, and chemoprophylaxis to prevent selected infections. JAMA 1987; 257:2264–70.DD

REFERENCES

1. Centers for Disease Control. Summary of notifiable diseases in the United States, 1987. MMWR 1988; 36:1–59.
2. Rose DN, Schechter CB, Silver AL. The age threshold for isoniazid chemoprophylaxis: a decision analysis for low-risk tuberculin reactors. JAMA 1986; 256:2709–13.
3. Centers for Disease Control. Tuberculosis, final data—United States, 1986. MMWR 1988; 36:817–20.
4. *Idem.* Tuberculosis in blacks—United States. MMWR 1987; 36:212–4,219–20.
5. *Idem.* Tuberculosis among Hispanics—United States, 1985. MMWR 1987; 36:568–9.
6. *Idem.* Tuberculosis among Asians/Pacific Islanders—United States, 1985. MMWR 1987; 36:331–4.
7. *Idem.* Tuberculosis among American Indians and Alaskan Natives—United States, 1985. MMWR 1987; 36:493–5.
8. *Idem.* Tuberculosis control among homeless populations. MMWR 1987; 36:257–60.
9. *Idem.* Tuberculosis and acquired immunodeficiency syndrome—New York City. MMWR 1987; 36:785–90,95.
10. Davidson PT. Routine screening for tuberculosis on hospital admission. Chest 1988; 94:228–30.
11. Murata P, Johnson RA. Tuberculosis screening. Am Fam Physician 1984; 29:247–53.
12. Tuberculin, PPD: generic statement. Fed Reg 1977; 42:52709–12.
13. Mellor J. False-positive results of Mantoux tests. Can Med Assoc J 1985; 132:1403.
14. Kendig EL. Tuberculin testing in the young. Compr Ther 1986; 12:66–70.
15. Rudd RM, Gellert AR, Venning M. Comparison of Mantoux, tine, and "Imotest" tuberculin tests. Lancet 1982; 2:515–8.
16. Bearman JE, Kleinman H, Glyer VV, et al. A study of variability in tuberculin test reading. Am Rev Resp Dis 1964; 90:913–9.
17. Catanzaro A. Multiple puncture skin test and Mantoux test in Southeast Asian refugees. Chest 1985; 87:346–50.
18. Hansen JP, Falconer JA, Gallis HA, et al. Inadequate sensitivity of tuberculin tine test for screening employee populations. J Occup Med 1982; 24:602–4.
19. Maqbool S, Asnes RS, Grebin B. Tine test compliance in a clinic setting. Pediatrics 1975; 55:388–91.
20. Weinberger HL, Terry C. Tuberculin testing in a pediatric outpatient clinic. J Pediatr 1969; 75:111–5.
21. Asnes RS, Maqbool S. Parent reading and reporting of children's tuberculin skin test results. Chest [Suppl 3] 1975; 68:459–62.
22. Comstock GW, Woolpert SF. Preventive therapy. In: Kubica GP, Wayne LG, eds. The mycobacteria: a source book. New York: Marcel Dekker, Inc., 1984:1071–81.
23. International Union Against Tuberculosis Committee on Prophylaxis. Efficacy of various durations of isoniazid preventive therapy for tuberculosis: five years of follow-up in the IUAT trial. Bull WHO 1982; 60:555–64.
24. Stead WW, Teresa T, Harrison RW, et al. Benefit-risk considerations in preventive treatment for tuberculosis in elderly persons. Ann Intern Med 1987; 107:843–5.
25. Centers for Disease Control. Multi-drug-resistant tuberculosis—North Carolina. MMWR 1987; 35:785–7.

26. Nolan CM, Aitken ML, Elarth AM, et al. Active tuberculosis after isoniazid chemoprophylaxis of Southeast Asian refugees. Am Rev Resp Dis 1986; 133:431–6
27. Mitchison DA, Nunn AJ. Influence of initial drug resistance on the response to short-course chemotherapy of pulmonary tuberculosis. Am Rev Resp Dis 1986; 133:423–30.
28. Barry MA, Wall C, Shirley L, et al. Tuberculosis screening in Boston's homeless shelters. Public Health Rep 1986; 101:487–94.
29. Kopanoff DE, Snider DE Jr, Caras GJ. Isoniazid-related hepatitis: a U.S. Public Health Service cooperative surveillance study. Am Rev Resp Dis 1978; 117:991–1001.
30. Comstock GW. Prevention of tuberculosis among tuberculin reactors: maximizing benefits, minimizing risks. JAMA 1986; 256:2729–30.
31. Taylor WC, Aronson MD, Delbanco TL. Should young adults with a positive tuberculin test take isoniazid? Ann Intern Med 1981; 94:808–13.
32. Cooper JK. Decision analysis for tuberculosis preventive treatment in nursing homes. J Am Geriatr Soc 1986; 34:814–7.
33. Tsevat J, Taylor WC, Wong JB, et al. Isoniazid for the tuberculin reactor: take it or leave it. Am Rev Resp Dis 1988; 137:215–20.
34. Comstock GW, Edwards PQ. The competing risks of tuberculosis and hepatitis for adult tuberculin reactors. Am Rev Resp Dis 1975; 111:573–7.
35. American Thoracic Society. Treatment of tuberculosis and tuberculosis infection in adults and children. Am Rev Resp Dis 1986; 134:355–63.
36. Snider DE Jr, Division of Tuberculosis Control, Centers for Disease Control. Personal communication, January 1989.

22

Screening for Syphilis

Recommendation: Routine screening for syphilis in asymptomatic persons is recommended for those in high-risk groups and for pregnant women (see *Clinical Intervention*).

Burden of Suffering

In 1987, over 35,000 cases of primary and secondary syphilis were reported in the United States.[1] Primary syphilis produces ulcers of the genitalia, pharynx, or rectum, and secondary syphilis produces complications such as contagious skin lesions, lymphadenopathy, and condylomalata. The disease then progresses into a latent phase in which syphilis may be clinically inapparent. If left untreated, one-third of cases progress to the potentially severe cardiovascular and neurologic complications of tertiary syphilis.[2] Cardiovascular syphilis produces aortic disease (insufficiency, aneurysms, aortitis), and neurosyphilis can result in meningitis, peripheral neuropathy (e.g., tabes dorsalis), meningovascular brain lesions, and psychiatric illness. Victims of tertiary syphilis have decreased life expectancy, and they often experience significant disability and diminished productivity as a result of their symptoms. Long-term hospitalization is often necessary for patients with severe neurologic deficits or psychiatric illness. Syphilis may also be associated epidemiologically with acquired immunodeficiency syndrome (AIDS); a possible relationship between diseases that cause genital ulcers, such as syphilis, and infection with human immunodeficiency virus (HIV) is being investigated.[3,4] The incidence of syphilis has increased in recent years and is currently at its highest rate since 1950.[1] The increase has been greatest among black and Hispanic persons.[1] A growing proportion of cases is also reported among prostitutes and persons who use illicit drugs.[5]

The incidence of syphilis in pregnant women is also increasing.[1] Transmission of the disease to the fetus results in congenital syphilis, a condition resulting in fetal or perinatal death in 40% of affected pregnancies as well as increased risk of medical complications in newborns who survive.[6] The incidence of congenital syphilis has been increasing steadily in the United States since 1978;[7] in late 1987 it was 10.5 cases per 100,000 live births.[1] The rate of increase escalated in 1987, and experts predict that, in the absence of intervention, this trend will continue in coming years.[1]

Efficacy of Screening Tests

The principal screening tests for syphilis are the VDRL (Venereal Disease Research Laboratory) and RPR (rapid plasma reagin) tests, which detect a rise in antibody titres following infection. The sensitivity of these tests is influenced by characteristic fluctuations in antibodies during the stages of the disease. Antibody titres are often not significantly elevated in the early primary stages of syphilis, and they may return to normal levels in latent and tertiary syphilis.[8] In secondary syphilis, when titres are often at their peak, the reported sensitivity of the VDRL approaches 100%. Sensitivity is lower, however, in primary syphilis (62–76%) and in late symptomatic syphilis (70%).[8] The VDRL and RPR can also produce false-positive reactions, primarily in persons with coexisting conditions (e.g., collagen vascular diseases, drug addiction, pregnancy, other infections) and through laboratory error.[8-10] The VDRL is therefore most specific (approaching 100%) in persons without coexisting illnesses and has lower specificity (75–85%) in those who are ill.[8,11] Due to this potential for false-positive results, persons with positive VDRL or RPR reactions require the FTA-ABS (fluorescent treponemal antibody absorption) test to confirm the diagnosis. The FTA-ABS technique is more sensitive and specific than either the VDRL or RPR, but it is too expensive to be used as a routine screening test.[8,10]

Effectiveness of Early Detection

Early detection of syphilis in asymptomatic persons permits the initiation of antibiotic therapy to eradicate the infection, thereby preventing both the disabling progression of the disease and its transmission to sexual contacts. Antibiotic therapy with penicillin G benzathine or tetracycline hydrochloride has been shown to be highly effective in eliminating *Treponema pallidum*, the organism responsible for syphilis. Early detection and penicillin treatment during pregnancy has the added benefit of reducing the risk to the fetus of acquiring congenital syphilis.[7] Prenatal antibiotic therapy is not completely effective in preventing congenital syphilis, however. Failures can occur, for example, if maternal penicillin allergy requires treatment with erythromycin, an antibiotic with limited efficacy in preventing congenital syphilis, or if antibiotic therapy is not started until the third trimester.[12,13]

Since the incidence of syphilis is only 15 cases per 100,000 persons,[1] routine screening of the general population is likely to have low yield. Screening may be reasonable, however, in certain populations at increased risk, such as prostitutes, persons who engage in sex with multiple partners in areas in which syphilis is prevalent, and contacts of persons with active syphilis. Pregnant women are generally at low risk for syphilis; depending on the exact prevalence, the positive predictive value of the VDRL in this population can be less than 1%.[8] Prenatal screening is considered worthwhile, however, because of the severe neonatal morbidity and mortality associated with congenital syphilis, as well as its potential preventability. Several studies have demonstrated that prenatal screening for syphilis is cost-effective, even when the prevalence of the disease among pregnant women is as low as 0.005%.[14,15] Currently, congenital syphilis occurs in 0.01% of all live births.[1]

Recommendations of Others

The Canadian Task Force recommends testing for syphilis in high-risk groups, such as persons with a history of multiple sexual partners, in all pregnant women at their first prenatal visit, and in high-risk gravidas at 34–36 weeks' gestation.[16] The American College of Obstetricians and Gynecologists also recommends routine prenatal screening for syphilis.[17] The Centers for Disease Control recommends obtaining serology for syphilis at the beginning of prenatal care and at delivery;

testing at 28 weeks is also recommended for women in high-risk groups.[6] The American Academy of Pediatrics recommends considering periodic screening for syphilis in sexually active adolescents.[18]

Clinical Intervention

Routine serologic testing is recommended for persons at increased risk for syphilis, such as prostitutes, persons who engage in sex with multiple partners in areas in which syphilis is prevalent, and sexual contacts of persons with active syphilis. The optimal frequency for such testing has not been determined and is left to clinical discretion. All pregnant women should be tested at their first prenatal visit and at delivery; an additional test at 28 weeks' gestation or later is recommended for women at increased risk of acquiring syphilis during pregnancy.

Note: See Appendix A for the U.S. Preventive Services Task Force Table of Ratings for this topic. See also the relevant Task Force background paper: Horsburgh CR, Douglas JM, LaForce FM. Preventive strategies in sexually transmitted diseases for the primary care physician. JAMA 1987; 258:814–21.

REFERENCES

1. Centers for Disease Control. Syphilis and congenital syphilis, United States, 1985–1988. MMWR 1988; 37:486–9.
2. Clark EG, Danbolt N. The Oslo study of the natural course of untreated syphilis: an epidemiologic investigation based on a restudy of the Boeck-Bruusgaard material. Med Clin N Am 1964; 48:613–23.
3. Stamm WE, Handsfield III H, Rompalo AM, et al. The association between genital ulcer disease and acquisition of HIV infection in homosexual men. JAMA 1988; 260: 1429–33.
4. Holmberg SD, Stewart JA, Gerber AR, et al. Prior herpes simplex virus type 2 infection as a risk factor for HIV infection. JAMA 1988; 259:1048–50.
5. Centers for Disease Control. Relationship of syphilis to drug use and prostitution— Connecticut and Philadelphia, Pennsylvania. MMWR 1988; 37:755–8,64.
6. Idem. Guidelines for the prevention and control of congenital syphilis. MMWR [Suppl 1] 1988; 37.
7. Idem. Congenital syphilis, United States, 1983–1985. MMWR 1986; 35:625–8.
8. Hart G. Syphilis tests in diagnostic and therapeutic decision making. Ann Intern Med 1986; 104:368–76.
9. Idem. Screening to control infectious diseases. Rev Infect Dis 1980; 2:701–12.
10. Feder HM, Manthous C. The asymptomatic patient with a positive VDRL test. Am Fam Physician 1988; 37:185–90.
11. Wentworth BB, Thompson MA, Peter CR, et al. Comparison of a hemagglutination treponemal test for syphilis (HATTS) with other serologic methods for the diagnosis of syphilis. Sex Transm Dis 1978; 5:103–11.
12. Hashisaki P, Wertzberger GG, Conrad GL, et al. Erythromycin failure in the treatment of syphilis in a pregnant woman. Sex Transm Dis 1983; 10:36–8.
13. Fenton LJ, Light IJ. Congenital syphilis after maternal treatment with erythromycin. Obstet Gynecol 1976; 47:492–4.
14. Stray-Pedersen B. Economic evaluation of maternal screening to prevent congenital syphilis. Sex Transm Dis 1983; 10:167–72.
15. Williams K. Screening for syphilis in pregnancy: an assessment of the costs and benefits. Community Med 1985; 7:37–42.

16. Canadian Task Force on the Periodic Health Examination. The periodic health examination. Can Med Assoc J 1979; 121:1–45.
17. American College of Obstetricians and Gynecologists. Standards for obstetric-gynecologic services. Washington, D.C.: American College of Obstetricians and Gynecologists, 1985:16.
18. American Academy of Pediatrics. Role of the pediatrician in management of sexually transmitted diseases in children and adolescents. Pediatrics 1987; 79:454–6.

23

Screening for Gonorrhea

Recommendation: Routine testing for gonorrhea in asymptomatic persons is recommended for persons at high risk (see *Clinical Intervention*) and for pregnant women. An ophthalmic antibiotic should be applied topically to the eyes of all newborns immediately after birth to prevent ophthalmia neonatorum.

Burden of Suffering

An estimated 2 million persons acquire gonococcal infections each year in the United States.[1] This disease is associated with considerable morbidity, producing urethritis, epididymitis, and proctitis in men and painful pelvic inflammatory disease (PID) in women.[2] The latter is an important risk factor for ectopic pregnancy and infertility; about 25% of women who have had PID are unable to conceive.[3] In 1979, U.S. costs for PID were $2.6 billion.[4] Pregnant women with active gonococcal infection are at increased risk for obstetrical complications and can give birth to infants with gonococcal conjunctivitis (ophthalmia neonatorum), a condition that often produces blindness if not treated.[2] Persons with gonorrhea are also at risk for a disseminated form of the disease in which skin, joints, and other sites become infected, producing complications such as tenosynovitis and septic arthritis. Sexual contacts of person with active disease are at risk for acquiring gonorrhea; a large proportion of carriers of gonorrhea are asymptomatic. The incidence of gonorrhea is highest in young adults under age 25, unmarried persons, persons of low socioeconomic status, and persons with multiple sexual contacts, such as prostitutes.[2]

Efficacy of Screening Tests

The most sensitive and reproducible test for detecting gonococcal infection in asymptomatic persons is direct culture. Other methods of screening have been proposed, such as Gram's stained urethral smears, serology, DNA hybridization, fluorescent antibody testing, and enzyme-linked immunoassay, but these tests currently lack the combination of speed, sensitivity, specificity, and low cost to be recommended as an alternative to culture.[2] Performing routine cultures for gonorrhea on all sexually active adults, however, is likely to be of low yield because the disease is relatively uncommon in the general population. In high-risk groups (see above), the incidence of gonorrhea may be high enough to justify routine cultures.

Effectiveness of Early Detection

Early detection of gonococcal infection in asymptomatic persons permits antibiotic therapy to eradicate the organism and prevent the complications of the disease. It also allows for notification of sexual contacts at risk of infection. Due to the ethical difficulties of performing controlled trials of gonorrhea treatment, there have been few studies examining whether early detection and treatment in asymptomatic persons results in improved outcome compared with delay until the appearance of symptoms. It is known, however, that most strains of *Neisseria gonorrhoea* are eradicated with appropriate antibiotic therapy. In the last decade, antimicrobial resistance to penicillins, tetracyclines, and aminoglycosides has become increasingly common. Over 16,000 infections with beta-lactamase-producing gonococci, the most common resistant strain, were reported in the United States in 1986.[5] These organisms are, however, currently sensitive to third-generation cephalosporins such as ceftriaxone.[5]

Recommendations of Others

The Canadian Task Force advises against routine screening for gonorrhea in the general population, but it does recommend obtaining cervical and urethral smears, cervical and urethral cultures, and first-voided urine cultures in high-risk women (history of multiple sexual partners) and pregnant women.[6] The Centers for Disease Control (CDC)[7] and the American College of Obstetricians and Gynecologists[8] recommend obtaining endocervical cultures for *Neisseria gonorrhoea* in all pregnant women during their first prenatal visit; a second culture is recommended late in the third trimester for women at high risk of acquiring sexually transmitted diseases. The American Academy of Pediatrics[9] and CDC[10] recommend administering ointment or drops containing tetracycline or erythromycin, or 1% silver nitrate solution, to the eyes of all infants shortly after birth. The Canadian Task Force recommends instilling silver nitrate solution.[6]

Discussion

A potential benefit of detecting gonorrhea during pregnancy is the prevention of ophthalmia neonatorum in the newborn. It has not been proved conclusively, however, that antibiotic treatment during pregnancy is effective in preventing this condition. Another strategy is the instillation of ophthalmic antibiotics immediately after birth. Erythromycin, silver nitrate, and tetracycline have all been shown to be effective in preventing gonococcal ophthalmia neonatorum in women infected with sensitive strains.[11,12] Silver nitrate, however, is chemically irritating, frequently causes chemical conjunctivitis, and has limited efficacy in preventing chlamydial ophthalmia neonatorum (see Chapter 25).

Clinical Intervention

Routine cultures for gonorrhea in asymptomatic persons should be obtained in high-risk groups, such as prostitutes, persons with multiple sexual partners or a sexual partner with multiple sexual contacts, sexual contacts of persons with culture-proven gonorrhea, and persons with a history of repeated episodes of gonorrhea. The optimal frequency of such testing has not been determined and is left to clinical discretion. Pregnant women should receive endocervical cultures for gonorrhea at their first prenatal visit. An additional test later in pregnancy is recommended for those at increased risk of acquiring gonorrhea during pregnancy. Erythromycin 0.5% ophthalmic ointment or tetracycline 1% ophthalmic ointment should be applied topically to the eyes of all newborns as soon as possible after birth and no later than 1 hour of age.

Note: See Appendix A for the U.S. Preventive Services Task Force Table of Ratings for this topic. See also the relevant Task Force background paper: Horsburgh CR, Douglas JM, LaForce FM. Preventive strategies in sexually transmitted diseases for the primary care physician. JAMA 1987; 258:814–21.

REFERENCES

1. Cates W Jr. Epidemiology and control of sexually transmitted diseases: strategic evolution. Infect Dis Clin N Am 1987; 1:1–23.
2. Hook EW, Holmes KK. Gonococcal infections. Ann Intern Med 1985; 102:229–43.
3. Westrom L. Effect of acute pelvic inflammatory disease on fertility. Am J Obstet Gynecol 1975; 121:707–13.
4. Washington AE, Arno PS. The economic cost of pelvic inflammatory disease. JAMA 1986; 255:1735–8.
5. Centers for Disease Control. Antibiotic-resistant strains of Neisseria gonorrhoeae: policy guidelines for detection, management, and control. MMWR [Suppl 5] 1987; 36.
6. Canadian Task Force on the Periodic Health Examination. The periodic health examination. Can Med Assoc J 1979; 121:1–45.
7. Centers for Disease Control. 1985 STD treatment guidelines. MMWR [Suppl 4] 1985; 34.
8. American College of Obstetricians and Gynecologists. Gonorrhea and chlamydial infections. ACOG Technical Bulletin No. 89. Washington, D.C.: American College of Obstetricians and Gynecologists, 1985.
9. American Academy of Pediatrics. Prophylaxis and treatment of neonatal gonococcal infections. Pediatrics 1980; 65:1047–8.
10. Centers for Disease Control. Chlamydia trachomatis infections: policy guidelines for prevention and control. MMWR [Suppl 3] 1985; 34.
11. Rothenberg R. Ophthalmia neonatorum due to Neisseria gonorrhoea. Sex Transm Dis 1979; 6:S187–91.
12. Bernstein GA, Davis JP, Katcher ML. Prophylaxis of neonatal conjunctivitis. Clin Pediatr 1982; 21:545–50.

24

Screening for Infection with Human Immunodeficiency Virus

Recommendation: Screening for infection with human immunodeficiency virus (HIV) should be offered periodically to persons seeking treatment for sexually transmitted diseases, intravenous drug users, homosexual and bisexual men, and others at increased risk of infection (see *Clinical Intervention*). Testing should also be offered to pregnant women (or women contemplating pregnancy) who are at increased risk for HIV infection. Testing should not be performed in the absence of informed consent and adequate pretest and posttest counseling. Clinicians should be careful to use proper tests and qualified laboratories. Seropositive persons require adequate posttest counseling, and sexual partners should be properly notified (see *Clinical Intervention*). Persons with negative test results also require counseling and repeat testing when appropriate. See also Chapter 53.

Burden of Suffering

It is estimated that 1–1.5 million persons in the United States are infected with the human immunodeficiency virus.[1,2] Within 10 years of infection with HIV, about 50% of persons develop acquired immunodeficiency syndrome (AIDS) and another 40% or more develop other clinical illnesses associated with HIV infection.[3] There is currently no available treatment that has been proved to prevent death in persons with AIDS. In a study performed before the licensure of AZT (azidothymidine, zidovudine; see below), only half of patients survived one year beyond diagnosis; the five-year survival rate was only 15%.[4] Of the 82,764 cases that had been reported to the Centers for Disease Control by the end of 1988, 56% (over 46,000 patients) had died, including over 80% of those diagnosed before 1985.[5] AIDS is the only major disease in the United States in which mortality is increasing.[6] Incidence is highest in young adults (aged 25–44), and therefore AIDS is an increasingly important cause of years of potential life lost (YPLL) in the United States. Between 1984 and 1987, AIDS rose in rank from the 13th to the 7th leading cause of YPLL before age 65.[6,7] AIDS is the leading cause of death in intravenous (IV) drug users and persons with hemophilia.[8]

Between its identification in 1981 and the end of 1988, 82,764 cases of AIDS had been reported.[5] By the end of 1992, it is projected that a total of 365,000 cases will have been diagnosed and 260,000 persons will have died of AIDS.[2] Currently, AIDS treatment costs the United States $2.2 billion per year;[9] these costs are expected to climb to as high as $13 billion per year by 1992.[2] HIV infection occurs primarily in homosexual and bisexual men, IV drug users, and persons with heterosexual contact with infected persons.[6] Other risk groups include blood transfusion recipients, persons with hemophilia, and infants born to infected mothers.[6] The prevalence of seropositivity ranges from 20% to 50% in homosexual and bisexual men living in various locations,[1] and from 5% to as high as 50–65% among IV drug users living in selected urban areas such as New York City.[10,11] Blacks account for 36% of all reported AIDS cases, and Hispanics account for another 16%.[2]

Depending on the geographic area, the proportion of childbearing women who are infected with HIV ranges from 0.02–3.0%.[6,12,13] There are some data suggesting that pregnant women with HIV infection have higher morbidity and mortality from viral diseases and increased risk of developing AIDS.[14,15] About 30–35% transmit the virus to their children.[16] Three-quarters of AIDS cases in children under age 13 result from perinatal transmission.[6]

Efficacy of Screening Tests

The initial screening test to detect antibodies to HIV is the enzyme-linked immunoassay (ELISA or EIA). The ELISA has a sensitivity and specificity of about 99% when licensed test kits are used under optimal laboratory conditions.[16-21] In actual practice, false-negative and false-positive results are probably more common.[22] False-negative results can occur for biological reasons in the first 6–12 weeks after infection, when persons exposed to HIV often have not yet developed detectable levels of antibody.[23] False-positive results can be caused by nonspecific serologic reactions in persons with immunologic disturbances or a history of multiple transfusions.[17] To reduce the likelihood of false-positive results, a reactive ELISA test is generally repeated. A reactive ELISA in sequential tests has a reported specificity of 99.8%.[17] Even this excellent specificity, however, yields a low positive predictive value when testing is performed in populations at low risk for HIV infection. It has been shown that three out of four persons with repeatedly reactive ELISA results are false positives when the prevalence is 30 per 100,000 (assuming ELISA test with 98% sensitivity and 99.8% specificity).[22]

It is therefore necessary to validate ELISA results by performing an independent test with high specificity (e.g., Western blot, radioimmunoprecipitation assays, and indirect immunofluorescence assays). The Western blot is the most common of these tests used in the United States.[17] When performed according to accepted performance standards, sequential ELISA tests followed by Western blot testing has a false-positive rate of less than 0.001%.[17,24] An important problem with this test, however, is that many laboratories do not use standardized methods or licensed Western blot products. Since the accuracy of this test is highly dependent on the choice of chemical reagents, the skill of technicians, and subjective interpretation,[25] laboratories lacking proper quality controls may generate a larger proportion of false-positive and false-negative results than has been observed under optimal conditions.[22,26-28] In addition, there remains some uncertainty about which combinations of reactive virus-specific protein bands should constitute a positive Western blot test.[22,25] Finally, there may be considerable delay in correcting false-positive ELISA results in cases with indeterminate Western blot results. This occurs in as many as 15–20% of tests performed on low-risk persons with reactive ELISA results.[17] In uninfected persons, the Western blot may remain indeterminate for months.[17] The future availability of viral cultures may provide a third tier of diagnostic tests to reduce the rate of diagnostic error.

Effectiveness of Early Detection

There is little direct evidence that asymptomatic HIV-infected individuals detected through screening have longer survival or lower morbidity than persons detected without screening. It is reasonable to assume, however, that early determination of HIV infection can be of clinical benefit to some individuals and of considerable public health value in preventing transmission to others. A major clinical benefit to the individual is the opportunity to modify personal behavior (e.g., high-risk sexual practices, sharing of IV drug needles) to reduce the risk of subsequent infection with other organisms, such as those causing syphilis and hepatitis B. In addition, through heightened awareness of the risk for opportunistic infections (e.g., *Pneumocystis carinii* pneumonia), the onset of illness may be recognized and treated earlier, perhaps leading to fewer complications. Some HIV-infected persons may also benefit from prophylactic measures, such as antimycobacterial treatment for persons who are tuberculin-positive. Antiviral agents such as AZT, although currently licensed only for the treatment of AIDS, are being investigated to determine their efficacy in preventing or delaying the onset of AIDS in asymptomatic seropositive persons.[29,30] Other antimicrobial agents, such as pentamidine, and vaccines for influenza, pneumococcal, and other infections may also be helpful.

Early detection of seropositivity is also of public health value in preventing HIV transmission to others. Partner notification programs (contact tracing) can alert unsuspecting persons of previous exposure to HIV and the need to be tested. Early reports from several states suggest that as many as 75% of sexual partners can be identified and given counseling as a result of organized partner notification programs.[31] Seropositive persons, by adopting new behaviors, can prevent subsequent HIV transmission to uninfected contacts such as sexual partners, transfusion recipients, and IV drug users. Health care workers (and others with potential parenteral contact with body fluids) can exercise special caution while caring for these infected persons. Women of childbearing age can avoid pregnancy, thereby preventing transmission of the virus to their children and perhaps reducing the risk to themselves of accelerating the development of AIDS. Testing is also of potential value for women who have already become pregnant. Knowledge of seropositivity may facilitate decisions on continuation of the pregnancy and may lead to fewer maternal complications through improved infection control techniques, the avoidance of breast-feeding, and early detection of HIV infection in the newborn and protection from potentially harmful vaccines.

There is little scientific evidence, however, that HIV testing actually achieves all of these potential benefits. It is not known, for example, whether infected persons change personal behavior on the basis of test results. Studies examining the effects of HIV testing on sexual behavior in homosexual men have found that high-risk practices decreased in all groups regardless of test results or the subjects' knowledge of the results.[32-34] Some studies have found that men who received seropositive results eliminated high-risk behaviors (i.e., numerous partners, unprotected insertive and receptive anal intercourse) significantly more than did those who received seronegative results.[32,33] Another study found that this information affected only certain sexual practices (unprotected insertive anal intercourse).[34] Personal behavior may be even more difficult to change in persons, such as prostitutes, who have special dependency on high-risk behaviors. In IV drug users, addiction to such agents as heroin and cocaine often interferes with advice to discontinue the use of intravenous drugs. Uncontaminated needles and syringes are frequently unavailable or prohibitively expensive, and access to health care for substance abuse counseling and medical treatment is often poor.

HIV testing has also been associated with intense anxiety, depression, somatization, or anger among those who receive reactive (positive) results.[35] If the meaning of reactive results is not properly explained, some may assume that a reactive test indicates the presence of AIDS, and suffer unnecessary (or premature) anxiety. Others, assuming that the presence of antibodies to HIV confers immunity to the organism, may disregard advice to discontinue high-risk behavior; complacency may also result from misinterpretation of nonreactive tests. Disclosure of test results to others can result in disrupted personal relationships, social ostracism, and discriminatory action, such as loss of employment, housing, health insurance, and educational opportunities.[36] These adverse effects can be minimized by providing adequate pretest and posttest counseling, by protecting confidentiality, by performing the proper sequence of ELISA and Western blot tests, and by other measures to reduce the frequency of false-positive results. This includes limiting routine testing in low-prevalence populations. Since false positives are more common under these conditions, it is possible for unfocused screening efforts in low-risk settings to result in frequent mislabeling, even when the most accurate laboratory tests are used. For example, a screening test with 99% sensitivity and specificity will generate 10 false positives for every case detected in a population with a prevalence of 0.1%.[36]

Recommendations of Others

The Centers for Disease Control (CDC) recommends offering counseling and HIV testing to persons seeking treatment for sexually transmitted diseases; IV drug users; persons who consider themselves at risk for HIV infection; women of childbearing age or pregnant women at increased risk (i.e., previous IV drug use; prostitution; sexual partners who were HIV infected, bisexual, or IV drug users; living or born in area with high prevalence of HIV infection in women; transfusion between 1978 and 1985); and prostitutes.[16] Pregnant women in the above categories should be tested as soon as the woman is known to be pregnant; if the initial test is negative, repeat testing may be indicated near delivery.[14] The CDC recommends that seropositive persons be instructed how to notify their partners. If it cannot be assured that partners will seek counseling, physicians or health department personnel should use confidential procedures to assure that partners are notified.

The American Medical Association (AMA) recommends offering counseling and testing to the same groups, as well as to high-risk persons receiving family planning services or undergoing surgical procedures.[37] The AMA also recommends that informed consent be obtained prior to testing; that persons with reactive test results be counseled regarding behavior to prevent transmission, strategies for health protection with a compromised immune system, and the necessity of alerting sexual contacts; that reactive results be reported to public health officials on an anonymous or confidential basis; and that public health officials be notified of sexual partners whom the physician believes would not otherwise be contacted. The American College of Physicians recommends selected screening on a case-by-case basis of persons whose personal conduct poses unique risks to others.[38] The American College of Obstetricians and Gynecologists recommends routine testing and counseling of women at increased risk for HIV infection and repeat testing for women who are found to be seronegative less than six months after the last potential exposure.[39]

Mandatory testing for HIV is currently required on entrance to the military; for donors of blood, organs, and tissue; federal prisoners; and persons seeking immigration to the United States. Clinicians are affected by legislation in a number of states regarding mandatory testing, confidentiality of results, informed consent, and reporting of HIV seropositivity to public health officials.[40]

Discussion

In summary, HIV testing is of potential benefit to the individual being tested and may be extremely important in preventing transmission of the virus to others, but direct evidence linking screening to these outcomes is lacking. It has not been proved that individuals who ultimately develop AIDS benefit personally by the early detection of seropositivity while asymptomatic. Past and future high-risk contacts may potentially benefit the most from the early detection of HIV-infected persons. However, although effective partner notification programs have been established, further data are needed to determine whether such programs are reproducible in the clinical setting or how often partner notification successfully prevents HIV transmission. It is also increasingly apparent that HIV testing, especially when performed in an inappropriate manner, can generate a variety of undesirable outcomes for many of those tested.

Despite these limitations, screening is important because of the extremely high mortality associated with AIDS and as a public health measure to help control the HIV pandemic. At the same time, it is also apparent from problems experienced to date that precautions must be taken in testing to minimize its potential harmful effects and to maximize its intended benefits. These measures include reducing the frequency of false-positive results by targeting screening to populations at increased risk; achieving optimal accuracy by using validated diagnostic tests and qualified medical laboratories; facilitating informed patient decision-making and accurate interpretation of results by providing complete information about potential benefits and risks before patients consent to testing; protecting the confidentiality of results; and taking appropriate measures to notify high-risk contacts, within the confines of the patient's wishes, the professional duty to warn, and existing legal requirements.

Clinical Intervention

Counseling and testing for HIV should be offered to persons seeking treatment for sexually transmitted diseases; homosexual and bisexual men; past or present IV drug users; persons with a history of prostitution or multiple sexual partners; women whose past or present sexual partners were HIV-infected, bisexual, or IV drug users; persons with long-term residence or birth in an area with high prevalence of HIV infection; and persons with a history of transfusion between 1978 and 1985. Counseling and testing should also be recommended for women in the above categories who are contemplating pregnancy. Pregnant women in these categories should be counseled and tested as soon as the woman is known to be pregnant; if the initial test is negative, repeat testing may be indicated near delivery. Testing should not be performed in the absence of informed consent and pretest counseling, which should include the purpose of the test, the meaning of reactive and nonreactive results, measures to protect confidentiality, and the need to notify persons at risk.

The diagnosis of seropositivity requires at least two reactive ELISAs and a follow-up Western blot test. Clinicians should have these tests performed only at qualified laboratories that perform frequent test runs, use appropriate controls, and receive regular external proficiency testing. Persons found to be seropositive should receive information regarding the meaning of the

results, the distinctions between casual nonsexual contact and proven modes of HIV transmission, measures to reduce risk to themselves and others, symptoms requiring medical attention, and the availability of community resources to provide psychological counseling, support groups, and other forms of assistance. Seropositive persons also should be evaluated for other infectious diseases such as tuberculosis. Arrangements for follow-up medical care are especially important for IV drug users, who may require assistance in achieving entrance to a drug treatment program (see Chapter 47). All seropositive individuals should be informed of the need to notify sexual partners, persons with whom intravenous drug needles have been shared, and others at risk of exposure. If it cannot be assured that partners will be properly notified, physicians or health department personnel should use confidential procedures to alert these individuals. All seropositive cases should be reported confidentially or anonymously to public health officials.

Persons with nonreactive test results should be informed that the risk of acquiring subsequent HIV infection can be prevented by maintaining monogamous sexual relationships with uninfected partners. Other measures to reduce the risk of infection, such as avoiding anal intercourse, using condoms, and not using unsterilized needles and syringes, should be specifically mentioned (see Chapter 53). The frequency of repeat testing of seronegative individuals is a matter of clinical discretion; persons with recent (less than three months) high-risk exposure are in greatest need of repeat testing to rule out false-negative results from low antibody titres.

Note: See Appendix A for the U.S. Preventive Services Task Force Table of Ratings for this topic. See also the relevant Task Force background paper: Horsburgh CR, Douglas JM, LaForce FM. Preventive strategies in sexually transmitted diseases for the primary care physician. JAMA 1987; 258:814–21.

REFERENCES

1. Centers for Disease Control. Human immunodeficiency virus infection in the United States: a review of current knowledge. MMWR [Suppl 6] 1987; 36:1–48.
2. *Idem*. Quarterly report to the Domestic Policy Council on the prevalence and rate of spread of HIV and AIDS, United States. MMWR 1988; 37:551–9.
3. Hessol NA, Rutherford GW, Lifson AR, et al. The natural history of HIV infection in a cohort of homosexual and bisexual men: a decade of follow-up. Proceedings of IV International Conference on AIDS, Stockholm, Sweden, June 14, 1988. Abstract 4096.
4. Rothenberg R, Woelfel M, Stoneburner R, et al. Survival with the acquired immunodeficiency syndrome: experience with 5833 cases in New York City. N Engl J Med 1987; 317:1297–1302.
5. Centers for Disease Control. AIDS Weekly Surveillance Report—United States. January 2, 1989.
6. *Idem*. Quarterly report to the Domestic Policy Council on the prevalence and rate of spread of HIV and AIDS in the United States. MMWR 1988; 37:223–6.
7. *Idem*. Years of potential life lost before age 65—United States, 1987. MMWR 1989; 38:27–9.
8. Curran JW, Jaffe HW, Hardy AM, et al. Epidemiology of HIV infection and AIDS in the United States. Science 1988; 239:610–6.
9. Hellinger FJ. Forecasting the personal medical care costs of AIDS from 1988 through 1991. Public Health Rep 1988; 103:309–19.
10. Lange WR, Snyder FR, Lozovsky D, et al. Geographic distribution of human immunodeficiency virus markers in parenteral drug abusers. Am J Public Health 1988; 78: 443–6.
11. Des Jarlais DC, Friedman SR, Novick DM, et al. HIV-1 infection among intravenous

drug users in Manhattan, New York City, from 1977 through 1987. JAMA 1989; 261:1008–12.

12. Holl H, Berardi VP, Welblen BJ, et al. Seroprevalence of human immunodeficiency virus among childbearing women: estimation by testing samples of blood from newborns. N Engl J Med 1988; 318:525–30.

13. Landesman S, Minkoff H, Holman S, et al. Serosurvey of human immunodeficiency virus infection in parturients: implications for human immunodeficiency virus testing programs of pregnant women. JAMA 1987; 258:2701–3.

14. Centers for Disease Control. Recommendations for assisting in the prevention of perinatal transmission of human T-lymphotrophic virus type III/lymphadenopathy-associated virus and acquired immunodeficiency syndrome. MMWR 1985; 34:721–6,731.

15. Minkoff HL. Care of pregnant women infected with human immunodeficiency virus. JAMA 1987; 258:2714–7.

16. Centers for Disease Control. Public Health Service guidelines for counseling and antibody testing to prevent HIV infection and AIDS. MMWR 1987; 36:509–15.

17. Idem. Update: serologic testing for antibody to human immunodeficiency virus. MMWR 1988; 36:833–40,845.

18. Burkhardt U, Mertens T, Eggers HJ. Comparison of two commercially available anti-HIV ELISAs: Abbott HTLV III EIA and Dupont HTLV III-ELISA. J Med Virol 1987; 23: 217–24.

19. Mortimer PP, Parry JV, Mortimer JY. Which anti-HTLV-III/LAV assays for screening and confirmatory testing? Lancet 1985; 2:873–7.

20. Reesink HW, Huisman JG, Gonsalves M, et al. Evaluation of six enzyme immunoassays for antibody against human immunodeficiency virus. Lancet 1986; 2:483–6.

21. Gurtler LG, Eberle J, Lorbeer B, et al. Sensitivity and specificity of commercial ELISA kits for screening anti-LAV/HTLV III. J Virol Methods 1987; 15:11–23

22. Schwartz LS, Dans PE, Kinosian BP. Human immunodeficiency virus test evaluation, performance, and use. JAMA 1988; 259:2574–9.

23. Kessler HA, Blaauw B, Spear J, et al. Diagnosis of human immunodeficiency virus infection in seronegative homosexuals presenting with an acute viral syndrome. JAMA 1987; 258:1196–9.

24. Burke DS, Brandt BL, Redfield RR, et al. Diagnosis of human immunodeficiency virus infection by immunoassay using a molecularly cloned and expressed virus envelope polypeptide: comparison to Western blot on 2707 consecutive serum samples. Ann Intern Med 1987; 106:671–6.

25. The Consortium for Retrovirus Serology Standardization. Serological diagnosis of human immunodeficiency virus infection by Western blot testing. JAMA 1988; 260:674–9.

26. Burke DS, Redfield RR. False-positive Western blot tests for antibodies to HTLV-III. JAMA 1986; 256:347.

27. Meyer KB, Pauker SG. Screening for HIV: can we afford the false positive rate? N Engl J Med 1987; 317:238–41.

28. Barnes DM. New questions about AIDS test accuracy. Science 1987; 238:884–5.

29. Food and Drug Administration. Drug treatment. FDA Drug Bull 1987; Sept:19–21.

30. Broder S, Fauci AS. Progress in drug therapies for HIV infection. Public Health Rep 1988; 103:224–9.

31. Centers for Disease Control. Partner notification for preventing human immunodeficiency virus (HIV) infection—Colorado, Idaho, South Carolina, Virginia. MMWR 1988; 37:393–6,401–2.

32. Fox R, Odaka NJ, Brookmeyer R, et al. Effect of HIV antibody disclosure on subsequent sexual activity in homosexual men. AIDS 1987; 1:241–6.

33. van Griensven GJP, de Vroome EMM, Tielman RAP, et al. Impact of HIV antibody testing on changes in sexual behavior among homosexual men in the Netherlands. Am J Public Health 1988; 78:1575–7.

34. McCusker J, Stoddard AM, Mayer KH, et al. Effects of HIV antibody test knowledge on subsequent sexual behaviors in a cohort of homosexually active men. Am J Public Health 1988; 78:462–7.

35. National Institute of Mental Health. Coping with AIDS: psychological and social consid-

erations in helping people with HTLV-III infection. Rockville, Md.: Alcohol, Drug Abuse, and Mental Health Administration, 1986. (Publication no. DHHS (ADM) 85–1432.)

36. Department of Health and Human Services. AIDS: A public health challenge. State issues, policies, and programs. Vol. 1. Assessing the problem. Washington, D.C.: Intergovernmental Health Policy Project, 1987.

37. American Medical Association. Board of Trustees Report. Prevention and control of acquired immunodeficiency syndrome: an interim report. JAMA 1987; 258:2097–103.

38. American College of Physicians. Health and Public Policy Committee. Acquired immunodeficiency syndrome. Ann Intern Med 1986; 104:575–81.

39. American College of Obstetricians and Gynecologists. Prevention of human immune deficiency virus infection and acquired immune deficiency syndrome. Statement of ACOG Committee on Obstetrics: Maternal and Fetal Medicine and Gynecologic Practice. Washington, D.C.: American College of Obstetricians and Gynecologists, 1987.

40. Lewis HE. Acquired immunodeficiency syndrome: state legislative activity. JAMA 1987; 258:2410–4.

25

Screening for Chlamydial Infection

Recommendation: Routine testing for *Chlamydia trachomatis* is recommended for asymptomatic persons at high risk of infection (see *Clinical Intervention*). Pregnant women in high-risk categories should be tested at the first prenatal visit. Ophthalmic antibiotics should be applied topically to the eyes of all newborns immediately after birth to help prevent ophthalmia neonatorum.

Burden of Suffering

An estimated 3–4 million persons acquire chlamydial infections each year in the United States.[1] This organism is responsible for about half of all cases of nongonococcal urethritis and acute epididymitis in men and about half of the cases of mucopurulent cervicitis in women.[1,2] It has been estimated that chlamydial infections are responsible for about 25–50% of the 1 million cases of pelvic inflammatory disease (PID) that are reported annually in the United States.[2] PID is an important cause of infertility and ectopic pregnancy in American women.[3] About half of the sexual partners of persons with chlamydial infection are also infected with this organism. The economic costs of chlamydial infection are estimated to be over $1 billion per year.[2] Chlamydial infection is more common in persons under age 25, especially adolescents.[2] Other risk factors for chlamydial infection in asymptomatic persons include having multiple sexual partners, a new sexual partner in the preceding two months, and a sexual partner with a chlamydial infection.[2]

About 8–12% of pregnant women have cervical chlamydial infections.[2] Infection during pregnancy can produce postpartum endometritis, and the organism is transmitted to the fetus in over half of deliveries. Each year more than 155,000 infants are born to *Chlamydia*-infected mothers.[2] Neonatal infection can result in ophthalmia neonatorum, nasopharyngeal colonization, and pneumonia.

Efficacy of Screening Tests

The most sensitive and specific test for detecting chlamydial infection in asymptomatic persons is direct culture. Urethral and endocervical cultures have been estimated to have a sensitivity of about 80–90% and a specificity of 100%.[4-9] Routine culture is not an ideal screening test, however, because the test is expensive, has limited availability, and requires special specimen storage procedures. Studies have shown that routine culture for *Chlamydia* is not a cost-effective strategy in asymptomatic persons.[10]

Recent technological developments have made available several screening tests that are potentially less expensive than cultures and have less complicated storage and transport requirements.[10,11] These include two methods for direct antigen testing (fluorescent antibody microscopy and enzyme-linked immunoassay) and serologic testing. Each test has important disadvantages, however, that currently limit its use as a routine screening test.[2,12] Fluorescent antibody microscopy has comparable sensitivity and specificity to chlamydial culture, but it is a labor-intensive procedure requiring special laboratory equipment and skilled technicians in order to produce reliable results. Enzyme-linked immunoassay (ELISA) does not require specially trained personnel and utilizes instruments that can produce standardized results in large volume, but its sensitivity and specificity for chlamydial infection are uncertain. Both tests, however, may be useful in areas where culture is not available or too costly. Serologic testing remains primarily a research tool due to difficulties associated with performing the laboratory procedure. Chlamydial cytology, once the only available test for detecting chlamydial infection, has been shown to be an insensitive screening test, except when evaluating newborn conjunctival scrapings, for which the sensitivity is 95% compared with culture.[2]

Effectiveness of Early Detection

Early detection of chlamydial infections in asymptomatic persons permits initiation of antibiotic therapy and prevention of complications. There have been few controlled studies examining whether early detection and treatment of asymptomatic persons result in improved outcome. It is thought, however, that occult infections, which may result in serious complications, account for a large proportion of chlamydial infections (up to 80% in women and 10–20% in men).[2] Over 95% of such infections can be cured with a seven-day course of an appropriate antibiotic.[2] Treatment failures are usually due to failure to treat sexual partners, noncompliance with therapy, reinfection, or laboratory error. There is also evidence that *Chlamydia* screening of pregnant women and treatment of positives with erythromycin can reduce the incidence of neonatal infections,[13,14] but a randomized controlled trial is needed to provide conclusive evidence of efficacy.

It is not known whether the yield of screening and the benefits of reduced morbidity are of sufficient magnitude to justify their considerable costs. In a recent study, the charge per test was $25 for culture and $12 for direct antigen testing.[10] Several centers have attempted to examine the cost-effectiveness of screening for *Chlamydia* under various conditions. They have found that routine testing is cost-effective for women attending clinics for sexually transmitted diseases who do not receive empirical antichlamydial therapy[4] or at routine gynecologic visits if the prevalence of *Chlamydia* in the patient population exceeds 7%.[15] Another study concluded that screening was cost-effective if the prevalence was 8% and if only direct antigen testing was used.[10] Others have disagreed with the assumptions used in such studies and have suggested that screening is appropriate in settings with lower prevalence.[16,17]

Recommendations of Others

The Centers for Disease Control (CDC) recommends chlamydial testing in asymptomatic persons who attend clinics for sexually transmitted diseases and who otherwise would not receive antichlamydial treatment; attenders of other high-risk health care facilities (e.g., adolescent and family planning clinics); and persons in urban settings who otherwise would not be offered chlamydial treatment and who are younger, of low socioeconomic status, or have multiple sexual partners.[2]

The CDC also recommends *Chlamydia* screening at the first prenatal visit of pregnant women who are less than 20 years of age, unmarried, have multiple sexual partners, or have a history of another sexually transmitted disease.[2] The Canadian Task Force also recommends screening high-risk groups and pregnant women.[18] The American College of Obstetricians and Gynecologists recommends chlamydial culture at the first prenatal visit and during the third trimester in pregnant women at increased risk (e.g., those who are single, less than 20 years old, reside in a socially disadvantaged community [e.g., inner city], have other sexually transmitted diseases, or begin prenatal care late).[19]

The CDC[2] and the American Academy of Pediatrics[20] recommend instilling erythromycin ophthalmic ointment, tetracycline ointment, or silver nitrate into the eyes of newborns as soon as possible after birth to prevent both gonococcal and chlamydial ophthalmia neonatorum.

Discussion

The efficacy of antibiotic therapy for maternal chlamydial infection in preventing neonatal complications requires further study, but there is some evidence that topical application of erythromycin ophthalmic ointment (and probably tetracycline) after birth can reduce the incidence of chlamydial ophthalmia neonatorum.[21,22] These topical antibiotics do not prevent nasopharyngeal chlamydial infection or pneumonia.[2] Silver nitrate, an agent that is effective against gonococcal ophthalmia neonatorum, does not prevent chlamydial conjunctivitis.[23]

Clinical Intervention

Routine testing for *Chlamydia trachomatis* is recommended for asymptomatic persons who attend clinics for sexually transmitted diseases, attend other high-risk health care facilities (e.g., adolescent and family planning clinics), or have other risk factors for chlamydial infection (e.g., age less than 20, multiple sexual partners, or a sexual partner with multiple sexual contacts). The optimal frequency of such testing has not been determined and is left to clinical discretion. Recent sexual partners of persons with positive cultures also require testing and treatment. Pregnant women in the high-risk categories listed above should be tested for *Chlamydia* at the first prenatal visit. Erythromycin 0.5% ophthalmic ointment or tetracycline 1% ophthalmic ointment should be applied topically to the eyes of all newborns as soon as possible after birth and no later than 1 hour of age.

Note: See Appendix A for the U.S. Preventive Services Task Force Table of Ratings for this topic. See also the relevant Task Force background paper: Horsburgh CR, Douglas JM, LaForce FM. Preventive strategies in sexually transmitted diseases for the primary care physician. JAMA 1987; 258:814–21.

REFERENCES

1. National Institutes of Health. NIAID Study Group on Sexually Transmitted Diseases: 1980 status report. Summaries and panel recommendations. Washington, D.C.: Government Printing Office, 1981: 215–64.
2. Centers for Disease Control. *Chlamydia trachomatis* infections: policy guidelines for prevention and control. MMWR [Suppl 3] 1985; 34.
3. Thompson SE, Washington AE. Epidemiology of sexually transmitted *Chlamydia trachomatis* infections. Epidemiol Rev 1983; 5:96–123.
4. Nettleman MD, Jones RB, Roberts SD, et al. Cost-effectiveness of serology and cell

culture for *Chlamydia trachomatis*: a study in a clinic for sexually transmitted diseases. Ann Intern Med 1986; 105:189–96.

5. Jones RB, Katz BP, Van Der Pol B, et al. Effect of blind passage and multiple sampling on recovery of *Chalmydia trachomatis* from urogenital specimens. J Clin Microbiol 1986; 24:1029–33.

6. Dunlop EM, Goh BT, Darougar S, et al. Triple-culture tests for diagnosis of chlamydial infection of the female genital tract. Sex Transm Dis 1985; 12:68–71.

7. Embil JA, Thiebaux HJ, Manuel FR, et al. Sequential cervical specimens and the isolation of *Chlamydia trachomatis*: factors affecting detection. Sex Transm Dis 1983; 10:62–6.

8. Uyeda CT, Welborn P, Ellison-Birang N, et al. Rapid diagnosis of chlamydial infection with the MicroTrak direct test. J Clin Microbiol 1984; 20:948–50.

9. Schachter J. Biology of *Chlamydia trachomatis*. In: Holmes KK, Mardh PA, Sparling PF, et al., eds. Sexually transmitted diseases. New York: McGraw Hill, 1984:243–57.

10. Nettleman MD, Jones RB. Cost-effectiveness of screening women at moderate risk for genital infections caused by *Chlamydia trachomatis*. JAMA 1988; 260:207–13.

11. Baselski VS, McNeeley SG, Ryan G, et al. A comparison of nonculture-dependent methods for detection of *Chlamydia trachomatis* infections in pregnant women. Obstet Gynecol 1987; 70:47–52.

12. Smith JW, Rogers RE, Katz BP, et al. Diagnosis of chlamydial infection in women attending antenatal and gynecologic clinics. J Clin Microbiol 1987; 25:868–72.

13. Schachter J, Sweet RL, Grossman M, et al. Experience with the routine use of erythromycin for chlamydial infections in pregnancy. N Engl J Med 1986; 314:276.

14. McMillan JA, Weiner LB, Lamberson HV, et al. Efficacy of maternal screening and therapy in the prevention of chlamydial infection of the newborn. Infection 1985; 13:263.

15. Phillips RS, Aronson MD, Taylor WC, et al. Should tests for *Chlamydia trachomatis* cervical infection be done during routine gynecologic visits? An analysis of the costs of alternative strategies. Ann Intern Med 1987; 107:188–94.

16. Handsfield HH, Jasman LL, Roberts PL, et al. Criteria for selective screening of *Chlamydia trachomatis* infection in women attending family planning clinics. JAMA 1986; 255:1730–4.

17. Rieger D. The predictive power and cost of screening for *Chlamydia* (letter). JAMA 1988; 260:3590.

18. Canadian Task Force on the Periodic Health Examination. The periodic health examination, 1984 update. Can Med Assoc J 1984; 130:1278–85.

19. American College of Obstetricians and Gynecologists. Gonorrhea and chlamydial infections. ACOG Technical Bulletin No. 89. Washington, D.C.: American College of Obstetricians and Gynecologists, 1985.

20. American Academy of Pediatrics. Prophylaxis and treatment of neonatal gonococcal infections. Pediatrics 1980; 65:1047–8.

21. Bernstein GA, Davis JP, Katcher ML. Prophylaxis of neonatal conjunctivitis. Clin Pediatr 1982; 21:545–50.

22. Hammerschlag MR, Chandler JW, Alexander ER, et al. Erythromycin ointment for ocular prophylaxis of neonatal chlamydial infection. JAMA 1980; 244:2291–3.

23. Treatment of sexually transmitted diseases. Medical Letter 1988; 30:5–10.

26

Screening for Genital
Herpes Simplex

Recommendation: Screening for genital herpes simplex virus (HSV) infection is recommended for pregnant women with active lesions (see *Clinical Intervention*).

Burden of Suffering

Primary episodes of genital herpes occur each year in approximately 200,000 to 500,000 Americans,[1] and as many as 20 million persons are already infected.[2] The chief morbidity associated with infection with the herpes simplex viruses (HSV-1 or HSV-2) are painful vesicular and ulcerative lesions that erupt in the anogenital and oral-facial areas.[0] About 4% of symptomatic primary episodes require hospitalization.[4] In most cases the virus establishes latent infections in spinal cord ganglia, and over a period of years the patient may experience periodic episodes of herpetic eruptions. Sexual contacts of persons with active and inactive disease are at risk of becoming infected. Pregnant women with genital herpes infection can transmit the infection to the newborn during vaginal delivery. An estimated 400 to 1000 cases of neonatal herpes occur each year in the United States.[5] Neonates have the highest frequency of visceral and central nervous system infection of any HSV-infected patient population.[3] If untreated, death occurs in 65% of infants; less than 10% of survivors with central nervous system infection have normal development.[3] Genital herpes costs the United States an estimated $500 million per year.[6]

Efficacy of Screening Tests

The sensitivity of all tests for herpes simplex depends primarily on the stage of the lesion at the time of testing and whether the patient is experiencing a primary or recurrent episode.[3] The principal test for detecting herpes simplex, viral culture, has excellent sensitivity (95%) during primary episodes and moderate sensitivity (65%) during recurrent episodes, but its sensitivity and specificity when performed on asymptomatic persons is uncertain. In addition, viral culture is expensive, not universally available, and results are often available only after two to four days.[3] More rapid diagnostic methods, such as cytology (Papanicolaou or Tzanck smear), immunoperoxidase tests, immunofluorescence, and enzyme immunoassay, have been proposed for screening, but they appear to be less sensitive than viral culture.[7]

Since an estimated 70–80% of infants with neonatal herpes are born to women with no history or physical findings of genital herpes at the time of delivery,[8,9] screening asymptomatic pregnant women has the potential of identifying undetected carriers and preventing neonatal transmission. Routine screening of pregnant women is likely to have low yield, however; even in women with a history of genital herpes predating the pregnancy, HSV can be isolated during asymptomatic intervals in only 1% of cultures.[10] In addition, a positive test result in an asymptomatic woman may be of limited value in predicting the risk of transmission during delivery, especially if active lesions are not present during labor.[11] Even for infants of mothers with a history of recurrent infection who are exposed to HSV at the time of delivery, the risk of infection is thought to be less than 10%.[12]

Effectiveness of Early Detection

The isolation of herpes virus in asymptomatic nonpregnant persons is of limited value. There is no effective treatment for eradicating latent herpes infections or completely preventing recurrences.[3,13] Oral acyclovir reduces the duration of painful episodes, viral shedding, and systemic symptoms in primary herpes infection;[13] it may also help prevent recurrent episodes in patients with very frequent or severe recurrent genital herpes.[14] Little information is available, however, on its effect on asymptomatic viral shedding. Further data are also needed on the long-term toxicity of this agent, the frequency with which resistant strains emerge, and the effects of long-term therapy on transmission.[3]

Early detection of herpes is of greater importance during pregnancy, however, because cesarean section can be performed to prevent transmission of the virus to the newborn. This has been shown to result in lower mortality. In one study, weekly cultures beginning at the 36th week were performed on 57 pregnant women with culture-verified HSV infection; cesarean section was performed if the culture preceding the onset of labor was positive or the disease became reactivated.[15] The investigators found very low neonatal mortality, with 58 of the 60 newborns surviving. This and similar studies, however, have lacked controls and randomization.

More definitive prospective studies are needed to determine the proper indications for operative delivery, especially when the risk of HSV transmission during delivery is reduced (e.g., in women without laboratory or clinical evidence of active disease in the week preceding delivery), or when the opportunity for preventing transmission has passed (e.g., long after rupture of membranes). In these situations, the potential benefits to the fetus may not outweigh the risk of potential maternal complications associated with cesarean section. Even when performed before rupture of membranes, cesarean section may not be completely effective in preventing neonatal infection. Randomized controlled trials to assess these issues may be difficult to perform for ethical reasons. Decision analysis models have shown that weekly cultures in pregnant women with recurrent herpes would, in a cohort of 3.6 million women, prevent 11.3 neonatal deaths and 3.7 cases of severe mental retardation, but 3.3 women would die as a result of operative deliveries necessitated by culture results.[16] The costs of screening and cesarean sections for maternal HSV infections in this scenario were estimated at $61 million, or about $2 million for each case prevented.

A second preventive maneuver in addition to cesarean section is prophylactic treatment of the mother with acyclovir. However, due to the lack of information on the clinical efficacy and adverse effects of this agent during pregnancy, acyclovir is generally not recommended for pregnant women in the absence of life-threatening infections.[13]

Recommendations of Others

The American College of Obstetricians and Gynecologists recommends performing cultures for HSV in pregnant women with active lesions. Vaginal delivery is considered acceptable if there are no visible lesions at the onset of labor. The College considers weekly surveillance cultures unnecessary in the absence of visible lesions.[17] The American Academy of Pediatrics is currently revising its recommendations[18] on the testing of pregnant women and neonates for HSV infection.

Clinical Intervention

All pregnant women should be asked at the first prenatal visit whether they or their sexual contacts have had genital herpetic lesions. Women with active lesions should be cultured, but cultures are not necessary in the absence of active disease.

Note: See Appendix A for the U.S. Preventive Services Task Force Table of Ratings for this topic. See also the relevant Task Force background paper: Horsburgh CR, Douglas JM, LaForce FM. Preventive strategies in sexually transmitted diseases for the primary care physician. JAMA 1987; 258:814–21.

REFERENCES

1. Chuang TY, Su WPD, Perry HO, et al. Incidence and trend of herpes progenitals: a 15–year population study. Mayo Clinic Proc 1983; 58:436–41.
2. Guinan ME, Wolinsky SM, Reichman RC. Epidemiology of genital herpes simplex virus infection. Epidemiol Rev 1985; 7:127–46.
3. Corey L, Spear PG. Infections with herpes simplex viruses. N Engl J Med 1986; 314:749–57.
4. Corey L, Adams HG, Brown ZA, et al. Genital herpes simplex virus infections: clinical manifestations, course, and complications. Ann Intern Med 1983; 98:958–72.
5. Nahmias AJ, Keyserling HL, Kerrick GM. Herpes simplex. In: Remington JS, Klein JO, eds. Infectious diseases of the fetus and newborn infant. Philadelphia: WB Saunders, 1983:636–78.
6. Cates W Jr. The "other STDs": do they really matter? JAMA 1988; 259:3606–8.
7. Whitley RJ, Hutto C. Neonatal herpes simplex virus infections. Pediatr Rev 1985; 7:119–26.
8. Jenista JA. Perinatal herpes virus infections. Semin Perinatol 1983; 7:9–15.
9. Stagno S, Whitley RJ. Herpes virus infections of pregnancy. Part II. Herpes simplex virus and varicella-zoster virus infections. N Engl J Med 1985; 313:1327–30.
10. Brown ZA, Vontver LA, Benedetti J, et al. Genital herpes in pregnancy: risk factors associated with recurrences and asymptomatic viral shedding. Am J Obstet Gynecol 1985; 153:24–30.
11. Arvin AM, Hensleigh PA, Prober CG, et al. Failure of antepartum maternal cultures to predict the infant's risk of exposure to herpes simplex virus at delivery. N Engl J Med 1986; 315:796–800.
12. Prober SG, Sullender WM, Yasukawa LL, et al. Low risk of herpes simplex virus infections in neonates exposed to the virus at the time of vaginal delivery to mothers with recurrent genital herpes simplex virus infections. N Engl J Med 1987; 316:240–4.
13. Baker DA, Milch PO. Acyclovir for genital herpes simplex virus infections: a review. J Reprod Med 1986; 31:433–8.
14. Straus SE, Croen KD, Sawyer MH, et al. Acyclovir suppression of frequently recurring genital herpes: efficacy and diminishing need during successive years of treatment. JAMA 1988; 260:2227–30.
15. Grossman JH III, Wallen WC, Sever JL. Management of genital herpes simplex virus infection during pregnancy. Obstet Gynecol 1981; 58:1–4.

16. Binkin NJ, Kaplan JP, Cates W. Preventing neonatal herpes: the value of weekly viral cultures in pregnant women with recurrent genital herpes. JAMA 1984; 251:2816–21.
17. American College of Obstetricians and Gynecologists. Perinatal herpes simplex virus infections. ACOG Technical Bulletin No. 122. Washington, D.C.: American College of Obstetricians and Gynecologists, 1988.
18. American Academy of Pediatrics. Perinatal herpes simplex virus infection. Pediatrics 1980; 66:147–8.

27

Screening for Asymptomatic Bacteriuria, Hematuria, and Proteinuria

Recommendation: Periodic urine testing of asymptomatic persons is recommended for those with diabetes mellitus and for pregnant women. In addition, it may also be clinically prudent to screen preschool children and persons aged 60 and older (see *Clinical Intervention*).

Burden of Suffering

A number of disorders that cause bacteriuria, hematuria, and proteinuria are associated with significant morbidity and mortality. Asymptomatic bacteriuria often precedes symptomatic urinary tract infection, which accounts for over 6 million outpatient visits each year.[1] (There are over 300,000 hospitalizations each year for urinary tract infections,[1] but these generally involve patients with indwelling urethral catheters.) In adults, bacteriuria and urinary tract infection may be associated with renal insufficiency, hypertension, and increased mortality. In pregnant women, bacteriuria is a risk factor for prematurity and low birthweight.[2] In children, about 13–17% of cases with recurrent bacteriuria develop chronic pyelonephritis, and 23–29% have evidence of vesicoureteral reflux.[3] Children with significant structural abnormalities are at increased risk of renal scarring, obstructive atrophy, hypertension, and renal insufficiency.

The risk of acquiring bacteriuria varies with age and sex. Asymptomatic bacteriuria during infancy is more common in boys (prevalence of 2–4%), but pediatric bacteriuria is considerably more common in girls after age 1.[4] Approximately 5–6% of girls have at least one episode of bacteriuria between first grade and their graduation from high school,and as many as 80% of these children experience recurrent infections.[4] Bacteriuria occurs in 4–7% of pregnant women and 10–20% of diabetic women.[5,6] The incidence of asymptomatic bacteriuria increases with age, and thus it is a common finding in the elderly, especially the very old and the institutionalized elderly.[4]

Hematuria and proteinuria are often the first detectable signs of urologic cancer and end-stage renal disease due to hypertension, diabetes, or glomerulonephritis. These diseases carry a significant burden of suffering. Kidney, bladder, and other urologic cancers will account for over 70,000 new cases and over 20,000 deaths in the United States in 1989.[7] Renal dysfunction of any form can contribute to the morbidity and mortality of diseases such as hypertension, heart failure, and liver disease, and it can limit the use of therapeutic drugs and contrast agents. About 92,000 Americans receive chronic dialysis for end-stage renal disease,[8] while an additional 175,000 acute dialyses are performed yearly on hospitalized patients.[1] Kidney transplantation is necessary in about 8400 persons each year.[8]

Efficacy of Screening Tests

Dipstick urinalysis is the most common test for detecting urinary tract disorders in asymptomatic persons. Multi-pad "dipstick" reagent strips can detect a variety of disorders, including bacteriuria (nitrite test), pyuria (leukocyte esterase test), hematuria (heme test), and proteinuria (tetrabromphenol test). Screening for bacteriuria may be impractical in infants, however, because positive dipstick tests are often contaminated (false positives) and require the collection of confirmatory sterile culture specimens by suprapubic aspiration. This procedure is too invasive and costly to be considered in a routine screening protocol for asymptomatic infants.

The most accurate test for bacteriuria is urine culture, but laboratory charges make this test too expensive for routine screening. Moreover, results are usually not available for at least 24 hours. The dipstick leukocyte esterase (LE) test, by detecting pyuria, is an indirect test for bacteriuria. When compared with culture (at least 100,000 organisms/mL), it has a sensitivity of 72–97% and a specificity of 64–82%.[9-14] The nitrite reduction test, which detects bacteriuria, has variable sensitivity (35–85%), but good specificity (92–100%).[9-13,15-23] The sensitivity of this test can be improved by obtaining first-morning specimens, preferably on consecutive days, rather than by performing random collection.[15] In detecting hematuria (more than two to five red blood cells per high-powered field in the sediment of centrifuged urine), dipstick urinalysis has a sensitivity of 91–100% and a specificity of 65–99%;[9,24-35] the sensitivity and specificity are 95–99% in detecting proteinuria.[36] False-positive and false-negative urinalysis results are due to a variety of factors, including specimen contamination, certain organisms, the timing of specimen collection, interfering substances (urobilinogen, glucose, ascorbic acid, drugs, urine cells and bacteria), other urine properties (specific gravity, pH, concentration), and biological factors (exercise, cold exposure, prolonged recumbency, medical illness). Examination of the sediment by microscopic urinalysis has limited value as a screening test for asymptomatic persons. Studies have reported a diagnostic yield of less than 3% in detecting clinically significant disorders by routine microscopic examination of urine that is grossly normal.[34,35]

In populations with a low prevalence of urinary tract disorders, most positive urinalyses are falsely positive. Thus, in asymptomatic men and in asymptomatic women under age 60, a dipstick test for bacteriuria has a positive predictive value of less than 10% (assuming a sensitivity of 85% and a specificity of 70%).[17,37-39] In groups at increased risk for urinary tract infection, the positive predictive value is higher: 13% in pregnant women, 18% in women over age 60, 33% in diabetic women, and 44% in the institutionalized elderly.[5,6,17,37,39-44] For similar reasons, the positive predictive value of a dipstick test for hematuria or proteinuria in the general population is 6–45% for disorders of possible clinical significance (e.g., asymptomatic bacteriuria, nonstaghorn calculi, mild glomerulonephritis) and less than 2% for serious urologic diseases (e.g., urogenital tumors, tuberculosis, staghorn calculi, vasculitis, nephritides, obstructive lesions).[45-50] In older men, a population at increased risk, studies have found that only 4–5% of men develop cancer or other urologic diseases in the first three years after the test.[48,49] A more recent study of men over age 50, however, reported a higher positive predictive value (26%), possibly due to the use of more sophisticated diagnostic follow-up studies to detect cancer.[32] Due to the frequently intermittent nature of hematuria and proteinuria in persons with urologic cancer, a single screening test for these abnormalities may have less sensitivity in detecting cases than periodic testing, but further comparative data are needed.

Effectiveness of Early Detection

The early detection of urinary tract malignancy may improve survival, and the detection of hematuria or proteinuria may be the first indication of disease in asymptomatic persons.[51] Survival from bladder cancer, for example, is directly related to the stage of the disease at diagnosis; the five-year survival rate is 72% for persons with localized disease but only 3% for those with advanced bladder cancer.[7] However, lead-time and length biases may contribute to these differences in survival. No controlled prospective studies have demonstrated that persons with bladder or other urologic cancers identified through screening have lower mortality than do those detected without screening. Primary prevention may offer a more effective strategy than screening in reducing mortality from urologic cancer; smoking accounts for 48% of all deaths from cancer of the kidney and 47% of all deaths from bladder cancer (see Chapter 48).

The early detection of asymptomatic bacteriuria may prevent symptomatic infection and its complications, but the evidence is inconsistent regarding the effectiveness of antibiotic treatment in preventing these outcomes.[37,52,53] Some studies suggest that persons with untreated asymptomatic bacteriuria are at increased risk of developing symptomatic urinary tract infection[52,54] and other complications (e.g., structural damage, renal insufficiency, hypertension, mortality).[38,40-44,55-57] There is little conclusive evidence, however, that these clinical outcomes are caused by bacteriuria (especially in the absence of a structural abnormality) or that they can be prevented by antibiotic therapy. The treatment of asymptomatic bacteriuria in the elderly, although associated with high recurrence rates in institutionalized patients, may be of benefit in the ambulatory setting. Two randomized controlled trials in elderly women have shown that treatment can reduce the incidence of subsequent bacteriuria (and possibly of symptomatic urinary tract infection).[53,54] It is not clear, however, whether this effect is of sufficient benefit to justify routine screening or the potential adverse effects of antibiotic therapy in the elderly, including drug toxicity and the development of resistant organisms while treating recurrent infections.

The early detection of asymptomatic bacteriuria is of greater potential value for pregnant women and children, in whom bacteriuria is an established risk factor for serious complications. About 20–40% of untreated pregnant women with asymptomatic bacteriuria develop symptomatic urinary tract infection.[58] These women are at increased risk of fetal prematurity and low birthweight, as well as of subsequent maternal chronic renal disease.[39,59,60] Several randomized controlled trials have shown that treatment of asymptomatic bacteriuria during pregnancy can reduce the incidence of symptomatic urinary tract infection and premature delivery.[39,61,62]

In children, detection of bacteriuria can lead to the detection of correctable abnormalities of the urinary tract and the prevention of renal scarring, obstructive atrophy, hypertension, and renal insufficiency. Most of these complications are thought to occur before children reach school age,[3,4] and therefore, screening would appear to be most effective in the preschool years. However, there have been few studies proving that preschool urinalyses result in lower morbidity from recurrent infection or less renal damage.[3,4,63,64] Screening during infancy might also be effective, but it is not currently feasible due to the unavailability of a screening test that is both accurate (not affected by bacterial contaminants) and noninvasive.

The effectiveness of detecting asymptomatic bacteriuria in patients with in-dwelling urethral catheters is not discussed in this report. This form of testing is considered within the domain of diagnostic studies for patients with underlying medical or surgical conditions, rather than of routine screening tests for asymptomatic persons.

Recommendations of Others

The American Academy of Pediatrics (AAP) recommends a single urinalysis during infancy.[65] Screening of preschool children has also been recommended by the AAP and the National Kidney Foundation.[3,64] Screening of schoolchildren is recommended by the AAP during late childhood and early adolescence.[65] Other authorities recommend screening only those in high-risk groups, such as children with diabetes or congenital defects of the urinary tract.[4]

Recommendations against routine screening urinalyses in asymptomatic adults have been issued by the Canadian Task Force[66] and other reviewers.[67-70] Urinalysis screening in adults is generally considered more appropriate for persons at risk for bladder cancer (e.g., persons with heavy exposure to cigarette smoke and other bladder carcinogens); the Canadian Task Force recommends urine cytologic screening in such persons.[66] The Canadian Task Force also recommends urine cultures during pregnancy. The American College of Obstetricians and Gynecologists recommends a urinalysis at each prenatal visit and urine culture for women with abnormal urinalysis or risk factors for urinary tract infection.[71,72]

Discussion

Screening urinalysis appears to be especially important during pregnancy, where there is strong evidence that treatment is efficacious. There are, however, inadequate data to determine the optimal frequency of urine testing during pregnancy or whether prenatal testing should be carried out by urine culture (rather than by urinalysis) to reduce the risk of false negatives. Screening for asymptomatic bacteriuria may also be beneficial in preschool children to help prevent permanent renal damage, but further studies are needed to establish its effectiveness. Screening urinalysis may be appropriate in high-risk groups, such as the elderly and persons with diabetes mellitus, but again firm evidence of benefit is limited. Screening is not justified in the general population because serious urinary tract disorders are relatively uncommon, the positive predictive value of screening urinalysis is low, and the effectiveness of early detection and treatment is unproved.

Clinical Intervention

Periodic testing for asymptomatic bacteriuria is recommended for persons with diabetes and for pregnant women, and it may also be clinically prudent in preschool children. The optimal frequency for urine testing in these groups has not been determined and is left to clinical discretion. The urine specimen should be obtained in a manner that minimizes contamination. Persons with abnormal results should receive further evaluation. In general, dipsticks combining the leukocyte esterase and nitrite tests should be used to detect asymptomatic bacteriuria. However, urine culture is a more accurate screening test than is dipstick urinalysis, and it is recommended for detecting asymptomatic bacteriuria during pregnancy.

Dipstick urinalysis for asymptomatic bacteriuria, hematuria, and proteinuria may also be clinically prudent in persons over age 60. Urinalysis is not

recommended as a screening test to detect diabetes mellitus (see Chapter 16) or preeclampsia (Chapter 35) in asymptomatic persons.

Note: See Appendix A for the U.S. Preventive Services Task Force Table of Ratings for this topic. See also the relevant Task Force background papers: Woolhandler S, Pels RJ, Bor DH, et al. Screening asymptomatic adults for hematuria and proteinuria: dipstick urinalysis; and Pels RJ, Bor DH, Woolhandler S, et al. Screening asymptomatic adults for bacteriuria. In: Goldbloom RB, Lawrence RS, eds. Preventing disease: beyond the rhetoric. New York: Springer-Verlag (in press).

REFERENCES

1. National Center for Health Statistics. Detailed diagnoses and procedures for patients discharged from short-stay hospitals: United States, 1985. Vital and Health Statistics, series 13, no. 90. Washington, D.C.: Government Printing Office, 1987. (Publication no. DHHS (PHS) 87–1751.)
2. Institute of Medicine, Division of Health Promotion and Disease Prevention. Preventing low birth weight. Washington, D.C.: National Academy Press, 1985.
3. American Academy of Pediatrics, Section on Urology. Screening school children for urologic disease. Pediatrics 1977; 60:239–43.
4. Kunin CM. Detection, prevention and management of urinary tract infections, 4th ed. Philadelphia: Lea and Febiger, 1987.
5. Norden CW, Kass EH. Bacteriuria of pregnancy: a critical appraisal. Ann Rev Med 1968; 19:431–70.
6. National Diabetes Data Group. Diabetes in America: diabetes data compiled 1984. Washington, D.C.: Government Printing Office, 1985. (Publication no. DHHS (NIH) 85–1468.)
7. American Cancer Society. Cancer statistics, 1989. CA 1989; 39:3–20.
8. Burton BT, National Institute of Diabetes and Digestive and Kidney Diseases. Personal communication, 1988.
9. Loo SY, Scottolini AG, Luangphinith S, et al. Urine screening strategy employing dipstick analysis and selective culture: an evaluation. Am J Clin Pathol 1984; 81:634–42.
10. Oneson R, Groschel DH. Leukocyte esterase activity and nitrite test as a rapid screen for significant bacteriuria. Am J Clin Pathol 1985; 83:84–7.
11. Pfaller MA, Koontz FP. Laboratory evaluation of leukocyte esterase and nitrite tests for the detection of bacteriuria. J Clin Microbiol 1985; 21:840–2.
12. Jones C, MacPherson DW, Stevens DL. Inability of the chemstrip LN compared with quantitative urine culture to predict significant bacteriuria. J Clin Microbiol 1986; 23:160–2.
13. Doern GV, Saubolle MA, Sewell DL. Screening for bacteriuria with the LN strip test. Diagn Microbiol Infect Dis 1986; 4:355–8.
14. Males BM, Bartholomew WR, Amsterdam D. Leukocyte esterase-nitrite and bioluminescence assays as urine screens. J Clin Microbiol 1985; 22:531–4.
15. Alwall N, Lohi A. Factors affecting the reliability of screening tests for bacteriuria I. Acta Med Scand 1973; 193:499–503.
16. James GP, Paul KL, Fuller JB. Urinary nitrite and urinary tract infection. Am J Clin Pathol 1978; 70:671–8.
17. Kunin CM, DeGroot JE. Self-screening for significant bacteriuria. JAMA 1975; 231:1349–53.
18. Czerwinski AW, Wilkerson RG, Merrill JA, et al. Further evaluation of the Griess test to detect significant bacteriuria. Am J Obstet Gynecol 1971; 110:677–81.
19. Finnerty FA, Johnson AC. A simplified accurate method for detecting bacteriuria. Am J Obstet Gynecol 1968; 101:238–43.
20. Kincaid-Smith P, Bullen M, Mills J, et al. The reliability of screening tests for bacteriuria in pregnancy. Lancet 1964; 2:61–2.

21. Takagi LR, Mruz RM, Vanderplow MG. Screening obstetric outpatients for bacteriuria. J Reprod Med 1975; 15:229–31.
22. Archbald FJ, Verma U, Tajani NA. Screening for asymptomatic bacteriuria with microstix. J Reprod Med 1984; 29:272–4.
23. Sleigh JD. Detection of bacteriuria by a modification of the nitrite test. Br Med J 1965; 1:765–7.
24. Sewell DL, Burt SP, Gabbert NJ, et al. Evaluation of the Chemstrip 9 as a screening test for urinalysis and urine culture in men. Am J Clin Pathol 1985; 83:740–3.
25. Mariani AJ, Luangphinith S, Loo S, et al. Dipstick chemical urinalysis: an accurate cost-effective screening test. J Urol 1984; 132:64–6.
26. Freedman SI. Routine microscopic examination of the urinary sediment (letter). Arch Pathol Lab Med 1984; 108:855.
27. Sarewitz SI. Routine microscopic examination of the urinary sediment (letter). Arch Pathol Lab Med 1984; 108:855.
28. Kiechle FL, Karcher RE, Epstein E. Routine microscopic examination of the urinary sediment (letter). Arch Pathol Lab Med 1984; 108:855–6.
29. Hearne CR, Donnell MG, Fraser CG. Assessment of new urinalysis dipstick. Clin Chem 1980; 26:170–1.
30. Shaw ST, Poon SY, Wong ET. Routine urinalysis: is the dipstick enough? JAMA 1985; 253:1596–1600.
31. Szwed JJ, Schaust C. The importance of microscopic examination of the urinary sediment. Am J Med Tech 1982; 48:141–3.
32. Messing EM, Young TB, Hunt VB, et al. The significance of asymptomatic microhematuria in men 50 or more years old: findings of a home screening study using urinary dipsticks. J Urol 1987; 137:919–22.
33. Smalley DL, Bryan JA. Comparative evaluation of biochemical and microscopic urinalysis. Am J Med Tech 1983; 49:237–9.
34. Schumann GB, Greenberg NF. Usefulness of macroscopic urinalysis as a screening procedure. Am J Clin Pathol 1979; 71:452–6.
35. Schumann GB, Greenberg NF, Henry JB. Microscopic look at urine often unnecessary. JAMA 1978; 239:13–4.
36. Simpson E, Thompson D. Routine urinalysis. Lancet 1977; 2:361–2.
37. Bengtsson C, Bengtsson U, Lincoln K. Bacteriuria in a population sample of women. Acta Med Scand 1980; 208:417–23.
38. Sussman M, Asscher AW, Waters WE, et al. Asymptomatic significant bacteriuria in the non-pregnant woman I. Description of a population. Br Med J 1969; 1:799–803.
39. Kass EH. Pyelonephritis and bacteriuria. Ann Intern Med 1962; 56:46–53.
40. Dontas AS, Papanayiotou P, Marketos S, et al. Bacteriuria in old age. Lancet 1966; 2:305–6.
41. Walkey FA, Judge TG, Thompson J, et al. Incidence of urinary tract infection in the elderly. Scott Med J 1967; 12:411–4.
42. Dontas AS, Papanayiotou P, Marketos SG, et al. The effect of bacteriuria on renal function patterns in old age. Clin Sci 1968; 34:73–81.
43. Alwall N, Lohi A. A population study on renal and urinary tract diseases I. Acta Med Scand 1973; 194:525–8.
44. Sourander LB, Kasanen A. A 5–year follow-up of bacteriuria in the aged. Gerontol Clin 1972; 14:274–81.
45. Froom P, Ribak J, Benbassat. Significance of microhaematuria in young adults. Br Med J 1984; 288:20–2.
46. Chen BTM, Ooi BS, Tan KK, et al. Comparative studies of asymptomatic proteinuria and hematuria. Arch Intern Med 1974; 134: 901–5.
47. Alwall N, Lohi A. A population study of renal and urinary tract diseases II. Acta Med Scand 1973; 194:529–35.
48. Mohr DN, Offord KP, Owen RA, et al. Asymptomatic microhematuria and urologic disease. JAMA 1986; 256:224–9.
49. Mohr DN, Offord KP, Melton LJ. Isolated asymptomatic microhematuria: a cross sectional analysis of test-positive and test-negative patients. J Gen Intern Med 1987; 2:318–24.

50. VonBonsdorff M, Koskenvuo K, Salmi HA, et al. Prevalence and causes of proteinuria in 20 your old Finnish men. Scand J Urol Nephrol 1981; 15:205–90.

51. Carter HB, Amberson JB, Bander NH, et al. Newer diagnostic techniques for bladder cancer. Urol Clin 1987; 14:763–9.

52. Asscher AW, Sussman M, Waters WE, et al. Asymptomatic significant bacteriuria in the non-pregnant woman II. Response to treatment and follow-up. Br Med J 1969; 1: 804–6.

53. Evans DA, Brauner E, Warren JW, et al. Randomized trial of vigorous antimicrobial therapy of bacteriuria in a community population. In: Program and Abstracts of the Twenty-Seventh Interscience Conference on Antimicrobial Agents and Chemotherapy. New York: American Society for Microbiology, 1987:148.

54. Boscia JA, Kobasa WD, Knight RA, et al. Therapy vs. no therapy for bacteriuria in elderly ambulatory nonhospitalized women. JAMA 1987; 257:1067–71.

55. Nordenstam GR, Branberg CA, Oden AS, et al. Bacteriuria and mortality in an elderly population. N Engl J Med 1986; 314:1152–6.

56. Dontas AS, Kasviki-Charvati P, Papanayiotou P, et al. Bacteriuria and survival in old age. N Engl J Med 1981; 304:939–43.

57. Evans DA, Kass EH, Hennekens CH, et al. Bacteriuria and subsequent mortality in women. Lancet 1982; 1:156–8.

58. Andriole VT. Advances in the treatment of urinary infections. J Antimicrob Chemother [Suppl A] 1982; 9:163–72.

59. Williams JD, Reeves DS, Condie AP, et al. Significance of bacteriuria during pregnancy. In: Kass EH, Brumfitt, eds. Infections of the urinary tract: proceedings of the Third International Symposium on Pyelonephritis. Chicago, Ill.: University of Chicago Press, 1978:8–18.

60. Zinner SH, Kass EH. Long-term (10 to 14 years) follow-up of bacteriuria of pregnancy. N Engl J Med 1971; 285:820–4.

61. Kass EH. Bacteriuria and pyelonephritis of pregnancy. Trans Assoc Am Physicians 1959; 72:257–64.

62. Kincaid-Smith P, Bullen M. Bacteriuria in pregnancy. Lancet 1965; 1:395–9.

63. Periodic Health Examination Monograph. Report of a Task Force to the Conference of Deputy Ministers of Health (cat.no.H39–3/1980E), Minister of Supply and Services, Ottawa, Canada, 1980:51.

64. Schwartz GJ, Edelmann CM. Screening for bacteriuria in children. Kidney 1975; 8: 11–4.

65. American Academy of Pediatrics, Committee on Practice and Ambulatory Medicine. Guidelines for health supervision of children and youth. Elk Grove, Ill.: American Academy of Pediatrics, 1981.

66. Canadian Task Force on the Periodic Health Examination. The periodic health examination. Can Med Assoc J 1979; 121:1–45.

67. Frame PS, Carlson SJ. A critical review of periodic health screening using specific screening criteria. Part 3. Selected diseases of the genitourinary system. J Fam Pract 1975; 2:189–94.

68. Kiel DP, Moskowitz MA. The urinalysis: a critical appraisal. Med Clin North Am 1987; 71.607–23.

69. Boscia JA, Abrutyn E, Kaye D. Asymptomatic bacteriuria in elderly persons: treat or do not treat? Ann Intern Med 1987; 106:764–6.

70. Akin BV, Hubbell FA, Frye EB, et al. Efficacy of routine admission urinalysis. Am J Med 1987; 82:719–22.

71. American College of Obstetricians and Gynecologists. Standards for obstetric-gynecologic services, 7th ed. Washington, D.C.: American College of Obstetricians and Gynecologists, 1989:17.

72. Kaminetzky HA, American College of Obstetricians and Gynecologists. Personal communication, September 1988.

28

Screening for Anemia

Recommendation: All infants and pregnant women·should be tested for anemia (see *Clinical Intervention*). Routine screening of other asymptomatic persons for anemia is not recommended in the absence of clinical indications.

Burden of Suffering

Anemia is not defined on the basis of clinical criteria but rather by the presence of a hemoglobin level that is below the normal range of values for the population. It is unclear whether low hemoglobin by itself produces significant health effects. Clearly, persons with markedly reduced levels are at risk for cardiopulmonary and other complications. However, the mild degree of anemia that is most often detected by screening asymptomatic persons may have little clinical impact. As early as the 1960s, researchers demonstrated that, in general, decreased hemoglobin by itself does not have readily apparent adverse effects unless it is below 10 g/dL (100 g/L).[1-3] Rather, the mortality and morbidity that are characteristically associated with anemia are more often the result of coexisting diseases, such as cancer.

Important exceptions occur in young children and pregnant women, who may suffer complications from anemia even in the absence of symptoms. Iron deficiency anemia during infancy and early childhood has been associated with impaired infant behavior and development.[4] Although mildly decreased hemoglobin during pregnancy is a normal physiologic response to expanded intravascular volume and increased demand for erythropoiesis, hemoglobin levels below what is considered normal for pregnancy have been associated with low birthweight, prematurity, and high perinatal mortality.[5-7]

The age groups in which anemia occurs most frequently are young children, women of reproductive age, and the elderly. The most common cause of anemia in the United States is iron deficiency. The prevalence of iron deficiency anemia during childhood has declined in recent years, due in part to iron fortification of food products,[8-10] but the prevalence of iron deficiency is currently estimated to be about 3% for children aged 1–5.[10] A hemoglobin below 12 g/dL (120 g/L) is present in about 9% of women aged 15–44[11] and is especially common during pregnancy. The prevalence of anemia (hemoglobin less than 12 g/dL [120 g/L]) in persons over age 65 is 2.3% in males and 5.5% in females.[11] Other populations at increased risk for anemia include blacks, some immigrants, and individuals of low socioeconomic status.[12]

Efficacy of Screening Tests

The hemoglobin concentration and hematocrit are the principal tests for detecting anemia. Studies have shown that automated electronic cell counters and chemical analyzers provide accurate and reliable data on red blood cell number and size and on the concentration of hemoglobin.[13,14] Although sampling of capillary blood is more convenient in ambulatory practice, and is especially useful for infant testing, results obtained from capillary blood specimens are less reliable than those from venous blood.[15,16] One study found the capillary microhematocrit to have a sensitivity of 90% and a specificity of 44% when compared with values obtained from venous blood with an automated cell counter.[16]

Tests for iron deficiency, the most common cause of anemia, include serum ferritin, transferrin saturation, and erythrocyte protoporphyrin. These tests are not suitable for primary screening due to their cost and the low prevalence of iron deficiency in the general population.[8,17]

Effectiveness of Early Detection

Evidence is lacking that early detection and treatment of anemia or iron deficiency in the absence of symptoms significantly reduces morbidity from these disorders.[1-3,18] Although the evaluation of anemia may disclose underlying diseases (e.g., occult malignancies) that benefit from early detection, there are no data to suggest that testing for anemia is an effective means of screening for these conditions. Infants with anemia do appear to benefit from early treatment. Prospective studies have documented improved developmental test scores among infants who have received enough supplemental iron to correct their iron deficiency.[4]

In addition, the early detection of anemia may also be of potential benefit during pregnancy. Epidemiologic studies have linked low maternal hemoglobin to intrauterine growth retardation, placental hypertrophy, prematurity, fetal distress, and perinatal death.[5-7] It is unclear from these largely retrospective studies, however, whether anemia causes these complications or is instead associated with other variables (e.g., poor nutrition, low socioeconomic status) that may be more directly responsible for poor outcome.[5,19] There is little firm evidence that maternal anemia causes anemia in the fetus.[20,21] In addition, most clinical trials have found that iron therapy, although efficacious in correcting red cell indices and iron stores, does not improve birthweight, length of gestation, or other outcome measures.[19] A moderate decline in maternal hemoglobin during pregnancy is a normal physiological response to increased intravascular volume; interventions to raise hemoglobin to normal nonpregnancy values may even have certain adverse effects.[22,23] On the other hand, the detection of anemia and the determination of its etiology may lead to the discovery of correctable obstetrical risks (e.g., poor nutritional status, medical illness) that might otherwise escape detection.

Recommendations of Others

A number of organizations recommend some form of anemia screening during infancy. The Canadian Task Force suggests hemoglobin measurement of infants who are premature, those born of a multiple pregnancy or of an iron-deficient woman, and those of low socioeconomic status. The test is recommended at birth or within the first week of life, followed by a measurement at age 9 months.[24] The American Academy of Pediatrics recommends a hemoglobin or hematocrit measurement at least once during infancy.[25] Similar recommendations for routine or selective screening of infants have been made by other experts.[18,26-29] Screening of older children and adolescents is advocated less consistently. The American Academy of Pediatrics recommends at least one measurement of hemoglobin or hematocrit at ages 1–4, 5–12, and 14–20.[26] The Canadian Task Force and other groups do not support anemia screening in children, with the exception of pregnant adolescents.[18,24,27-29]

Screening for anemia in adults has been the subject of inconsistent recommendations. Breslow and Somers advocate screening for anemia every five years;[27] the Institute of Medicine recommends measuring the hematocrit at least once during ages 40 to 59, 60 to 74, and beyond age 75;[30] and the Canadian Task Force describes adult screening as discretionary.[24] Other authorities have argued against screening nonpregnant adults unless they are immigrants from underdeveloped countries or the institutionalized elderly.[18,31,32] Prenatal screening for anemia is, however, recommended by the Canadian Task Force,[24] the American College of Obstetricians and Gynecologists,[33] and other reviewers.

Discussion

The burden of suffering of anemia in the general population is relatively low. Although it is prevalent in certain high-risk groups, mild anemia in the absence of symptoms has only subtle health consequences. Thus, although an accurate screening test for anemia may be available, there is relatively little evidence to suggest that early detection is beneficial. Treatment of some forms of anemia not caused by iron deficiency (e.g., vitamin B_{12} or folate deficiency) can produce dramatic results, but these disorders are too rare to justify mass screening. Finally, current evidence does not support the practice of screening for anemia in all asymptomatic individuals to detect coexisting diseases. There is therefore little basis for large-scale efforts to screen for anemia. Screening is reasonable for infants and pregnant women who appear to benefit from early correction of anemia.

Clinical Intervention

Except for pregnant women and infants, routine testing for anemia is not recommended for asymptomatic persons in the absence of clinical indications. A hemoglobin analysis should be obtained on all pregnant women at their first prenatal visit. Further prenatal testing for anemia is not necessary for asymptomatic women lacking evidence of medical or obstetrical complications. All infants should also be screened once for anemia. Although capillary blood specimens are easier to obtain in infants, a venous blood count provides more accurate and reliable data. Appropriate hematological studies and nutritional counseling should be provided for all persons with evidence of anemia.

REFERENCES

1. Elwood PC, Waters WE, Greene WJ, et al. Symptoms and circulating hemoglobin level. J Chron Dis 1969; 21:615–28.
2. Elwood PC. Evaluation of the clinical importance of anemia. Am J Clin Nutr 1973; 26: 958–64.
3. Elwood PC, Waters WE, Benjamin IT, et al. Mortality and anemia in women. Lancet 1974; 1:891–4.
4. Lozoff B, Brittenham GM, Wolf AW, et al. Iron deficiency anemia and iron therapy effects on infant developmental test performance. Pediatrics 1987; 79:981–95.

5. Harrison KA. Anaemia, malaria and sickle cell disease. Clin Obstet Gynecol 1982; 9: 445–77.
6. Kuizon MD, Cheong RL, Ancheta LP, et al. Effect of anaemia and other maternal characteristics on birthweight. Hum Nutr Clin Nutr 1985; 39C:419–26.
7. Murphy JF, O'Riordan J, Newcombe RG, et al. Relation of haemoglobin levels in first and second trimester to outcome of pregnancy. Lancet 1986; 1:992–4.
8. Expert Scientific Working Group. Summary of a report on assessment of the iron nutritional status of the United States population. Am J Clin Nutr 1985; 42:1318–30.
9. Vazquez-Seoane P, Windom R, Pearson HA. Disappearance of iron-deficiency anemia in a high-risk infant population given supplemental iron. N Engl J Med 1985; 313: 1239–40.
10. Yip R, Binkin NJ, Fleshood L, et al. Declining prevalence of anemia among low-income children in the United States. JAMA 1987; 258:1619–23.
11. National Center for Health Statistics. Hematological and nutritional biochemistry reference data for persons 6 months—74 years of age: United States, 1976–80. Vital and Health Statistics, series 11, no. 232. Washington, D.C.: Government Printing Office, 1982. (Publication no. DHHS (PHS) 83–1682.)
12. Life Sciences Research Office. Assessment of the iron nutritional status of the U.S. population based on data collected in the second National Health and Nutrition Examination Survey, 1976–1980. FDA contract no. 223–83–2384. Rockville, Md.: Food and Drug Administration, August 1984:50.
13. Mayer K, Chin B, Baisley A. Evaluation of the S-plus IV. Am J Clin Pathol 1985; 83: 40–6.
14. Cox CJ, Habermann TM, Payne BA, et al. Evaluation of the Coulter counter model S-Plus IV. Am J Clin Pathol 1985; 84:297–306.
15. Thomas WJ, Collins TM. Comparison of venipuncture blood counts with microcapillary measurements in screening for anemia in one-year-old infants. J Pediatr 1982; 101:32–5.
16. Young PC, Hamill B, Wasserman RC, et al. Evaluation of the capillary microhematocrit as a screening test for anemia in pediatric office practice. Pediatrics 1986; 78:206–9.
17. Dallman PR. New approaches to screening for iron deficiency. J Pediatr 1977; 90: 678–81.
18. Shapiro MF, Greenfield S. The complete blood count and leukocyte differential count: an approach to their rational application. Ann Intern Med 1987; 106:65–74.
19. Hemminki E, Starfield B. Routine administration of iron and vitamins during pregnancy: review of controlled clinical trials. Br J Obstet Gynecol 1978; 85:404–10.
20. Anonymous. Do all pregnant women need iron? Br Med J 1978; 2:1317.
21. Agrawal RM, Tripathi AM, Agarwal KN. Cord blood haemoglobin, iron and ferritin status in maternal anaemia. Acta Paediatr Scand 1983; 72:545–8.
22. Goodlin RC. Why treat "physiologic" anemias of pregnancy? J Reprod Med 1982; 27:639–46.
23. Lind T. Nutrient requirements during pregnancy. Am J Clin Nutr 1981; 34:669–78.
24. Canadian Task Force on the Periodic Health Examination. The periodic health examination. Can Med Assoc J 1979; 121:1194–254.
25. American Academy of Pediatrics, Committee on Practice and Ambulatory Medicine. Recommendations for preventive pediatric health care. Chicago, Ill.: American Academy of Pediatrics, 1987.
26. Dallman PR. Has routine screening of infants for anemia become obsolete in the United States? Pediatrics 1987; 80:439–41.
27. Breslow L, Somers A. The lifetime health monitoring program. N Engl J Med 1977; 296:601–8.
28. Lifecycles: a framework for developing a clinical strategy for primary care. Rockville, Md.: Bureau of Health Care Delivery and Assistance, 1986.
29. College of Family Physicians of Canada, Patterns of Practice and Health Care Delivery Committee. Health maintenance guide. Willowdale, Ontario: College of Family Physicians of Canada, 1983.
30. National Academy of Sciences, Institute of Medicine. Ad Hoc Advisory Group on Pre-

ventive Services. Preventive services for the well population. Washington, D.C.: National Academy of Sciences, 1978.

31. Frame PS, Carlson SJ. A critical review of periodic health screening using specific screening criteria. Part 4. Selected miscellaneous diseases. J Fam Pract 1975; 2: 283–9.

32. Berwick DM. Screening in health fairs: a critical review of benefits, risks, and costs. JAMA 1985; 254:1492–8.

33. American College of Obstetricians and Gynecologists. Standards for obstetric-gynecologic services, 6th ed. Washington, D.C.: American College of Obstetricians and Gynecologists, 1985.

29

Screening for Hemoglobinopathies

Recommendation: Hemoglobin analysis is recommended for all newborns at risk for hemoglobin disorders. Hemoglobin analysis should also be discussed and offered to adolescents and young adults at risk for hemoglobinopathies and should be performed routinely at the first prenatal visit on all pregnant black women. All screening efforts should be accompanied by comprehensive counseling and treatment services (see *Clinical Intervention*).

Burden of Suffering

Some of the abnormal hemoglobins detected by electrophoresis include hemoglobin S, C, and E. Hemoglobin S and hemoglobin C are found in sickle cell disease. This disease affects an estimated 50,000 black Americans.[1,2] It occurs in 1 out of every 625 black infants born in the United States.[2] The case fatality rate of sickle cell disease during infancy can be as high as 30–35% with inadequate or delayed treatment of infections.[3] The principal causes of infant death are bacterial sepsis and acute splenic sequestration crisis.[3] Persons surviving beyond infancy are usually anemic and may experience sickling crises and other complications.[4] The severity of the symptoms and life expectancy vary considerably, with some patients surviving beyond middle age and others dying in infancy or childhood. Treatment for this chronic illness can be expensive and places a large psychosocial burden on both patient and caretakers.[4]

About 2 million Americans have sickle cell trait. It is present in about 8% of the black population.[2] Although sickle cell carriers themselves experience negligible morbidity (microscopic hematuria, hyposthenuria, and possibly exercise limitations under extreme hypoxic conditions),[5,6] parents who both are carriers have a 25% probability with each pregnancy of having offspring with sickle cell disease. One in every 150 black couples in the United States (about 3000 pregnancies per year) are at risk of giving birth to a child with sickle cell disease.[7,8]

Beta-thalassemia occurs primarily among individuals of Mediterranean or Southeast Asian descent. Fewer than 1000 Americans have beta-thalassemia major, or Cooley's anemia.[9] Although some victims of this disease suffer from severe anemia and are transfusion-dependent, modern transfusion and iron chelation therapy have greatly improved the prognosis; some patients now survive past the third decade of life.[10] Beta-thalassemia trait, the heterozygous carrier state, is present in about 1.5% of American blacks, 3–4% of Italian Americans, 5% of Greek Americans, and about 3–9% of Southeast Asians.[9,11] There is a 25%

probability with each pregnancy that offspring of two heterozygous parents will have thalassemia major.

Alpha-thalassemia occurs primarily among individuals of Asian, African, or Mediterranean origin. The disease consists of four different syndromes, depending on the number of alpha globin gene deletions. Infants with hydrops fetalis, which is due to a four-gene deletion, suffer from severe anemia and die before or immediately after birth. Their mothers are at risk for toxemia during the pregnancy, an operative delivery, and postpartum hemorrhage.[12] Hemoglobin H disease, in which three alpha genes are affected, is present in about 1% of Southeast Asians.[13] These individuals experience hemolytic anemia that may be worsened by exposure to oxidant agents and that may require blood transfusion. The exact prevalence of alpha-thalassemia minor or trait (one or two genes affected) is uncertain, but it is estimated to be 5–30% among blacks and 15–30% among Southeast Asians.[11,13,14] These individuals often have mild microcytosis and require genetic counseling.

Hemoglobin E trait is the third most common hemoglobinopathy in the world and the most common hemoglobinopathy in Southeast Asia, where its prevalence is estimated to be 30%.[13] Although associated with no morbidity, the offspring of these individuals may develop severe thalassemia major (hemoglobin E/beta-thalassemia) if the other parent has beta-thalassemia trait. This combination is the most common cause of transfusion-dependent thalassemia in areas of Southeast Asia.[13] The recent immigration to the United States of over 630,000 Indochinese refugees, more than half of whom are under 18 years of age, is expected to result in the doubling or tripling of severe thalassemic disorders in this country.[11,15,16]

Efficacy of Screening Tests

Cellulose acetate/citrate agar hemoglobin electrophoresis or isoelectric focusing are the preferred screening tests for hemoglobin disorders. Routine testing of all newborns, in contrast to selective screening of specified ethnic groups, detects a relatively small proportion of clinically significant hemoglobinopathies. In a recent report from a community with a large at-risk population, routine cord-blood testing of 84,663 newborns detected 89 babies (0.11%) with sickle cell disease and 20 babies (0.02%) with clinically significant thalassemia (i.e., hemoglobin FE, F, H).[17] Although the yield can be poor, electrophoresis is highly specific in the detection of certain hemoglobin disorders, such as sickle cell disease. In one study, each of the 138 children with hemoglobin S, identified in screening 3976 black newborns, was found to have a sickling disorder when retested at age 3–5 years.[18] Another study of 131 infants detected by screening found only nine instances in which the sickling disorder required reclassification and no instance in which a child originally diagnosed as having sickle cell disease was found to have sickle cell trait.[19]

The yield of screening pregnant women for hemoglobin disorders depends on the risk profile of the population being tested. In one study, electrophoresis in combination with a complete blood count was performed on 298 black and Southeast Asian prenatal patients; 94 women (31.5%) had a hemoglobin disorder (including hemoglobin E, alpha-thalassemia trait, beta-thalassemia trait, hemoglobin H, hemoglobin C, or sickle cell disease and trait).[11] In a larger study in a different community, similar tests were performed on 6641 prenatal patients selected without regard to race or ethnic origin.[20] The yield was 185 women (3%) with sickle cell trait, 68 (1%) with hemoglobin C, 30 (0.5%) with beta thalassemia trait, and 17 (0.3%) with other disorders (hemoglobin E, alpha-thalassemia trait, hemoglobin H, hemoglobin E/beta-thalassemia disease). These results were obtained by combining electrophoresis with red cell indices; when low mean corpuscular volume

(MCV) is used as the only screening test (to detect thalassemia), the yield is only 0.3–0.5%.[21]

In recent years, new diagnostic techniques have become available to detect sickle cell disease and other hemoglobinopathies in the fetus when carrier status has been confirmed in both parents. Early tests involved the analysis of fetal blood obtained by fetoscopy or placental aspiration.[22] Recent genetic advances, however, have provided a safer[8] and more practical technique in which amniocytes are obtained by amniocentesis and chromosomal mutations are identified directly through recombinant DNA technology.[7] These techniques are highly accurate (error rate of less than 1%) in detecting sickle cell disease and certain forms of thalassemia.[8,22-25] The principal disadvantage, however, is that amniocentesis cannot be performed safely until about 16 weeks' gestation, thereby delaying diagnosis and potential interventions until late in the second trimester. A new technique, chorionic villus sampling, offers promise as a means of obtaining tissue for DNA analysis as early as 8–10 weeks of gestation.[26,27] (See also Chapter 38.)

Effectiveness of Early Detection

Screening for hemoglobin disorders is usually discussed with respect to two target populations: neonates and adults of reproductive age. In newborns with sickle cell disease, early detection allows prevention of septicemia with prophylactic antibiotics and prompt clinical intervention for infection and sequestration crises. In addition, the family can be educated to detect suspicious symptoms and bring the child to medical attention. A randomized controlled multicenter trial demonstrated that screening followed by the administration of prophylactic oral penicillin to infants and young children with sickle cell disease reduced the incidence of pneumococcal septicemia by 84%.[28] A seven-year longitudinal study recently reported lower mortality in children with sickle cell disease identified in the newborn period than in children diagnosed after 3 months of age (2% vs. 8%), but the investigators did not account for confounding variables in the control group.[17] A briefer longitudinal study (8–20 months) reported no deaths in 131 newborns detected through screening.[19]

Screening older children and adolescents is designed to detect carriers with sickle cell trait, beta-thalassemia trait, and other hemoglobin disorders that often escape detection during the first years of life. Although it is unlikely that these heterozygous individuals will become ill,[5,6] their carrier status has direct implications for their offspring. Identification of carriers before conception permits genetic counseling about partner selection and the availability of diagnostic tests in the event of pregnancy. There is some evidence that individuals who receive certain forms of counseling may retain this information and may have other individuals, such as partners, tested.[20,29-31] A prospective study of 142 coroonees found that 62 (43%) encouraged other persons to be screened.[29] Compared with controls, those who had received counseling demonstrated significantly better understanding of thalassemia when tested immediately after the session. There is no direct evidence, however, that individual genetic counseling by itself significantly alters reproductive behavior or the birth rate of infants with hemoglobin disorders.[4,32]

Detection of carrier status is especially important during pregnancy to provide prospective parents with the option of testing the fetus for a hemoglobinopathy. If the test is positive, they have the time to discuss continuation of the pregnancy and to plan optimal care for their newborn. Parents appear to act on this genetic information. Studies indicate that about half of pregnant women with positive tests for thalassemia refer their partners for testing, and if the father is positive, about 60% consent to amniocentesis.[20] If sickle cell disease is diagnosed in the fetus, about 50% of parents elect therapeutic abortion.[24,33] There is evidence from some European communities with a high prevalence of beta-thalassemia that the birth rate of affected infants has declined significantly following the implementation of routine prenatal screening,[22] and there are data suggesting a similar trend in some North American communities that have introduced community education and testing for thalassemia.[9] Time-series studies do not, however, provide direct evidence that such trends are due specifically to prenatal screening rather than other concurrent variables.

Recommendations of Others

Universal screening of newborns for sickle cell disease, regardless of their race or ethnic origin, was recommended by the National Institutes of Health Consensus Development Conference on Newborn Screening for Sickle Cell Disease and Other Hemoglobinopathies.[3] Screening of high-risk infants has been recommended by the World Health Organization[34] and the British Society for Haematology.[35] Newborn screening for sickle cell disease, coupled with comprehensive counseling, is also advocated in the medical literature.[1,18,28,32,36] Newborn screening for hemoglobinopathies is mandatory in many states.[19,37]

Screening of older children and young adults is not universally recommended. Some states require sickle cell screening of schoolchildren, but many medical authorities have advised against this practice.[1,36-38] The Canadian Task Force found poor evidence for performing thalassemia screening in the general population but added there was fair evidence for discussing screening with Asians, Africans, and Mediterraneans of childbearing age, including an explanation of the pertinent facts and an invitation to participate in screening.[39] The British Society for Haematology has recently recommended measuring red cell indices routinely on all pregnant women and performing hemoglobin electrophoresis on women at risk.[35] Similar recommendations for prenatal testing have been issued by the American College of Obstetricians and Gynecologists[40] and other leading experts.[11]

Discussion

Although hemoglobinopathies occur almost exclusively among defined ethnic and racial groups, some experts advocate universal newborn screening to insure the detection of persons whose ethnicity is uncertain.[3] Proponents of selective, high-risk screening emphasize that, especially in geographic areas with a small population at risk, cost-effectiveness is compromised and considerable expense incurred in screening large numbers of low-risk newborns to identify the rare individuals with sickle cell disease or other uncommon hemoglobin disorders.

There has been considerable debate over the value of screening for sickle cell disease and other hemoglobinopathies in persons of reproductive age. Critics cite evidence that sickle cell screening programs in the past have failed to demonstrate to the patient and the public the significant differences between sickle cell trait and the disease. This has resulted in unnecessary anxiety for carriers and inappropriate labeling by insurers and employers. In addition, there is no evidence that counseling, however comprehensive, will be remembered throughout the individual's reproductive life, influence partner selection, alter use of prenatal testing, or ultimately reduce the birth rate of affected children.[4,21] Proponents argue that these outcomes should not be used as measures of effectiveness since the goal of genetic counseling is to facilitate informed decisionmaking by prospective parents.[4,14,21] In this regard, clinicians are responsible for making the individual aware of the diagnosis, the risk to future offspring, and the recommended methods to reduce that risk, regardless of the strength of the evidence that such counseling reduces the birth rate of affected offspring.

Clinical Intervention

Umbilical cord or heel prick blood specimens should be obtained on all newborns at risk for hemoglobin disorders (those of Caribbean, Latin American, Asian, Mediterranean, and African descent). These samples should be tested for hemoglobin disorders by electrophoresis or other tests of comparable accuracy. In geographic areas with a large proportion of persons at risk for hemoglobin disorders, routine screening of all newborns may be more efficient than selective screening. Infants with sickle cell disease should receive appropriate follow-up testing, immunizations, antibiotic prophylaxis, and regular clinical evaluations of growth and nutritional status. Their families should receive genetic counseling regarding family testing and future offspring, information about the disease, early warning signs of serious complications, and advice and referrals for health care management, peer groups, and sources of medical and mental health services.

Hemoglobin testing should also be discussed with adolescents and young adults at risk for sickle cell trait, thalassemia, and other hemoglobinopathies (see above). The counseling should include a description of the significance of the disease, how it is inherited, the availability of a screening test, and the implications to the individual and offspring of having a positive result. Hemoglobin electrophoresis should be performed at the first prenatal visit of all pregnant black women. Carriers should be urged to have the father tested and should receive information on the availability of prenatal diagnosis if the father is positive.

REFERENCES

 1. Scott RB, Castro O. Screening for sickle cell hemoglobinopathies. JAMA 1979; 241: 1145–7.
 2. Motulsky AG. Frequency of sickling disorders in U.S. blacks.N Engl J Med 1973; 288: 31–3.
 3. National Institutes of Health Consensus Development Conference Statement. Newborn screening for sickle cell disease and other hemoglobinopathies. JAMA 1987; 258: 1205–9.
 4. Bowman JE. Is a national program to prevent sickle cell disease possible? Am J Ped Hem Onc 1983; 5:367–72.
 5. Sears DA. The morbidity of sickle cell trait: a review of the literature. Am J Med 1978; 64:1021–36.
 6. Sullivan LW. The risks of sickle-cell trait: caution and common sense. N Engl J Med 1987; 317:830–1.
 7. Embury SH, Scharf SJ, Saiki RK, et al. Rapid prenatal diagnosis of sickle cell anemia by a new method of DNA analysis. N Engl J Med 1987; 316:656–61.
 8. Kazazian HH Jr, Boehm CD, Dowling CE. Prenatal diagnosis of hemoglobinopathies by DNA analysis. Ann NY Acad Sci 1985; 445:337–48.
 9. Pearson HA, Guiliotis DK, Rink L, et al. Patient age distribution in thalassemia major: changes from 1973 to 1985. Pediatrics 1987; 80:53–7.
10. Giardina PJ, Ehlers K, Lesser M, et al. Improved survival in beta thalassemia major. Pediatric Res 1987; 21:299a.
11. Stein J, Berg C, Jones JA, et al. A screening protocol for a prenatal population at risk

for inherited hemoglobin disorders: results of its application to a group of Southeast Asians and blacks. Am J Obstet Gynecol 1984; 150:333–4l.

12. Wasi P. Hemoglobinopathies including thalassemia. Part 1. Tropical Asia. Clin Haematol 1981; 10:707–29.

13. Hurst D, Tittle B, Kleman KM, et al. Anemia and hemoglobinopathies in Southeast Asian refugee children. J Pediatr 1983; 102:692–7.

14. Steinberg MH, Embury SH. Alpha-thalassemia in blacks: genetic and clinical aspects and interactions with the sickle hemoglobin gene. Blood 1986; 68:985–90.

15. Pickwell S. Health screening for Indochinese refugees. Nurs Pract 1983; 8:20–5.

16. Fitzpatrick S, Johnson J, Shragg P, et al. Health care needs of Indochinese refugee teenagers. Pediatrics 1987; 79:118–24.

17. Vichinsky E, Hurst D, Earles A, et al. Newborn screening for sickle cell disease: effect on mortality. Pediatrics 1988; 81:749–55.

18. Kramer MS, Rooks Y, Johnston D, et al. Accuracy of cord blood screening for sickle hemoglobinopathies: three- to five-year follow-up. JAMA 1979; 241:485–6.

19. Grover R, Shahidi S, Fisher B, et al. Current sickle cell screening program for newborns in New York City, 1979–1980. Am J Public Health 1983; 73:249–51.

20. Rowley PT, Loader S, Walden ME. Toward providing parents the option of avoiding the birth of the first child with Cooley's anemia: response to hemoglobinopathy screening and counseling during pregnancy. Ann NY Acad Sci 1986; 445:408–16.

21. Gehlbach DL, Morgenstern LL. Antenatal screening for thalassemia minor. Obstet Gynecol 1988; 71:801–3.

22. Alter BP. Advances in the prenatal diagnosis of hematologic diseases. Blood 1984; 64:329–40.

23. Weatherall DJ, Mold J, Thein SL, et al. Prenatal diagnosis of the common haemoglobin disorders. J Med Genet 1985; 22:422–30.

24. Boehm CD, Antonarakis SE, Phillips JA III, et al. Prenatal diagnosis using DNA polymorphisms: report on 95 pregnancies at risk for sickle-cell disease or beta-thalassemia. N Engl J Med 1983; 308:1054–8.

25. Orkin SH. Prenatal diagnosis of hemoglobin disorders by DNA analysis. Blood 1984; 63:249–53.

26. Goosens M, Dumez Y, Kaplan L, et al. Prenatal diagnosis of sickle-cell anemia in the first trimester of pregnancy. N Engl J Med 1983; 309:831–3.

27. Old JM, Fitches A, Heath C, et al. First-trimester fetal diagnosis for haemoglobinopathies: report on 200 cases. Lancet 1986; 2:763–7.

28. Gaston MH, Verter JI, Woods G, et al. Prophylaxis with oral penicillin in children with sickle cell anemia: a randomized trial. N Engl J Med 1986; 314:1593–9.

29. Lipkin M, Fisher L, Rowley PT, et al. Genetic counseling of asymptomatic carriers in a primary care setting: the effectiveness of screening and counseling for beta-thalassemia trait. Ann Intern Med 1986; 105:115–23.

30. Whitten CF, Thomas JF, Nishiura EN. Sickle cell trait counseling: Evaluation of counselors and counselees. Am J Hum Genet 1981; 33:802–16.

31. Scriver CR, Bardanis M, Cartier L, et al. Beta-thalassemia disease prevention: genetic medicine applied. Am J Hum Genet 1984; 36:1024–38.

32. Rucknagel DL. A decade of screening in the hemoglobinopathies: is a national program to prevent sickle cell anemia possible? Am J Ped Hem Onc 1983; 5:373–7.

33. Driscoll MC, Lerner N, Anyane-Yeboa K, et al. Prenatal diagnosis of sickle hemoglobinopathies: the experience of the Columbia University Comprehensive Center for Sickle Cell Disease. Am J Hum Genet 1987; 40:548–58.

34. Treatment of haemoglobinopathies and allied disorders: report of a WHO scientific group. World Health Organization Technical Report Series No. 509. Geneva: World Health Organization, 1972:33.

35. British Society for Haematology. Guidelines for haemoglobinopathy screening. Clin Lab Hematol 1988; 10:87–94.

36. Pearson HA, O'Brien RT. Sickle cell testing programs. J Pediatr 1972; 81:1201–4.

37. Andrews LB. State laws and regulations governing newborn screening. Chicago, Ill.: American Bar Foundation, 1985:147–55.

38. Beutler E, Boggs DR, Heller P, et al. Hazards of indiscriminate screening for sickling. N Engl J Med 1971; 285:1405–6.
39. Canadian Task Force on the Periodic Health Examination. The periodic health examination. Can Med Assoc J 1979; 121:1194–254.
40. American College of Obstetricians and Gynecologists. Standards for obstetric-gynecologic services, 6th ed. Washington, D.C.: American College of Obstetricians and Gynecologists, 1985:17–9.

30

Screening for Lead Toxicity

Recommendation: Annual lead screening is recommended for all children aged 9 months to 6 years who are at high risk for lead toxicity (see *Clinical Intervention*), especially those who live in or frequently visit older housing that is dilapidated or undergoing renovation.

Burden of Suffering

Data collected in the late 1970s suggested that about 2% of Americans had elevated blood lead levels (30 ug/dl [1.45 umol/L] or greater).[1] Prolonged exposure to lead can produce serious renal, hematologic, and neurologic complications.[2] Elevated blood lead levels can affect all age groups, including adults with occupational exposure to lead. The developing fetus, infant, and young child, however, are at special risk, since lead can produce irreversible effects on intelligence and behavior at this age.[2,3] Even low blood lead levels can result in subtle long-term effects on intelligence, fine motor skills, electrophysiological function, heme synthesis, psychological development, and behavior.[4-8] Lead toxicity (blood lead of 30 ug/dL [1.45 umol/L] or greater) affects nearly 700,000 American children between the ages of 6 months and 5 years.[2] There are a number of sources of environmental lead exposure, including contaminated air and water supplies. A very important route of exposure in children is the ingestion of lead-based paint chips, lead-impregnated plaster, or contaminated dust or dirt found in dilapidated homes built before 1950.[2] These building conditions are found most commonly in low-income urban neighborhoods. As a result, about 19% of black children who are poor or who live in the center of large American cities have lead levels above 30 ug/dL (1.45 umol/L).[1,2] In recent years, a growing body of evidence suggests that lead is toxic for children at levels previously thought to be harmless (10–15 ug/dL [0.50–0.70 umol/L]).[9] The expanding definition of lead toxicity suggests that the burden of suffering from this disorder is considerably higher than previously assumed, affecting 17% of American children (about 2–3 million). Fully 55% of poor black children have blood lead levels greater than 15ug/dL (0.70 umol/L).[9,10]

Efficacy of Screening Tests

The principal tests for detecting lead toxicity are blood lead and free erythrocyte protoporphyrin (EP) levels. Blood lead is the more accurate test, but it is not ideal for screening purposes due to its cost and the potential for sample contamination with environmental lead, especially when collecting finger-stick specimens.[11] In addition, while blood lead indicates recent lead absorption, it does not provide evidence of chronic exposure or total body burden of lead. Blood lead is therefore generally performed as a confirmatory test in persons with an elevated erythrocyte protoporphyrin. The EP test is less expensive than the blood lead, and it is unaffected by contamination with environmental lead.[11,12] It is easily performed on capillary blood specimens and is therefore more acceptable for use with young patients.[11] An elevated EP level is also a better indicator of chronic lead exposure than is a blood lead measurement. However, EP is often unaffected by modest elevations in blood lead levels; the sensitivity of the test is 50% or less in detecting blood lead levels below 50 ug/dL (2.40 umol/L).[13,14] In light of recent evidence that blood lead levels as low as 10–15 ug/dL (0.50–0.70 umol/L) may be toxic,[9] this limitation in sensitivity may affect the usefulness of EP testing in the early detection of lead toxicity. In addition, the test lacks specificity, since an elevated EP is commonly seen in persons with iron deficiency.[14] The positive predictive value of the EP test is thus limited. In one study, EP measurements were taken on 47,230 suburban and rural children; although 4.7% of the children had an elevated EP level, only 0.6% had elevated blood lead levels.[15]

Routine lead screening may be of greater predictive value when performed selectively in high-risk groups. Children at increased risk of lead exposure include children who live in older, dilapidated housing; children living near lead processing plants and other sources of lead exposure (e.g., busy highways); and children with parents or other household members who work in a lead-related occupation. Screening of adults with occupational exposure to lead is also likely to have greater yield.

Effectiveness of Early Detection

Early detection of lead toxicity before the development of potentially irreversible complications permits the clinician to recommend environmental measures to limit further exposure to lead and, when necessary, to begin medical treatment with chelating agents.[16] Few controlled studies, however, have demonstrated the efficacy of these measures in preventing the complications of lead toxicity, and ethical and logistical considerations may limit the performance of such studies in the future. Chelating agents can lower blood lead levels,[16] but there have been few studies comparing the benefits of chelation therapy in asymptomatic persons with its potential adverse effects and nephrotoxicity. In addition, recommendations to make environmental changes, such as removing lead-based materials from the home, limiting a child's access to neighborhood areas with these materials, and reducing the occupational exposure of adults to lead, may also be ineffective due to circumstances outside the control of the clinician. Many homeowners are unable to afford or arrange extensive home repairs, removal of lead from water supplies, or a change in residence, and it is often difficult to prevent children from playing outside the home in areas with lead-based materials. Persons with occupational exposure may be unable to modify conditions at the worksite or to change jobs.

Nonetheless, the potentially irreversible effects of lead exposure in young children justify making a special effort to detect lead toxicity in this population. Modest elevations in lead, which often escape detection in the absence of screening, have been associated with the development of abnormal intelligence and behavior,[6-8] and high lead levels produce severe neuropsychological impairment and mental retardation.[3] Thus, although direct evidence of efficacy is lacking, most experts consider the toxicity of chelation therapy to be a reasonable risk for all children with marked elevations of lead (above 55–60 ug/dL [2.65–2.90 umol/L]) and for children with only moderate elevations who have adequate renal function.[11,16,19] In addition, although lead removal from the home may be beyond the means of some parents, others may be able to take corrective action; providing information to these parents may therefore be beneficial in preventing further exposure.

Recommendations of Others

The Centers for Disease Control (CDC) has issued lead screening guidelines for children between the ages of 9 months and 6 years,[11] and similar recommendations have recently been adopted by the American Academy of Pediatrics.[20] The guidelines specify that an EP test should be performed on all children aged 12–36 months who live in or frequently visit old, dilapidated housing. When possible, EP testing should be carried out annually from age 9 months to 6 years in children with specific risk factors. These include, in decreasing order of importance: children who come in close contact with other children with known lead toxicity; children who live in older, dilapidated housing; children living near lead processing plants or whose parents or other household members work in a lead-related occupation; and children living near busy highways or hazardous waste sites.

There are no screening recommendations for asymptomatic older children or for adults without known or suspected exposure to lead. The Occupational Safety and Health Administration (OSHA) has published screening recommendations for workers with occupational exposure to lead.[21]

Clinical Intervention

Erythrocyte protoporphyrin should be measured annually in all children aged 9 months to 6 years who are at high risk for lead toxicity, especially those who live in or frequently visit housing built before 1950 that is dilapidated or undergoing renovation. Other high-risk children include those who come in close contact with other children with known lead toxicity, those living near lead processing plants or whose parents or other household members work in a lead-related occupation, and those living near busy highways or hazardous waste sites. Children with EP levels greater than 35 ug/dL (0.60 umol/L) should receive confirmatory blood lead determination. A blood lead level of 25 ug/dL (1.20 umol/L) or greater is considered abnormally elevated. [These criteria and the role of EP testing may change in the near future as new evidence emerges regarding the toxic effects of low levels of blood lead.] The EP sample may be obtained by capillary tube, but the blood lead sample should only be obtained by venipuncture. Although screening of asymptomatic older children and adults is not necessary, clinicians should follow existing guidelines for screening patients with possible occupational lead exposure.[21]

REFERENCES

1. Mahaffey KR, Annest JL, Roberts J, et al. National estimates of blood lead levels: United States, 1976–1980. Association with selected demographic and socioeconomic factors. N Engl J Med 1982; 307:573–9.
2. National Center for Health Statistics. Blood lead levels for persons ages 6 months—74 years: United States, 1976–80. Data from the National Health and Nutrition Examination Survey. Vital and Health Statistics, series 11, no. 233. Washington, D.C.: Government Printing Office, 1984. (Publication no. DHHS (PHS) 84–1683.)
3. Bellinger D, Leviton A, Waternaux C, et al. Longitudinal analyses of prenatal and postnatal lead exposure and early cognitive development. N Engl J Med 1987; 316:1037–43.
4. Otto D, Robinson G, Baumann S, et al. 5–year follow-up study of children with low-to-

moderate lead absorption: electrophysiological evaluation. Environ Res 1985; 38: 168–86.

5. Piomelli S, Seaman C, Zullow D, et al. Threshold for lead damage to heme synthesis in urban children. Proc Nat Acad Sci USA 1982; 79:3335–9.

6. Needleman HL, Gunnoe C, Leviton A, et al. Deficits in psychologic and classroom performance of children with elevated dentine lead levels. N Engl J Med.1979; 300: 689–95.

7. de la Burde B, Choate MS. Early asymptomatic lead exposure and development at school age. J Pediatr 1975; 87:638–42.

8. Schroeder SR, Hawk B, Otto DA, et al. Separating the effects of lead and social factors on IQ. Environ Res 1985; 38:144–54.

9. Mushak P, Crochetti A. The nature and extent of lead poisoning in children in the United States: a report to Congress. Washington, D.C.: Department of Health and Human Services, Agency for Toxic Substances and Disease Registry, 1987.

10. Needleman HL. The persistent threat of lead: a singular opportunity. Am J Public Health 1989; 79:643–5.

11. Centers for Disease Control. Preventing lead poisoning in young children: a statement by the Centers for Disease Control—January 1985. Atlanta, Ga.: Centers for Disease Control, 1985.

12. Berwick DM, Komaroff AL. Cost effectiveness of lead screening. N Engl J Med 1982; 306:1392–8.

13. Piomelli S, Davidow B, Guinee VF, et al. The FEP (free erythrocyte porphyrins) test: a screening micromethod for lead poisoning. Pediatrics 1973; 51:254–9.

14. Mahaffey KR, Annest JL. Association of erythrocyte protoporphyrin with blood lead level and iron status in the second National Health and Nutrition Examination Survey, 1976–1980. Environ Res 1986; 41:327–38.

15. Guthrie R, Orfanos A, Widger K, et al. Screening suburban/rural children for lead exposure, iron deficiency. Am J Public Health 1988; 78:856–7.

16. Piomelli S, Rosen JF, Chisolm JJ Jr, et al. Management of childhood lead poisoning. J Pediatr 1984; 105:523–32.

17. Amitai Y, Graef JW, Brown MJ, et al. Hazards of "deleading" homes of children with lead poisoning. Am J Dis Child 1987; 141:758–60.

18. Fischbein A, Anderson KE, Sassa S, et al. Lead poisoning from "do-it-yourself" heat guns for removing lead-based paint: report of two cases. Environ Res 1981; 24: 425–31.

19. Graef JW. Clinical outpatient management of childhood lead poisoning. In: Chisolm JJ Jr, O'Hara DM, eds. Lead absorption in children: management, clinical, and environmental aspects. Baltimore, Md.: Urban and Schwarzenberg, 1982.

20. American Academy of Pediatrics. Statement on childhood lead poisoning. Committee on Environmental Hazards, Committee on Accident and Poison Prevention. Pediatrics 1987; 79:457–65.

21. Occupational Safety and Health Administration. Occupational exposure to lead: final standard. Fed Regist 1978; 43:52952–3014.

31

Screening for Diminished Visual Acuity

Recommendation: Vision screening is recommended for all children once before entering school, preferably at age 3 or 4 (see *Clinical Intervention*). Routine vision testing is not recommended as a component of the periodic health examination of asymptomatic schoolchildren. Clinicians should be alert for signs of ocular misalignment when examining all infants and children. Vision screening of adolescents and adults is not recommended, but it may be appropriate in the elderly. Screening for glaucoma is discussed in Chapter 32.

Burden of Suffering

About 2–5% of American children suffer from amblyopia ("lazy eye") and strabismus (ocular misalignment), and nearly 20% have simple refractive errors by age 16.[1-4] Amblyopia and strabismus usually develop between infancy and ages 5–7.[3] Since normal vision from birth is necessary for proper eye development, failure to treat amblyopia and strabismus before school age may later result in irreversible visual deficits, permanent amblyopia, loss of depth perception and binocularity, cosmetic defects, and educational and occupational restrictions.[1,4,5] In contrast, refractive errors such as myopia become common during school age but rarely carry serious prognostic implications.[1,3,6,7] Experts disagree on whether uncorrected refractive errors cause diminished academic performance among schoolchildren.[1,3,5,7,8]

The majority of vision disorders occur in adults; over 8.5 million Americans suffer from visual impairment.[9] Visual disorders such as presbyopia (decreased ability to focus on near objects) become more common with age,[10] and therefore the prevalence of visual impairment is highest in those over age 65. Preliminary statistics from recent surveys suggest that nearly 13% of Americans age 65 and older have some form of visual impairment, and almost 8% of this age group suffer from severe impairment: blindness in both eyes or inability to read newsprint even with glasses.[11] Vision disorders in the elderly may be associated with injuries due to falls and motor vehicle accidents, diminished productivity, and loss of independence.[12] Many older adults are unaware of changes in their visual acuity, and up to 25% of them may be using an incorrect lens prescription.[12]

Efficacy of Screening Tests

Although screening for strabismus and amblyopia is most critical at an early age, screening tests to detect occult vision disorders in children under age 3 have generally been unsuccessful due to the child's inability to cooperate, the time required for testing, and the inaccuracy of the tests.[13-15] Promising techniques such as alternate stimulation (cover testing), preferential-looking, grating acuity cards, and refractive screening are currently being developed for this age group.[14,16,17] Although refractive errors detected during infancy can predict some cases of amblyopia and strabismus, the sensitivity of this form of screening is quite poor.[2]

Screening tests for detecting strabismus and amblyopia in preschool children over age 3 include simple inspection, visual acuity tests, and stereograms. Visual acuity tests include the Snellen eye chart, the Landolt C, the tumbling E, the Sheridan-Gardner STYCAR test, Allen picture cards, grating cards, and other techniques.[15] The specificity of most acuity tests, however, is imperfect for detecting strabismus and amblyopia because diminished visual acuity can occur in other conditions, such as simple refractive error or visual immaturity.[2] In addition, many children with nonamblyopic strabismus often have normal visual acuity but are at risk for serious complications.[2,18] Thus, although simple acuity tests are inexpensive and easy to administer, they may miss many cases. Snellen letters, for example, are estimated to have a sensitivity of only 25–37%.[2,18,19] Refractive screening has also been criticized as not being a direct test for either amblyopia or strabismus.[2]

Stereograms such as the Random Dot E (RDE) have been proposed as more effective than visual acuity tests in detecting strabismus and amblyopia in preschool children.[2,18,20,21] The test, in which the patient views test cards through Polaroid glasses, requires about one minute to perform.[18,20] When compared with a battery of visual tests, the RDE has an estimated sensitivity of 64%, specificity of 90%, positive predictive value of 57%, and negative predictive value of 93%.[18]

A more effective but less efficient strategy is the combination of more than one visual test.[2,19] The Modified Clinical Technique (MCT), for example, includes retinoscopy, cover and Hirschberg tests, the Snellen acuity test, a color vision test, and external observation of the eye. The MCT has gained acceptance among optometrists since its introduction in the Orinda Study of 1959.[18,22-24] Sensitivity and specificity in excess of 90% were found in that study and have since been reproduced in screening programs involving as many as 50,000 children.[18] The MCT cannot be used routinely by primary care physicians for screening purposes, however, because it requires about 12 minutes to perform and the examiner must be a skilled eye care specialist.[18,23]

Vision screening of older children and adults is a means of detecting unrecognized refractive errors. Tests of visual acuity are often used for this purpose, but few studies have examined the sensitivity, specificity, and predictive value of these tests in adult age groups.

Effectiveness of Early Detection

There is convincing evidence that early detection and treatment of vision disorders in infants and young children improve the prognosis for normal eye development.[21] A prospective study has demonstrated that preschool children who receive visual acuity screening have significantly less visual impairment than controls when reexamined 6–12 months later.[25] Detection and treatment of strabismus and amblyopia by age 1–2 can increase the likelihood of developing normal or near-normal binocular vision and may improve fine motor skills.[2,4] Interventions for amblyopia and strabismus are significantly less effective if started after age 5, and such a delay increases the risk of irreversible amblyopia, ocular misalignment, and other visual deficits.[1,3] It is widely held that clinical screening tests can detect these disorders earlier than parents or teachers; only about 50% of children with ocular misalignment have a cosmetically noticeable defect.[2,8]

There is little evidence that bilaterally equal refractive errors among older children and adolescents are associated with significant morbidity, such as diminished academic performance.[1,3,6,7] This is true in young adults as well, and, in addition, uncorrected vision disorders are quite uncommon among young adults.[26] Vision screening for older adults is defended on the grounds that the prevalence of abnormal visual acuity is considerably greater among the elderly[10] and these deficits are more commonly left uncorrected.[26] Among persons aged 65–74, a visual acuity of 20/50 or less has been measured in 11% of those who wear glasses and in 26% of those who do not.[26] Some forms of visual impairment in the elderly are associated with difficulties in ambulation,[27] and early correction of refractive errors may serve a role in preventing injuries and facilitating the performance of daily living functions. However, there have been no prospective studies documenting these benefits in an elderly cohort receiving vision screening.

Recommendations of Others

The American Academy of Ophthalmology recommends an ophthalmological examination of newborns who are premature or at risk for eye disease; an examination of fixation preference and ocular alignment by age 6 months; an examination of visual acuity, ocular alignment, and ocular disease at age 3–4; annual screening of schoolchildren for visual acuity and ocular alignment; occasional examinations from puberty to age 40; and an examination for presbyopia at age 40 and every two to five years thereafter.[1] The American Academy of Pediatrics recommends external examination and tests of following ability and the pupillary light reflex in the newborn period and once during the first six months.[5] Testing of visual acuity, ocular alignment, and ocular disease is recommended by the Academy at ages 4, 5–6, and at less frequent intervals thereafter.[5] The Canadian Task Force recommends an eye examination and cover test at ages 1 week, 2 months, and, along with a vision chart test, at age 2–3 years and 5–6 years. Testing at age 10–11 is considered discretionary, and no adult screening is recommended.[28] The American Optometric Association recommends screening schoolchildren every three years and annual eye examinations in adults after age 35.[29] Screening guidelines have also been issued by other organizations, such as the National Society to Prevent Blindness, the National Association of Vision Program Consultants, Volunteers for Vision, and the American Public Health Association.[2,8] Vision screening of preschool and school children is also required by law in some states and in a number of Federal programs.[2,22]

Discussion

Although it is established that early detection of strabismus and amblyopia is most beneficial for children under age 3, a practical and effective screening test is not yet available for this age group. Clinicians should, of course, be alert to signs of ocular misalignment when examining infants and young children. Screening tests for preschool children are available but, with the exception of a comprehensive battery (e.g., the MCT), most tests for amblyopia and strabismus lack the sensitivity, specificity, and predictive value that are expected of good screening tests. Of these, the Random Dot E stereogram appears to have the best performance and is recommended by many experts.[2,21] Due to the high rate of false-negative results with this test, however, it would need to be repeated throughout the preschool period to achieve optimal effectiveness.

Screening of schoolchildren by primary care clinicians is not recommended because the procedure is usually performed by the public school system, and there is little scientific evidence that early detection of myopia is of greater benefit than detection when symptoms first become apparent. Similarly, there is no basis for screening asymptomatic adolescents or adults below age 40 who lack specific risk factors for vision disorders. With increasing age, there is a stronger argument for the early detection of uncorrected visual impairment to help prevent injury and improve independent living. The performance characteristics of acuity tests at this age are poorly described, and the claimed benefits of screening have not been proved. Repeated acuity testing can, however, improve sensitivity with presumably little cost or inconvenience to the patient. There are no available data for any age group on the optimal interval for vision screening; recommended frequencies are selected arbitrarily on the basis of expert opinion.

Clinical Intervention

Testing for amblyopia and strabismus is recommended for all children once before entering school, preferably at age 3 or 4. Stereotesting (e.g., Random Dot E stereogram) is more effective than visual acuity testing (e.g., Snellen optotype cards) in detecting these conditions. Routine screening for refractive errors is not recommended as a component of the periodic health examination of asymptomatic schoolchildren. Clinicians should be alert for signs of ocular misalignment when examining all infants and children. Vision screening of asymptomatic adolescents and adults is not recommended. It may be appropriate in the elderly, but there is insufficient evidence to recommend an optimal interval. All patients with abnormal test results should be referred to an eye specialist for further evaluation. Screening for glaucoma is discussed in Chapter 32.

REFERENCES

1. American Academy of Ophthalmology. Infants and children's eye care. Statement by the American Academy of Ophthalmology to the Select Panel for the Promotion of Child Health, Department of Health and Human Services. San Francisco, Calif.: American Academy of Ophthalmology, 1980.
2. Ehrlich MI, Reinecke RD, Simons K. Preschool vision screening for amblyopia and strabismus: programs, methods, guidelines, 1983. Surv Ophthalmol 1983; 28:145–63.
3. Cross AW. Health screening in schools. Part I. J Pediatr 1985; 107:487–94.
4. Sanke RF. Amblyopia. Am Fam Physician 1988; 37:275–8.
5. American Academy of Pediatrics. Vision screening and eye examination in children. Committee on Practice and Ambulatory Medicine. Pediatrics 1986; 77:918–9.
6. Rosner J, Rosner J. Comparison of visual characteristics in children with and without learning difficulties. Am J Optom Physiol Opt 1987; 64:531–3.
7. Helveston EM, Weber JC, Miller K, et al. Visual function and academic performance. Am J Ophthalmol 1985; 99:346–55.
8. APHA resolution number 8203: children's vision screening. Am J Public Health 1983; 73:329.
9. National Center for Health Statistics. Prevalence of selected chronic conditions, United States, 1979–81. Vital and Health Statistics, series 10, no. 155. Washington, D.C.: Government Printing Office, 1986. (Publication no. DHHS (PHS) 86–1583.)
10. Idem. Monocular visual acuity of persons 4–74 years, United States, 1971–1972. Vital and Health Statistics, series 11, no. 201G. Washington, D.C.: National Center for Health Statistics, 1977:60. (Publication no. DHEW (HRA) 77–1646.)

11. Nelson KA. Visual impairment among elderly Americans: statistics in transition. J Vis Impair Blind 1987; 81:331 4.

12. Stults BM. Preventive health care for the elderly. West J Med 1984, 141.832–45.

13. Hall SM, Pugh AG, Hall DMB. Vision screening in the under-5s. Br Med J 1982; 285: 1096–8.

14. Jenkins PL, Simon JW, Kandel GL, et al. A simple grating visual acuity test for impaired children. Am J Ophthalmol 1985; 99:652–8.

15. Fern KD, Manny RE. Visual acuity of the preschool child: a review. Am J Optom Physiol Opt 1986; 63:319–45.

16. Jacobson SG, Mohindra I, Held R. Visual acuity of infants with ocular diseases. Am J Ophthalmol 1982; 93:198–209.

17. Brown AM, Yamamoto M. Visual acuity in newborn and preterm infants measured with grating acuity cards. Am J Ophthalmol 1986; 102:245–53.

18. Hammond RS, Schmidt PP. A Random Dot E stereogram for the vision screening of children. Arch Ophthalmol 1986; 104:54–60.

19. Lieberman S, Cohen AH, Stolzberg M, et al. Validation study of the New York State Optometric Association (NYSOA) vision screening battery. Am J Optom Physiol Opt 1985; 62:165–8.

20. Simons K. A comparison of the Frisby, Random-Dot E, TNO, and Randot Circles stereotests in screening and office use. Arch Ophthalmol 1981; 99:446–52.

21. Reinecke RD. Screening 3–year-olds for visual problems: are we gaining or falling behind? Arch Ophthalmol 1986; 104:33.

22. Nussenblatt H. Symposium on optometry's obligation in vision screening. Opening remarks. Am J Optom Physiol Opt 1984; 61:357–8.

23. Peters HB. The Orinda Study. Am J Optom Physiol Opt 1984; 61:361 3.

24. Woodruff ME. Vision and refractive status among grade 1 children of the province of New Brunswick. Am J Optom Physiol Opt 1986; 63:545–52.

25. Feldman W, Milner R, Sackett B, et al. Effects of preschool screening for vision and hearing on prevalence of vision and hearing problems 6–12 months later. Lancet 1980; 2:1014–6.

26. National Center for Health Statistics. Refraction status and motility defects of persons 4–74 years, United States, 1971–1972. Vital and Health Statistics, series 11, no. 206. Washington, D.C.: National Center for Health Statistics, 1978: 89–93. (Publication no. DHEW (PHS) 78–1654.)

27. Idem. Aging in the eighties, impaired senses for sound and light in persons age 65 and over. Advance Data from Vital and Health Statistics, no. 125. Hyattsville, Md.: National Center for Health Statistics, 1986:4–5. (Publication no. DHHS (PHS) 86–1250.)

28. Canadian Task Force on the Periodic Health Examination. The periodic health examination. Can Med Assoc J 1979; 121:1194–254.

29. Miller SC, American Optometric Association. Personal communication, October 1988.

32

Screening for Glaucoma

Recommendation: There is insufficient evidence to recommend routine performance of tonometry by primary care physicians as an effective screening test for glaucoma. It may be clinically prudent, however, to advise patients at high risk, such as those aged 65 and older, to be tested periodically for glaucoma by an eye specialist.

Burden of Suffering

Glaucoma, the second leading cause of new cases of blindness in the United States, affects over 1.4 million Americans and accounts for over 3 million visits to ophthalmologists each year.[1,2] Of the various forms of glaucoma (e.g., congenital, open-angle, closed-angle, secondary), open-angle glaucoma (OAG) is the most common (90% of cases) and insidious form, usually progressing in the absence of symptoms until irreversible visual field loss occurs.[3] The proportion of persons with OAG who develop blindness is not known with certainty, but studies suggest that over the course of 20 years blindness develops in as many as 75% of persons with severe disease.[4] In addition to blindness (diminished acuity), an unknown number of individuals with OAG also suffer from other visual deficits, such as decreased peripheral vision. Glaucoma occurs in less than 1% of persons under age 70 but is more common in the elderly: the prevalence is 2–4% in those over age 75.[5] In blacks, a population at increased risk for the disease, glaucoma is the leading cause of blindness.[2] In addition to age and race, other risk factors for glaucoma include diabetes mellitus, myopia, and a family history of glaucoma.[2,6]

Efficacy of Screening Tests

The three most common screening tests for glaucoma are tonometry, ophthalmoscopy, and perimetry. Tonometers, which include Schiotz, applanation, and noncontact (air puff) devices, are used to measure intraocular pressure. The accuracy and reliability of tonometry is affected to some extent by the choice of device, the experience of the examiner, and physiological variables in the patient.[7-9] The more fundamental problem with this screening test, however, is the limited specificity of ocular hypertension (OH), which is usually defined as an intraocular pressure (IOP) exceeding 21 mm Hg. Although OH often precedes glaucomatous visual field loss by months or years and is an important risk factor for glaucoma (which is five to six times more likely if IOP exceeds 21 mm Hg),[2] mild OH is also a common finding in persons who do not appear to have glaucoma.

The population prevalence of glaucoma, about 1% or less, is much lower than that of OH (between 5% and 13% in various studies); OH occurs in nearly 25% of persons over age 65.[2,10] Thus, although OH predisposes to glaucoma, a large proportion of persons with it, perhaps as many as 70–97%, are unlikely to ever develop the signs and symptoms of glaucoma.[4,8,11-18]

The risk of glaucoma increases with higher levels of intraocular pressure so that a threshold pressure of 35 mm Hg, for example, offers greater specificity but lower sensitivity in predicting glaucoma than the more conventional cutoff of 21 mm Hg.[19] A single measurement of IOP has limited negative predictive value in ruling out glaucoma. Indeed, OAG often develops in persons with normal IOP ("low tension" glaucoma).[20-22] Even in persons with documented glaucoma, only 50% have evidence of OH (IOP greater than 21 mm Hg) on random measurement,[23] due in part to fluctuations in IOP over time.[24] The limited specificity of tonometry combined with the low prevalence of OAG results in a positive predictive value of only 5% in asymptomatic populations such as persons participating in glaucoma screening programs.[23,25]

A second screening test for OAG is ophthalmoscopy. It can be used to detect glaucomatous abnormalities of the optic nerve head (e.g., cupping, pallor, hemorrhage), which often precede the development of irreversible visual field deficits. Although rarely performed solely to screen for glaucoma, the ophthalmoscopic examination is for several reasons an imperfect screening test for this condition. First, it has low sensitivity; even with confirmed visual field loss, cupping and other fundoscopic findings are apparent in only 50–60% of cases.[26,27] Second, it has limited specificity for detecting current glaucomatous visual field loss; the ophthalmoscopic findings of glaucoma are seen in about 15% of persons lacking the visual field deficits characteristic of glaucoma.[27] Some of these individuals may eventually develop OAG over time, but the exact proportion in whom this will occur has not been determined. Third, these data have been obtained by ophthalmologists, often with expertise in glaucoma. Primary care clinicians with less skill in ophthalmoscopy and less time to dilate pupils would be expected to have poorer accuracy.[27] Fourth, the interpretation of fundoscopic findings is subject to considerable interobserver variation, even among experts using standardized criteria.[28,29] Finally, ophthalmoscopic techniques such as the cup-disc ratio and stereoscopic optic disc photography, which can increase sensitivity and specificity to 95%, are too difficult, impractical, or expensive to be used for routine screening in primary care.[23,25,30,31]

The third method of screening for OAG is perimetry, the measurement of visual fields. This procedure is most likely to detect glaucomatous visual field deficits, offering greater accuracy than either tonometry or ophthalmoscopy in detecting OAG. The problems once encountered in performing manual perimetry have in recent years been overcome by automated perimetry devices that produce more uniform and reproducible measurements. Recent evaluations of these devices report a sensitivity in excess of 90% and a specificity of 70–88%.[32-34] Despite the superiority of this technology in expert hands, however, automated perimetry is currently too expensive and impractical to be used routinely by primary care clinicians. Moreover, the detection of visual field deficits may not be useful as an early detection tool since visual field loss is often a late event in the natural history of glaucoma.[35]

Effectiveness of Early Detection

It has long been believed that early detection and treatment of ocular hypertension are important means of preventing progression to open-angle glaucoma and visual loss. While it is well accepted that the reduction of extremely high levels of intraocular pressure (e.g., greater than 35 mm Hg) can be of significant benefit in preventing visual loss, such levels occur infrequently in the general population. The magnitude of benefit from treating mild to moderate OH, the more common finding detected through screening, is less clear. Research studies to date have produced conflicting results. Five controlled trials have indicated that treatment of OH can reduce the incidence of OAG,[13,36-39] but others have observed no effect or, in some cases, a paradoxical increase in OAG.[14,40-44]

Serious methodological problems affect most of these studies. In only two trials have the observed benefits of treating OH been statistically significant.[36,37] One study, in which subjects treated only one eye with epinephrine for one to five years, found that OAG developed in 32% of the untreated eyes but in none of the treated eyes.[36] However, the small sample size (19 subjects) and a strong selection bias limit the usefulness of these results.[45] The second study, a randomized controlled trial, reported a lower incidence of OAG in persons receiving timolol than in those receiving placebo.[37] However, these results achieved statistical significance only after a subsequent data analysis classified patients who discontinued the drug as "lost to follow-up." Three additional trials have reported a beneficial effect from treating OH,[13,38,39] but they suffered from design problems such as failure to randomize by subject, high attrition rates, and the absence of statistically significant results. (Two of the above studies have not been completed, and their results are currently available only in abstract form.[37,39]) Thus, while it is likely that the treatment of mild to moderate OH is of some value in reducing the risk of progression to open-angle glaucoma, the potential magnitude and clinical significance of this effect remain uncertain. The difficulty in demonstrating a significant effect in clinical studies may be due in part to the length of time (an estimated 18 years) required for mild OH to produce detectable damage.[46]

A second issue is whether treatment of open-angle glaucoma itself prevents or delays visual loss. Despite years of experience with this disease, there have been few properly controlled studies examining the efficacy of treatment. Clinical intervention is considered the standard of care for glaucoma, and therefore most controlled studies of treatment compare different modes of therapy with each other rather than comparing treatment to no treatment. A few studies have reported outcomes in persons not receiving treatment,[40,44,47,48] but their designs are inadequate and most report a higher incidence of disease progression in those receiving treatment. Thus, the treatment of OAG to prevent blindness is based primarily on expert opinion rather than on firm evidence that medical intervention improves prognosis.

The adverse effects of glaucoma treatment are not insignificant. Antiglaucoma medications (e.g., timolol, pilocarpine, epinephrine, acetazolamide) must be taken for life and are accompanied by a variety of ocular and systemic side effects. In one study of topical epinephrine, for example, 80% of the subjects were unable to complete the study due to reactive hyperemia, irritation, and tearing.[38] Several agents, such as beta-adrenergic antagonists, can have important systemic side effects.[49] There are also potential risks and costs associated with surgical treatment. Filtering surgery, which is often performed if patients are unresponsive to antiglaucoma medications, may be followed by serious postoperative ophthalmologic complications.[50] Argon laser trabeculoplasty may offer a safer alternative to surgery, but its efficacy and long-term effects remain uncertain.[50,51]

Recommendations of Others

The American Academy of Ophthalmology recommends that ophthalmoscopy and tonometry be performed annually on all persons over age 40.[52] A complete ocular examination by an ophthalmologist is recommended at least once between the ages of 35 and 45 and should be repeated every five years after age 50.[52] The American Optometric Association recommends annual tonometry of persons over age 35 as part of a complete eye and vision examination.[53] Routine screening for glaucoma is also advocated by the National Society to Prevent Blindness.[54] Other groups, however, have expressed concern about the lack of definitive evidence of efficacy. The lack of convincing evidence was the principal finding of a recent examination of glaucoma screening in the elderly by the Office of Technology Assessment of the U.S. Congress.[55] The Canadian Task Force has concluded that there is poor justification on scientific grounds to screen for OAG.[56] Other experts have also recommended omitting glaucoma screening from the periodic health examination.[57,58]

Discussion

Although scientific evidence is lacking that early treatment of OH and OAG improves outcome, it is widely held on the basis of clinical experience that early intervention is important in the prevention of visual loss. Prompt initiation of treatment has been the standard of care for many years, and thus it is unlikely for ethical reasons that definitive studies of efficacy will be carried out in which the control groups do not receive immediate therapy. Therefore, in the absence of further evidence, there are insufficient grounds for discouraging the current practice of early treatment of OH and glaucoma once these conditions are detected. It is important, however, that glaucoma detection procedures be carried out in ways that maximize accuracy and minimize the frequency of false-positive errors. To achieve the latter, it is necessary to target screening to populations at increased risk (e.g., the elderly). Accurate glaucoma screening is best performed by eye specialists (ophthalmologists, optometrists). Primary care physicians often lack the time and equipment available to eye specialists to perform tonometry correctly, to dilate the pupils for thorough fundoscopy, and to carry out precise visual field measurements. Combinations of more than one test, which are known to improve the sensitivity and specificity of glaucoma screening, are also impractical in the busy primary care setting.

Clinical Intervention

There is insufficient evidence to recommend routine performance of tonometry by primary care physicians as an effective screening test for glaucoma. It may be clinically prudent to advise persons at high risk, such as those aged 65 and older, to be tested for glaucoma by an eye specialist. The optimal frequency for glaucoma screening has not been determined and is left to clinical discretion.

REFERENCES

1. National Center for Health Statistics. Prevalence of selected chronic conditions, United States, 1979–81. Vital and Health Statistics, series 10, no. 155. Washington, D.C.: Government Printing Office, 1986. (Publication no. DHHS (PHS) 86–1583.)
2. Leske MC. The epidemiology of open-angle glaucoma: a review. Am J Epidemiol 1983; 118:166–91.
3. National Institutes of Health. Vision research—a national plan: 1983–1987 (vol. 2, part 4: Report of the Glaucoma Panel). Bethesda, Md.: Department of Health and Human Services, 1984. (Publication no. DHHS (NIH) 84–2474.)

4. Grant WM, Burke JF. Why do some people go blind from glaucoma? Ophthalmology 1982; 89:991–8.

5. Podgor MJ, Leske MC, Ederer F. Incidence estimates for lens changes, macular changes, open-angle glaucoma, and diabetic retinopathy. Am J Epidemiol 1983; 118:206–12.

6. Daubs JG, Crick PP. The effect of refractive error on the risk of ocular hypertension and primary open angle glaucoma. Trans Ophthalmol Soc UK 1981; 101:121–6.

7. Spector R, Lightfoot JB, Cohen P, et al. Should tonometry screening be done by technicians instead of physicians? Arch Intern Med 1975; 135:1260–3.

8. Armaly MF. Ocular pressure and visual fields. Arch Ophthalmol 1969; 81:25–40.

9. Thorburn W. The accuracy of clinical applanation tonometry. Acta Ophthalmol 1978; 56:1–5.

10. Kahn HA, Leibowitz HM, Ganley JP, et al. The Framingham Eye Study. Am J Epidemiol 1977; 106:17–32.

11. Lundberg L, Wettrell K, Linner E. Ocular hypertension. Acta Ophthalmol 1987; 65: 705–8.

12. Hovding G, Aasved H. Prognostic factors in the development of manifest open angle glaucoma. Acta Ophthalmol 1986; 64:601–8.

13. Kitazawa Y. Prophylactic therapy of ocular hypertension: a prospective study. Trans Ophthal Soc NZ 1981; 33:30–2.

14. David R, Livingston DG, Luntz MH. Ocular hypertension—a long-term follow-up of treated and untreated patients. Br J Ophthalmol 1977; 61:668–74.

15. Cockburn DM. The prevalence of ocular hypertension in patients of an optometrist and the incidence of glaucoma occurring during long-term follow-up of ocular hypertensives. Am J Optom Physiol Opt 1982; 59:330–7.

16. Linner E. Diagnostic and therapeutic aspects of early chronic simple glaucoma. Israel J Med Sci 1972; 8:1394–6.

17. Perkins ES. The Bedford Glaucoma Survey. I. Long-term follow-up of borderline cases. Br J Ophthalmol 1973; 57:179–85.

18. Wilensky JT, Podos SM, Becker B. Prognostic indicators in ocular hypertension. Arch Ophthalmol 1974; 91:200–2.

19. Daubs JG, Crick PP. Epidemiological analysis of the Kings College Hospital glaucoma data. Res Clin Forums 1980; 2:41–59.

20. Drance SM. Low tension glaucoma: enigma and opportunity. Arch Ophthalmol 1985; 103:1131–3.

21. Abedin S, Simmons RJ, Grant WM. Progressive low-tension glaucoma: treatment to stop glaucomatous cupping and field loss when these progress despite normal intraocular pressure. Ophthalmology 1982; 89:1–6.

22. Armaly MF. Lessons to be learned from the Collaborative Glaucoma Study. Surv Ophthalmol 1980; 25:139–44.

23. Leske MC, Podgor M, Ederer F. An evaluation of glaucoma screening methods. Invest Ophthalmol Vis Sci [Suppl] 1982; 22:128. abstract.

24. Kolker AE, Hetherington J Jr. Diagnosis and therapy of the glaucomas. St. Louis, Mo.: CV Mosby Company, 1970.

25. Ford VJ, Zimmerman TJ, Kooner K. A comparison of screening methods for the detection of glaucoma. Invest Ophthalmol Vis Sci [Suppl] 1982; 22:257. abstract.

26. Shutt HKR, Boyd TAS, Salter AB. The relationship of visual fields, optic disc appearances and age in non-glaucomatous and glaucomatous eyes. Can J Ophthalmol 1967; 2: 83–90.

27. Wood CM, Bosanquet RC. Limitations of direct ophthalmoscopy in screening for glaucoma. Br Med J 1987; 1587–8.

28. Schwartz JT. Methodologic differences and measurement of cup-disc ratio: an epidemiologic assessment. Arch Ophthalmol 1976; 94:1101–5.

29. Holmin C. Optic disc evaluation versus the visual field in chronic glaucoma. Acta Ophthalmologica 1982; 60:275–83.

30. Hoskins HD, Gelber EC. Optic disk topography and visual field defects in patients with increased intraocular pressure. Am J Ophthalmol 1975; 80:284–90.

31. Hitchings RA, Spaeth GL. The optic disc in glaucoma. II. Correlation of the appearance of the optic disc with the visual field. Br J Ophthalmol 1977; 61:107–13.
32. Keltner JL, Johnson CA. Screening for visual field abnormalities with automated perimetry. Surv Ophthalmol 1983; 28:175–83.
33. Sommer A, Enger C, Witt K. Screening for glaucomatous visual field loss with automated threshold perimetry. Am J Ophthalmol 1987; 103:681–4.
34. Douglas GR. The Peritest automatic perimeter in screening for glaucomatous visual field deficits. Can J Ophthalmol 1983; 18:318–20.
35. Read RM, Spaeth GL. The practical clinical appraisal of the optic disc in glaucoma: the natural history of cup progression and some specific disc-field correlations. Trans Am Acad Ophthalmol Otol 1974; 78:255–74.
36. Shin DH, Kolker AE, Kass MA, et al. Long-term epinephrine therapy of ocular hypertension. Arch Ophthalmol 1976; 94:2059–60.
37. Krug JH, Hertzmark E, Remis LL, et al. Long term study of timolol vs. no treatment in the management of glaucoma suspects. Invest Ophthalmol Vis Sci [Suppl] 1987; 28:148. abstract.
38. Becker B, Morton RW. Topical epinephrine in glaucoma suspects. Am J Ophthalmol 1966; 62:272–7.
39. Hoff M, Parkinson JM, Kass MA, et al. Long-term trial of unilateral timolol treatment in ocular hypertensive subjects. Invest Ophthalmol Vis Sci [Suppl] 1988; 29:16. abstract.
40. Norskov K. Routine tonometry in ophthalmic practice. II. Five-year follow-up. Acta Ophthalmol 1970; 48:873–95.
41. Levene RZ. Uniocular miotic therapy. Trans Am Acad Ophthalmol Otol 1975; 79: 376–80.
42. Kass MA, Kolker AE, Becker B. Prognostic factors in glaucomatous visual field loss. Arch Ophthalmol 1976; 94:1274–6.
43. Sorensen PN, Nielsen NV, Norskov K. Ocular hypertension: a 15–year follow-up. Acta Ophthalmol 1978; 56:363–72.
44. Bengtsson B. Manifest glaucoma in the aged. I. Occurrence nine years after a population survey. Acta Ophthalmol 1981; 59:321–31.
45. Becker B, Shin S. Response to topical epinephrine: a practical prognostic test in patients with ocular hypertension. Arch Ophthalmol 1976; 94:2057–8.
46. Goldman H. Some basic problems of simple glaucoma. Am J Ophthalmol 1959; 48: 213–9.
47. Hildreth HR, Becker B. Routine tonometry. Trans Am Ophthalmol Soc 1956; 54:55–61.
48. Harbin TS, Podos SM, Kolker AE, et al. Visual field progression in open-angle glaucoma patients presenting with monocular field loss. Trans Am Acad Ophthalmol Otol 1976; 81:253–7.
49. Fraunfelder FT, Meyer SM. Systemic reactions to ophthalmic drug preparations. Med Toxicol Adverse Drug Exp 1987; 2:287–93.
50. Johnson DH, Brubaker RF. Glaucoma: an overview. Mayo Clin Proc 1986; 61:59–67.
51. Wishart PK, Nagasubramanian S, Hitchings RA. Argon laser trabeculoplasty in narrow angle glaucoma. Eye 1987; 1(pt 5):567–76.
52. Aiken-O'Neill P, American Academy of Ophthalmology. Personal communication, January 1989.
53. Miller SC, American Optometric Association. Personal communication, October 1988.
54. National Society to Prevent Blindness. A guide for community control of glaucoma. Schaumburg, Ill.: National Society to Prevent Blindness, 1978.
55. Power EJ, Wagner JL, Duffy BM. Screening for open-angle glaucoma in the elderly. Washington, D.C.: Office on Technology Assessment, Congress of the United States, 1988.
56. Canadian Task Force on the Periodic Health Examination. The periodic health examination: 1985 update. Can Med Assoc J 1986; 134:721–9.
57. Frame PS. A critical review of adult health maintenance. Part 4. Prevention of metabolic, behavioral, and miscellaneous conditions. J Fam Pract 1986; 23:29–39.
58. Eddy DM, Sanders LE, Eddy JF. The value of screening for glaucoma with tonometry. Surv Ophthalmol 1983; 28:194–205.

33

Screening for Hearing Impairment

Recommendation: Screening should be performed on all neonates at high risk for hearing impairment (see *Clinical Intervention*). High-risk children not tested at birth should be screened before age 3, but there is insufficient evidence of accuracy to recommend routine audiologic testing of all children in this age group. There is also insufficient evidence of benefit to recommend for or against hearing screening of asymptomatic children beyond age 3. Screening is not recommended for asymptomatic adolescents or adults not exposed routinely to excessive noise. Elderly patients should be evaluated regarding their hearing, counseled regarding the availability and use of hearing aids, and referred appropriately for any abnormalities.

Burden of Suffering

Over 17 million Americans suffer some hearing impairment.[1] An estimated 1–2% of infants and children are hearing impaired, and half of these cases are congenital or acquired during infancy.[2-4] If left uncorrected, hearing impairment at this age may interfere with the development of speech and language skills. Infants at greatest risk for hearing loss include those with low birthweight, congenital infection with rubella or other infections, malformations, trauma, perinatal asphyxia, prematurity, and hospitalization in the intensive care nursery.[2,4-6] Temporary hearing loss is common among schoolchildren. At any given time, about 5–7% of children aged 5–8 have a 25 dB hearing loss, usually a self-limited complication of otitis media with middle ear effusion.[7] Only a small proportion of new school-aged cases result in serious long-term complications, usually due to chronic middle ear effusion or previously undetected sensorineural deficits.[7] In addition to its effects during childhood on language development, hearing impairment creates added difficulties during adulthood. The hearing impaired suffer from poor communication and have less desirable jobs, incomes, and housing conditions than those with normal hearing.[4,8,9] The development of hearing loss between adolescence and age 50 can have diverse etiologies (e.g., Meniere's disease, ototoxicity, head trauma), but the incidence of these forms of hearing impairment in the general population is low. Exceptions occur in certain high-risk groups, such as the estimated 5 million Americans with occupational exposure to hazardous noise levels (e.g., factory, maintenance, and farm workers).[10] Presbycusis, the hearing loss that occurs with aging, becomes increasingly common after age 50.[7] Hearing impairment is reported by 23% of persons aged 65–74, 33% of those aged 75–

84, and 48% of persons aged 85 and over.[11] Older persons with hearing impair ment may suffer from reduced interpersonal communication, social isolation, depression, reduced mobility, and exacerbation of coexisting psychiatric conditions.[12,13] Hundreds of millions of dollars are spent annually to provide the hearing impaired with communication skills training and hearing aid devices.[4,14]

Efficacy of Screening Tests

The detrimental effect of hearing loss on language development occurs before age 3, but the abnormality is often not detected until age 2–6.[2,3,5,8,9] Therefore, screening tests have been recommended during infancy, preferably during the neonatal period. Because infants cannot cooperate with standard tests such as pure-tone and visual reinforcement audiometry, specialized neonatal tests have been developed.[2] An accurate noninvasive newborn screening test is the measurement of auditory brainstem responses.[3,4] Although the published sensitivity of this test is 97–100%,[4,15,16] the infants examined in these studies may not be representative of the general population. Technical problems with the procedure also result in a high false-positive rate of 10–40%,[2-4,6,15] and further testing is often necessary to confirm abnormal results. Other electrophysiologic tests for hearing impairment (e.g., electrocochleography) are not appropriate for routine screening because they are invasive, require general anesthesia, or have poor sensitivity and specificity.[2,3,9]

A traditional method of examining hearing in children under age 2 is behavioral testing: evoking body movements in response to auditory stimuli.[17] The body movements are recorded by a human observer, however, and thus results are influenced by observer bias, lack of standardization, the skill of the examiner, and irregularities in the examining conditions.[4,9,17,18] This method fails to detect between 22% and 76% of infants with hearing impairment.[2,3] In recent years, automated devices, such as the auditory response cradle (ARC) and crib-o-gram (COG), have been used to record body movements objectively.[17] The reported sensitivity and specificity of the COG are 60–91% and 64–77%, respectively.[4,5] The specificity of the ARC is also limited; studies suggest that most infants with abnormal ARC results have normal hearing when follow-up testing is performed.[17,19]

Hearing tests for preschool and school-aged children generally involve some combination of conventional audiometry, tympanometry, and otoscopic examination. Most cases of hearing loss in schoolchildren are transient and due to serous otitis media with middle ear effusion. This causes a conductive hearing loss that is often detectable by audiometry. Although precise data on sensitivity are lacking, it is known that audiometry does not detect all cases of middle ear effusion.[7] One study found that 55% of children with reduced middle ear pressure passed the routine audiometric sweep test at the 25 dB level.[20] Audiometric accuracy is also affected by background noise, cooperation of the child, and instrument calibration.[7,14] Otoscopic examination is also a poor screening test for conductive hearing loss because the findings of opaque tympanic membrane and loss of light reflex correlate poorly with middle ear effusion.[14,20]

The most accurate screening test for serous otitis media is impedance testing by tympanometry, which detects reduced middle ear pressure. The test has a reported sensitivity of 65–99% and a specificity of 77% in detecting reduced middle ear pressure.[7,14] Abnormal tympanometry is a common finding in healthy children. In one prospective study, between 24% and 39% of healthy children had abnormal results when screening tympanometry was performed periodically between ages 4 and 7.[21] Another limitation of tympanometry, in contrast to audiometry, is its limited ability to detect sensorineural impairment. The latter is an uncommon finding in schoolchildren, however, since most cases are diagnosed earlier in childhood.[20]

I learing function in adults is often assessed by simple clinical techniques, such as the whisper or watch-tick tests, but the validity and reliability of these maneuvers have not been adequately studied.[22] Free-field voice testing (whispering at a distance of 60 cm [2 feet]) has been reported to have a sensitivity of 100% and a specificity of about 85% in detecting audiometry-confirmed hearing loss.[23,24] These data have been criticized, however, because the study populations were not asymptomatic and because the studies provide little information on the test-retest reliability of free-field voice testing; the whisper of different examiners would presumably differ to some extent in terms of frequency and loudness.[25]

Pure-tone audiometry is a more accurate and reproducible screening test for hearing impairment. With pure-tone thresholds in audiometric test booths used as a reference criterion, pure-tone audiometry has a reported sensitivity of 92% and a specificity of 94% in detecting sensorineural impairment.[26] Some hand-held audiometers for physicians have achieved comparable results in recent studies.[22,26] Audiometry results are subject to error, however, due to improper technique, ambient noise in the test area, and accidental or intentional misreporting by the subject.[14] In addition, routine audiometry may be costly when applied to a large population. A careful history and examination by an alert clinician may be a more practical means of evaluating hearing in most adults, but there are insufficient data on the accuracy (sensitivity, specificity, predictive value) of the history and physical examination in detecting adult hearing loss.

Effectiveness of Early Detection

Auditory thresholds in hearing-impaired persons can be improved through sound amplification with hearing aids and frequency modulation radio devices.[1,8,9,14,18] Auditory and language training can also improve communication skills.[9] Although, on theoretical grounds, early detection and treatment of hearing loss would therefore appear to be beneficial, there have been few prospective studies comparing the outcome of hearing-impaired persons identified through screening and those who are not screened. Theoretically, the greatest benefit from being screened comes from the detection of hearing impairment due to sensorineural deficits or recurrent otitis media between birth and age 3. It is during this period that speech and language skills develop, and auditory stimuli appear to be critical to this process.[4,17] It is believed that early treatment of hearing loss may permit the development of normal language and psychosocial skills, and most experts recommend screening infants beginning at birth.[1-4,9,14,15,17] There is little evidence, however, regarding the efficacy of these measures. Studies of conductive hearing loss suggest an association between hearing impairment during early childhood and poor performance on speech and language tests,[8,27,28] but the methodologic design of these studies has been criticized.[29,30] A recent prospective study of children enrolled at birth found that many otitis-prone children had mild or moderate hearing loss when tested at age 2, but their hearing was normal when tested at age 3–4 and there was no evidence of language delay.[31] Correction of sensorineural impairment is also thought to be beneficial, but reliable data on the effectiveness of early detection are lacking. Randomized and controlled prospective studies of both forms of hearing impairment are needed to determine whether children receiving early intervention have better language skills than untreated children or those whose treatment is delayed. In the meantime, it is reasonable to assume on the basis of existing evidence that early correction of hearing impairment before age 3 is of some clinical value, especially for children with signs of marked hearing impairment.

In older children, hearing screening detects a larger proportion of conductive hearing loss due to serous otitis media with middle ear effusion.[5] Once again, there are few studies demonstrating that screened children have a better outcome than those who are not screened. In fact, a controlled cohort study found that kindergarten children who received audiometric screening had the same prevalence of hearing disorders 6–12 months after the test as the children who were not screened.[32] Most cases detected at this age are self-limited episodes of acute otitis media with effusions that resolve spontaneously or within 6–8 weeks.[5,7,14,18] Since the critical period of language development has passed at this age, these episodes appear to have little impact on educational performance; some studies suggest a subtle effect on verbal skills and scholastic performance but definitive evidence is lacking.[29] Detection of such cases is more likely to generate parental anxiety and visits to pediatricians.[7,32,33] However, a small proportion of the screened population, children with protracted hearing impairment that has escaped detection, is more likely to benefit from screening. Some studies suggest that schoolchildren with undetected subtle sensorineural hearing deficits, recurrent otitis media, or chronic middle ear effusions are at increased risk for educational and language problems[1,3,34] or inappropriate labeling by adults and peers,[14] but the quality of this evidence is poor.[29] Those with unresolved serous otitis media may also develop middle ear fibrosis, adhesions, and cholesteatoma.[7,20] Early detection of these cases through screening provides an opportunity to prevent some of these complications through such measures as hearing aids, communication training, and medical or surgical treatment,[18] but there have been few studies examining whether early intervention does, in fact, prevent complications. Studies have been unable to provide consistent evidence that clinical interventions for chronic otitis media (e.g., antibiotics, myringotomy, tympanostomy tubes) are able to achieve sufficient long-term improvement in hearing and language skills to justify the risk of complications.[30,32,34,35]

Among adults, hearing impairment is too rare and the value of early detection too small to justify hearing screening, with the exception of high-risk groups such as persons in occupations at risk for noise-induced hearing loss.[36] The elderly are the most likely to benefit from screening, because of the prevalence of presbycusis and because significant limitations in independent activity and functional status are more common among older persons with hearing loss.[12,13] In addition, hearing impairment in the elderly is probably more likely to escape detection and to receive inadequate treatment. In the National Health Interview Survey, 23–48% of persons over age 65 reported that they were hearing impaired but only 8% used a hearing aid.[11] Older persons often view hearing loss as an uncorrectable consequence of aging, and they may be unaware of their impairment due to its gradual onset or coexisting cognitive deficits.[22,37] Some may benefit from simple clinical interventions such as the removal of cerumen obstructing the external ear canal, but the exact prevalence of this cause of hearing impairment in the elderly is uncertain. Other measures, such as hearing aids, patient and family communication training, and environmental structuring, have not been formally tested for efficacy[22] but are believed by many to enhance the functional status and quality of life of hearing-impaired elderly.[37]

Recommendations of Others

Many groups recommend hearing screening during infancy. The American Speech-Language-Hearing Association (ASHA) recommends electrophysiological testing between birth and 6 months of age (preferably before hospital discharge) of all infants meeting selected risk criteria related to family history, congenital infection, anatomic malformations, low birthweight, hyperbilirubinemia, bacterial meningitis, and severe asphyxia.[38] A joint policy statement by ASHA, the American Academy of Otolaryngology, Head and Neck Surgery, the American Academy of Pediatrics (AAP), and the American Nurses Association is currently being developed to replace earlier (1982) joint recommendations by these groups.[39]

Differing recommendations have been issued on screening of preschool and schoolchildren. The Canadian Task Force recommends a clinical examination of hearing at ages 2–3, 5–11, and 16.[40] The Institute of Medicine recommends hearing testing for preschool children and during ages 6–11 and 12–17.[41] The AAP recommends periodic historical inquiry regarding hearing throughout infancy and childhood and objective hearing testing at ages 4, 5, 12, and 18.[42] The AAP opposes the use of tympanometry in mass screening programs for the detection of hearing loss or middle ear effusion and recommends pure-tone audiometry as the primary method for detecting hearing loss in schoolchildren.[33] ASHA recommends annual audiometry for all children functioning at a developmental level of 3 years through grade 3 and for all children in high-risk groups.[43]

Recommendations for adults also vary. The Canadian Task Force recommends risk assessment for hearing loss by history and physical examination at age 16 and thereafter during clinical visits for other reasons.[40,44] Breslow and Somers recommend audiometry for adults every five years.[45] The Institute of Medicine recommends hearing testing once during ages 40–59, 60–74, and 75 and over.[41] Most employers are required by Federal law to perform baseline and annual audiometry on workers exposed to hazardous noise levels.[46] Guidelines on referral criteria for such workers and on hearing conservation programs are published elsewhere.[47,48]

Discussion

The detection of hearing loss during infancy appears to be worthwhile, but the auditory brainstem response (ABR) is currently the only test with sufficient accuracy and validation for screening. Routine ABR testing on all neonates is not feasible because the procedure is expensive and time-consuming.[2,4,5,9] Each test costs over $100 and, because of the expense of confirmatory testing of false-positive results, about $10,600 would be spent for each case of hearing loss correctly identified by ABR.[4] ABR screening is likely to be more cost-effective among high-risk neonates, where a higher prevalence of hearing impairment has been documented. Other devices such as the crib-o-gram and auditory response cradle are faster and less expensive to perform, but their inaccuracy makes them even less cost-effective than ABR.[4,9,19] More economical and practical screening tests are available for children over age 3, but the correction of hearing impairment is most important before this age. It is unclear whether the early detection of infrequent cases of sensorineural or persistent hearing loss after this age outweighs the costs of referrals and false-positive labeling for the vast majority of children with conductive losses due to self-limited acute otitis media. At the same time, there is insufficient evidence of harm to discourage current clinical practice or hearing screening efforts by local school systems and private organizations.

In adolescents and young adults, however, there is little basis for screening, except for selected high-risk groups with occupational or recreational exposure to excessive noise. The elderly may benefit the most from screening because of the increased prevalence of presbycusis at this age and the reluctance of many patients to bring their symptoms to medical attention. It is unclear, however, that these benefits are of sufficient magnitude to justify the substantial cost of audiometric screening of the nearly 30 million Americans over age 65.[49] A more practical but unproven strategy might include a careful historical evaluation of hearing in older patients, a simple otoscopic examination for cerumen and other findings, and patient education regarding the availability of efficacious hearing aid devices.

Clinical Intervention

Screening for hearing impairment should be performed on all high-risk neonates. Risk factors include family history of childhood hearing impairment; congenital perinatal infection with herpes, syphilis, rubella, cytomegalovirus, or toxoplasmosis; malformations involving the head or neck (e.g., dysmorphic and syndromal abnormalities, cleft palate, abnormal pinna); birthweight below 1500 g; bacterial meningitis; hyperbilirubinemia requiring exchange transfusion; or severe perinatal asphyxia (Apgar scores of 0–3, absence of spontaneous respirations for 10 minutes, or hypotonia at 2 hours of age).[39] High-risk children not tested at birth should be screened before age 3, but there is insufficient evidence of accuracy to recommend routine audiologic testing of all children in this age group.

Although there is insufficient evidence of benefit to recommend hearing screening of asymptomatic children beyond age 3, it is recognized that such testing often occurs outside of the clinical setting. When this occurs, abnormal test results should be confirmed by repeat testing at appropriate intervals, and all confirmed cases identified through screening should be referred for ongoing audiological assessment, selection of hearing aids, family counseling, psychoeducational management, and periodic medical evaluation.

Hearing screening is not necessary for asymptomatic adolescents and young adults, except for those who are exposed regularly to excessive noise (e.g., in recreational or occupational settings). Screening of workers for noise-induced hearing loss should be performed in the context of existing worksite programs and occupational medicine guidelines. Elderly patients should be evaluated periodically regarding their hearing, counseled regarding the availability of hearing aid devices, and referred appropriately for any abnormalities. The optimal frequency of hearing examinations has not been determined and is left to clinical discretion. An otoscopic examination and audiometric testing should be performed on all persons with evidence of impaired hearing.

REFERENCES

1. National Center for Health Statistics. Prevalence of selected chronic conditions, United States, 1979–81. Vital and Health Statistics, series 10, no. 155. Washington, D.C.: Government Printing Office, 1986. (Publication no. DHHS (PHS) 86–1583.)
2. Parving A. Hearing disorders in childhood: some procedures for detection, identification and diagnostic evaluation. Int J Pediatr Otorhinolaryngol 1985; 9:31–57.
3. Riko K, Hyde ML, Alberti PW. Hearing loss in early infancy: incidence, detection and assessment. Laryngoscope 1985; 95:137–45.
4. Prager DA, Stone DA, Rose DN. Hearing loss screening in the neonatal intensive care unit: auditory brain stem response versus crib-o-gram; a cost-effectiveness analysis. Ear Hear 1987; 8:213–6.
5. Calogero B, Giannini P, Marciano E. Recent advances in hearing screening. Adv Otorhinolaryngol 1987; 37:60–78.
6. Duara S, Suter CM, Bessard KK, et al. Neonatal screening with auditory brainstem

responses: results of follow-up audiometry and risk factor evaluation. J Pediatr 1986; 108.276–81.

7. Cross AW. Health screening in schools. Part I. J Pediatr 1985; 107:487–94.

8. Ruben RJ, Levine R, Fishman G, et al. Moderate to severe sensorineural hearing impaired child: analysis of etiology, intervention, and outcome. Laryngoscope 1982; 92:38–46.

9. Stewart IF. After early identification—what follows? A study of some aspects of deaf education from an otolaryngological viewpoint. Laryngoscope 1984; 94:784–99.

10. Department of Labor, Occupational Safety and Health Administration. Occupational noise exposure: hearing conservation amendment. Fed Reg 1981; 46:4078–180.

11. Havlik RJ. Aging in the eighties: impaired senses for sound and light in persons age 65 years and over. Preliminary data from the supplement on aging to the National Health Interview Survey: United States, January–June 1984. Advance Data from Vital and Health Statistics, no. 125. Hyattsville, Md.: National Center for Health Statistics, 1986. (Publication no. DHHS (PHS) 86–1250.)

12. Herbst KRG. Psychosocial consequences of disorders of hearing in the elderly. In: Hinchcliffe R, ed. Hearing and balance in the elderly. Edinburgh: Churchill Livingstone, 1983.

13. Bess FH, Lichtenstein MJ, Logan SA, et al. Hearing impairment as a determinant of function in the elderly. J Am Geriatr Soc 1989; 37:123–8.

14. Brooks DN. Audiology: state of the art. J Med Eng Technol 1986; 10:167–79.

15. Dennis JM, Sheldon R, Toubas P, et al. Identification of hearing loss in the neonatal intensive care unit population. Am J Otol 1984; 5:201–5.

16. Nield TA, Schrier S, Ramos AD, et al. Unexpected hearing loss in high-risk infants. Pediatrics 1986; 78:417–22.

17. Bhattacharya J, Bennett MJ, Tucker SM. Long term follow up of newborns tested with the auditory response cradle. Arch Dis Child 1984; 59:504–11.

18. Bellman S. Hearing screening in infancy. Arch Dis Child 1986; 61:637–8.

19. Shepard NT. Newborn hearing screening using the Linco-Bennett auditory response cradle: a pilot study. Ear Hear 1983; 4:5–10.

20. Ferrer HP. The use of impedance measurements in the diagnosis of serous otitis media. Int J Pediatr Otorhinolaryngol 1983; 5:243–50.

21. Tos M, Strangeup SE, Holms-Jensen S, et al. Spontaneous course of secretory otitis media and changes in the ear drum. Arch Otolaryngol 1984; 110:281–9.

22. Lichtenstein MJ, Bess FH, Logan SA. Validation of screening tools for identifying hearing-impaired elderly in primary care. JAMA 1988; 259:2875–8.

23. Swan IRC, Browning GG. The whispered voice as a screening test for hearing impairment. J R Coll Gen Pract 1985; 35:197.

24. Macphee GJA, Crowther JA, McAlpine CH. A simple screening test for hearing impairment in elderly patients. Age Ageing 1988; 17:347–51.

25. Lichtenstein MJ, Bess FH, Logan SA. Screening for impaired hearing in the elderly (letter). JAMA 1988; 260:3589–90.

26. Frank T, Petersen DR. Accuracy of a 40 dB HL audioscope and audiometer screening for adults. Ear Hear 1987; 8:180–3.

27. Bess FH, Tharpe AM. Unilateral hearing impairment in children. Pediatrics 1984; 74: 206–16.

28. Teele DW, Klein JO, Rosner BA, Greater Boston Otitis Media Study Group. Otitis media with effusion during the first three years of life and development of speech and language. Pediatrics 1984; 74:282–7.

29. Rapin I. Conductive hearing loss effects on children's language and scholastic skills: a review of the literature. Ann Otol Rhinol Laryngol [Suppl 60] 1979; 88(5 pt 2):3–12.

30. Paradise JL. Otitis media during early life: how hazardous to development? A critical review of the evidence. Pediatrics 1981; 68:869–73.

31. Wright PF, Sell SH, McConnell KB, et al. Impact of recurrent otitis media on middle ear function, hearing and language. J Pediatr 1988; 113:581–7.

32. Feldman W, Sackett B, Milner R, et al. Effects of preschool screening for vision and

hearing on prevalence of vision and hearing problems 6–12 months later. Lancet 1980; 2:1014–6.

33. American Academy of Pediatrics. Impedance bridge (tympanometer) as a screening device in schools. Policy statement of Committee on School Health. Pediatrics 1987; 79:472.

34. Callahan CW, Lazoritz S. Otitis media and language development. Am Fam Physician 1988; 37:186–90.

35. Barfoed C, Rosborg J. Secretory otitis media: long-term observations after treatment with grommets. Arch Otolaryngol 1980; 106:553–6.

36. Berwick DM. Screening in health fairs. JAMA 1985; 254:1492–8.

37. Stults BM. Preventive health care for the elderly. West J Med 1984; 141:832–45.

38. American Speech-Language-Hearing Association. Audiologic screening of newborn infants who are at risk for hearing impairment. ASHA 1989; 31:89–92.

39. *Idem*. Joint Committee on Infant Hearing position statement. ASHA 1982; 24:1017–8.

40. Canadian Task Force on the Periodic Health Examination. The periodic health examination. Can Med Assoc J 1979; 121:1193–254.

41. National Academy of Sciences, Institute of Medicine. Ad Hoc Advisory Group on Preventive Services. Preventive services for the well population. Washington, D.C.: National Academy of Sciences, 1978.

42. American Academy of Pediatrics. Recommendations for preventive pediatric health care. Committee on Practice and Ambulatory Medicine. Chicago, Ill.: American Academy of Pediatrics, 1987.

43. American Speech-Language-Hearing Association. Guidelines for identification audiometry. ASHA 1985; 27:49–52.

44. Canadian Task Force on the Periodic Health Examination. 1984 Update. Can Med Assoc J 1984; 130:1–16.

45. Breslow L, Somers AR. The lifetime health-monitoring program. A practical approach to preventive medicine. N Engl J Med 1977; 296:601–8.

46. Department of Labor, Occupational Safety and Health Administration. Occupational noise exposure, hearing conservation amendment, final rule. Fed Reg 1983; 48: 9738–85.

47. American Occupational Medicine Association. Guidelines for the conduct of an occupational hearing conservation program. Report of the Noise and Hearing Conservation Committee of the Council on Scientific Affairs. J Occup Med 1987; 29:981–2.

48. American Academy of Otolaryngology, Head and Neck Surgery. Otologic referral criteria for occupational hearing conservation programs. Washington, D.C.: American Academy of Otolaryngology, Head and Neck Surgery, 1983.

49. National Center for Health Statistics. Health, United States, 1988. Washington, D.C.: Government Printing Office, 1989:41. (Publication no. DHHS (PHS) 89–1232.)

34

Screening for Intrauterine Growth Retardation

Recommendation: Women at increased risk for delivering a growth-retarded infant (see *Clinical Intervention*) should receive ultrasound examinations early in the second trimester to determine gestational age and in the third trimester to measure the size of critical fetal structures. Routine ultrasound screening is otherwise not recommended in normal pregnancies, although physicians may wish to consider ultrasound dating in pregnant women with uncertain menstrual histories. All pregnant women should receive appropriate counseling regarding smoking (see Chapter 48), alcohol and other drug abuse (Chapter 47), and nutrition (Chapter 50).

Burden of Suffering

Fetal growth retardation occurs in about 3–10% of all pregnancies[1] and is associated with approximately 20% of all fetal deaths.[2] Growth-retarded fetuses are at increased risk for fetal distress during labor,[1] and their perinatal mortality is as much as 10 times higher than that of fetuses with normal growth.[1,3] At birth, affected infants are characteristically small for gestational age and at risk for serious complications in the nursery. Low birthweight, along with short gestation, is the third leading cause of death among newborns in the United States and accounts for over 3200 neonatal deaths each year, usually in the first 24 hours of life.[4] Common complications of intrauterine growth retardation (IUGR) include meconium aspiration, peripartum asphyxia and acidosis, pneumonia, hypoglycemia, hypocalcemia, hypothermia, and polycythemia/hyperviscosity syndrome.[1,3] IUGR may also be associated with increased risk of sudden infant death syndrome[5] and long-term neurologic and developmental sequelae.[6]

Efficacy of Screening Tests

Screening tests for IUGR include physical examination of the abdomen, biochemical studies, and ultrasound examination. Physical examination by inspection and palpation of the abdomen detects only 30–50% of fetuses with IUGR.[2,7,8] Most clinicians supplement the examination with serial measurements of the symphysis-fundus height (SFH), the distance between the symphysis pubis and the superior aspect of the uterine fundus; an SFH 4 cm less than the gestational age has been described as abnormal.[1] The published sensitivity and specificity of this test are 65–85%[1,9-13] and 80–93%,[1,10,12,13] respectively, although the sensitivity of SFH measurement in a large study of over 2900 women was only 27%.[14] Some researchers believe SFH measurement is as accurate as an ultrasound examination in detecting IUGR;[15] others caution that most studies of this test are not generalizable due to small samples and selection biases.[16] Other concerns about this test include the large proportion of pregnancies that would be identified as abnormal (8–28%),[9,15] its low positive predictive value (21–45%),[9,15,16] and measurement error in identifying anatomic landmarks. In one study, the SFH reported by one of the examiners differed by as much as 3–4 cm when the test was repeated on the same patient.[11]

A variety of biochemical methods have been advocated for detecting IUGR. These include measurement of estriols, human placental lactogen, amniotic fluid C-amino peptide, serum cystine aminopeptidase, Schwangerschafts protein 1, and the foam stability index. Most of these tests are not thought to have a role as screening tests for normal pregnancies[1,9] because of their limited sensitivity.[17] For example, human placental lactogen and estrogens reportedly detect less than 10% of fetuses with IUGR.[18]

The most accurate means of detecting IUGR is the ultrasound examination. Measurements of the fetal abdomen and head, and indices that compare the relative size of these structures, have proved to be highly accurate in assessing fetal growth.[3,9,15,19-22] A small abdominal circumference, for example, the most commonly affected anatomical measurement,[23] has a sensitivity of 80–96% and a specificity of 80–90% in detecting growth-retarded fetuses.[9,23-25] The product of the crown-rump length and the trunk area has a sensitivity of 94% and a specificity of 90%.[17] The generalizability of these studies has been questioned, however; many had small samples, used expert ultrasonographers, and/or suffered from methodologic limitations.[9,26] In addition, the equipment that is necessary for certain measurements (e.g., static B-mode scanners for measuring crown-rump length) may be impractical for routine screening. It is also likely that routine scanning would yield a greater proportion of false positives than true cases of IUGR, because of the relatively low risk of IUGR in the general population. The positive predictive value of the most accurate ultrasound parameter, an abnormal abdominal circumference at 34–36 weeks' gestation, is only 40–50%[9,27] and may be as low as 21% in some populations.[24]

Most recommendations for ultrasound screening in the third trimester to detect IUGR also advise an ultrasound examination early in the second trimester to determine gestational age. Accurate information on gestational age is necessary to determine the appropriate size and growth rate of fetal structures in the third trimester.[9] Ultrasound is the recommended test because measurement of the biparietal diameter, when performed early in the second trimester, has been shown to be significantly more accurate in determining gestational age than the dates of the last menstrual period.[28,29] About 25–45% of women are unable to provide an accurate menstrual history;[23,28,29] the estimated date of confinement derived from the last menstrual period differs by more than two weeks from the actual date of birth in nearly one-quarter of pregnancies.[28] Clinical estimation of gestational age by bimanual palpation does not improve accuracy;[30] errors of up to eight weeks are not uncommon.[9] In contrast, 90% of patients deliver within two weeks of the due date when gestational age is determined by ultrasound measurement of the biparietal diameter.[28]

Indirect benefits often attributed to ultrasound screening for IUGR include the early sonographic detection of multiple gestations and low-lying placentas. Ultrasound is an accurate screening test for multiple gestations, which are missed by clinical examination in nearly one-third of cases.[31] One center that provided the only maternity services in its community[29] reported that 98% of all twins were detected when routine ultrasound screening was performed.[32] The average gestational age at detection fell from 27 weeks to 20 weeks.[29] False-positive ultrasound diagnoses also occur, however; over 20% of multiple fetuses identified in the first trimester are either artifacts or abort spontaneously early in pregnancy.[00] There is little information on the accuracy of ultrasound in detecting a low-lying placenta. Early identification is probably of limited predictive value, however, since only 0.5% of low-lying placentas remain in this location until the third trimester.[32,34]

Effectiveness of Early Detection

It is believed that at least some of the complications of IUGR can be prevented if growth disorders are discovered early in the third trimester and certain interventions are implemented promptly.[1,3,35] Examples of commonly recommended interventions include diagnostic studies to determine the cause (viral antibodies, karyotyping), behavior modification counseling (cigarette smoking, substance abuse, nutrition), fetal assessment (evaluation of fetal lung maturity, electronic fetal monitoring, periodic ultrasound examination), antenatal therapy (bedrest), and intrapartum precautions (optimizing the timing and mode of delivery, and preparing the delivery room with appropriate resuscitation equipment and personnel).[35]

Evidence is limited that these measures are successful in changing the outcome of IUGR, however. Few controlled prospective studies have examined morbidity or mortality outcomes in either the mother or fetus.[35] Those that have examined specific treatment practices, such as bedrest, have been unable to demonstrate significant benefits.[36] Four recent randomized controlled trials have specifically examined the effectiveness of routine ultrasound screening. Two of these trials were unable to demonstrate statistically significant benefits in lowering perinatal mortality, morbidity (as measured by birthweight and Apgar scores), postterm induction, or maternal hospitalization.[17,37] The third trial found that providing the obstetrician with ultrasound evidence of IUGR at the 34th week increased the incidence of induced labor but did not improve the outcome for the baby.[38]

The fourth trial, which provides the strongest evidence for ultrasound screening, compared routine ultrasound examination at the 18th and 32nd weeks with ultrasound only for clinical indications.[39] Screened pregnancies had a statistically significant reduction in interventions for postterm pregnancy, maternal hospital admissions, and the hospital length of stay of some newborns. Perinatal mortality was also lower in the screened group, but the difference was not statistically significant. No trial to date has demonstrated a statistically significant reduction in perinatal mortality associated with the use of routine ultrasound.[40] Data from several trials were pooled in an attempt to increase statistical power, but the combined reduction in neonatal mortality did not reach statistical significance.[40]

For the assessment of fetal structures in the third trimester to be meaningful, it is first necessary to obtain an accurate determination of gestational age early in pregnancy;[9,10] an ultrasound examination early in the second trimester is the most accurate method of dating the pregnancy. By providing improved information on gestational age, the benefits of ultrasound screening can extend beyond the prevention of IUGR. Accurate dates may help prevent the induction of preterm fetuses thought to be postterm on the basis of erroneous dating.[9,23,32] In one community, the incidence of postterm inductions fell from 8% to 2.6% after ultrasound screening was instituted,[32] but it was not proved that this trend was due specifically to improved dating. A randomized controlled trial found that providing ultrasound-derived dates to obstetricians did not significantly lower perinatal mortality or morbidity (as measured by birthweight and Apgar scores).[41] The investigators[41] and others[23,37,40] have questioned these findings, however, because ultrasound dates were released for medical reasons in 30% of the control group pregnancies.

One recent randomized controlled trial did find that a one-stage screening program, in which ultrasound was offered at about 15 weeks' gestation, resulted in a statistically significant reduction in the rate of induction for suspected postterm pregnancy when compared with controls, who were dated in the customary manner.[42] Moreover, babies born to screened women had a significantly greater mean birthweight (3521 g vs. 3479 g) than did those born to controls. The investigators found that the difference in birthweight was noted primarily among screened women who reported smoking at their first prenatal visit; there was no significant difference in birthweight between controls and screened women who did not smoke. This led the authors to hypothesize that viewing the fetus on ultrasound examination may have motivated women to reduce tobacco use during pregnancy.

Other indirect benefits of prenatal ultrasound are often cited in support of screening for IUGR. These include the detection of congenital anomalies, multiple gestations, and low-lying placentas. Ultrasound screening for congenital anomalies is discussed in Chapter 38. The early detection of multiple gestations, a risk factor for intrapartum and neonatal complications,[23] was shown to be of some benefit in a randomized controlled trial.[29] A large community study also found that perinatal complica tions in twins decreased significantly after ultrasound screening was instituted.[32] However, there are limitations to this evidence. The results of the clinical trial were not statistically significant, and the community study, which relied on historical controls, did not provide evidence that the outcome was due specifically to ultrasound screening. A recent randomized controlled trial reported that early detection of twins through ultrasound screening had no significant effect on neonatal outcome.[42] Detection of low-lying placenta by ultrasound, although of little value early in pregnancy,[43] may be of potential benefit in the second or third trimester in counseling patients about physical activity and sexual intercourse, in avoiding speculum and manual examinations of the vagina, and in making informed decisions at term about the safety of vaginal delivery.[23] The efficacy of these measures in preventing complications has not been proved, however.

Recommendations of Others

Some authors recommend measuring fundal height at each prenatal visit to detect growth disorders and then performing ultrasound examinations on women with abnormal results.[15,23] In Britain, the Royal College of Obstetricians and Gynaecologists has recommended routine ultrasound examinations.[44] In the United States, a National Institutes of Health consensus development conference has recommended that ultrasound imaging during pregnancy be performed only in response to a specific medical indication and not for routine screening.[45] This position has also been endorsed by the American College of Obstetricians and Gynecologists.[46,47] A number of authors, however, have recommended routine ultrasound during weeks 16–18 as a means of determining gestational age.[9,28] Some perform this test only in women with uncertain menstrual histories.[43] The Canadian Task Force has recently concluded that there is insufficient evidence to recommend the inclusion (or exclusion) of routine serial ultrasound screening for IUGR in normal pregnancies.[48]

Discussion

Although evidence to date is not conclusive, some recent clinical trials suggest that obtaining ultrasound data on gestational age and fetal size may result in improved fetal outcome. Even a single ultrasound examination early in the second trimester may improve birthweight and lower the rate of induction for presumed postterm pregnancy (see above). These findings need further confirmation through additional clinical research, and the significant economic implications of widespread testing also require careful study. Until conclusive evidence becomes available on the clinical effectiveness of scanning all pregnant women, ultrasound screening should be considered primarily for those women with uncertain menstrual histories, who may benefit from an examination early in the second trimester; it also should be considered for those with established risk factors for IUGR or other complications identifiable by ultrasound, for whom an examination may be especially important in the third trimester.

Clinical Intervention

Maternal risk factors for IUGR should be assessed in all pregnancies. These include hypertension, renal disease, short maternal stature, low prepregnancy weight, failure to gain weight during pregnancy, smoking, alcohol and other drug abuse, and history of a previous fetal death or growth-retarded baby. Women with these risk factors should receive ultrasonic cephalometry during weeks 16–18 to determine gestational age, serial fundal height measurements, and an additional ultrasound examination in the third trimester (34–36 weeks) to evaluate fetal growth parameters such as abdominal circumference. Routine ultrasound screening is not recommended in pregnancies at low risk for IUGR, although physicians may wish to consider ultrasound dating in pregnant women with uncertain menstrual histories. Counseling to reduce behavioral risk factors (e.g., cigarette smoking [see Chapter 48], alcohol and other drug abuse [Chapter 47], poor nutrition [Chapter 50]) should be provided routinely to all pregnant women.

REFERENCES

1. Lockwood CJ, Weiner S. Assessment of fetal growth. Clin Perinatol 1986; 13:3–35.
2. Tejani N, Mann LI. Diagnosis and management of the small-for gestational age fetus. Clinical Obstet Gynecol 1977; 20:943–55.
3. Mintz MC, Landon MB. Sonographic diagnosis of fetal growth disorders. Clinical Obstet Gynecol 1988; 31:44–52.
4. National Center for Health Statistics. Vital statistics of the United States, 1985, Vol. II, Mortality, Part A. Washington, D.C.: Government Printing Office, 1988. (Publication no. DHHS (PHS) 88–1101.)
5. Hoffman HJ, Bekketeig LS. Heterogeneity of intrauterine growth retardation and recurrence risk. Semin Perinatol 1984; 8:15–24.
6. Fitzhardinge PM, Stevens EM. The small-for-dates infant. II. Neurological and intellectual sequelae. Pediatrics 1972; 50:50–7.
7. Hall MH, Chng PK, MacGillivray I. Is routine antenatal care worthwhile? Lancet 1980; 2:78–80.
8. Rosenberg K, Grant JM, Hepburn M. Antenatal detection of growth retardation: actual practice in a large maternity hospital. Br J Obstet Gynecol 1982; 89:12–5.
9. Geirsson RT, Persson PH. Diagnosis of intrauterine growth retardation using ultrasound. Clin Obstet Gynecol 1984; 11:457–79.
10. Belizan JM, Villar J, Nardin JC, et al. Diagnosis of intrauterine growth retardation by a simple clinical method: measurement of uterine height. Am J Obstet Gynecol 1978; 131:643–6.
11. Calvert JP, Crean EE, Newcombe RG, et al. Antenatal screening by measurement of symphysis-fundus height. Br Med J 1982; 285:846–9.

12. Cnattingius S, Axelsson O, Lindmark G. Symphysis-fundus measurements and intrauterine growth retardation. Acta Obstet Gynecol 1984; 63:335–40.
13. Mathai M, Jairaj P, Muthurathnam S. Screening for light-for gestational age infants: a comparison of three simple measurements. Br J Obstet Gynecol 1987; 94:217–21.
14. Persson B, Stangenberg M, Lunell NO, et al. Prediction of size of infants at birth by measurement of symphysis fundus height. Br J Obstet Gynecol 1986; 93:206–11.
15. Pearce JM, Campbell S. A comparison of symphysis-fundal height and ultrasound as screening tests for light-for-gestational-age infants. Br J Obstet Gynecol 1987; 94: 100–4.
16. Rosenberg K, Grant JM, Tweedie I, et al. Measurement of fundal height as a screening test for fetal growth retardation. Br J Obstet Gynecol 1982; 89:447–50.
17. Neilson JP, Munjanja SP, Whitfield CR. Screening for small for dates fetuses: a controlled trial. Br Med J 1984; 289:1179–82.
18. Persson PH, Grennert L, Gennser G, et al. Fetal biparietal diameter and maternal plasma concentration of placental lactogen, chorionic gonadotrophin, oestriol and alphafetoprotein in normal and pathological pregnancies. Br J Obstet Gynecol 1980; 87:25–32.
19. Eik-Nes SH, Persson PH, Grottum P, et al. Prediction of fetal growth deviation by ultrasonic biometry. II. Clinical application. Acta Obstet Gynecol 1983; 62:117–23.
20. Campbell S, Kurjak A. Comparison between urinary oestrogen assay and serial ultrasonic cephalometry in assessment of fetal growth retardation. Br Med J 1972; 2: 336–40.
21. Campbell S, Dewhurst CJ. Diagnosis of the small-for-dates fetus by serial ultrasonic cephalometry. Lancet 1971; 2:1002–6.
22. Persson PH, Grennert L, Gennser G. Diagnosis of intrauterine growth retardation by serial ultrasonic cephalometry. Acta Obstet Gynecol Scand [Suppl] 1978; 78:40–8.
23. Warsof SL, Pearce JM, Campbell S. The present place of routine ultrasound screening. Clin Obstet Gynecol 1983; 10:445–57.
24. Brown HL, Miller JM, Gabert HA, et al. Ultrasonic recognition of the small-for-gestational-age fetus. Obstet Gynecol 1987; 69:631–5.
25. Neilson JP, Whitfield CR, Aitchison TC. Screening for the small-for-dates fetus: a two-stage ultrasonic examination schedule. Br Med J 1980; 280:1203–6.
26. Deter RL, Harrist RB, Hadlock FP, et al. The use of ultrasound in the detection of intrauterine growth retardation: a review. J Clin Ultrasound 1982; 10:9–16.
27. Warsof SL, Cooper DJ, Little D, et al. Routine ultrasound screening for antenatal detection of intrauterine growth retardation. Obstet Gynecol 1986; 67:33.
28. Campbell S, Warsof SL, Little D, et al. Routine ultrasound screening for the prediction of gestational age. Obstet Gynecol 1985; 65:613–20.
29. Grennert L, Persson PH, Gennser G. Benefits of ultrasonic screening of a pregnant population. Acta Obstet Gynecol 1978; 78:5–14.
30. Campbell S. Fetal growth. Clin Obstet Gyencol 1974; 1:41.
31. Farooqui MD, Grossman JH, Shannon RA. A review of twin pregnancies. Obstet Gynecol Surv 1973; 28:144–52.
32. Persson PH, Kullander S. Long-term experience of general ultrasound screening in pregnancy. Am J Obstet Gynecol 1983; 146:942–7.
33. Landy HJ, Weiner S, Corson SL, et al. The "vanishing twin": ultrasonographic assessment of fetal disappearance in the first trimester. Am J Obstet Gynecol 1986; 155: 14–9.
34. Rizos N, Doran TA, Miskin M, et al. Natural history of placenta praevia ascertained by diagnostic ultrasound. Am J Obstet Gynecol 1979; 133:287–91.
35. Simpson GF, Creasy RK. Obstetric management of the growth retarded baby. Clin Obstet Gynecol 1984; 11:481–97.
36. Laurin J, Persson PH. The effect of bedrest in hospital on fetal outcome in pregnancies complicated by intrauterine growth retardation. Acta Obstet Gynecol 1987; 66:407–11.
37. Bakketeig LS, Eik-Nes SH, Jacobsen G, et al. Randomised controlled trial of ultrasonographic screening in pregnancy. Lancet 1984; 2:207–11.
38. Secher NJ, Hansen PK, Lenstrup C, et al. A randomized study of fetal abdominal

diameter and fetal weight estimation for detection of light-for-gestation infants in low-risk pregnancies. Br J Obstet Gynecol 1987; 94:105–9.

39. Eik-Nes SH, Okland O, Aure JC, et al. Ultrasound screening in pregnancy: a randomised controlled trial. Lancet 1984; 1:1347.

40. Thacker SB. Quality of controlled clinical trials. The case of imaging ultrasound in obstetrics: a review. Br J Obstet Gynecol 1985; 92:437–44.

41. Bennett MJ, Little G, Dewhurst J, et al. Predictive value of ultrasound measurement in early pregnancy: a randomized controlled trial. Br J Obstet Gynecol 1982; 89:338–41.

42. Waldenstrom U, Axelsson O, Nilsson S, et al. Effects of routine one-stage ultrasound screening in pregnancy: a randomised controlled trial. Lancet 1988; 2:585–8.

43. Imoedemhe DAG, Mitford E, Chan R, et al. An evaluation of routine early pregnancy ultrasonography. Acta Obstet Gynecol Scand 1985; 64:427–31.

44. Royal College of Obstetricians and Gynaecologists Working Party. Routine ultrasound examination in pregnancy. London: Royal College of Obstetricians and Gynaecologists, 1984.

45. National Institutes of Health Consensus Development Conference. The use of diagnostic ultrasound imaging during pregnancy. JAMA 1984; 252:669–72.

46. American College of Obstetricians and Gynecologists. Ultrasound in pregnancy. ACOG Technical Bulletin No. 116. Washington, D.C.: American College of Obstetricians and Gynecologists, 1988.

47. Kaminetzky HA, American College of Obstetricians and Gynecologists. Personal communication, September 1988.

48. Anderson GM, Allison D. Intrauterine growth retardation and the routine use of serial ultrasound. In: Goldbloom RB, Lawrence RS. Preventing disease: beyond the rhetoric. New York: Springer-Verlag (in press).

35

Screening for Preeclampsia

Recommendation: All pregnant women should receive systolic and diastolic blood pressure measurements at the first prenatal visit and periodically throughout the third trimester (see *Clinical Intervention*).

Burden of Suffering

Hypertension is the most common medical complication of pregnancy, occurring in about 6–8% of all pregnancies.[1,2] It is seen in a group of disorders that include preeclampsia-eclampsia, latent or chronic essential hypertension, a variety of renal diseases, and gestational (transient) hypertension. The definitions used to discriminate these disorders are a matter of debate, leading to uncertainty about their exact prevalence, natural history, and response to treatment.[3,4]

Preeclampsia, or toxemia of pregnancy, is the most dangerous of these disorders. Although definitions differ, many describe preeclampsia as acute hypertension (over 140/90; or a rise of 15 mm Hg or 30 mm Hg above the usual diastolic and systolic pressures, respectively) presenting after the 20th week of gestation, accompanied by abnormal edema, proteinuria (more than 0.3 g/24 h), or both.[5] Women with preeclampsia are at increased risk for such complications as abruptio placentae, acute renal failure, cerebral hemorrhage, disseminated intravascular coagulation, pulmonary edema, circulatory collapse, and eclampsia.[6] The fetus may become hypoxic, increasing its risk for low birthweight, premature delivery, or perinatal death.[7] Eclampsia, the advanced stage of this disorder characterized by seizures, is the leading cause of maternal deaths in the United States.[2] Women with preeclampsia are not at increased risk of developing chronic hypertension.[5,8] Those at increased risk of developing preeclampsia and eclampsia include primigravidas and women with multiple gestations, chronic hypertension or diabetes, or a family history of eclampsia or preeclampsia.[6]

Other causes of hypertension during pregnancy include gestational and essential hypertension. Gestational, or transient, hypertension is the acute onset of hypertension in pregnancy or the early puerperium without proteinuria or abnormal edema and resolving within 10 days after delivery.[2] Essential hypertension that had been latent prior to the pregnancy may become evident during gestation. Gravidas with latent essential hypertension are also at increased risk for stillbirth, neonatal death, and other fetal complications, but the risk is much lower than that of women with preeclampsia. Women with latent essential hypertension are also more likely to develop chronic hypertension in later years.[9]

Efficacy of Screening Tests

Screening tests for preeclampsia are difficult to evaluate due to the absence of a "gold standard" to confirm the diagnosis. Glomerular endotheliosis, the renal lesion characteristic of preeclampsia, is present in only 54% of patients who meet the clinical criteria for the disease.[8] In addition, the glomerular lesions of preeclampsia are not specific for preeclampsia, having been observed in association with other conditions, such as abruptio placentae and chronic renal disease.[8,10] For practical reasons, most studies of potential screening tests for preeclampsia have relied on clinical criteria to confirm the diagnosis.

Many proposed screening tests have been found unsuitable for early detection of preeclampsia. The appearance of edema and proteinuria alone is unreliable, because edema is common in normal pregnancies[11] and therefore lacks specificity. Measurable proteinuria usually occurs late in the course of the illness and therefore is not useful for early detection.[2] In a prospective study of women between 24 and 34 weeks of gestation, a urine albumin concentration equal to or greater than 11 mcg/mL had a sensitivity of 50% in predicting subsequent preeclampsia.[12] The conventional dipstick test is unreliable in detecting the moderate and highly variable elevations in albumin that occur early in the course of preeclampsia.[4,13,14] The definitive test for proteinuria, the 24-hour urine collection, is not practical for screening.[14] Other tests that have been suggested include the angiotensin II infusion test and the supine pressor "rollover" examination, but these have also been found to be unsuitable, as the former is impractical and the latter lacks adequate sensitivity, specificity, and positive predictive value.[1,14]

The most promising screening test for preeclampsia is blood pressure measurement to detect elevated readings, although there are several problems in relying on blood pressure readings as an accurate predictor. There are the usual sources of measurement error associated with sphygmomanometry, such as instrument defects and examiner technique (see Chapter 3). In addition, maternal posture can significantly affect blood pressure in pregnant women;[14] the results can be erroneous, for example, if blood pressure is measured with the woman in the supine position. Most important, a single elevated blood pressure reading is neither diagnostic of nor a good predictor for preeclampsia.[1,15] The trend in blood pressure over time may be more important than a single isolated measurement.

As mentioned above, the usual screening criteria for preeclampsia recommended by authorities are a blood pressure greater than 140 mm Hg systolic or 90 mm Hg diastolic, or a rise of 15 mm Hg above baseline diastolic blood pressure or 30 mm Hg above baseline systolic pressure. The latter criteria, however, require at least two elevated measurements, thereby increasing the margin of error, and have been shown to have limited sensitivity (21–52% and 7–23% for the diastolic and systolic criteria, respectively) in predicting preeclampsia.[16] A combination of these blood pressure criteria may be more effective in identifying women at risk for preeclampsia.[17]

In the middle trimester, the normal decline in blood pressure is often dampened or absent in women who develop preeclampsia. This finding or an observed increase in blood pressure during the second trimester may be an early indicator of increased risk for preeclampsia.[7,18] Some experts recommend using the middle trimester mean arterial pressure—MAP, equal to (systolic pressure + [2 × diastolic pressure])/3)—as a screening test.[7] Studies indicate that a middle trimester MAP in excess of 90 mm Hg has a sensitivity of 61–71% and a specificity of 62–74% in predicting preeclampsia,[7,19] and even higher values have been reported by some researchers.[20] More recent reports suggest the sensitivity of this test in detecting preeclampsia may actually be much lower (22–35%) and is of little value in predicting eclampsia itself.[21] A recent review concluded that due to inconsistencies in the definition of "preeclampsia" as used in most of these studies (e.g., failure to require proteinuria for the diagnosis), elevations in second trimester blood pressure may be a better predictor of transient or essential hypertension than of true preeclampsia.[22]

Effectiveness of Early Detection

The early detection of hypertension during pregnancy permits clinical monitoring and prompt therapeutic intervention should severe preeclampsia or eclampsia develop. Although some studies support the use of bedrest, pharmacologic agents, and early delivery of the fetus to prevent complications, there is little conclusive evidence that these measures improve outcome.[14,23,24] A randomized controlled trial found that antihypertensive therapy and hospitalization, when compared with hospitalization alone, did not improve maternal or fetal outcome.[25] There have been no clinical trials to determine whether hypertensive women treated early in pregnancy have a better prognosis than those who are not detected early.

Nonetheless, most obstetrical experts believe, on the basis of clinical experience, that early detection and treatment of preeclampsia is beneficial to the patient and fetus.[1,26] This is based in part on inferences drawn from the apparent effectiveness of regular prenatal care in reducing the risk of preeclampsia-eclampsia. Studies conducted as early as the 1940s suggested an inverse relationship between the extent of prenatal care and the incidence of eclampsia, perhaps reflecting a beneficial effect due to early detection.[27] These findings do not provide direct evidence, however, that improved outcome is due solely to blood pressure measurement itself, rather than to other components of prenatal care or to the characteristics of women who receive regular prenatal care.

Recommendations of Others

The American College of Obstetricians and Gynecologists recommends blood pressure measurements at the initial visit, every 4 weeks until 28 weeks' gestation, every 2–3 weeks until 36 weeks' gestation, and weekly thereafter.[28] The Canadian Task Force recommends one blood pressure measurement during each of the following time periods: weeks 1–13, 14–27, 28–30, 31–33, 34–36, 37–40, and postpartum.[29] The National Institute of Child Health and Human Development is currently considering recommendations to perform blood pressure measurement less frequently during pregnancy.[30]

Discussion

The most efficacious screening strategy for preeclampsia is the early detection of an abnormal blood pressure trend over time. Serial measurements during the second and third trimester increase the likelihood that a pathological pattern or overt hypertension will be detected.[7,15,19,31] There is no conclusive proof that these efforts will result in reduced maternal or perinatal morbidity and mortality. However, screening may be justified because there is widespread expert opinion that these benefits occur, it is unlikely that a study will be conducted in which a control group is not permitted to receive blood pressure screening or treatment, the target condition is the most common medical complication of pregnancy, and the screening test is fast, inexpensive, and acceptable to patients. Consistent attention should be given to using proper measurement technique to collect reliable blood pressure data. Although the use of isolated specific blood pressure levels (e.g., above

140/90) for diagnosing preeclampsia has an important role in evaluating patients, it may be inappropriate for use as a screening test until more definitive data are obtained on its positive predictive value.[17] Measurement of blood pressure and calculation of the MAP during the second trimester may also provide useful information prior to the development of preeclampsia-eclampsia, but more reliable data are needed to determine the positive predictive value of second trimester blood pressure and whether acting on this information results in improved clinical outcome.

Clinical Intervention

Systolic and diastolic pressures should be measured on all obstetric patients at the first prenatal visit and periodically throughout the third trimester of pregnancy. The optimal frequency for measuring blood pressure in pregnant women has not been determined and is left to clinical discretion. Although blood pressure screening of all pregnant women during the second trimester is not specifically recommended, it is clinically prudent during this period to measure blood pressure on women who are being seen by their clinicians for other reasons. The collection of meaningful blood pressure data requires consistent use of correct technique and a cuff of appropriate size. In addition to the guidelines listed in Chapter 3, the patient should be in the lateral recumbent position and the blood pressure should be measured in the superior arm after the patient has rested for several minutes. Further diagnostic evaluation and clinical monitoring, including frequent blood pressure monitoring and urinalysis, are indicated if blood pressure does not decrease normally during the middle trimester, if the diastolic pressure increases 15 mm Hg above baseline or the systolic pressure increases 30 mm Hg above baseline, or if the blood pressure exceeds 140/90.[5] Medical interventions should not be prescribed until the diagnosis of preeclampsia is confirmed.

REFERENCES

1. DeVoe SJ, O'Shaughnessy RW. Clinical manifestations and diagnosis of pregnancy-induced hypertension. Clin Obstet Gynecol 1984; 27:836–53.
2. Chesley LC. History and epidemiology of preeclampsia-eclampsia. Clin Obstet Gynecol 1984; 27:801–20.
3. Chesley LC. Diagnosis of preeclampsia. Obstet Gynecol 1985; 65:423–5.
4. Davey DA, MacGillivray I. The classification and definition of the hypertensive disorders of pregnancy. Am J Obstet Gynecol 1988; 158:892–8.
5. Chesley LC. Hypertension in pregnancy: Definitions, familial factor, and remote prognosis. Kidney Intern 1980; 18:234–40.
6. Wynn RM. Obstetrics and gynecology: the clinical core, 3rd ed. Philadelphia: Lea & Febiger, 1983:143.
7. Page EW, Christianson R. The impact of mean arterial pressure in the middle trimester upon the outcome of pregnancy. Am J Obstet Gynecol 1976; 125:740–6.
8. Fisher KA, Luger A, Spargo BH, et al. Hypertension in pregnancy: clinical-pathological correlations and remote prognosis. Medicine 1981; 60:267–76.
9. World Health Organization. The hypertensive disorders of pregnancy: report of a WHO Study Group. Technical Report Series No. 758. Geneva: World Health Organization, 1987.
10. Thomson D, Paterson WG, Smart GE, et al. The renal lesions of toxaemia and abruptio placentae studied by light and electron microscopy. J Obstet Gynecol Br Commonwealth 1972; 79:311–20.

11. Vollman RF. Study design, population and data characteristics. In: Friedman EA, ed. Blood pressure, edema and proteinuria in pregnancy. New York: Alan R. Liss, 1976:00.

12. Rodriguez MH, Masaki DI, Mestman J, et al. Calcium/creatinine ratio and microalbuminuria in the prediction of preeclampsia. Am J Obstet Gynecol 1988; 159:1452–5.

13. Irgens-Moller L, Hemmingsen L, Holm J. Diagnostic value of microalbuminuria in preeclampsia. Clin Chim Acta 1986; 157:295–8.

14. Sibai BM. Pitfalls in diagnosis and management of preeclampsia. Am J Obstet Gynecol 1988; 159:1–5.

15. Reiss RE, O'Shaughnessy RW, Quilligan TJ, et al. Retrospective comparison of blood pressure course during preeclamptic and matched control pregnancies. Am J Obstet Gynecol 1987; 156:894–8.

16. Moutquin JM, Giroux L, Rainville C, et al. Does a threshold increase in blood pressure predict preeclampsia? Proceedings of 5th Congress International Society for the Study of Hypertension in Pregnancy. Nottingham, England, July 1986:108.

17. Redman CW, Jefferies M. Revised definition of pre-eclampsia. Lancet 1988; 1:809–12.

18. Fallis NE, Langford HG. Relation of second trimester blood pressure to toxemia of pregnancy in the primigravid patient. Am J Obstet Gynecol 1963; 87:123–5.

19. Moutquin JM, Rainville C, Giroux L, et al. A prospective study of blood pressure in pregnancy: prediction of preeclampsia. Am J Obstet Gynecol 1985; 151:191–6.

20. Oney T, Kaulhausen H. The value of the mean arterial blood pressure in the second trimester (MAP-2 value) as a predictor of pregnancy-induced hypertension and preeclampsia. Clin Exp Hypertens 1983; 2:211–6.

21. Chesley LC, Sibai BM. Blood pressure in the midtrimester and future eclampsia. Am J Obstet Gynecol 1987; 157:1258–61.

22. Chesley LC, Sibai BM. Clinical significance of elevated mean arterial pressure in the second trimester. Am J Obstet Gynecol 1988; 159:275–9.

23. Mathews DD, Shuttleworth TP, Hamilton EFB. Modern trends in management of non-albuminuric hypertension in late pregnancy. Br Med J 1978; 2:623–5.

24. Gilstrap LC, Cunningham FG, Whalley PG. Management of preg nancy-induced hypertension in the nulliparous patient remote from term. Semin Perinatol 1978; 2:73.

25. Sibai BM, Gonzalez AR, Mabie WC, et al. A comparison of labetalol plus hospitalization versus hospitalization alone in the management of preeclampsia remote from term. Obstet Gynecol 1987; 70:3237.

26. Chamberlain GVP, Lewis PJ, De Swiet M, et al. How obstetricians manage hypertension in pregnancy. Br Med J 1978; 1:626–9.

27. Chesley LC. Eclampsia at the Margaret Hague Maternity Hospital. Bull Marg Hague Mat Hosp 1953; 6:2–11.

28. American College of Obstetricians and Gynecologists. Standards for obstetric-gynecologic services, 6th ed. Washington, D.C.: American College of Obstetricians and Gynecologists, 1985:17–8.

29. Canadian Task Force on the Periodic Health Examination. The periodic health examination. Can Med Assoc J 1979; 121:1194–254.

30. Hill JG, National Institute of Child Health and Human Development. Personal communication, February 1989.

31. Page EW, Christianson R. Influence of blood pressure changes with and without proteinuria upon outcome of pregnancy. Am J Obstet Gynecol 1976; 126:821–33.

36

Screening for Rubella

Recommendation: Serologic testing for rubella antibodies should be performed at the first clinical encounter with all pregnant and nonpregnant women of childbearing age lacking evidence of immunity (see *Clinical Intervention*). Susceptible nonpregnant women who agree not to become pregnant for three months should be vaccinated. Susceptible pregnant women should not be vaccinated until immediately after delivery.

Burden of Suffering

Rubella is generally a minor illness, but it can result in serious fetal complications when women become infected during pregnancy. Between 30% and 80% of fetuses of women with rubella become infected, depending on when during the pregnancy maternal infection occurs.[1] Fetal infection increases the risk of miscarriage, abortion, and stillbirth. Infected infants are at risk of developing congenital rubella syndrome (CRS), especially if maternal infection occurs during the first 16 weeks of pregnancy.[2] Hearing loss is the most common manifestation of CRS. In first trimester infections, it is often accompanied by mental retardation, cardiac malformations, and ocular defects (cataracts, microphthalmos).[1,3-5] Some manifestations of CRS, such as retarded growth, diabetes mellitus, thyroid disease, and glaucoma, do not appear until after infancy.[1] The lifetime costs of treating a patient with CRS exceed $220,000.[6]

Rubella has become an uncommon illness, with only 221 infections and one reported case of CRS occurring in the United States in 1988.[7] Incidence has decreased 99% since 1969, when rubella vaccine first became available in this country.[7-9] In the prevaccine years, rubella epidemics occurred on a regular six- to nine-year cycle; major pandemics occurred in 1935, 1943, and 1964.[10] The 1964 pandemic in the United States resulted in over 12 million rubella infections, with over 11,000 fetal losses and about 20,000 infants born with CRS.[6,10] The introduction of rubella vaccine led to the eradication of major periodic epidemics and dramatic reductions in the incidence of the disease. Although the risk of rubella infection is highest in children under age 5, nearly 60% of all infections occur in persons aged 15 and older.[7,8] About 10–20% of this population (including women of childbearing age) lack antibodies to rubella.

Efficacy of Screening Tests

One method of preventing rubella infection and reducing the incidence of CRS is to identify susceptible individuals through serologic screening and to administer rubella vaccine. For many years, hemagglutination inhibition (HI) was the principal serologic test for rubella antibodies. Nonspecific inhibitors occasionally interfere with this test, however, and produce false-positive HI results.[11] In one study, 8 out of 895 prenatal patients with positive HI tests during pregnancy were later found to be seronegative when they returned for further antenatal care.[12] Faster and more convenient laboratory methods (e.g., latex agglutination, enzyme-linked immunosorbent assay, indirect immunofluorescence, and radioimmunoassay) have become available in recent years.[13] The enzyme-linked immunosorbent assay (ELISA or EIA), in particular, has a sensitivity and specificity of 95–99% when compared with HI methods.[13,14]

Effectiveness of Early Detection

Rubella vaccination is recommended for all children (see Chapter 56), and therefore routine screening for antibodies is not necessary in this age group. Testing may be appropriate, however, in postpubertal adolescents and adults (especially women of childbearing age), because this population currently accounts for about 60% of all cases of rubella and 10–20% of this age group lack immunity.[7,8] Since identification and vaccination of these individuals may help prevent subsequent rubella infection and transmission to childbearing women, a nationwide effort was launched in 1977 to increase vaccinations of adolescents and adults.[8] This effort has been accompanied by a 95% reduction in the incidence of rubella and CRS. It is unclear, however, to what extent vaccination of adolescents and young adults, rather than children, has been responsible for this outcome. In fact, susceptibility to rubella among adults in the United States does not appear to have declined appreciably since rubella vaccine became available in 1969.[8] In Britain, an intensive campaign in the early 1980s led to a reduction in the susceptibility of pregnant women,[15] but this trend did not continue beyond 1984.[16]

A number of factors can limit the effectiveness of serologic testing and vaccination. False-positive serologic results erroneously suggesting the presence of antibodies can result in failure to recognize the need for vaccination. Even when susceptible persons are identified, many may be unable or unwilling to receive the vaccine. Investigators have shown that vaccination occurs in only 55–85% of seronegative persons identified in screening programs for nonpregnant women[16] and health care workers;[17] only 37–39% of susceptible persons identified through premarital screening are vaccinated.[18,19]

The rubella vaccine, once administered, is efficacious. The current RA27/3 live attenuated vaccine produces an antibody response in 95–98% of recipients;[20-26] 87–99% of persons who received older vaccines in the late 1960s remain seropositive 16–18 years after vaccination.[27-29]

There are often limited opportunities to evaluate antibody status in women of childbearing age before they become pregnant. Once a woman becomes pregnant, the principal value of rubella testing is in the prevention of maternal infection during subsequent pregnancies. The vaccine is contraindicated during pregnancy because of the potential teratogenicity of the vaccine virus, although to date there have been no reported cases of rubella vaccine-related birth defects in nearly 400 studied infants born to susceptible women who were vaccinated during pregnancy.[7,30-32] Vaccination of susceptible women identified during pregnancy is therefore recommended during the immediate postpartum period. However, about 13–18% of susceptible women fail to receive postpartum immunization,[15,16,33] perhaps due to the time interval between prenatal testing and the puerperium. Even in programs emphasizing compliance with postpartum immunization, 10 out of 100 women lack evidence of antibodies at a subsequent pregnancy.[12]

Another limitation of postpartum vaccination is the potential for adverse effects. Although further evidence is needed regarding the risks of transmitting rubella to breast-fed infants, the virus has been isolated in the breast milk of up to two-thirds of vaccinated women.[34] Postpartum immunization also produces transient arthritis and arthralgia in 4–18% of women, and persistent arthritis or arthropathy has also been reported.[8,35] Finally, postpartum immunization often occurs too late to prevent CRS; over one-half of cases occur with the first live birth.[9] Nonetheless, although rubella screening is clearly most effective in identifying susceptible women in clinical encounters occurring before conception, for many women prenatal care may provide the first opportunity for the clinician to evaluate antibody status. Even if the first pregnancy of a susceptible woman is missed, postpartum vaccination may help prevent the nearly 50% of CRS cases that occur in infants born to women with previous live births.[9]

Recommendations of Others

The Centers for Disease Control (CDC) and the American Academy of Pediatrics (AAP) recommend offering rubella vaccine to all women of childbearing age whose immunity is uncertain, are not pregnant, and agree not to become pregnant for the next three months.[7,36,37] Serologic screening is recommended when practical but is not a requirement for vaccination; it may be useful to collect a blood specimen at the time of vaccination. The CDC does not recommend routine pregnancy testing prior to vaccination.[8] The American College of Obstetricians and Gynecologists recommends routine screening for rubella during pregnancy.[38] The AAP recommends routine prenatal or antepartum rubella serology and administration of vaccine to susceptible women in the immediate postpartum period prior to hospital discharge.[37] The CDC and AAP also recommend offering serologic testing and vaccination to susceptible health care workers (lacking proof of vaccination or laboratory evidence of immunity) who have exposure to rubella, college students, or military trainees.[36,37]

Discussion

The incidence of rubella and CRS is likely to decrease dramatically and perhaps be eliminated as an indigenous problem in the United States when the current cohort of highly immunized children and adolescents passes through its childbearing years. In the intervening 10–30 years, however, a large number of childbearing women in the United States will probably remain inadequately immunized and susceptible to infection. Although CRS is a rare complication of pregnancy, it is largely preventable through maternal vaccination; therefore, clinical efforts to assess susceptibility through serologic screening are justified. At the same time, it is clear from current evidence that prenatal screening is a less effective and efficient means of preventing CRS than are screening and vaccination prior to pregnancy. It is therefore important for clinicians to emphasize the assessment of rubella susceptibility at their earliest clinical encounters with women of childbearing age. Women who are first seen for prenatal care also require testing, and specific arrangements must be made by the clinician to ensure that susceptible women receive postpartum immunization on schedule.

Clinical Intervention

Serologic testing for rubella antibodies should be performed at the first clinical encounter with pregnant and nonpregnant women of childbearing

age lacking evidence of immunity (proof of vaccination after the first birthday or laboratory evidence of immunity). Susceptible nonpregnant women who agree not to become pregnant for three months should be immunized with RA27/3 live attenuated vaccine. Susceptible pregnant women should be informed of the risks of fetal damage should they develop infection. They should be vaccinated in the immediate postpartum period, before discharge from the hospital.

Note: See also the relevant U.S. Preventive Services Task Force background paper: LaForce FM. Immunizations, immunoprophylaxis, and chemoprophylaxis to prevent selected infections. JAMA 1987; 257:2464–70.

REFERENCES

1. Freij BJ, South MA, Sever JL. Maternal rubella and the congenital rubella syndrome. Clin Perinatol 1988; 15:247–57.
2. Peckham CS, Marshall WC. The epidemiology of pregnancy. In: Barron SL, Thomson AM, eds. Obstetrical epidemiology. London: Academic Press, 1983:210.
3. Munro ND, Sheppard S, Smithells RW, et al. Temporal relations between maternal rubella and congenital defects. Lancet 1987; 2:201–4.
4. Miller E, Cradock-Watson JE, Pollock TM. Consequences of confirmed maternal rubella at successive stages of pregnancy. Lancet 1982; 2:781–4.
5. Peckham CS. Rubella and cytomegalovirus infection in pregnancy. Clin Exp Obstet Gynecol 1986; 13:97–107.
6. Orenstein WA, Bart KJ, Hinman AR, et al. The opportunity and obligation to eliminate rubella from the United States. JAMA 1984; 251:1988–94.
7. Centers for Disease Control. Rubella and congential rubella syndrome—United States, 1985–1988. MMWR 1989; 38:173–8.
8. *Idem*. Rubella and congenital rubella—United States, 1984–1986. MMWR 1987; 36:664.
9. *Idem*. Rubella and congenital rubella syndrome—New York City. MMWR 1986; 35: 770–9.
10. Witte JJ, Karchmer AW, Case G, et al. Epidemiology of rubella. Am J Dis Child 1969; 118:107–11.
11. Morgan-Capner P, Pullen HJM, Pattison JR, et al. A comparison of three tests for rubella antibody screening. J Clin Pathol 1979; 32:542–5.
12. Griffiths PD, Baboonian C. Is post partum rubella vaccination worthwhile? J Clin Pathol 1982; 35:1340–4.
13. Skendzel LP, Edson DC. Evaluation of enzyme immunosorbent rubella assays. Arch Pathol Lab Med 1985; 109:391–3.
14. Steece RS, Talley MS, Skeels MR, et al. Comparison of enzyme-linked immunosorbent assay, hemagglutination inhibition, and passive latex agglutination for determination of rubella immune status. J Clin Microbiol 1985; 21:140–2.
15. Miller CL, Miller E, Sequeira PJL, et al. Effect of selective vaccination on rubella susceptibility and infection in pregnancy. Br Med J 1985; 291:1398–401.
16. Miller CL, Miller E, Waight PA. Rubella susceptibility and the continuing risk of infection in pregnancy. Br Med J 1987; 294:1277–8.
17. Hartstein AI, Quan MA, Williams ML, et al. Rubella screening and immunization of health care personnel: critical appraisal of a voluntary program. Am J Infect Control 1983; 11:1–9.
18. Vogt RL, Clark SW. Premarital rubella vaccination program. Am J Public Health 1985; 75:1088–9.
19. Lieberman E, Faich GA, Simon PR, et al. Premarital rubella screening in Rhode Island. JAMA 1981; 245:1333–5.
20. Hillary IB, Meenan PN, Griffity AH, et al. Rubella vaccine trial in children. Br Med J 1969; 2:531–2.

21. Buser F, Nicolas A. Vaccination with RA27/3 rubella vaccine. Am J Dis Child 1971; 122:53–6.

22. Schiff GM, Linnemann CC, Shea L, et al. Evaluation of RA27/3 rubella vaccine. J Pediatr 1974; 85:379–81.

23. Balfour HH, Balfour CL, Edelman CK, et al. Evaluation of Wistar RA27/3 rubella virus vaccine in children. Am J Dis Child 1976; 130:1089–91.

24. Weibel RE, Villarejos VM, Klein EB, et al. Clinical and laboratory studies of live attenuated RA27/3 and HPV-77DE rubella virus vaccines. Proc Soc Exp Biol Med 1980; 165: 44–9.

25. Plotkin SA, Farquhar JD, Katz M, et al. Attenuation of RA27/3 rubella virus in WI-38 human diploid cells. Am J Dis Child 1969; 118:178–85.

26. Plotkin SA, Farquhar JD, Ogra PL. Immunologic properties of RA27/3 rubella virus vaccine. JAMA 1973; 225:585–90.

27. Chu SY, Bernier RH, Stewart JA, et al. Rubella antibody persistence after immunization: sixteen-year follow-up in the Hawaiian Islands. JAMA 1988; 259:3133–6.

28. Just M, Just V, Berger R, et al. Duration of immunity after rubella vaccination: a long-term study in Switzerland. Rev Infect Dis [Suppl] 1985; 7:91–4.

29. Shea S, Best JM, Banatvala JE, et al. Persistence of rubella antibody eight to 18 years after vaccination. Br Med J Clin Res 1984; 288:1043.

30. Centers for Disease Control. Rubella vaccination during pregnancy—United States, 1971–1986. MMWR 1987; 36:457–61.

31. Sheppard S, Smithells RW, Dickson A, et al. Rubella vaccination and pregnancy: preliminary report of a national survey. Br Med J 1986; 292:727.

32. Enders G. Rubella antibody titers in vaccinated and nonvaccinated women and results of vaccination during pregnancy. Rev Infect Dis [Suppl 1] 1985; 7:S103–7.

33. Edmond E, Zealley H. The impact of a rubella prevention policy on the outcome of rubella in pregnancy. Br J Obstet Gynecol 1986; 93:563–7.

34. Losonsky GA, Fishaut JM, Strussenberg J, et al. Effect of immunization against rubella on lactation products. II. Maternal-neonatal interactions. J Infect Dis 1982; 145:661–6.

35. Tingle AJ, Chantler JK, Pot KH, et al. Postpartum rubella immunization: association with development of prolonged arthritis, neurological sequelae, and chronic rubella viremia. J Infect Dis 1985; 152:606–12.

36. Recommendations of the Public Health Service Advisory Committee on Immunization Practices, rubella vaccine. MMWR 1978; 27:452–9.

37. American Academy of Pediatrics. Revised recommendations on rubella vaccine. Pediatrics 1980; 65:1182–4.

38. American College of Obstetricians and Gynecologists. Standards for obstetric-gynecologic services, 7th ed. Washington, D.C.: American College of Obstetricians and Gynecologists, 1989:15.

Screening for Rh Incompatibility

Recommendation: All pregnant women should receive ABO/ Rh blood typing and testing for anti-Rh(D) antibody at their first prenatal visit. Unsensitized Rh-negative women should receive Rh(D) immune globulin at 28–29 weeks' gestation and within 72 hours after delivery, as well as after spontaneous or therapeutic abortion, ectopic pregnancy, amniocentesis, antepartum placental hemorrhage, or a transfusion of Rh-positive blood products (see *Clinical Intervention*).

Burden of Suffering

Rh incompatibility occurs when an Rh-negative woman is pregnant with an Rh-positive fetus. This occurs in 9–10% of pregnancies.[1] If no preventive measures are taken, 0.7–1.8% of Rh-negative women with an Rh-positive fetus will become isoimmunized antenatally, developing Rh(D) antibody through exposure to fetal blood; 8–15% will become isoimmunized at birth, 3–5% after abortion (spontaneous or therapeutic), and 2.1–3.4% after amniocentesis.[1-4] Rh(D) isoimmunization currently occurs at a rate of about 1.5 per 1000 births.[5] Its effects on the fetus or newborn include hemolytic anemia, hyperbilirubinemia, kernicterus, or intrauterine deaths due to hydrops fetalis.[6] About 45% of cases require intrauterine or exchange transfusions to survive,[7] and there are about four deaths from this disease per 100,000 total births.[8] The prevalence of Rh(D) isoimmunization has declined significantly following the introduction of new modes of treatment in the 1960s. Between 1970 and 1979, the crude incidence fell from 40.5 cases to 14.3 cases per 10,000 total births.[9] Rh disease now accounts for only 0.33% of the combined stillbirth and perinatal mortality rates.[10]

Efficacy of Screening Tests

Determination of Rh(D) blood type by hemagglutination is considered the established reference standard for blood group assessment, and the indirect Coomb's test for detecting anti-Rh(D) antibody is highly accurate in identifying women who are sensitized to Rh-positive blood. Antibody titers by themselves, however, are not good indicators of the severity of erythroblastosis.[6]

Effectiveness of Early Detection

The early detection of Rh incompatibility is of substantial benefit if the patient is unsensitized (having no evidence of anti-Rh(D) antibody). The administration of Rh(D) immune globulin (RhIG) to these women prevents maternal sensitization and subsequent hemolytic disease in Rh-positive infants. RhIG must be administered after abortion, amniocentesis, ectopic pregnancy, and antepartum hemorrhage, as well as after delivery.[2,9,11] The efficacy of RhIG prophylaxis was convincingly demonstrated in a series of clinical trials in the early 1960s. Despite a variety of flaws in study designs, these trials clearly demonstrated that isoimmunization did not occur in any of the women who received a full dose of RhIG and who were unsensitized when it was administered.[3,12-14] These findings led to the introduction of routine postpartum RhIG prophylaxis following licensure of RhIG in the late 1960s. Time series studies have since shown a dramatic decline in the incidence of Rh isoimmunization, from 13–17% in the mid-1960s to 0.3–1.9% in the mid-1970s.[1-3,8,12] In Canada, where compliance with prophylaxis was maximized, Rh isoimmunization fell from 10.3 per 1000 births and 55 deaths in 1964 to 3.4 per 1000 births and 1 death in 1975.[8]

The decline in mortality cannot be attributed entirely to prevention, however, since it was already occurring before the introduction of RhIG. Prior to 1945, about half of all babies with erythroblastosis died; by 1963, mortality had declined to 2%.[12] These early improvements were due to a trend towards smaller families and to the introduction of new interventions, such as amniotic fluid spectrophotometry, exchange transfusion, amniocentesis, intrauterine fetal transfusion, early induction of labor, and improved care of the premature erythroblastotic infant.[8,10]

It is clear, however, that postpartum prophylaxis has been extremely effective in the prevention of isoimmunization. There is additional evidence that antenatal administration of RhIG, when combined with postpartum prophylaxis, is effective in preventing isoimmunization during the third trimester.[9,10] This form of isoimmunization occurs in only 0.7–1.8% of women at risk[1-4] but is the most frequent cause of apparent failure of postpartum prophylaxis.[2,3] Clinical trials have demonstrated that the administration of RhIG at 28 weeks' gestation, when combined with postpartum administration, reduces the incidence of isoimmunization to 0.07–0.18% of total births.[1,8,15-17] Although sample selection and other design features in these trials were not optimal, the evidence for antepartum prophylaxis was conclusive.

The combination of antenatal and postnatal prophylaxis will therefore prevent isoimmunization in 95–99% of persons at risk.[8,18] The remainder of cases are due to failure to give RhIG when indicated, isoimmunization from previous pregnancies before the availability of RhIG, administration of an insufficient dose, or treatment failure.[2,5,18] At least 20–30% of these cases result from human error.[10-12] While clinicians almost always administer postpartum doses in accordance with recommendations, compliance rates are 88–94% for abortion, 31% for antepartum hemorrhage, and 14% for amniocentesis.[1]

Rh immune globulin is safe,[2] and although some fetuses will become weakly direct-antiglobulin-positive following antenatal administration, anemia and hyperbilirubinemia in the newborn are exceedingly rare.[3] The evidence is therefore quite compelling that early detection of the unsensitized Rh-negative woman is highly effective in preventing isoimmunization.

For women who have already become isoimmunized, the risk of Rh disease is considerably greater. Even under these conditions early detection is beneficial because it permits prompt intervention through intrauterine transfusion or early delivery. Intrauterine transfusion is technically difficult and has been associated with increased fetal mortality, but technical advances such as real-time ultrasound guidance and direct fetal blood sampling have increased perinatal survival of the fetus to 50–74%[5] and to 90% in expert hands.[10,19] More commonly, the fetus can be delivered early and exchange transfusion performed with only 1% mortality.[10]

Recommendations of Others

The American College of Obstetricians and Gynecologists (ACOG) recommends ABO/Rh blood typing and testing for anti-Rh(D) antibody at the initial prenatal visit; a repeat antibody determination at 28–29 weeks' gestation for unsensitized Rh-negative women; administration of RhIG at 28–29 weeks for unsensitized Rh-negative women; and administration of RhIG postpartum, preferably within 72 hours after delivery. The ACOG also recommends RhIG administration to unsensitized Rh-negative women who have an abortion, ectopic pregnancy, amniocentesis, or receive a transfusion of Rh-positive blood products.[20] To identify women needing larger postpartum doses of RhIG, testing for excess fetal-maternal transfusion by measuring fetal blood cell levels after high-risk deliveries (e.g., abruptio placenta, placenta previa) is recommended. Others have urged testing for fetal blood cells in all Rh-negative women who have delivered Rh-positive babies.[21] Administration of RhIG at 28 weeks is recommended by the American Academy of Pediatrics[22] and the Canadian College of Obstetricians and Gynecologists.[1] The Canadian Task Force recommends determination of blood type at 1–13 weeks, screening for anti-D antibodies every two weeks beginning at 20 weeks, and administration of RhIG to unsensitized Rh-negative women at 28 weeks and postpartum.[23]

Discussion

Although the burden of suffering from this disease is currently low, the incidence was at least 10 per 1000 live births prior to the introduction of preventive measures in the 1960s.[5,8] There is excellent evidence for the efficacy and effectiveness of screening and postpartum RhIG prophylaxis. Although antepartum prophylaxis offers some additional benefit, some critics argue that the total impact of antepartum prophylaxis on the incidence of Rh disease is relatively small, making it approximately 16 times less cost-effective than a program consisting only of postpartum treatment.[1,2,10] Other studies support the cost-effectiveness of antepartum prophylaxis.[18,24]

Clinical Intervention

All pregnant women should receive ABO/Rh blood typing and testing for anti-Rh(D) antibody at their first prenatal visit. A repeat Rh(D) antibody test should be performed at about 28 weeks' gestation on all unsensitized Rh-negative women, followed by the administration of 300 mcg of RhIG. The dose should be repeated postpartum, preferably within 72 hours after delivery. RhIG should also be administered to all unsensitized Rh-negative women who have an abortion (50 mcg before 13 weeks), ectopic pregnancy (50 mcg before 13 weeks), amniocentesis, antepartum placental hemorrhage, or a transfusion of Rh-positive blood products (10 mcg/mL whole blood transfused).[20] ABO/Rh antibody screening should be performed before patients are admitted for elective procedures, such as amniocentesis and therapeutic abortions, and RhIG should then be administered when these procedures are performed.

REFERENCES

1. Huchcroft S, Gunton P, Bowen T. Compliance with postpartum Rh isoimmunization prophylaxis in Alberta. Can Med Assoc J 1985; 133:871–5.

2. Nusbacher J, Bove JR. Rh immunoprophylaxis: is antepartum therapy desirable? N Engl J Med 1980; 303:935–7.
3. Bowman JM, Chown B, Lewis M. Rh isoimmunization during pregnancy: antenatal prophylaxis. Can Med Assoc J 1978; 118:623–7.
4. McMaster Conference on Prevention of Rh Immunization, 28–30 September 1977. Vox Sang 1979; 36:50–64.
5. Baskett RF, Parsons ML, Peddle LJ. The experience and effectiveness of the Nova Scotia Rh program, 1964–1984. Can Med Assoc J 1986; 134:1259–61.
6. Wynn RM. Obstetrics and gynecology: the clinical core, 3rd ed. Philadelphia: Lea & Febiger, 1983:143.
7. Creasy RK, Resnik R, eds. Maternal-fetal medicine: principles and practice. Philadelphia: WB Saunders, 1984.
8. Bowman JM, Pollock J. Rh immunization in Manitoba: progress in prevention and management. Can Med Assoc J 1983; 129:343–5.
9. Centers for Disease Control. Rh hemolytic disease—Connecticut, United States, 1970–1979. MMWR 1981; 30:13–5.
10. Urbaniak SJ. Rh(D) haemolytic disease of the newborn: the changing scene. Br Med J 1985; 291:4–6.
11. Wysoski DK, Flynt JW, Goldberg MF, et al. Rh hemolytic disease: epidemiologic surveillance in the United States, 1968 to 1975. JAMA 1979; 242:1376–9.
12. Bowman JM, Chown B, Lewis M. Rh isoimmunization, Manitoba, 1963–75. Can Med Assoc J 1977; 116:282–4.
13. Freda VJ, Gorman JG, Pollack W. Prevention of Rh hemolytic disease: ten years' clinical experience with Rh immune globulin. N Engl J Med 1975; 292:1014–6.
14. Prevention of primary Rh immunization: first report of the Western Canadian Trial, 1966–1968. Can Med Assoc J 1969; 100:1021–4.
15. Bowman JM, Pollock JM. Antenatal prophylaxis of Rh isoimmunization: 28 weeks gestation service program. Can Med Assoc J 1978; 118:627–30.
16. Tovey LA, Stevenson BJ, Townley A. The Yorkshire antenatal anti-D immunoglobulin trial in primigravidae. Lancet 1983; 2:244–6.
17. Clarke CA, Mollison PL, Whitfield AG. Deaths from rhesus haemolytic disease in England and Wales in 1982 and 1983. Br Med J 1985; 291:17–9.
18. Bowman JM, Pollack JM. Failures of intravenous Rh immune globulin prophylaxis: an analysis of the reasons for such failures. Transfus Med Rev 1987; 1:101–12.
19. Parer JT. Severe Rh isoimmunization: current methods of in utero diagnosis and treatment. Am J Obstet Gynecol 1988; 158:1323–9.
20. American College of Obstetricians and Gynecologists. Prevention of Rho(D) isoimmunization. ACOG Technical Bulletin No. 79. Washington, D.C.: American College of Obstetricians and Gynecologists, 1984.
21. Ness PM, Baldwin ML, Niebyl JR. Clinical high-risk designation does not predict excess fetal-maternal hemorrhage. Am J Obstet Gynecol 1987; 156:154–8.
22. Lockhart JD, American Academy of Pediatrics. Personal communication, November 1987.
23. Canadian Task Force on the Periodic Health Examination. The periodic health examination. Can Med Assoc J 1979; 121:1194–254.
24. Torrance GW, Zipursky A. Cost-effectiveness of antepartum prevention of Rh immunization. In: Zipursky A, ed. Clinics in perinatology. Philadelphia: WB Saunders, 1984: 267–81.

38

Screening for Congenital Birth Defects

Recommendation: Amniocentesis for karyotyping should be offered to pregnant women aged 35 and older. Maternal serum alpha-fetoprotein should be measured on all pregnant women during weeks 16–18 in locations that have adequate counseling and follow-up services (see *Clinical Intervention*). Ultrasound examination is not recommended as a routine screening test for congenital defects.

Burden of Suffering

Congenital malformations occur in about 3% of all newborns. Although most such malformations are minor and do not threaten life, over 6300 infants died in 1985 as a result of congenital anomalies.[1] They rank as the leading cause of infant mortality in the United States[1] and the fifth leading cause of years of potential life lost.[2] Congenital anomalies are also responsible for over three-fourths of physical handicaps.[3] The most common defects that can be detected through antenatal screening are those caused by chromosomal aneuploidy, such as Down's syndrome (trisomy 21), and those caused by neural tube defects. Down's syndrome occurs in 1 in 660 live births.[4] Affected children are characterized by physical abnormalities that include congenital heart disease and varying degrees of mental retardation. Women aged 35 and over are more likely to give birth to children with this and other aneuploidies.[5]

Neural tube defects, which include anencephaly and spina bifida, occur in about 1 out of every 1000 births in the United States.[6,7] Anencephaly is a fatal anomaly, resulting either in stillbirth or death within hours or days of birth. The manifestations of severe spina bifida include infectious complications, hydrocephalus, Arnold Chiari malformations, and, often as a complication of hydrocephalus, diminished intelligence.[7] Aggressive surgical and medical care is often necessary for severely affected cases, along with special schooling and rehabilitative services for patients with permanent disabilities. Families with a previous child with neural tube defects are at increased risk of having an affected child,[8] but about 90–95% of cases occur in the absence of a prior history.[6,8]

Efficacy of Screening Tests

Screening tests for Down's syndrome include karyotyping of specimens obtained by amniocentesis or chorionic villus sampling, measurement of maternal serum alpha-fetoprotein (MSAFP), and ultrasound imaging. Amniocentesis is now offered routinely to pregnant women aged 35 and older. The efficacy of this approach is limited by the fact that older mothers, although at exponentially increased risk for having a trisomic child, have low birth rates and thus give birth to only 20% of all children with Down's syndrome.[9] The vast majority of children of older mothers are normal; the incidence of Down's syndrome is about 1 out of 375 births at age 35, 1 out of 100 births at age 40, and 1 out of 30 births at age 45.[10,11] It can be predicted from available data (odds of Down's syndrome during second trimester) that a program offering amniocentesis to all pregnant women at age 35 has the potential of exposing 200–300 normal fetuses to this procedure for every case detected.[11] With an estimated iatrogenic fetal loss rate of about 0.5%, one normal fetus would be lost by amniocentesis for every one to two chromosomal anomalies detected. With increasing maternal age, the ratio of fetal loss to affected fetuses becomes more favorable.

As an alternative to performing routine amniocentesis on older women, screening of younger women, who give birth to 80% of children with Down's syndrome,[9] has been discussed as a potentially more effective means of detecting the disorder. Two proposed approaches are the measurement of MSAFP and ultrasonography. MSAFP screening for Down's syndrome is based on evidence that this and other trisomies are more common in women with *low* levels of MSAFP.[12-14] (MSAFP screening is also used to detect neural tube defects, in which the level is usually *high*; see below.) Studies suggest that routine screening for low levels of MSAFP could detect about 20–30% of fetuses with Down's syndrome.[15,16] Although this sensitivity is low, the absolute number of cases detected would be equivalent to that currently achieved by routine screening of older women by amniocentesis. The specificity of the test is about 90%.[15,16] There are disadvantages to this form of screening, however. These include the high false-positive rate associated with routine screening; a positive predictive value as low as 1–2% is reported in some series.[13,17] Since amniocentesis is required to evaluate each positive test, the ratio of amniocenteses performed on healthy fetuses for every proven case of Down's syndrome could be quite high.[18] The false-positive rate has been decreased in recent years by using adjusted cutoff values for low MSAFP that vary with maternal age. Using this approach, the odds of finding a chromosomal abnormality in a woman with low MSAFP are equivalent to those of a 35-year-old woman.[10,11]

Ultrasonography has been proposed as another potential screening test for Down's syndrome. Researchers at one center have shown that the sonographic finding of a thickened nuchal skin fold has a sensitivity of up to 45%[19] and the measurement of a short femur has a sensitivity of 51–70% in detecting affected fetuses.[20] A recent study by the same group found the combination of both findings to have a sensitivity of 75% and a specificity of 98%.[21] It will be important for researchers at other centers to reproduce these findings. The use of ultrasound as a screening test for Down's syndrome faces other limitations, including its low positive predictive value and the technical difficulty of producing a reliable sonographic image of critical fetal structures.[20,21] Incorrect positioning of the transducer, for example, can produce artifactual images resembling a thickened nuchal skin fold in a normal fetus.[22] Sonographic indices are therefore subject to considerable variation. Imaging techniques require further standardization before routine screening by ultrasound can be considered for the general population.[20,23]

Chorionic villus sampling (CVS), a new technique for obtaining trophoblastic tissue, offers promise as a method of detecting chromosomal anomalies. The advantages of this procedure include the ability to perform karyotyping as early as the 9th to 11th week and more rapid cytogenetic analysis. Its potential disadvantages include apparent discrepancies between the karyotype of villi and the fetus due to contamination or placental mosaicism, miscarriage, chorioamnionitis, and the complications of membrane damage.[24] Available data indicate that these adverse effects occur infrequently.[24-27] Preliminary results from a large multicenter trial indicate that the complication rate is low in expert hands but may be slightly higher than that of amniocentesis.[28] Pending the final results of this trial, CVS may be appropriate as a routine alternative to amniocentesis for screening in the general population.

Screening tests for neural tube defects include measurement of MSAFP and ultrasound. An *elevated* MSAFP is a good predictor of neural tube defects. Depending on the cutoff used to define an "elevated" level (usually 2.5 times the median value), screening can detect between 56% and 90% of affected fetuses (if followed by ultrasonography and measurement of amniotic alpha-fetoprotein).[14,29-34] The reported specificity approaches 100%.[30,35] Although the test is intended primarily to detect neural tube defects, the finding of elevated MSAFP is also a predictor of other congenital anomalies, intrauterine growth retardation, multiple gestations, preterm labor, and fetal demise.[6]

In comparison with the number of women who must be tested, however, the actual number of neural tube defects detected through screening the general population is relatively small (0.06–0.16% of pregnancies).[6,13,14,35] This low yield is due to several factors. First, a positive test (i.e., elevated MSAFP) occurs in only about 1–7% of pregnant women.[6,13,35] Second, about one-third of these are false positives and are not confirmed by a second MSAFP measurement.[6,13] Third, 90–95% of cases of elevated MSAFP are caused by conditions other than neural tube defects,[8,14,35] such as underestimated gestational age or twins. An ultrasound examination is often necessary to rule out these explanations for an elevated MSAFP (as well as anencephaly and fetal demise). If the ultrasound is unremarkable (about 50%), an amniocentesis is then performed to measure amniotic alpha-fetoprotein levels. Less than 10% of these lead to the discovery of a neural tube or abdominal wall defect; the majority of the fetuses are normal.[6] Some have expressed concern that the relatively small number of defects detected through screening may not justify the potential risks of amniocentesis and parental anxiety for the large majority of normal fetuses.[36]

Some authors have predicted that ultrasound may replace MSAFP measurement as the primary screening test for neural tube defects.[35,37] Virtually all cases of anencephaly can be detected by ultrasound alone,[38] as well as many closed neural tube defects that often escape detection by MSAFP measurement. However, current ultrasound techniques are less sensitive in detecting other neural tube defects, such as small meningomyeloceles.[29] In addition, although the published sensitivity and specificity of sonographic detection of spina bifida are good (79–96% and 90–100%, respectively),[37-40] investigators have emphasized that these data were obtained from centers with special expertise.[38] They may overestimate the sensitivity that would be expected when prenatal ultrasound is performed by those with less complete training, which has become increasingly common as more physicians perform their own ultrasound examinations.[41]

Effectiveness of Early Detection

The early detection of congenital defects in utero provides as its principal benefit the opportunity to inform prospective parents of the likelihood of giving birth to an affected child. Parents may be counseled about the consequences of the malformation and can make more informed decisions about optimal care for their newborn or continuation of the pregnancy. The usefulness of this information depends to a large extent on the personal preferences and abilities of the parents.[36] The diagnosis of a severe and/or fatal malformation (e.g., anencephaly) may spare unsuspecting parents some of the trauma associated with delivering a grossly deformed infant. Early detection of congenital defects may be beneficial in helping parents to prepare emotionally. It may also enable clinicians to provide more intensive obstetrical care and to better prepare for the delivery and care of the baby. Studies are lacking, however, regarding the impact of these measures on neonatal morbidity and mortality.

An indirect benefit of screening for congenital malformations is the discovery during testing of abnormalities other than the target condition. The ultrasound evaluation that follows the detection of raised MSAFP, for example, may lead to a diagnosis of twins or a more accurate assessment of gestational age, and some studies suggest that acting on this information may improve neonatal outcome (see Chapter 34). Raised levels of MSAFP, even in the absence of a congenital defect, is a risk factor for low birthweight and premature labor,[6] and early obstetrical intervention for these problems may be beneficial (Chapter 34). Other congenital anomalies, such as diaphragmatic hernia, gastroschisis, nonimmune fetal hydrops, and obstructive uropathy, may be detected. These discoveries will permit antenatal treatment as well as delivery and neonatal care planning. Controlled trials proving that early detection of these anomalies improves outcome, however, have not been published. Indeed, studies suggest that fetuses in which diaphragmatic hernia is detected in utero have poorer outcomes than those detected after birth,[42,43] perhaps in part because larger defects are more likely to be detected by ultrasound.

The benefits of early detection of congenital defects must be weighed against the potential risks of screening. The most important risks include those to the fetus from amniocentesis and the psychological effects on the parents of a positive test. The risks of amniocentesis include puncture of the fetus, bleeding, infection, and possibly isosensitization; orthopedic injuries and respiratory distress syndrome following amniocentesis have been reported but not confirmed.[6,16] The exact rate of fetal loss with current technique is uncertain but appears to be very low, about 0.5–1.0%.[6] Despite the safety of amniocentesis, the target conditions for which amniocentesis is performed are relatively uncommon, and in certain low-prevalence populations, it is possible for the complication rate to equal or exceed the detection rate for the target condition. It has been suggested, for example, that amniocenteses performed to detect Down's syndrome in women with low MSAFP could result in iatrogenic miscarriages in normal fetuses equal to the number of trisomic cases detected.[44-46] While some authors view these findings as adequate grounds to discourage routine testing,[44,46,47] others emphasize that the increased risk may be acceptable to parents with strong fears of having an abnormal child.[45,48,49]

Another risk of screening is the harmful psychological effect on parents of a positive test result. This is especially important because the large majority of positive screening tests in normal pregnancies are false positives. There is evidence that prospective parents with normal fetuses who are informed of an abnormal MSAFP test suffer significant anxiety during the weeks of diagnostic testing and waiting for definitive cytology results.[50,51] However, most women screened will have normal results, and this may have psychological benefits for the reassured parents.

The most serious consequence of false-positive results, the termination of a normal pregnancy on the basis of erroneous amniocentesis results, appears to be extremely uncommon with current assay techniques. The estimated rate is 1 in 10,000–50,000 screened pregnancies.[6,29]

Recommendations of Others

A statement by the American Medical Association in 1982 advised against routine measurement of MSAFP in pregnant women.[52] In recent years, however, a consensus has emerged among experts that MSAFP screening can be appropriate, provided that it is accompanied by adequate counseling and follow-up and is performed in areas with qualified diagnostic centers (level II ultrasound, amniocentesis) and standardized laboratories. Statements to this effect have recently been issued by the American College of Obstetricians and Gynecologists,[53] the American Society of Human Genetics,[54] the American Academy of Pediatrics,[55] and an international expert consensus conference.[29] Although no groups have called for universal MSAFP screening, a recent alert from the legal department of the American College of Obstetricians and Gynecologists (advising members to discuss the test with every patient and to document the discussion in the chart)[56] has been interpreted by some as requiring physicians to perform MSAFP screening in all pregnancies for medicolegal reasons.[54,57] Others have urged physicians not to adopt this legal statement as a medical standard.[23]

The currently accepted practice for detecting Down's syndrome and other chromosomal abnormalities is to offer amniocentesis to all women aged 35 and older. Screening for trisomy by testing for low MSAFP is considered investigational by most groups, including the American College of Obstetricians and Gynecologists,[58] the American Society of Human Genetics,[54] the American Academy of Pediatrics,[55] and others.[6,8] When MSAFP is measured for other reasons, clinicians are advised to counsel women with low values regarding the risk of aneuploidy. There are no official recommendations to perform routine screening for congenital defects by ultrasound; a National Institutes of Health consensus development conference has recommended that ultrasound imaging be performed during pregnancy only in response to a specific medical indication.[59]

Clinical Intervention

Amniocentesis for karyotyping should be offered to pregnant women aged 35 and older. Counseling before the procedure should include a comparison of the risks to the fetus from the procedure and the probability of a chromosomal defect at the patient's age. Maternal serum alpha-fetoprotein should be measured on all pregnant women during gestational weeks 16–18, except where the patient does not have access to counseling and follow-up services, skilled high-resolution ultrasound and amniocentesis capabilities, and reliable, standardized laboratories. Women with elevated MSAFP levels should receive a second confirmatory test and ultrasound examination before amniocentesis is performed. Women with low values should receive information comparing the increased risk of trisomy and the risks of fetal loss from amniocentesis. Testing for low MSAFP, however, is not recommended as a primary screening test for chromosomal anomalies. Routine ultrasound examination in normal pregnancies is not recommended as a screening test for congenital defects.

REFERENCES

1. National Center for Health Statistics. Vital statistics of the United States, 1985. Vol. II, mortality, part A. Washington, D.C.: Government Printing Office, 1988. (Publication no. DHHS (PHS) 88–1101.)
2. Centers for Disease Control. Years of potential of life lost before age 65--United States, 1987. MMWR 1989; 38:27–9.
3. Galjaard H. Early diagnosis and prevention of genetic disease. In: Galjaard H, ed. Aspects of human genetics. Basel: Karger, 1984.

4. Donnenfeld AE, Mennuti MT. Sonographic findings in fetuses with common chromosome abnormalities. Clin Obstet Gynecol 1988; 31:80–96.
5. Hansen JP. Older maternal age and pregnancy outcome: a review of the literature. Obstet Gynecol 1986; 41:726–42.
6. Campbell TL. Maternal serum alpha-fetoprotein screening: benefits, risks, and costs. J Fam Pract 1987; 25:461–7.
7. Hoffman HJ. Spinal dysraphism. Am Fam Physician 1987; 36:129–36.
8. Macri JN. Critical issues in prenatal maternal serum alpha-fetoprotein screening for genetic anomalies. Am J Obstet Gynecol 1986; 155: 240–6.
9. National Center for Health Statistics. Advance report of final natality statistics, 1983. Monthly Vital Statistics Report [Suppl], vol. 34, no. 6. Hyattsville, Md.: Public Health Service. (Publication no. DHHS (PHS) 85–1120.)
10. Cuckle HS, Wald NJ, Thompson SG. Estimating a woman's risk of having a pregnancy with Down's syndrome using her age and serum alpha-fetoprotein level. Br J Obstet Gynecol 1987; 94:387–402.
11. Palomaki GE, Haddow JE. Maternal serum alpha-fetoprotein, age, and Down syndrome risk. Am J Obstet Gynecol 1987; 156:460–3.
12. Merkatz IR, Nitowsky HM, Macri JN, et al. An association between low maternal serum alpha-fetoprotein and fetal chromosomal abnormalities. Am J Obstet Gynecol 1984; 148:886–94.
13. Simpson JL, Baum LD, Marder R, et al. Maternal serum alpha-fetoprotein screening: low and high values for detection of genetic abnormalities. Am J Obstet Gynecol 1986; 155:593–7.
14. Milunsky A, Alpert E. Results and benefits of a maternal serum alpha-fetoprotein screening program. JAMA 1984; 252:1438–42.
15. DiMaio MS, Baumgarten A, Greenstein RM, et al. Screening for fetal Down's syndrome in pregnancy by measuring maternal serum alpha-fetoprotein levels. New Engl J Med 1987; 317:342–6.
16. Cuckle HS, Wald NJ, Lindenbaum RH. Maternal serum alpha-fetoprotein measurement: a screening test for Down syndrome. Lancet 1984; 1:926–9.
17. Pueschel SM. Maternal alpha-fetoprotein screening for Down's syndrome. New Engl J Med 1987; 317:376–8.
18. Seller MJ. Prenatal screening for Down syndrome (letter). Lancet 1984; 1:1359.
19. Benacerraf BR, Frigoletto FD, Laboda LA. Sonographic diagnosis of Down syndrome in the second trimester. Am J Obstet Gynecol 1985; 153:49.
20. Lockwood C, Benacerraf B, Krinsky A, et al. A sonographic screening method for Down syndrome. Am J Obstet Gynecol 1987; 157:803–8.
21. Benacerraf BR, Gelman R, Frigoletto FD. Sonographic identification of second-trimester fetuses with Down's syndrome. New Engl J Med 1987; 317:1371–6.
22. Toi A, Simpson GF, Filly RA. Ultrasonically evident fetal nuchal skin thickening: is it specific for Down syndrome? Am J Obstet Gynecol 1987; 156:150–3.
23. Elias S, Annas GJ. Routine prenatal genetic screening. New Engl J Med 1987; 317: 1407–9.
24. Hogge WA, Schonberg SA, Golbus MS. Chorionic villus sampling: experience of the first 1000 cases. Am J Obstet Gynecol 1986; 154: 1249–52.
25. Brambati B, Oldrini A, Ferrazzi E, et al. Chorionic villus sampling: an analysis of the obstetric experience of 1000 cases. Prenat Diag 1987; 7:157–69.
26. Jackson LG, Wapner RA, Barr MA. Safety of chorionic villus biopsy. Lancet 1986; 1: 674–5.
27. Sachs ES, Jahoda MGJ, Kleijer WJ, et al. Impact of first-trimester chromosome, DNA, and metabolic studies on pregnancies at high genetic risk: experience with 1000 cases. Am J Med Genet 1988; 29:293–303.
28. Rhoads GG, Jackson LG, Schlesselman SE, et al. The safety and efficacy of chorionic villus sampling for early prenatal diagnosis of cytogenetic abnormalities. N Engl J Med 1989; 320:609–17.
29. Maternal serum alpha-fetoprotein screening for neural tube defects: results of a consensus meeting. Prenat Diagn 1985; 5:77–83.

30. United Kingdom collaborative study on alpha-fetoprotein in relation to neural tube defects: maternal serum alpha-fetoprotein measurement in antenatal screening for anencephaly and spina bifida in early pregnancy. Lancet 1977; 1:1323–32.
31. Haddow JE, Kloza EM, Smith DE, et al. Data from an alpha-fetoprotein pilot screening program in Maine. Obstet Gynecol 1983; 62:556–60.
32. Macri JN, Weiss RR. Prenatal serum alpha-fetoprotein screening for neural tube defects. Obstet Gynecol 1982; 59:633–9.
33. Burton BK, Sowers SG, Nelson LH. Maternal serum alpha-fetoprotein screening in North Carolina: experience with more than twelve thousand pregnancies. Am J Obstet Gynecol 1983; 146:439–44.
34. Brock DJH, Barron L, Watt M, et al. Maternal plasma alpha-fetoprotein and low birthweight: a prospective study throughout pregnancy. Br J Obstet Gynecol 1982; 89: 348–51.
35. Hooker JG, Lucas M, Richards BA, et al. Is maternal alpha-fetoprotein screening still of value in a low-risk area for neural tube defects? Prenat Diagn 1984; 4:29–33.
36. Reed BD, Ratcliffe S, Sayres W. Maternal serum alpha-fetoprotein screening. J Fam Pract 1988; 27:20–3.
37. Tyrrell S, Howel D, Bark M, et al. Should maternal alpha-fetoprotein estimation be carried out in centers where ultrasound screening is routine? A sensitivity analysis approach. Am J Obstet Gynecol 1988; 158:1092–9.
38. Roberts CJ, Evans KT, Hibbard BM, et al. Diagnostic effectiveness of ultrasound in detection of neural tube defect: the South Wales experience of 2509 scans (1977–1982) in high-risk mothers. Lancet 1983; 2:1068–9.
39. Sabbagha RE, Sheikh Z, Tamura RK, et al. Predictive value, sensitivity, and specificity of ultrasonic targeted imaging for fetal anomalies in gravid women at high risk for birth defects. Am J Obstet Gynecol 1985; 152:822–7.
40. Robinson HP, Hood VD, Adam AH, et al. Diagnostic ultrasound: early detection of fetal neural tube defects. Obstet Gynecol 1980; 56:705–10.
41. Sack RA, Maharry JM. Misdiagnoses in obstetric and gynecologic ultrasound examinations: causes and possible solutions. Am J Obstet Gynecol 1988; 158:1260–6.
42. Benacerraf BR, Adzick NS. Fetal diaphragmatic hernia: ultrasound diagnosis and clinical outcome in 19 cases. Am J Obstet Gynecol 1987; 156.573–6.
43. Adzick NS, Harrison MR, Glick PL, et al. Diaphragmatic hernia in the fetus: prenatal diagnosis and outcome in 94 cases. J Pediatr Surg 1985; 20:357–61.
44. Ager RP, Oliver RWA. Screening for Down syndrome (letter). Lancet 1987; 2:566–7.
45. Brock DJH. Screening for Down syndrome (letter). Lancet 1987; 2:1083–4.
46. Spencer K, Carpenter P. Screening for Down's syndrome using serum alpha fetoprotein: a retrospective study indicating caution. Br Med J 1985; 290:1940–3.
47. Wu LR. Maternal serum alpha-fetoprotein screening and Down's syndrome. Am J Obstet Gynecol 1986; 155:1362–3.
48. Thornton JG, Lilford RJ, Howell D. Safety of amniocentesis. Lancet 1986; 2:225–6.
49. Hershey DW. Screening for Down's syndrome. New Engl J Med 1988; 318:927–8.
50. Robinson JO, Hibbard BM, Laurence KM. Anxiety during a crisis: emotional effects of screening for neural tube defects. J Psychosom Res 1984; 28:163–9.
51. Burton BK, Dillard RG, Clark EN. The psychological impact of false positive elevations of maternal serum alpha-fetoprotein. Am J Obstet Gynecol 1985; 151:77–82.
52. Council on Scientific Affairs. Maternal serum alpha-fetoprotein monitoring. JAMA 1982; 247:1478–81.
53. American College of Obstetricians and Gynecologists. Prenatal detection of neural tube defects. Technical Bulletin No. 99. Washington, D.C.: American College of Obstetricians and Gynecologists, 1986.
54. American Society of Human Genetics. Policy statement for maternal serum alpha-fetoprotein screening programs and quality control for laboratories performing maternal serum and amniotic fluid alpha-fetoprotein assays. Am J Hum Genet 1987; 40:75–82.
55. American Academy of Pediatrics. Alpha-fetoprotein screening. Pediatrics 1987; 80: 444–5.
56. American College of Obstetricians and Gynecologists. Professional liability implications

232 I. Screening

of AFP tests. DPL alert. Washington, D.C.: American College of Obstetricians and Gynecologists, 1985.

57. Schwager EJ, Weiss BD. Prenatal testing for maternal serum alpha-fetoprotein. Am Fam Physician 1987; 35:169–74.

58. Committee on Obstetrics. Maternal and fetal medicine: newsletter. Washington, D.C.: American College of Obstetricians and Gynecologists, 1987.

59. National Institutes of Health Consensus Development Conference. The use of diagnostic ultrasound imaging during pregnancy. JAMA 1984; 252:669–72.

39

Screening for Fetal Distress

Recommendation: Fetal heart rate should be measured by auscultation on all women in labor to detect signs of fetal distress. Electronic fetal monitoring should not be performed routinely on all women in labor. It should be reserved for pregnancies at increased risk for fetal distress.

Burden of Suffering

Intrapartum fetal distress is an important cause of stillbirth and neonatal death. Although the exact incidence of fetal distress is uncertain, over 1100 infant deaths each year in the United States are attributed to intrauterine hypoxia and birth asphyxia.[1] Although most fetuses tolerate intrauterine hypoxia during labor and are delivered without complication, some require resuscitation and other aggressive medical interventions for such complications as acidosis and seizures. Fetal distress during labor has also been implicated as a cause of cerebral palsy, which can be accompanied by mental retardation or epilepsy. Recent evidence suggests, however, that most cases of cerebral palsy occur in persons with no evidence of birth asphyxia or other intrapartum events.[2,3] Risk factors earlier in pregnancy, rather than intrapartum events, are now considered the principal causes of cerebral palsy and mental retardation.[4,5]

Efficacy of Screening Tests

Although antepartum fetal well-being can be evaluated through nonstress tests and contraction stress tests,[6] the principal screening technique for fetal distress during labor is the measurement of fetal heart rate. Abnormal decelerations and decreased beat-to-beat variability during uterine contractions, as measured by auscultation or by continuous electronic monitoring (cardiotocography), are common fetal heart rate patterns observed during periods of fetal distress. The detection of these patterns during monitoring increases the likelihood that the fetus is in distress, but the patterns are not diagnostic. In addition, normal or equivocal heart rate patterns do not exclude the diagnosis of fetal distress.[5] Precise information on the frequency of false-negative and false-positive results is lacking, however, due in large part to the absence of an accepted definition of fetal distress.[7] For many years, acidosis and hypoxemia as determined by fetal scalp pH were used for this purpose in research and clinical practice, but it is now clear that neither finding is diagnostic of fetal distress.[5,6,8,9] Newborn health indices, such as Apgar scores, also appear to be inadequate criteria for fetal distress.[10] Nonetheless, it has become apparent in recent years that electronic fetal heart rate monitoring can detect at least some cases of fetal distress, and it is often used for routine monitoring of women in labor. It should be noted, however, that the published performance characteristics of this technology, derived largely from research at major academic centers, may overestimate the accuracy that would be expected were this test to be performed for routine screening in typical community settings. Two factors in particular that might limit the accuracy and reliability achievable in actual practice are the method used to measure fetal heart activity and the variability associated with cardiotocogram interpretations.

The measurement of fetal heart activity is performed most accurately by attaching an electrode directly to the fetal scalp, an invasive procedure requiring amniotomy and associated with occasional complications. This has been the technique used in most clinical trials of electronic fetal monitoring. Other noninvasive techniques of monitoring fetal heart rate, which include external Doppler ultrasound and periodic auscultation of heart sounds by clinicians, are more appropriate for widespread screening but provide less precise data than the direct electrocardiogram using a fetal scalp electrode. In studies comparing external ultrasound with the direct electrocardiogram, about 20–25% of tracings differed by at least five beats per minute.[11,12] Second-generation ultrasound instruments are currently being developed to improve the reliability of external ultrasound technology.[12]

A second factor influencing the reliability of widespread fetal heart rate monitoring is inconsistency in interpreting results. Several studies have documented significant intraobserver and interobserver variation in assessing cardiotocograms even when tracings are read by experts in electronic fetal monitoring.[13-15] It would be expected that routine performance of electronic monitoring in the community with interpretations by less experienced clinicians would generate a higher proportion of inaccurate results and potentially unnecessary interventions than has been observed in the published work of major research centers.

Effectiveness of Early Detection

A potentially more important issue is whether electronic evidence of fetal distress during labor is of benefit to either the fetus or mother. Research in the 1960s suggested that electronic fetal monitoring during labor reduced the risk of intrapartum stillbirth, neonatal death, and developmental disability, but methodologic problems in these largely retrospective studies left the issue unsettled.[4,7] Eight randomized controlled trials of electronic fetal monitoring have since been published, however, and they have shown that continuous electronic monitoring does not alter outcome when compared with intermittent auscultation. Three trials,[16-18] the largest of which involved nearly 13,000 patients,[18] compared both approaches in low-risk pregnancies and found no significant difference in neonatal deaths, maternal and neonatal morbidity, Apgar scores, umbilical cord blood gases, the need for assisted ventilation, or admission to the intensive care nursery. Similar findings were reported in a recent prospective study of nearly 35,000 pregnancies in which routine monitoring was compared with a policy of monitoring only high-risk pregnancies.[19]

The benefits of electronic fetal monitoring, both before and during labor, have also been examined in high-risk pregnancies. Four clinical trials found that electronic fetal heart rate monitoring in high-risk pregnancies was of limited benefit when compared with intermittent auscultation during labor.[20-23] Neonatal death, Apgar scores, cord blood gases, and neonatal nursery morbidity were unchanged in three of the four trials;[21-23] in two of these trials, intermittent auscultation of women in the control groups was performed systematically: every 15 minutes in the first stage of labor and every 5 minutes in the second stage.[21,22] The fourth trial found that continuous monitoring was associated with improved umbilical cord blood gases and neurologic status; also, the need for intensive care was ~~reduced.~~[?] This study has been criticized, however, because monitoring techniques in the control group were poorly described and one physician withdrew his patients from the control group after the trial began.[7,24] Studies have also found little benefit from cardiotocography performed prior to labor (e.g., nonstress tests, contraction stress tests). To date, four randomized controlled trials of antenatal electronic screening in high-risk pregnancies have failed to demonstrate significant effects.[25-28]

Although most outcome measures in these studies have not been influenced by electronic fetal monitoring, there is evidence that the incidence of neonatal seizures can be reduced by monitoring. This was suggested in early research[20,29] and was recently confirmed in a large clinical trial.[18] This study reported a statistically significant reduction in the rate of neonatal seizures and other neurological findings when continuous intrapartum fetal monitoring was compared with intermittent auscultation. What remains unclear is the extent to which infants benefit from the prevention of neonatal seizures. Seizures have been viewed by many as a poor prognostic indicator; in the above trial, death occurred in 23% of the babies who experienced seizures, and autopsy confirmed that at least two-thirds of these deaths were due to asphyxia during labor.[18] There are, however, few prospective data on whether the prevention of neonatal seizures reduces the risk of neonatal death or long-term neurologic sequelae. In the above trial, a physical examination performed on the infants at 12 months of age found the same number of children with neurologic complications in the monitored group as in the control group.[18] These children will be reevaluated at 4 years of age; in the meantime, further study has been recommended to assess the long-term implications of neonatal seizures.[24]

The benefits of intrapartum monitoring must be weighed against the potential risks associated both with diagnostic procedures and operative interventions for fetal distress. The insertion of fetal scalp electrodes, for example, is generally a safe procedure, but it may occasionally cause umbilical cord prolapse or infection due to early amniotomy; electrode or pressure catheter trauma to the eye, fetal vessels, umbilical cord, or placenta; and scalp infections with Herpes hominis type 2 or group B streptococcus.[6] Similarly, fetal scalp blood sampling can sometimes result in infection, blade breakage, and bleeding.[6] Perhaps the most important complication of screening for fetal distress, however, is the unnecessary performance of cesarean section, an operation with a small but measurable complication rate and operative mortality. Fetal distress is the second most common indication for cesarean section, and there is evidence from randomized controlled trials that the operation is performed more frequently in association with electronic fetal monitoring.[16,17,20-22] These studies were carried out in the 1970s. In recent years, an effort has been made to lower the frequency of operative delivery; findings from earlier trials may therefore not be generalizable to current practice. Thus, two of three trials carried out in the 1980s found that the cesarean section rate was not increased with electronic fetal monitoring[18,23] (forceps deliveries, however, were increased[18]). The third trial reported a very small increase that was statistically but not clinically significant.[19]

Recommendations of Others

A National Institutes of Health consensus development conference recommended in 1979 that electronic fetal monitoring be strongly considered in high-risk pregnancies but stated that periodic auscultation of fetal heart rate is an acceptable alternative in women at low risk for fetal distress.[30] The Canadian Task Force recently advised against routine electronic fetal monitoring in normal pregnancies but recommended it in high-risk pregnancies.[31] Similarly, most authors recommend performing electronic fetal monitoring only on women at increased risk of fetal distress.[6,7] The American College of Obstetricians and Gynecologists considers electronic fetal monitoring equivalent to intermittent auscultation, but it advises hospitals to tailor their policies to the availability of skilled nursing to monitor tracings.[32]

Discussion

Electronic fetal monitoring has become an accepted standard of care in the United States for the management of labor.[4] A national survey in 1980 found that this technology was used in nearly half of all live births;[33] in certain academic centers the rate may be as high as 86–100%.[4] In addition to the risks associated with electronic fetal monitoring mentioned above, increased use of this technology is associated with increased costs of labor care.

As discussed above, there are important questions regarding the definition of fetal distress, as well as about the accuracy and reliability of electronic fetal monitoring in discriminating accurately between pregnancies with and without this disorder. It is also unclear whether the use of this technology results in significantly improved outcome for either the baby or the mother. The widespread use of electronic fetal monitoring in low-risk pregnancies in the face of these uncertainties has been attributed to concerns about litigation.[7,34] It has been estimated that nearly 40% of all obstetrical malpractice losses are due to fetal monitoring problems,[35] and this may be a major motivating factor behind the widespread use of electronic fetal monitoring during labor.

Clinical Intervention

Clinicians should auscultate and record the fetal heart rate for signs of fetal distress on a frequent basis throughout labor. An auscultation schedule of every 15 minutes in the first stage of labor and every 5 minutes in the second stage has proved effective in clinical trials. Electronic fetal monitoring should not be performed routinely on all women in labor. It should be reserved for pregnancies at risk for fetal distress, such as those with suspected intrauterine growth retardation, abnormal fetal heart rates, dysfunctional labor, meconium-stained amniotic fluid, oxytocin administration, or a history of previous obstetric complications.

REFERENCES

1. National Center for Health Statistics. Vital statistics of the United States, 1985. Vol. II. Mortality, part A. Washington, D.C.: Government Printing Office, 1988. (Publication no. DHHS (PHS) 88–1101.)
2. Freeman JM, Nelson KB. Intrapartum asphyxia and cerebral palsy. Pediatrics 1988; 82:240–9.
3. Nelson KB, Ellenberg JH. Antecedents of cerebral palsy. N Engl J Med 1986; 315:81.
4. Shy KK, Larson EB, Luthy DA. Evaluation of a new technology: the effectiveness of electronic fetal heart rate monitoring. Ann Rev Public Health 1987; 8:165–90.
5. Goodlin RC, Haesslein HC. When is it fetal distress? Am J Obstet Gynecol 1977; 128:440–5.
6. Pritchard JA, MacDonald PC, Gant NF. Williams obstetrics, 17th ed. Norwalk, Conn.: Appleton-Century-Crofts, 1985:281–93.

7. Prentice A, Lind T. Fetal heart rate monitoring during labour: too frequent intervention, too little benefit? Lancet 1987; 2:1375–7.
8. Perkins RP. Perinatal observations in a high-risk population managed without intrapartum fetal pH studies. Am J Obstet Gynecol 1984; 149:327–34.
9. Clark SL, Paul RH. Intrapartum fetal surveillance: the role of fetal scalp blood sampling. Am J Obstet Gynecol 1985; 153:717–20.
10. Sykes GS, Johnson P, Ashworth F, et al. Do Apgar scores indicate asphyxia? Lancet 1982; 1:494.
11. Suidan JS, Young BK, Hochberg HM, et al. Observations on perinatal heart rate monitoring. II. Quantitative unreliability of Doppler fetal heart rate variability. J Reprod Med 1985; 30:519–22.
12. Boehm FH, Fields LM, Hutchison JM, et al. The indirectly obtained fetal heart rate: comparison of first- and second-generation electronic fetal monitors. Am J Obstet Gynecol 1986; 155:10–4.
13. Cohen AB, Klapholz H, Thompson MS. Electronic fetal monitoring and clinical practice: a survey of obstetric opinion. Med Decis Making 1982; 2:79.
14. Beaulieu MD, Fabia J, Leduc B, et al. The reproducibility of intrapartum cardiotocogram assessments. Can Med Assoc J 1982; 127:214–6.
15. Nielsen PV, Stigsby B, Nickelsen C, et al. Intra- and inter-observer variability in the assessment of intrapartum cardiotocograms. Acta Obstet Gynecol Scand 1987; 66: 421–4.
16. Kelso IM, Parsons RJ, Lawrence GF, et al. An assessment of continuous fetal heart rate monitoring in labor: a randomized trial. Am J Obstet Gynecol 1978; 131:526–31.
17. Wood C, Renou P, Oats J, et al. A controlled trial of fetal heart rate monitoring in a low-risk obstetric population. Am J Obstet Gynecol 1981; 141:527–34.
18. MacDonald D, Grant A, Sheridan-Pereira M, et al. The Dublin randomized controlled trial of intrapartum fetal heart rate monitoring. Am J Obstet Gynecol 1985; 152:524–39.
19. Leveno KJ, Cunningham FG, Nelson S, et al. A prospective comparison of selective and universal electronic fetal monitoring in 34,995 pregnancies. N Engl J Med 1986; 315:615–9.
20. Renou P, Chang A, Anderson I, et al. Controlled trial of fetal intensive care. Am J Obstet Gynecol 1976, 126:470–6.
21. Haverkamp AD, Thompson HE, McFee JG, et al. The evaluation of continuous fetal heart rate monitoring in high-risk pregnancy. Am J Obstet Gynecol 1976; 125:310–7.
22. Haverkamp AD, Orleans M, Langendoerfer S, et al. A controlled trial of the differential effects of intrapartum fetal monitoring. Am J Obstet Gynecol 1979; 134:399–409.
23. Luthy DA, Shy KK, van Belle G, et al. A randomized trial of electronic fetal monitoring in preterm labor. Obstet Gynecol 1987; 69:687–95.
24. Thacker SB. The efficacy of intrapartum electronic fetal monitoring. Am J Obstet Gynecol 1987; 156:24–30.
25. Brown VA, Sawers RS, Parsons RJ, et al. The value of antenatal cardiotocography in the management of high-risk pregnancy: a randomized controlled trial. Br J Obstet Gynecol 1982; 89:716–22.
26. Flynn AM, Kelly J, Mansfield H, et al. A randomized controlled trial of non-stressed antepartum cardiotocography. Br J Obstet Gynecol 1982; 89:434–40.
27. Lumley J, Lester A, Anderson I, et al. A randomized trial of weekly cardiotocography in high-risk obstetric patients. Br J Obstet Gynecol 1983; 90:1018–26.
28. Kidd LC, Patel NB, Smith R. Non-stress antenatal cardiotocography: a prospective randomized clinical trial. Br J Obstet Gynecol 1985; 92:1156–9.
29. Chalmers I. Randomized controlled trials of intrapartum monitoring. In: Thalhammer O, Baumgarten KV, Pollak A, eds. Perinatal medicine. Stuttgart: Georg Thieme 1979: 260–5.
30. Task Force on Predictors of Fetal Distress. Consensus development conference of the National Institute of Child Health and Human Development. Reported in: Clin Pediatrics 1979; 18:585–98.
31. Allison DJ, Anderson GM. Intrapartum electronic fetal monitoring: a review of current status for the Task Force on the Periodic Health Examination. In: Goldbloom RB, Law-

rence RS, eds. Preventing disease: beyond the rhetoric. New York: Springer-Verlag (in press).

32. Kaminetzky HA. Personal communication, September 1988.
33. Placek PJ, Keppel KG, Taffel S, et al. Electronic fetal monitoring in relation to cesarean section delivery, for live births and stillbirths in the U.S., 1980. Public Health Rep 1984; 99:173–83.
34. Cunningham AS. Electronic fetal monitoring in labour. J R Soc Med 1987; 80:783.
35. Frigoletto FD Jr, Nadel AS. Electronic fetal heart rate monitoring: why the dilemma? Clinic Obstet Gynecol 1988; 31:179–83.

40

Screening for
Postmenopausal
Osteoporosis

Recommendation: Routine radiologic screening to detect low bone mineral content is not recommended (see *Clinical Intervention*). Estrogen replacement therapy is discussed in Chapter 59.

Burden of Suffering

An estimated 1.3 million osteoporosis-related fractures occur each year in the United States.[1] Up to 70% of fractures in persons aged 45 or older are attributable to osteoporosis.[2] Most of these injuries occur in postmenopausal women. Over half of all postmenopausal women will develop a spontaneous fracture as a result of osteoporosis.[3] It has been estimated that about one-quarter of all women over age 60 have spinal compression fractures and about 15% of women sustain hip fractures during their lifetime.[4,5] The annual cost of osteoporosis-related fractures in the United States has been estimated to be over $7 billion in direct and indirect costs.[6] The most common osteoporosis-related fractures are those involving the proximal femur, vertebral body, and distal forearm. Of these sites, the proximal femur (hip) has the greatest effect on morbidity and mortality; there is a 15–20% reduction in expected survival in the first year following a hip fracture.[7] Hip fractures are associated with significant pain, disability, and decreased functional independence. Among persons living at home at the time of a hip fracture, about one-half experience a deterioration in social function within 2.5 years.[8] The principal risk factors for osteoporosis are advanced age, female gender, Caucasian race, slender build, and bilateral oophorectomy before menopause.[1,4] Low bone mineral content (BMC) is another important risk factor for osteoporosis,[1,4] and it serves as the basis for radiologic screening tests.

Efficacy of Screening Tests

A number of radiologic screening tests are available to detect osteoporotic bone loss in asymptomatic persons. These include conventional skeletal radiographs, radiogrammetry, photodensitometry, single photon absorptiometry, quantitated computerized tomography, dual photon absorptiometry, and dual energy x-ray absorptiometry. Many of these tests are not suitable for routine screening in asymptomatic persons. Conventional radiography is not a sensitive detector of reduced mineral content. Although skeletal x-rays can detect focal bone disorders and advanced osteoporosis, they do not reliably detect bone loss of less than 20%, and they are therefore of limited value in detecting early disease.[9] Radiogrammetry, which involves the measurement of the cortex of peripheral tubular bones (e.g., metacarpals) as viewed on x-ray, provides little information on absolute BMC, the condition of trabecular bone, or cortical porosity. The test has an intraobserver error rate of 3–10% and an interobserver error rate of 8–11%.[10,11] Photodensitometry, the measurement of the optical density of the bone image appearing on x-ray, is affected by soft-tissue interference, as well as by other aspects of radiographic technique and film processing.[12,13] Single photon absorptiometry, in which radioisotope techniques are used to measure bone density, is only useful to evaluate appendicular bones (those of the extremities).[14]

The most sophisticated and accurate noninvasive techniques are quantitated computerized tomography (CT), dual photon absorptiometry (DPA), and dual energy x-ray absorptiometry (DEXA). These techniques are most useful in evaluating the bone mineral density of skeletal structures with large amounts of overlying soft tissue (e.g., lumbar vertebrae, proximal femur). Quantitated CT is highly accurate in examining the anatomy and BMC of transverse sections, but it is not appropriate as a routine screening test due to its cost and the level of radiation exposure associated with the procedure.

DPA and DEXA, which are more appropriate for screening, use radioisotopes (DPA) or x-rays (DEXA) to emit photons at two different energy levels, thereby correcting for the effect produced by layers of soft tissue.[15,16] DEXA has only recently been introduced in the clinical setting, but preliminary data suggest that this technology provides a more reliable measure of BMC than does DPA.[16] Whereas the precision of DPA (i.e., variation in results on repeated measurement) is about 2–5%, the precision of DEXA is estimated to be 1–2%.[16,17] DEXA also appears to require shorter scan times, to emit less radiation, and to be less expensive than DPA.[16] Current data on the performance of these devices have been obtained at specialized research centers; further evaluations will be necessary to determine whether inter- and intraobserver variation increases under typical practice conditions as a result of differences in equipment, technique, and length of follow-up.

Effectiveness of Early Detection

There is little evidence from randomized controlled trials that asymptomatic women who are screened for low BMC have fewer complications from osteoporosis (e.g., fractures) than women who are not screened. However, there is good evidence that, once identified, postmenopausal women with low BMC are at increased risk for subsequent fractures of the hip, vertebrae, and wrist;[17-26] recent prospective cohort studies have demonstrated the dose-response characteristics of this relationship.[27] Moreover, a number of observational and nonrandomized experimental studies suggest that this risk can be reduced by estrogen replacement therapy (see Chapter 59). Exogenous estrogen may also have important cardiovascular benefits.

Estrogen replacement therapy is not recommended routinely for all women because many at low risk for osteoporosis and treatment can produce menstrual bleeding, endometrial hyperplasia, and perhaps endometrial cancer (see Chapter 59). Treatment may be more appropriate in women who are at increased risk for osteoporosis, such as those with low bone mass. Thus, BMC data can be useful in making decisions about therapy, and this serves as the principal basis for recommendations to perform routine bone mineral screening on perimenopausal women. It has not been determined, however, whether the routine assessment of BMC in such women results in improved outcome or whether the benefit is of sufficient magnitude to justify the costs, diagnostic errors, and potential radiation exposure that may occur with widespread screening. Moreover, should estrogen replacement therapy be recommended in the future for all women, regardless of BMC, the clinical usefulness of routine bone mineral screening is likely to become quite limited.[28]

Recommendations of Others

In 1984, a National Institutes of Health consensus development conference concluded that no tests could be recommended to identify persons with mild osteoporosis.[1] More recently, recommendations against routine radiologic screening for osteoporosis have been issued by the Canadian Task Force[9] and other reviewers.[28-30] In a 1984 report, the American College of Physicians discussed the performance limitations of these tests but did not issue a definitive recommendation.[12] The National Osteoporosis Foundation advises that bone density measurements of the spine may be useful in assessing risk in perimenopausal women, but cautions that the results are not reliable predictors of subsequent bone loss and fractures.[31] The National Center for Health Services Research and Health Care Technology Assessment has recommended that further research into methods of predicting fracture risk be carried out before techniques such as DPA are recommended for widespread use.[15] Recommendations of others on exercise, calcium supplementation, and estrogen replacement therapy appear in Chapters 49, 50, and 59, respectively.

Discussion

Routine radiologic screening of asymptomatic women is likely to be very expensive. Both DPA and quantitated CT are time-consuming procedures that require considerable technical expertise.[15,29] Charges range from $40–$120 for a single examination by single photon absorptiometry to $100–$400 for DPA and quantitated CT.[15,29] The cost of screening may be reduced with the advent of DEXA. These costs of screening may be justified if the burden of suffering from osteoporosis can be reduced, but further research is necessary to demonstrate both the clinical effectiveness and cost-effectiveness of this strategy.

Although routine screening may not be appropriate for all asymptomatic women, measurement of BMC may be useful in selected cases, such as perimenopausal women at increased risk for osteoporosis who are considering long-term estrogen replacement therapy. An assessment of the level of risk of osteoporosis based on the measured BMC may help both the patient and the clinician make more informed decisions about the potential benefits and risks of therapy. Periodic tests to measure BMC may also be appropriate in patients with established osteoporosis to monitor response to therapy. There is little basis for screening, however, if the information is not likely to influence decisions by the patient or provider.

Clinical Intervention

Routine radiologic screening for decreased BMC is not recommended for asymptomatic women. In perimenopausal women who are at increased risk for osteoporosis and for whom estrogen therapy would otherwise not be recommended, a measurement of BMC may help the patient and clinician determine whether such therapy is appropriate (see Chapter 59). Women should also receive counseling regarding dietary calcium supplementation (Chapter 50) and weight-bearing exercise (Chapter 49). Elderly persons should also receive counseling regarding preventive measures to reduce the risk of falls and the severity of fall-related injuries (Chapter 52).

Note: See Appendix A for the U.S. Preventive Services Task Force Table of Ratings for this topic. See also the relevant Task Force background paper: Mann K, Wiese WH, Stachencko S. Preventing postmenopausal osteoporosis and related fractures. In: Goldbloom RB, Lawrence RS, eds. Preventing disease: beyond the rhetoric. New York: Springer-Verlag (in press).

REFERENCES

1. National Institutes of Health. Consensus conference: osteoporosis. JAMA 1984; 252:799–802.
2. Iskrant AP, Smith RW Jr. Osteoporosis in women 45 and over related to subsequent fractures. Public Health Rep 1969; 84:33–8.
3. Christiansen C, Riis BJ, Ridbro P. Prediction of rapid bone loss in postmenopausal women. Lancet 1987; 1:1105–8.
4. Cummings SR, Kelsey JL, Nevitt C, et al. Epidemiology of osteoporosis and osteoporotic fractures. Epidemiol Rev 1985; 7:178–208.
5. Melton LJ III. Epidemiology of fractures. In: Riggs BL, Melton LJ III. Osteoporosis: etiology, diagnosis, and management. New York: Raven Press, 1988.
6. Holbrook TL, Grazier K, Kelsey JL, et al. The frequency of occurrence, impact, and cost of selected musculoskeletal conditions in the United States. Chicago, Ill.: American Academy of Orthopedic Surgeons, 1984.
7. Jensen GF, Christiansen C, Boesen J, et al. Epidemiology of postmenopausal spinal and long bone fractures: a unifying approach to postmenopausal osteoporosis. Clin Orthoped 1982; 166:75–81.
8. Jensen JS, Baggar J. Long term social prognosis after hip fractures. Acta Orthop Scand 1982; 53:97–101.
9. Canadian Task Force on the Periodic Health Examination. The periodic health examination: 2. 1987 update. Can Med Assoc J 1988; 138:621–6.
10. Wahner HW, Dunn WL, Riggs BL. Assessment of bone mineral. Part 1. J Nucl Med 1984; 25:1134–41.
11. Idem. Assessment of bone mineral. Part 2. J Nucl Med 1984; 25:1241–53.
12. American College of Physicians. Radiologic methods to evaluate bone mineral content. Ann Intern Med 1984; 100:908–11.
13. Mazess RB. The noninvasive measurement of skeletal mass. In: Peck WA, ed. Bone and mineral research: annual 1. Amsterdam: Excerpta Medica, 1983:223–79.
14. National Center for Health Services Research and Health Care Technology Assessment. Single photon absorptiometry for measuring bone mineral density. Health Technology Assessment Report No. 7. Rockville, Md.: Department of Health and Human Services, 1986.
15. Idem. Dual photon absorptiometry for measuring bone mineral density. Health Technology Assessment Report No. 6. Rockville, Md.: Department of Health and Human Services, 1986.
16. Wahner HW, Dunn WL, Brown ML, et al. Comparison of dual energy absorptiometry and dual photon absorptiometry for bone mineral measurements of the lumbar spine. Mayo Clin Proc 1988; 63:1075–84.
17. Riggs BL, Wahner HW, Seeman E, et al. Changes in bone mineral density of the proximal femur and spine with aging: differences between the postmenopausal and senile osteoporosis syndromes. J Clin Invest 1982; 70:716–23.
18. Bohr H, Schaadt O. Bone mineral content of femoral bone and the lumbar spine measured in women with fracture of the femoral neck by dual photon absorptiometry. Clin Orthop 1983; 179:240–5.
19. Krolner B, Nielsen SP. Bone mineral content of the lumbar spine in normal and osteoporotic women: cross sectional and longitudinal studies. Clin Sci 1982; 62:329–36.
20. Cann CE, Genant HK, Folb FO, et al. Quantitated computed tomography for prediction of vertebral fracture risk. Bone 1985; 6:1–7.
21. Firooznia H, Golimbu C, Rafii M, et al. Quantitated computed tomography assessment

of spinal trabecular bone. II. In osteoporotic women with and without vertebral fractures. J Comput Tomogr 1984; 8:99–103.

22. Wasnich RD, Ross PD, Heilbrun LK, et al. Prediction of postmenopausal fracture risk with use of bone mineral measurements. Am J Obstet Gynecol 1985; 153:745–51.

23. Nillson BE, Westlin NE. The bone mineral content in the forearm of women with Colles' fracture. Acta Orthop Scand 1974; 45:836–44.

24. Cummings S. Are patients with hip fractures more osteoporotic? Review of the evidence. Am J Med 1985; 78:487–94.

25. Melton W, Wahner HW, Richelson LS, et al. Osteoporosis and the risk of hip fracture. Am J Epidemiol 1986; 124:254–61.

26. Riggs BL, Wahner HW, Dunn WL, et al. Differential changes in bone mineral density of the appendicular and axial skeleton with aging. J Clin Invest 1981; 67:328–35.

27. Hui SL, Slemenda CW, Johnston CC Jr. Age and bone mass as predictors of fracture in a prospective study. J Clin Invest 1988; 81:1804–9.

28. Hall FM, Davis MA, Baran DT. Bone mineral screening for osteoporosis. N Engl J Med 1987; 316:212–4.

29. Cummings SR, Black D. Should perimenopausal women be screened for osteoporosis? Ann Intern Med 1986; 104:817–23.

30. Frame PS. A critical review of adult health maintenance. Part 4. Prevention of metabolic, behavioral, and miscellaneous conditions. J Fam Pract 1986; 23:29–39.

31. National Osteoporosis Foundation. Physician's resource manual on osteoporosis. Washington, D.C.: National Osteoporosis Foundation, 1987.

41

Screening for Risk of Low Back Injury

Recommendation Screening asymptomatic persons for risk of low back injury is not recommended. Routine spinal radiographs of asymptomatic persons are also not recommended (see *Clinical Intervention*).

Burden of Suffering

The annual incidence of low back pain is 5–14%, and the lifetime reported prevalence ranges from 60–90%.[1-4] Impairment of the back is the most frequent cause of activity limitation in persons less than 45 years old.[5-7] Low back pain disables 5.4 million Americans and costs at least $16 billion each year.[1] Risk factors for low back injury include occupations that require repetitive lifting (particularly in a forward bent and twisted position), exposure to vibration produced by vehicles or industrial machinery, and cigarette smoking.[1-3,8,9] Certain sports activities (e.g., cross-country skiing) and prolonged vehicle driving are also associated with an increased incidence of back pain, as are spinal osteochondrosis, spondylolisthesis, and spinal stenosis. Osteoporosis increases the risk of vertebral compression, and this may account for the increase in reported low back pain symptoms in older women.[4,10] Increased age is also associated with back pain.[11]

Some studies have shown that certain psychosocial characteristics are common in persons disabled by low back pain. High rates of depression, anxiety, and alcoholism as well as increased divorce rates have been reported.[12-14] It is not known whether these problems are the cause or the result of the disability, or if they are simply associated with it.

Occupational back injury is clearly related to lifting activities. The injury rate is about 3 to 5 per 1000 in light industry compared with 200 per 1000 in heavy industry.[15] One study found that nurses who frequently lift patients are four times more likely to report back injuries than are nurses whose jobs require less lifting.[16] The prognosis for back injury is generally favorable. Ninety percent of patients with low back pain improve with minimal or no medical intervention.[15]

Efficacy of Screening Tests

Low back injury is usually immediately detected by the affected individual; there is no asymptomatic period that delays detection of the condition. Because of this, prevention of low back injury requires the identification by screening tests of those at increased risk of injury before they are injured. Three types of screening tests have been suggested to identify those at risk for low back injury: occupational and medical history, physical examination, and diagnostic imaging.

Persons with a history of bending over frequently or lifting heavy objects are more likely to report low back injuries.[15] A history of previous back problems can also be used to identify a subset of the population at increased risk for back injury. In a survey of over 5000 nurses, those reporting previous low back injury were significantly more likely to experience injury than were those without any prior back problems.[16] Another study showed that workers suffering a low back problem during a one-year study period had a mean rate of past problems that was three times greater than their fellow workers'.[17] None of these studies calculated the sensitivity, specificity, or predictive value of a history of back injury, however.

Physical examination of the low back—testing lumbar flexibility, trunk muscle strength, and hamstring elasticity—may also be useful in predicting back problems. In a prospective study of 928 inhabitants of Glostrup, Denmark, it was shown that men with good isometric endurance of the back muscles were less likely to have a first-time occurrence of low back trouble and that those with hypermobile backs were more likely to develop low back pain.[7] Again, the sensitivity and specificity of these findings were not calculated.

Conventional radiographic imaging of the spine is not useful as a screening test to predict low back injury. Several studies since 1958 have shown that there is no greater incidence of radiographic abnormalities in individuals who have symptoms of low back problems than in those who do not.[18] Other imaging technologies may be effective, however. There is evidence that time lost from work because of low back problems is inversely correlated with the diameter of the lumbar spinal canal, measurable by computed tomographic, magnetic resonance, or ultrasound imaging.[19-21] One study found that persons with a central canal measurement below the 10th percentile as measured by ultrasound were four times more likely to have nerve root entrapment symptoms.[19] In a small case-control study of hospital workers, those who were in the lowest 10th percentile (canal diameter 1.4 cm or less) were 10 times more likely to have missed time from work because of low back pain.[20] The sensitivity and specificity of spinal canal diameter screening have not been evaluated, however.

Effectiveness of Early Detection

Two types of interventions could be applied if persons at increased risk for low back injury were identifiable by screening: physical conditioning and educational programs. In a study of 1652 firefighters participating in a program that emphasized health education (proper diet, control of smoking, blood pressure control, and cardiovascular health) and strength and endurance training, subjects who achieved the highest levels of physical fitness had much lower back injury costs than did the least fit group.[22] Because of the multiple interventions in this trial, attributing the results to improved physical conditioning alone is inappropriate; the results are, however, suggestive.

Training in proper lifting techniques has been emphasized as an important preventive measure in reducing the incidence of low back injury. Since 1930, it has been recommended to lift with the back straight and the knees bent. The adoption of this lifting method, however, has not produced any great change in the incidence of low back injuries.[7,23] Other studies have questioned the validity and the practical utility of a single recommended lifting technique.[7,24,25] In a study in which a computer-controlled lifting stress calculator was used to determine the optimum method of lifting given the characteristics of the human body and the load, no single proper lifting technique could be demonstrated.[7] The different postures one can take to lift an object are relatively limited once the physical characteristics of the load are determined. The physical characteristics of the load are a more significant predictor of joint stresses than is the lifting technique. This may explain the lack of success of training for proper lifting technique and the greater success in preventing injuries when the task or workplace itself is redesigned.[7]

Education through "back school" training has been effective in reducing employment-related injuries and relieving chronic low back pain.[14,26] A back school program usually includes education, lifestyle analysis, and exercise. These schools can be individualized for each industry, with the educational program customized and jobs evaluated from an ergonomic point of view. Back schools for a plastics-related manufacturer with 800 employees and a woodworking firm with 400 employees are said to have reduced the incidence of back injuries by 49% and 68%, respectively.[15]

Recommendations of Others

There are no official recommendations for physicians to routinely screen their patients for susceptibility to low back injury. The National Institute for Occupational Safety and Health (NIOSH) has produced a standard for manual lifting by workers that specifies safe load weight, size, location, and frequency of handling.[27] Other factors, such as worker training, physical fitness, and selection criteria, are also discussed.

Discussion

Effective prevention of low back injury in the general population is difficult because there is usually no consistent association between common activities and injury. While certain specific activities such as repetitive lifting, cross-country skiing, and prolonged driving probably increase the risk of low back injury,[2] screening by history, physical examination, or diagnostic imaging to find those at increased risk has not been proved to be sensitive or specific.

The severity, or even the frequency, of low back injury among those at risk may be reduced by general improvement in physical fitness,[22] but conclusive studies of this have not been reported. Back schools have been effective in preventing injury, but there is insufficient evidence to recommend a single, universally correct lifting technique.[7,28]

Clinical Intervention

Screening asymptomatic persons for risk of low back injury is not recommended. All individuals should receive appropriate counseling about exercise (see Chapter 49) and dietary measures (Chapter 50) to maintain ideal body weight. Individuals at increased risk for low back injury because of past history, body configuration, or specific activity may benefit from a program of conditioning exercises. For individuals planning to enter an occupation known to have a high incidence of low back injuries, preemployment screening and selective placement may be useful. The screening procedure used should be appropriate for the degree of risk exposure on the job. Spinal radiographs should not be used as a screening procedure. Worksite screening and job placement practices should be carried out in accordance with existing occupational medicine guidelines.

Note: See also the relevant U.S. Preventive Services Task Force background paper:

Gross G. Preventing low-back pain. In: Goldbloom RB, Lawrence RS, eds. Preventing disease: beyond the rhetoric. New York: Springer-Verlag (in press).

REFERENCES

1. Frymoyer JW. Back pain and sciatica. N Engl J Med 1988; 318:291–300.
2. Frymoyer JW, Pope MH, Clements JH, et al. Risk factors in low-back pain: an epidemiological survey. J Bone Joint Surg 1983; 65:213–8.
3. Svensson HO, Anderson GBJ. Low-back pain in 40– to 47–year old men: work history and work environment factors. Spine 1983; 8:272–6.
4. Biering-Sorensen F. Physical measurements as risk indicators for low-back trouble over a one year period. Spine 1984; 9:106–19.
5. Kelsey JL, White AA, Pastides H, et al. The impact of musculoskeletal disorders on the population of the United States. J Bone Joint Surg 1979; 61:959–64.
6. Anderson GBJ. Epidemiological aspects of low back pain in industry. Spine 1981; 6:53–60.
7. Parnianpour M, Bejjani FJ, Pavlidis L. Worker training: the fallacy of a single, correct lifting technique. Ergonomics 1987; 30:331–4.
8. Kelsey JL, Githens PB, White AA III, et al. An epidemiologic study of lifting and twisting on the job and risk for acute, prolapsed lumbar vertebral disc. J Orthop Res 1984; 2:61–6.
9. Kelsey JL, Githens PB, O'Conner T, et al. Acute prolapsed lumbar intervertebral disc: an epidemiologic study with special reference to driving automobiles and cigarette smoking. Spine 1984; 9:608–13.
10. Buchanan JR, Myers C, Greer RB III, et al. Assessment of the risk of vertebral fracture in menopausal women. J Bone Joint Surg 1987; 69:212–8.
11. Reisbord LA, Greenland S. Factors associated with self-reported back pain: a population-based study. J Chron Dis 1985; 38:691–702.
12. Anderson GBJ, Svensson HO, Oden A. The intensity of work recovery in low back pain. Spine 1983; 8:880–4.
13. Vallfors B. Acute, subacute and chronic low back pain: clinical symptoms, absenteeism and working environment. Scand J Rehabil Med [Suppl] 1985; 11:1–98.
14. Frymoyer JW, Rosen JC, Clements J, et al. Psychologic factors in low-back-pain disability. Clin Orthop 1985; 195:178–84.
15. Schuchmann JA. Low back pain: a comprehensive approach. Compr Ther 1988; 14:14–8.
16. Venning PJ, Walter SD, Stitt LW. Personal and job-related factors as determinants of incidence of back injuries among nursing personnel. J Occup Med 1987; 29:820–5.
17. Chaffin DB, Park KS. A longitudinal study of low-back pain as associated with occupational weight lifting factors. Am Ind Hyg Assoc J 1973; 34:513–24.
18. Montgomery CH. Preemployment back x-rays. J Occup Med 1976; 18:495–8.
19. Porter RW, Hibbert C, Wellman P. Backache and the lumbar spinal canal. Spine 1980; 5:99–105.
20. Anderson DJ, Adcock DF, Chovil AC, et al. Ultrasound lumbar canal measurement in hospital employees with back pain. Br J Ind Med 1988; 45:552–5.
21. Macdonald EB, Porter R, Hibbert C, et al. The relationship between spinal canal diameter and back pain in coal miners. J Occup Med 1984; 26:23–8.
22. Cady LD, Thomas PC, Karwasky RJ. Progam for increasing health and physical fitness of fire fighters. J Occup Med 1985; 27:110.
23. Brown JR. Lifting as an industrial hazard. Ontario: Labour Safety Council of Ontario, Ontario Department of Labor, 1972.
24. Chaffin DB, Park KS. A longitudinal study of low back pain as associated with occupational weight lifting factors. Am Ind Hyg Assoc J 1973; 34:513–25.
25. Graveling RA, Simpson GC, Sims MT. Lift with your legs, not with your back: a realistic directive? In: Brown ID, Goldsmith R, Coombes K, et al., eds. Ergonomics international 1985: proceedings of the Ninth Congress of the International Ergonomics Association. London: Taylor and Francis, 1985:910–2.

26. Klaber-Moffett JA, Chase SM, Portek BS, et al. A controlled, prospective study to evaluate the effectiveness of a back school in the relief of chronic low back pain. Spine 1986, 11.120–2.
27. National Institute for Occupational Safety and Health. Work practices guide for manual lifting: NIOSH standard 81–122. Cincinnati, Ohio: National Institute for Occupational Safety and Health, 1981.
28. Lankhorst GJ, Van de Stadt RJ, Vogelaar TW, et al. The effect of the Swedish Back School in chronic idiopathic low back pain: a prospective controlled study. Scand J Rehab Med 1983; 15:141–5.

42

Screening for Dementia

Recommendation: Screening for cognitive impairment among asymptomatic persons is not recommended.

Burden of Suffering

About 3 million Americans above age 65 suffer from dementia, which has been defined as global impairment of cognitive function.[1,2] Between 50% and 75% of these persons have dementia of the Alzheimer type. The remainder of cases are secondary to multiple infarcts, alcoholism, and other causes.[1,3] The prevalence of dementia is about 5% in persons over age 65, and it rises dramatically to about 20% by age 80.[2] Cognitive impairment is present in one-half to two-thirds of the 1.3 million American nursing home residents.[3,4]

Dementia is a leading cause of death in the United States. Mortality due to dementia is estimated to be 5.2 per million, accounting for about 120,000 deaths annually.[2,5] Alzheimer's disease progresses over a period of 2 to 20 years, and it is frequently accompanied by acute medical illnesses, functional disability, depression, wandering, incontinence, adverse drug reactions, poor personal hygiene, and unintentional injuries (e.g., falls).[6,7] Care of the demented patient imposes an enormous psychosocial and economic burden on family and other caretakers.[2,4] The disease is estimated to cost society about $30 billion annually.[8] This burden of suffering is expected to increase as the number of Americans over age 65 grows at a rate of 600,000 per year.[3] This population, which is at greatest risk for dementia, is expected to double by the year 2020.[9]

Efficacy of Screening Tests

Clinicians fail to detect between 21% and 72% of patients with dementia, especially when the disease is early in its course.[10-12] Conversely, many persons without the disease incorrectly receive a diagnosis of dementia.[11] The principal reasons for this are the insidious presentation of the disease and the absence, until recently,[13] of standardized criteria that could be applied to the common diagnostic methods: medical history, physical examination, and specialized screening tools.

The medical history can offer the most meaningful evidence of cognitive impairment.[14] It has not been possible to identify specific interview questions regarding behavioral or physical symptoms that reliably discriminate between dementia and other conditions. Rather, a thorough behavioral interview is often necessary to detect subtle changes in functional status at home or at work.[13] Such an evaluation cannot be standardized for screening purposes because techniques must be tailored to the individual patient and the clinician's interview style. Furthermore, the significance of historical information is often misinterpreted by those physicians who confuse cognitive impairment with "normal aging."[15,16]

Physical examination procedures, such as the abbreviated mental status examination that is typically performed by clinicians, are highly insensitive.[17] Neurologic findings, such as release signs, gait disorders, and impaired stereognosis, can have significant interobserver variation, high false-negative rates, and poor specificity.[10,14,18] Sensitivity can be markedly improved by combining various psychometric tests,[15,19-22] but these are often too lengthy to permit patient cooperation or to be practical for primary care practitioners.[3,23,24]

A promising approach is the use of brief screening tools that require only about five minutes to complete. A large number of tests have been described and evaluated in the medical literature.[25] Some of the most widely studied include the Mini-Mental State Exam (MMSE), the Short Portable Mental Status Questionnaire (SPMSQ), the Blessed Information-Memory-Concentration test, and the Mental Status Questionnaire (MSQ).[23,26,27] These tests generally provide good specificity at the expense of sensitivity, which is often below 50%.[21,23,26,28] No single instrument is generally considered to be adequate to detect mild impairment in populations with differing premorbid levels of education and intelligence and varied cultural backgrounds.[25] Rather, such tests are generally recommended to corroborate other clinical evidence of dementia.[3,15] Although the accuracy of such tests is uncertain, prospective studies suggest that providing test results to the physician at the patient interview has the effect of increasing the rate of the detection of dementia. For example, in one controlled study it was shown that among persons over age 65, the detection of mental morbidity, including dementia, was significantly greater when the physicians were given the results of the patient's score on the General Health Questionnaire.[16]

Effectiveness of Early Detection

The early detection of dementia is of potential benefit to the patient and care providers.[12] The greatest benefit occurs among the 10–20% of dementias and pseudodementias that are potentially reversible, such as those caused by drug toxicity, metabolic disorders, depression, and hypothyroidism.[1,3,29] Correction of the underlying disorder does not guarantee a reduction in cognitive impairment; however, studies suggest that between 11% and 69% of these patients will improve with treatment.[24,30] It is believed that the extent of reversibility depends in part on the clinician's ability to reach a prompt diagnosis and begin treatment.[15]

At the present time, early detection is probably ineffective in preventing the neurologic consequences of irreversible dementia, such as that caused by Alzheimer's disease or multiple infarcts.[12] Nonetheless, early detection in Alzheimer's patients is defended on the grounds that early treatment of secondary medical and psychiatric complications and attention to social, psychological, and environmental needs may reduce the morbidity experienced by the patient.[1,6,24,31] There is prospective evidence of periods of improved cognition in "irreversible dementia" following treatment of coexisting disorders.[24,32] About one-half of elderly demented patients manifest at least one such coexisting illness.[33] Most of them experience transient improvement for at least one month with appropriate treatment, and about one-quarter continue the improvement for at least a year.[33] The psychiatric symptoms accompanying dementia are treatable with psychotropic drugs and/or counseling.[34]

An early diagnosis also permits care providers, especially family and friends of the patient, to benefit from support and self-help strategies in order to prepare for and minimize the financial, emotional, and medicolegal pressures that will occur throughout the patient's illness.[1,4,6,12,34,31,35] Rather than making pressured decisions late in the course of the illness, early attention can be devoted to such issues as nutrition and hydration, treatment of infections, transfers, and resuscitation.[36] These benefits of early detection are intuitive and based on clinical experience. There is to date no scientific evidence that patients who receive an early diagnosis of dementia are less likely to experience these complications than are those diagnosed at later stages.

Recommendations of Others

There are no official recommendations to screen patients for dementia. A recent National Institutes of Health consensus development conference concluded that no single test can diagnose dementia and urged clinicians to take the time necessary to conduct a thorough clinical evaluation.[15] Both the World Health Organization[12] and the Institute of Medicine[37] have outlined a broad dementia research agenda, but no screening measures have been recommended. A consensus on the diagnostic criteria for Alzheimer's disease has been developed by a work group of the National Institute of Neurological and Communicative Disorders and Stroke and the Alzheimer's Disease and Related Disorders Association.[13]

Discussion

Dementia is responsible for an enormous burden of suffering that has an impact on patients and their social support network. An effective test for the early detection of this disease is not yet available. Promising strategies are currently being developed and published, but they have been insufficiently tested to be recommended for screening. Furthermore, the claimed benefits of early detection of dementia have not been proved through rigorous research. Nonetheless, a growing number of reports describe the value of interventions to reduce excess morbidity that can occur during the clinical course of dementia. Since cognitive impairment is marked by changes in the patient's functional status at home, clinicians familiar with the patient's baseline abilities should be alert to evidence of deterioration reported by the patient, family, and friends.[15]

Clinical Intervention

Routine screening tests for dementia are not recommended for elderly persons with no evidence of cognitive impairment. Clinicians should, however, periodically inquire into the functional status of elderly patients at home and at work, and they should remain alert to changes in performance with age.

REFERENCES

1. American Medical Association. Dementia. Council on Scientific Affairs. JAMA 1986; 256:2234–8.
2. Weiler PG. The public health impact of Alzheimer's disease. Am J Public Health 1987; 77:1157–8.
3. Beck JC, Benson DF, Scheibel AB, et al. Dementia in the elderly: the silent epidemic. Ann Intern Med 1982; 97:231–41.
4. Rabins PV. Psychosocial aspects of dementia. J Clin Psychiatry [Suppl] 1988; 49: 29–31.

5. Jordan BD, Schoenberg BS. Mortality from presenile and senile dementia in the United States. South Med J 1986; 79:529–31.
6. Larson EB, Buchner DM, Uhlmann RF, et al. Caring for elderly patients with dementia. Arch Intern Med 1986; 146:1909.
7. Teri L, Larson EB, Reifler BV. Behavioral disturbance in dementia of the Alzheimer's type. J Am Geriatr Soc 1988; 36:1–6.
8. Hay JW, Ernst RL. The economic costs of Alzheimer's disease. Am J Public Health 1987; 77:1169–75.
9. Plum F. Epidemiology of aging and its effects on the nervous system. Gerontology [Suppl 1] 1986; 32:3–5.
10. Pinholt EM, Kroenke K, Hanley JF, et al. Functional assessment of the elderly: a comparison of standard instruments with clinical judgement. Arch Intern Med 1987; 147: 484–8.
11. Roca RP, Klein LE, Kirby SM, et al. Recognition of dementia among medical patients. Arch Intern Med 1984; 144:73–5.
12. World Health Organization. Dementia in later life: research and action: report of a WHO scientific group on senile dementia. Technical Report Series 730. Geneva: World Health Organization, 1986:40–7.
13. McKhann G, Drachman D, Folstein M, et al. Clinical diagnosis of Alzheimer's disease: a report of the NINCDS-ADRDA Work Group under the auspices of the Department of Health and Human Services Task Force on Alzheimer's Disease. Neurology 1984; 34:939–44.
14. McIntyre L, Frank J. Evaluation of the demented patient. J Fam Pract 1987; 24:399–404.
15. National Institutes of Health Consensus Development Conference. Differential diagnosis of dementing diseases. JAMA 1987; 258:3411–6.
16. German PS, Shapiro S, Skinner EA, et al. Detection and management of mental health problems of older patients by primary care providers. JAMA 1987; 257:489–93.
17. Klein LE, Roca RP, McArthur J, et al. Diagnosing dementia: univariate and multivariate analyses of the mental status examination. J Am Geriatr Soc 1985; 33:483–8.
18. Huff FJ, Boller F, Lucchelli F, et al. The neurologic examination in patients with probable Alzheimer's disease. Arch Neurol 1987; 44:929–32.
19. Storandt M, Botwinick J, Danziger WL, et al. Psychometric differentiation of mild senile dementia of the Alzheimer type. Arch Neurol 1984; 41:497–9.
20. Eslinger PJ, Damasio AR, Benton AL, et al. Neuropsychologic detection of abnormal mental decline in older persons. JAMA 1985; 253:670–4.
21. Pfeiffer RI, Kurosaki TT, Harrah CH, et al. A survey diagnostic tool for senile dementia. Am J Epidemiol 1981; 114:515–27.
22. Huff FJ, Becker JT, Belle SH, et al. Cognitive deficits and clinical diagnosis of Alzheimer's disease. Neurology 1987; 37:1119–24.
23. Pfeiffer E. A short portable mental status questionnaire for the assessment of organic brain deficit in elderly patients. J Am Geriatr Soc 1975; 23:433–41.
24. Larson EB, Reifler BV, Featherstone HJ, et al. Dementia in elderly outpatients: a prospective study. Ann Intern Med 1984; 100:417–23.
25. Ritchie K. The screening of cognitive impairment in the elderly: a critical review of current methods. J Clin Epidemiol 1988; 41:635–43.
26. Folstein MF, Folstein SE, McHugh PR. Mini-Mental State: a practical method for grading the cognitive state of patients for the clinician. J Psychiat Res 1975; 12:189–98.
27. Katzman R, Brown T, Fuld P, et al. Validation of a short orientation-memory-concentration test of cognitive impairment. Am J Psychiatry 1983; 140:734–9.
28. Fillenbaum GG. Comparison of two brief tests of organic brain impairment, the MSQ and the Short Portable MSQ. J Am Geriatr Soc 1980; 28:381–4.
29. Caine ED. Pseudodementia. Arch Gen Psychiatry 1981; 38:1359–64.
30. Clarfield AM. The reversible dementias: do they reverse? Ann Intern Med 1988; 109: 476–86.
31. National Institute on Aging Task Force. Senility reconsidered: treatment possibilities for mental impairment in the elderly. JAMA 1980; 244:259–63.

32. Larson EB, Reifler BV, Sumi SM, et al. Diagnostic evaluation of 200 elderly outpatients with suspected dementia. J Gerontol 1085; 40:536–43.
33. Reifler BV, Larson E. Excess disability in demented elderly outpatients. the rule of halves. J Am Geriatr Soc 1988; 36:82–3.
34. Small GW. Psychopharmacological treatment of elderly demented patients. J Clin Psychiatry [Suppl] 1988; 49:8–13.
35. Mann SH. Practical management strategies for families with demented victims. Neurol Clin 1986; 4:469–78.
36. Lynn J. Dying and dementia. JAMA 1986; 256:2244–5.
37. Institute of Medicine. Research on mental illness and addictive disorders: progress and prospects: report of the Board on Mental Health and Behavioral Medicine. Am J Psychiatry 1985; 142:28–9.

43

Screening for Abnormal Bereavement

Recommendation: Clinicians aware of the impending or recent death of a patient's loved one should assess potential risk factors for abnormal grieving and should provide emotional support for mourning (see *Clinical Intervention*). Clinicians should also remain alert for the signs and symptoms of pathological bereavement.

Burden of Suffering

A large number of Americans experience the loss of a relative or close friend. Over 2.1 million deaths were registered in the United States in 1986.[1] It has been estimated that about 8 million Americans experience the death of a family member each year.[2] Over 920,000 spouses became widows or widowers in 1986.[1] In the same year, deaths occurred in over 95,000 children and adults under age 25.[1] As part of a normal grief reaction, about half of the bereaved become depressed at some point during the year following the death. Although precise prevalence data are lacking, a significant proportion of mourners experience abnormal bereavement reactions, with about 16% remaining depressed for a year or more after the death.[3]

Persons who experience abnormal bereavement may suffer both psychological and physical morbidity and mortality. Potential complications include depression, social isolation, and alcohol or other drug abuse. Some children who experience bereavement may manifest emotional difficulties in later years.[2] There is evidence from a number of studies that mortality may be increased in some bereaved persons.[4-12] Suicide is more common among widowed men, the bereaved elderly, and men who lose their mothers. Risk factors for abnormal bereavement are poorly defined but may include persons with inadequate social support, widowed men who do not remarry or who live alone, persons with preexisting psychiatric disorders, and those who abuse alcohol or other drugs.[2]

Efficacy of Screening Tests

Grief after the death of a loved one is normal, and therefore it is often difficult for clinicians to distinguish accurately between normal sadness and abnormal bereavement until a year or more after the death has occurred. By the time the diagnosis is certain, the patient may have experienced considerable psychological morbidity and may be less likely to benefit from clinical and social support measures. A better understanding of the risk factors for abnormal bereavement might help clinicians develop screening strategies to identify and assist such individuals immediately after (or before) the death has occurred. A number of possible risk factors have been proposed. These include characteristics of the bereaved person (e.g., inadequate support systems, physical or mental illness, alcohol abuse, financial difficulties); the relationship with the deceased (e.g., those characterized by ambivalence or dependency); and the timing of the death itself (e.g., unexpected death). Unfortunately, these nonspecific characteristics are not unique to persons experiencing abnormal bereavement. Screening strategies based on these risk factors are likely to have poor positive predictive value. Thus, a large number of mourners identified as "high-risk" would, in fact, be experiencing normal grief reactions. Special clinical involvement with the grieving process under these circumstances might be unnecessary and perhaps inappropriate.

Effectiveness of Early Detection

Detection of a problem in the grieving process early in the mourning period is of potential value in minimizing the psychological and physical morbidity associated with abnormal bereavement. In theory, counseling and social support measures may help the mourner advance through the natural stages of grieving.[13] Evidence that such interventions are successful is limited, however. The effectiveness of clinical interventions prior to the death of the loved one, such as providing emotional support, information, and practical assistance, has also been examined, with mixed results. A study of children of terminally ill patients showed some benefit,[14] while another study that involved families of children with terminal leukemia reported no major differences in outcome.[15]

In a clinical trial evaluating interventions in the early weeks after death, widows considered to be at risk for postbereavement morbidity were randomly assigned to an intervention group, which received support for grief and encouragement of mourning for the first three months, or to a control group, which received no intervention.[16] A survey conducted 13 months later suggested that morbidity was lower in the intervention group. A nonrandomized controlled study found that pairing widows with other widows to provide social support helped the bereaved progress through the stages of mourning more rapidly than controls.[17] In addition, clinical studies have shown that intervention after overt signs of abnormal bereavement have developed can also be beneficial.

Counseling can reduce symptomatic distress levels,[18] and professional psychotherapy or cognitive-behavioral counseling may be of special value. Some bereaved patients with clinical depression may benefit from antidepressant medication.[19] Others may receive needed emotional support from self-help groups, hospices, and other community resources.

Recommendations of Others

There are no official recommendations for physicians to routinely screen for abnormal bereavement reactions in persons having experienced a recent death.

Discussion

Further research into the characteristics of abnormal bereavement is needed, but it is clear from available evidence that a significant proportion of mourners suffers considerable psychological and physical morbidity during grieving. It is also apparent that supportive measures in general, and clinical interventions in particular, can help deal with the stresses of grief reactions. There is no reliable screening test to accurately discriminate between mourners who are in need of such interventions and those who are not. Nonetheless, it is important for clinicians to be alert for the signs of pathological bereavement, especially in persons who are likely to have difficulty advancing normally through the stages of mourning.[10]

Clinical Intervention

Clinicians aware of the impending or recent death of a patient's loved one should assess potential risk factors for abnormal grieving (e.g., inadequate social support, living alone, preexisting psychiatric disorders, alcohol or other drug abuse) and should help patients prepare emotionally for mourning. Although methods of providing emotional support for grieving persons must be individualized to the patient's situation and stage of mourning, clinicians should help bereaved persons accept the loss of the deceased, experience the pain of grief, adjust to life without the deceased, and reinvest emotional energy into new relationships. Clinicians should also remain alert for the subtle signs and symptoms of pathological bereavement, such as delayed progression through the natural stages of mourning,[13] depression or suicidal ideation, and increased use of alcohol or other drugs. Patients with evidence of abnormal bereavement may benefit from counseling by a mental health professional.

Note: See also the relevant U.S. Preventive Services Task Force background paper: Medalie JH. Bereavement: health consequences and preventive strategies. In: Goldbloom RB, Lawrence RS, eds. Preventing disease: beyond the rhetoric. New York: Springer-Verlag (in press).

REFERENCES

1. National Center for Health Statistics. Advance report of final mortality statistics, 1986. Monthly Vital Statistics Report, vol. 37, no. 6. Hyattsville, Md.: Public Health Service, 1988. (Publication no. DHHS (PHS) 88-1120.)
2. Osterweis M, Solomon F, Green M, eds. Bereavement: reactions, consequences and care. A report of the Institute of Medicine. Washington, D.C.: National Academy Press, 1984.
3. Bornstein PE, Clayton PJ, Halikas JA, et al. The depression of widowhood after 13 months. Br J Psychiatry 1973; 122:561-6.
4. Kraus AS, Lilienfeld AM. Some epidemiological aspects of the high mortality rate in the young widowed group. J Chron Dis 1959; 10:207-17.
5. Cox PR, Ford JR. The mortality of widows shortly after widowhood. Lancet 1964; 1: 163-4.
6. Rees W, Lutkins SG. Mortality of bereavement. Br Med J 1967; 4:13-6.
7. Clayton PJ. Mortality and morbidity in the first year of widowhood. Arch Gen Psychiatry 1974; 125:747-50.
0. Gerber I, Rusalem R, Hannon N, et al. Anticipatory grief and aged widows and widowers. J Gerontol 1975; 30:225-9.
9. Ward AWM. Mortality of bereavement. Br Med J 1976; 1:700-2.
10. Helsing KJ, Szklo M. Mortality after bereavement. Am J Epidemiol 1981; 114:41-52.
11. Levav I. Mortality and psychopathology following the death of an adult child. Isr Ann Psychiatry 1982; 19:23-38.
12. Levav I, Friedlander Y, Kark JD, et al. An epidemiologic study of mortality among bereaved parents. N Engl J Med 1988; 319:457-61.
13. Kubler-Ross E. On death and dying. London: MacMillan, 1969.
14. Rosenheim E, Ichilov Y. Short-term preventive therapy with children of fatally-ill parents. Isr Ann Psychiatry 1979; 17:67-73.
15. Kupst MJ, Tylke L, Thomas L, et al. Strategies of intervention with families of pediatric leukemia patients: a longitudinal perspective. Soc Work Health Care 1982; 8:31-47.

16. Raphael B. Preventive intervention with the recently bereaved. Arch Gen Psychiatry 1977; 34:1450–4.
17. Vachon ML, Lyall WA, Rogers J, et al. A controlled study of self-help intervention for widows. Am J Psychiatry 1980; 137:1380–4.
18. Horowitz MJ, Weiss DS, Kaltreider N, et al. Reactions to the death of a parent: results from patients and field subjects. J Nerv Ment Dis 1984; 172:383–92.
19. Jacobs SC, Nelson JC, Zisook S. Treating depressions of bereavement with antidepressants: a pilot study. Psychiatr Clin North Am 1987; 10:501–10.

44

Screening for Depression

Recommendation: The performance of routine screening tests for depression in asymptomatic persons is not recommended. Clinicians should maintain an especially high index of suspicion for depressive symptoms in those persons at increased risk for depression (see *Clinical Intervention*).

Burden of Suffering

Depression is the most common psychiatric disorder and one of the most common problems seen in general medicine,[1] occurring in up to 30% of the patients seen by primary care physicians.[2-7] The prevalence of this disease in the general population is about 3–5%.[8] Up to 30% of the population may develop depression at some point during their lifetime,[3] and the direct and indirect costs incurred by persons with depression in the United States exceed $16 billion annually.[9] The incidence of depression is greater among persons who are young, female, single, divorced, separated, seriously ill, or have a family history of depression.[10] It is also more common among the recently bereaved (see Chapter 43).

Depression can result in serious complications. About half of those who suffer from major depression will develop recurrent episodes, and some of these persons will become overtly suicidal. The suicide rate in depressed persons is considerably higher than that of the general population. It is estimated that 50,000–70,000 suicides occur annually,[11] 30–70% of these among people previously diagnosed with major depression.[4,11] The incidence of suicides by adolescents and young adults has tripled in the last 25 years, with 5000 youths committing suicide each year and 500,000–1,000,000 making an unsuccessful attempt[11,12] (see Chapter 45). In addition to the risk of suicide, depression has a significant effect on the victim's quality of life and productivity.[2] Finally, depressed persons frequently present with a variety of physical symptoms.[1] If their depression is not recognized, they may experience iatrogenic morbidity due to unnecessary diagnostic testing and treatment.[2,3]

Efficacy of Screening Tests

The prevailing standard for the diagnosis of depression is the opinion of an examining psychiatrist that a patient's symptoms meet the criteria described in the third revised edition of the *Diagnostic and Statistical Manual of Mental Disorders* (DSM-III-R).[13] However, the routine assessment of these diagnostic criteria is not an effective means of screening for early depression in asymptomatic persons. The majority of persons with depression are seen by nonpsychiatrist physicians.[2]

These practitioners often lack the skills and time to make a definitive diagnosis and may therefore fail to diagnose depression.[2-4] Also, the early diagnosis of depression is difficult to make on clinical grounds. In its early stages, symptoms of depression may be confused with symptoms of physical illness. Even when the classical findings of dysphoric mood, anorexia, anxiety, insomnia, fatigue, and reduced interest in normal activities are present, these symptoms are not pathognomonic for depression.

As an alternative to using standardized clinical criteria, specialized laboratory tests and short questionnaires have been proposed to predict a patient's risk of depression. Subtle changes in endocrine function may occur in depressed persons, and it has been suggested that the dexamethasone suppression test or thyroid stimulating hormone level might make useful diagnostic tools. These tests are generally not considered appropriate for screening, however, because of their invasiveness, cost, and poor sensitivity. Several validated depression screening questionnaires have been proposed for routine use by primary care practitioners.[3,4] These include the Beck Depression Inventory and the Zung Self-Rating Depression Scale (SDS), which is the most widely used screening tool for depression.[2,3] The Beck Depression Inventory has a reported sensitivity of 86%, a specificity of 82%, and a positive predictive value of 30%.[14] About 82% of persons with a Zung Self-Rating Depression Scale greater than 55 have major depression by DSM-III criteria.[15]

Effectiveness of Early Detection

It has been repeatedly documented that primary care physicians often overlook the diagnosis of depression.[2-4] Although validated depression screening instruments have been available for many years,[4,16] only recently has their effectiveness been studied in prospective randomized trials. These studies suggest that providing the test results to the physician at the patient interview will increase the index of suspicion and the detection of depression.[2,6,14] In addition, a randomized controlled trial showed that providing physicians with the results of the General Health Questionnaire (GHQ) improved the detection of mental disorders in older persons, blacks, and men; overall detection in the entire population and clinical management decisions were not affected by the information.[17]

It is, however, unclear whether providing the results of depression screening questionnaires to physicians leads to improved patient outcome. A prospective controlled study found that providing SDS scores to the physician and prescribing a four-week course of antidepressants resulted in lower patient depression scores than in controls in whom SDS results were withheld and who received unspecified care.[15] Chart review revealed that depression had been diagnosed in only one member of the control group. The study had certain design limitations, however, involving confounding variables, different data collection techniques for controls, short follow-up, and the use of questionnaire scores as outcome measures. A randomized controlled trial demonstrated short-term reductions in the duration of depression when results of the GHQ were made available to the physician, but one year after the intervention, a benefit remained only for those with severe depression.[5] Limited improvements have also been reported in other studies.[18,19]

There is no conclusive evidence that the initiation of treatment in the early stages of depression has greater long-term effectiveness than intervention when the traditional symptoms of depression become conspicuous.[4,14] Additional factors complicate the assessment of the effectiveness of early detection. The natural history of depression is characterized by spontaneous remission in at least 50% of depressed persons.[16] Thus, symptoms may not be apparent during the clinical encounter. Conversely, the improvement that occurs with spontaneous remission may be attributed erroneously to the presumed benofits of early intervention.[5,14] Finally, due to the negative societal implications of psychiatric referral, some authors have expressed concern about the harmful effect of false-positive labeling.[14]

Recommendations of Others

The Canadian Task Force found little evidence to support screening for affective disorders.[20] Although screening for depression is favored by some authors,[2,4,6,21] others have reviewed the evidence and concluded that screening is inappropriate.[14,22]

Discussion

At present, available diagnostic tests for depression lack the evidence necessary to support their application as widespread screening tools. Future research may change this situation. Nonetheless, the enormous burden of suffering from this disease argues for better awareness of depressive symptoms by primary care physicians so that fewer cases of depression will escape detection. It is also important that depressed persons identified through screening receive adequate follow-up care. Although the treatment of depression using antidepressant medication and counseling has proven efficacy,[24,12] there is evidence that depressed persons do not always receive recommended medication, counseling, or referrals from primary care physicians.[14,22]

Clinical Intervention

The performance of routine screening tests for depression in asymptomatic persons is not recommended. Clinicians should, however, maintain an especially high index of suspicion for depressive symptoms in adolescents and young adults, persons with a family or personal history of depression, those with chronic illnesses, and those who perceive or have experienced a recent loss (see Chapter 43). Other persons in whom depression should be considered are those with sleep disorders or multiple unexplained somatic complaints.

REFERENCES

1. Katon W. The epidemiology of depression in medical care. Int J Psychiatry Med 1987; 17:93–112.
2. Prestidge BR, Lake CR. Prevalence and recognition of depression among primary care outpatients. J Fam Pract 1987; 25:67–72.
3. Rosenthal MP, Goldfarb NI, Carlson BL, et al. Assessment of depression in a family practice center. J Fam Pract 1987; 25:143–9.
4. Kamerow DB. Controversies in family practice: is screening for mental health problems worthwhile? J Fam Pract 1987; 25:181–4.
5. Johnstone A, Goldberg D. Psychiatric screening in general practice: a controlled trial. Lancet 1976; 1:605–8.
6. Rucker L, Frye EB, Cygan RW. Feasibility and usefulness of depression screening in medical outpatients. Arch Intern Med 1986; 146:729–31.
7. Kessler JG, Cleary PD, Burke JD. Psychiatric disorders in primary care. Arch Gen Psychiatry 1985; 42:583–7.
8. Myers JK, Weissman MM, Tischler GE, et al. Six-month prevalence of psychiatric disorders in three communities. Arch Gen Psychiatry 1984; 41:959–70.

9. Stoudemire A, Frank R, Hedemark N, et al. The economic burden of depression. Gen Hosp Psychiatry 1986; 8:387–94.
10. Weissman MM. Advances in psychiatric epidemiology: rates and risks for depression. Am J Public Health 1987; 77:445–51.
11. National Institute of Mental Health. Depression: what we know. Washington, D.C.: Department of Health and Human Services, 1985. (Publication no. DHHS (ADM) 85–1318.)
12. Greydanus DE. Depression in adolescence: a perspective. J Adolesc Health Care 1986; 7:109S-20S.
13. American Psychiatric Association. Diagnostic and statistical manual of mental disorders, 3rd ed., revised. Washington, D.C.: American Psychiatric Association, 1987.
14. Campbell TL. Controversies in family medicine: why screening for mental health problems is not worthwhile in family practice. J Fam Pract 1987; 25:184–7.
15. Zung WWK, King RE. Identification and treatment of masked depression in a general medical practice. J Clin Psychiatry 1983; 44:365–8.
16. Hankin JR, Locke BZ. The persistence of depressive symptomatology among prepaid group practice enrollees; an exploratory study. Am J Public Health 1982; 72:1000–7.
17. Shapiro S, German PS, Skinner EA, et al. An experiment to change detection and management of mental morbidity in primary care. Med Care 1987; 25:327–39.
18. Hoeper EW, Nycz GR, Kessler LG, et al. The usefulness of screening for mental illness. Lancet 1984; 1:33–5.
19. Zung WWK. Personal communication, 1988.
20. Canadian Task Force on the Periodic Health Examination. The periodic health examination. Can Med Assoc J 1979; 121:1194–254.
21. Anonymous. Treatment of depression in medical patients. Lancet 1986; 2:949–50.
22. Frame PS. A critical review of adult health maintenance. Part 4. J Fam Pract 1986; 23:29–39.

45

Screening for Suicidal Intent

Recommendation: Routine screening for suicidal intent is not recommended. Clinicians should be alert to signs of suicidal ideation in persons with established risk factors (see *Clinical Intervention*). Persons suspected of suicidal intent should be questioned regarding the extent of preparatory actions and referred for further evaluation if evidence of suicidal behavior is detected. Clinicians should be alert to symptoms of depression (see Chapter 44) and should routinely ask patients about their use of alcohol and other drugs (Chapter 47).

Burden of Suffering

It is estimated that over 30,000 Americans died from suicide in 1986.[1] The actual incidence is uncertain because suicidal intent is often difficult to prove after the fact; uniform criteria for declaring a death due to suicide have only recently been developed.[2] An estimated 210,000 persons attempt suicide each year, resulting in over 10,000 permanent disabilities, 155,500 physician visits, 259,200 hospital days, over 630,000 lost work days, and over $115 million in direct medical expenses.[3] The suicide rate in American teenagers has increased significantly in recent years[4-6] and is currently one of the highest in the world.[7] Suicide is the third leading cause of death in young persons[1] and the fourth leading cause of years of potential life lost.[8] Suicides among young persons may also lead to suicide clusters, in which a number of other adolescents or young adults in the same community commit suicide.[9]

The most important risk factor for suicide is psychiatric illness. A large majority of adult suicide victims suffer from affective disorders, substance abuse, or schizophrenia.[7,10] Other important risk factors for suicide include divorce, separation, unemployment, serious medical illnesses, living alone, and recent bereavement.[7] Firearms are the suicide weapon used by over 60% of men, adolescents, and young adults[5,7,10,11] and by over one-third of women. Poisoning (e.g., drug overdose) is the second most common means of suicide.[3] Alcohol intoxication is associated with 25–50% of all suicides[7] and is especially common in suicides involving firearms.[5]

Efficacy of Screening Tests

About one-half to two-thirds of persons who commit suicide visit physicians less than one month before the incident, and 10–40% visit in the preceding week.[7,12] However, it is often difficult for physicians to accurately identify suicidal patients.

Direct questions about suicidal intent may have low yield; only 3–5% of persons threatening suicide express unequivocal certainty that they want to die.[13] Although the clinician can identify persons at risk by identifying established risk factors in the medical history (e.g., living alone, recent death or divorce, substance abuse, psychiatric illness), the majority of patients with these characteristics are false positives and do not intend to kill themselves.[14,15] Researchers have attempted to identify specific risk factors that are the strongest predictors of subsequent suicidal behavior,[16-18] but early evidence suggests that instruments to systematically assess these risk factors in the clinical setting would have low positive predictive value as screening tests. One scoring system,[18] based on four to six years of longitudinal data from 4800 psychiatric patients, was able to identify correctly 35 of 63 (56%) subsequent suicides, but it generated 1206 false positives (positive predictive value less than 3%).

Also, physicians may not effectively assess certain risk factors for suicide, such as previous suicide attempts or psychiatric illness. In one study of completed suicides,[19] over two-thirds of victims had made previous attempts or threats, but only 39% of their physicians were aware of this history. Although psychological autopsy studies reveal that many suicide victims have evidence of previous psychiatric diagnoses (e.g., depression, bipolar disorder, alcohol or other drug abuse, schizophrenia) and previous psychiatric treatment,[12,20] many primary care clinicians fail to recognize the presence of mental illness. A number of studies have shown that depression, the most common psychiatric disorder, is frequently overlooked as a diagnosis (see Chapter 44), and similar difficulties exist in detecting substance abuse (Chapter 47). Improved early detection of these conditions might help identify persons at risk for suicide, but further research is needed.

Effectiveness of Early Detection

Clinical interventions for suicidal persons include psychiatric counseling and hospitalization, limitation of access to potential instruments of suicide, and treatment of underlying conditions.[13] Although these measures are clinically prudent, there is limited direct evidence that they alter outcome. Suicide is a rare event, and large samples and lengthy follow-up are needed for studies to demonstrate significant reduction in suicide rates. Thus, in the few studies that have examined the effectiveness of psychiatric treatment, suicide rates are rarely lowered. Only effects on less specific outcome measures, such as feelings of hopelessness,[21] have been reported. Studies involving treatment of persons who have attempted suicide unsuccessfully may not be generalizable because of potential differences between this population and those who complete suicide. Even in the setting of attempted suicide, there is limited evidence that intervention is beneficial. Surveys indicate that patients receiving psychiatric consultation for attempted suicide find the therapy to be of limited benefit[22] and over 40% choose not to remain in treatment.[23] One study of hospitalized patients admitted for poisoning or self-inflicted injury reported fewer subsequent suicide attempts in persons who received psychiatric counseling than in controls who were discharged prematurely before seeing a psychiatrist.[24] A number of potential selection biases, however, were apparent in this study, thereby limiting the generalizability of its results. Finally, involuntary hospitalization can be of immediate benefit to persons planning suicide and is often required for medicolegal reasons in persons with suspected suicidal ideation,[25,26] but there are few reliable data on the long-term effectiveness of this measure.

Another potential intervention is limiting access to potential instruments of suicide, such as firearms and drugs. Firearms are used in over half of all suicides.[5,7,10,11] Although there is no direct evidence that removal of firearms can prevent suicide, studies have shown that locations with reduced availability of these weapons have lower suicide rates.[10] Poisoning, the second most common means of suicide,[3] often involves prescription drugs made available by the physician. Studies of deaths by overdose have found that, in over half of cases, the ingested drugs were either prescribed by a physician within the preceding week or were provided in a refillable prescription.[27] There is limited information, however, on how the physician can best identify persons who require nonlethal quantities of prescription drugs or whether these measures will prevent subsequent suicide. Legislation in one country restricting the prescription of sedatives may have been associated with a reduced rate of suicide, but the evidence was not conclusive.[28]

Since over 90% of persons who commit suicide suffer from psychiatric disorders, it is possible that treatment of these underlying illnesses may prevent suicide.[21] Indirect evidence suggests that patients with affective disorders who receive comprehensive psychiatric care have lower suicide rates than most persons with psychiatric illnesses,[29,30] but studies with control groups are needed to exclude the possibility of selection bias in these results. As many as half of persons who kill themselves are intoxicated by alcohol or other drugs,[7] and a significant proportion also suffer from a substance abuse disorder.[10] Early detection and treatment of alcohol or other drug abuse thus has the potential of preventing suicide, but firm evidence to this effect is lacking.

Recommendations of Others

The American Academy of Pediatrics recommends asking all adolescents about suicidal thoughts during the routine medical history.[31]

Clinical Intervention

Routine screening of asymptomatic persons for suicidal intent is not recommended. Clinicians should assess the emotional well-being of patients when the history reveals risk factors for suicide, such as recent divorce, separation, unemployment, depression, alcohol or other drug abuse, serious medical illnesses, living alone, and recent bereavement. Patients with evidence of suicidal ideation should be questioned regarding the extent of preparatory actions (e.g., obtaining a weapon, making a plan, putting affairs in order, giving away prized possessions, preparing a suicide note). Those with evidence of serious suicidal intent should be referred for psychiatric counseling and possible hospitalization. Clinicians should be alert to signs of depression (see Chapter 44) and should routinely ask patients about their use of alcohol and other drugs (Chapter 47).

Patients with suicidal ideation, or patients who suspect suicidal thoughts in their relatives or friends, should be made aware of available community resources such as local mental health agencies and crisis intervention centers. Parents and homeowners should also be counseled to restrict unauthorized access to potentially lethal prescription drugs and firearms within the home (see Chapter 52).

Note: See also the relevant U.S. Preventive Services Task Force background paper: Haynes MA. Preventing suicide: the physician's role. In: Goldbloom RB, Lawrence RS, eds. Preventing disease: beyond the rhetoric. New York: Springer-Verlag (in press).

REFERENCES

1. National Center for Health Statistics. Advance report of final mortality statistics, 1986. Monthly Vital Statistics Report, vol. 37, no. 6. Hyattsville, Md.: Department of Health and Human Services, 1988.
2. Centers for Disease Control. Operational criteria for determining suicide. MMWR 1988; 37:773–4,779–80.
3. Rosenberg ML, Gelles RJ, Holinger PC, et al. Violence: homicide, assault, and suicide. In: Amler RW, Dull BH, eds. Closing the gap: the burden of unnecessary illness. New York: Oxford University Press, 1987:164–78.
4. Fingerhut LA, Kleinman JC. Suicide rates for young people. JAMA 1988; 259:356.
5. Brent DA, Perper JA, Allman CJ. Alcohol, firearms, and suicide among youth: temporal trends in Allegheny County, Pennsylvania, 1960 to 1983. JAMA 1987; 257:3369–72.
6. Centers for Disease Control. Youth suicide in the United States, 1970–1980. Atlanta, Ga.: Centers for Disease Control, 1986.
7. Blumenthal SJ. Suicide: a guide to risk factors, assessment, and treatment of suicidal patients. Med Clin North Am 1988; 72:937–71.
8. Centers for Disease Control. Years of potential life lost before age 65—United States, 1987. MMWR 1989; 38:27–9.
9. Idem. Cluster of suicides and suicide attempts—New Jersey. JAMA 1988; 259: 2666–8.
10. Monk M. Epidemiology of suicide. Epidemiol Rev 1987; 9:51–69.
11. Moscicki EK, Boyd JH. Epidemiologic trends in firearm suicides among adolescents. Pediatrician 1985; 12:52–62.
12. Robins E, Murphy GE, Wilkinson RH Jr, et al. Some clinical considerations in the prevention of suicide based on a study of 134 successful suicides. Am J Public Health 1959; 49:888–99.
13. Pfeffer CR. Suicide prevention: current efficacy and future promise. Ann NY Acad Sci 1986; 487:341–50.
14. Mann JJ. Psychobiologic predictors of suicide. J Clin Psychiatry [Suppl 12] 1987; 48: 39–43.
15. Murphy GE. On suicide prediction and prevention. Arch Gen Psychiatry 1983; 40: 343–4.
16. Motto JA, Heilbron DC, Juster RP. Development of a clinical instrument to estimate suicide risk. Am J Psychiatry 1985; 142:680–6.
17. Erdman HP, Greist JH, Gustafson DH, et al. Suicide risk prediction by computer interview: a prospective study. J Clin Psychiatry 1987; 48:464–7.
18. Pokorny AD. Prediction of suicide in psychiatric patients: report of a prospective study. Arch Gen Psychiatry 1983; 40:249–57.
19. Murphy GE. The physician's responsibility for suicide. II. Errors of omission. Ann Intern Med 1975; 82:305–9.
20. Barraclough B, Bunch J, Nelson B, et al. A hundred cases of suicide: clinical aspects. Br J Psychiatry 1974; 125:355–73.
21. Blumenthal SJ, Kupfer DJ. Generalizable treatment strategies for suicidal behavior. Ann NY Acad Sci 1986; 487:327–39.
22. Hengleveld MW, Kerkhof AJFM, van der Wal J. Evaluation of psychiatric consultations with suicide attempters. Acta Psychiatr Scand 1988; 77:283–9.
23. Morgan HG, Barton J, Pottle S, et al. Deliberate self-harm: a follow-up study of 279 patients. Br J Psychiatry 1976; 128:361–8.
24. Greer S, Bagley C. Effect of psychiatric intervention in attempted suicide: a controlled study. Br Med J 1971; 1:310–2.
25. Waltzer H. Malpractice liability in a patient's suicide. Am J Psychother 1980; 34:89–98.
26. Wise TN, Berlin R. Involuntary hospitalization: an issue for the consultation-liaison psychiatrist. Gen Hosp Psychiatry 1987; 9:40–4.
27. Murphy GE. The physician's responsibility for suicide. I. An error of commission. Ann Intern Med 1975; 82:301–4.

28. Goldney RD, Katsikitas M. Cohort analysis of suicide rates in Australia. Arch Gen Psychiatry 1983; 40:71–4,

29. Martin RL, Cloninger R, Guze SB, et al. Mortality in a follow-up of 500 psychiatric outpatients. Arch Gen Psychiatry 1985; 42:58–66.

30. Jamison KR. Suicide and bipolar disorders. Ann NY Acad Sci 1986; 487:301–15.

31. American Academy of Pediatrics Committee on Adolescence. Suicide and suicide attempts in adolescents and young adults. Pediatrics 1988; 81:322–4.

46

Screening for Violent Injuries

Recommendation: Routine screening interviews or examinations for evidence of violent injuries are not recommended. Children and adults presenting with unusual injuries should be examined with attention to possible abuse or neglect, and efforts should be made to prevent subsequent violent injury. Counseling and referral should be offered to those persons at high risk of becoming victims or perpetrators of violence (see *Clinical Intervention*).

Burden of Suffering

Violent injury is a serious public health problem in the United States. Millions of violent incidents occur each year, but because many cases are unreported the true magnitude of the problem can only be estimated. In 1986 there were over 830,000 reported incidents of aggravated assault alone.[1] Victims of violence suffer psychological trauma, physical injuries, disability, and death. In one year, aggravated assaults accounted for 355,000 hospitalizations, 4 million lost workdays, and $638 million in medical costs.[2] In addition to medical injuries, violence can also produce fear, anxiety, and isolation in its victims.[2] Assailants risk disrupted personal lives, damaging criminal records, extended imprisonment, and, in some cases, capital punishment.

Women are frequent victims of violence. About 90,000 rapes are reported to the police each year, and 2–4 million women are abused each year by their spouses.[1-6] Battering may occur in as many as 25% of couples, and it is the cause of trauma injuries in 6% of women who visit the emergency room.[7] Due to underreporting, the actual number of attacks on women is thought to be considerably larger. In addition to the physical injuries produced by such attacks, victims of spouse abuse can also suffer psychological complications; they are more likely than are other women to abuse alcohol and drugs, attempt suicide, and transfer their aggression to children. Pregnant women are three times as likely as nonpregnant women to be victims of abuse, and severe beatings can endanger both mother and fetus.[8]

Between 1 and 2 million cases of child abuse are reported each year; many additional cases are not reported.[4,5,9] Abused children experience physical injuries such as bruises, burns, fractures, and neurological and abdominal trauma. As many as 5000 die from their injuries each year.[10] Child sexual abuse, which occurs in 100,000 to 500,000 children each year,[11] often results in severe psychological trauma as well as in medical complications such as sexually transmitted diseases. Children who have been victims or witnesses of violence often experience abnormal physical, social, and emotional development, and many manifest violent behavior as adolescents and adults.[2,8] Elderly persons are often as vulnerable as children; it is estimated that over 1.1 million persons over age 65 are victims of elder abuse, and in 86% of cases the abuser is a relative.[12]

The most serious manifestation of violent behavior is homicide. Over 20,000 Americans were murdered during 1986.[1] Homicide is most common in the young; along with suicide, it ranks fourth in causes of potential years of life lost.[13] Studies indicate that about 56% of all murders are committed by relatives (16%), friends (9%), or acquaintances (31%).[1] In about 25% of homicides, either the victim or the killer has a previous arrest record.[6,14] Persons at greatest risk of death by homicide include minorities, young males, and those living in poor urban communities.[4] Blacks are at especially increased risk. One in 21 black males dies from homicide.[1] It is the leading cause of death in black males aged 15–24.[4]

Efficacy of Screening

The clinician can identify victims of violence through the patient interview and the physical examination. The interview provides an opportunity to ask the patient about previous experiences with violent behavior, either as a perpetrator or victim, and about the presence of risk factors for violence (e.g., firearms in the home). It has been suggested that victims are more comfortable sharing this information with physicians than with other professionals,[8] but the sensitivity and specificity of such questions are not known. Many victims of violence may be reluctant to expose details for fear of humiliation, criticism, or punitive action directed at themselves or their loved ones. Battered women may be fearful of terminating their relationship with the abusive partner.[8] Children may be afraid of punishment, and both young children and adults with cognitive impairment may be unable to provide accurate details. Other victims of violence may reveal problems common in abused persons (e.g., substance abuse, headache, fatigue, insomnia, and indigestion) which are not in themselves specific for physical abuse. Some progress has been made in recent years in the development of questionnaires to assess more precisely the risk of child abuse,[15,16] but further validation of these instruments is needed.

The physical examination is a second means of detecting evidence of abuse. Burns, bruises, and other lesions can be suggestive by their appearance (e.g., patterns resembling hands, belts, cords, and other weapons) or location (e.g., corporal punishment of children on buttocks, lower back, upper thighs, and face). Multiple traumatic injuries without a plausible explanation are also suspicious. The sensitivity and specificity of this form of screening are not known, however. Physical findings may not be apparent in many victims of abuse, such as sexually abused children, and persons with suspicious injuries may not have been victims of intentional injury. Errors in suspecting abuse are of great concern because of the serious emotional, legal, and societal implications of either failing to take action in cases of abuse or of incorrectly accusing innocent persons.

Thus, there is currently no evidence on which to evaluate the accuracy of the interview or the physical examination in detecting victims of violence. Some studies report that less than 10% of battered women are accurately diagnosed by physicians, even in hospitals with an established protocol for this problem.[6,8] It is not known, however, how much of this high failure rate is due to patient reluctance to disclose incidents, the types of questions or examination procedures used, and/ or physician failure to consider violence as a possible etiology.

Effectiveness of Early Detection

In addition to medical and psychiatric treatment for previous injuries, potential victims of violence can be given information and counseling from the clinician in an attempt to prevent future injuries or killings. Specifically, patients can be advised about risk factors, such as possession of firearms and substance abuse, that increase the likelihood of serious harm in intentional injuries. About 60% of all homicides are committed with firearms,[1] and at least 50% are associated with alcohol use.[5] Psychological counseling, by either the primary care clinician or a mental health professional, may help the patient terminate personal relationships with violent individuals. The patient can also be provided with telephone numbers and encouraged to contact community resources such as crisis centers, shelters, protective service agencies, or the police department if there is fear of injury. The clinician may also identify individuals who are at increased risk of committing intentional injuries in the future. Such persons may be referred for psychiatric counseling or family therapy to learn nonviolent alternatives to conflict resolution and stress management. Finally, the clinician is able (and, in many instances, required) to report suspected cases of abuse and neglect to appropriate protective service and foster care agencies. The efficacy of these measures is largely unstudied, however, and the available evidence is inadequate to determine whether any of these strategies are successful in preventing subsequent violent injury.

Recommendations of Others

Although many groups advise counseling by clinicians to prevent unintentional injuries (see Chapter 52), there are no specific recommendations to screen patients for evidence of violent injury. Legislation in all states requires health care professionals to report suspected cases of child abuse,[10] and failure to report is a prosecutable offense in 37 states.[9] Many states also require reporting of abuse of elders and other adults. In addition to these regulatory guidelines, recommendations for physicians on the detection and treatment of child abuse have been issued by the American Medical Association.[10] Guidelines for the prevention of sexual abuse have been issued by the National Institute of Mental Health.[3] Recommendations for clinicians on the identification of battered women have recently been issued by the American College of Obstetricians and Gynecologists and have been supported by the U.S. Surgeon General.[17] Finally, recommendations for improved training of health care professionals in the identification, treatment, and follow-up of victims of violence were included in the 1986 report of the Secretary's Task Force on Black and Minority Health.[4]

Discussion

The etiology of violent behavior is multifactorial; it is a function of such variables as cultural attitudes toward violence, socioeconomic conditions, biological factors, and the availability of weapons.[4] Therefore, the clinician, as a single agent of change, will have difficulty in preventing violent injury. There are also few data to suggest that proposed interventions are efficacious in preventing violence. Nonetheless, efforts by clinicians to prevent violence are justified because intentional injury and homicide are serious public health problems in the United States; in young black males, homicide is the leading cause of death. Although there is insufficient evidence to support routine screening of all patients, it is important for clinicians to maintain a high index of suspicion when examining persons at increased risk of physical abuse (young children, pregnant women, and the elderly), to assess potential risk factors for violent injury, and to refer potential victims and perpetrators to other professionals and community services to help prevent future incidents.

Clinical Intervention:

Routine screening interviews or examinations for evidence of violent injuries are not recommended. Clinicians examining children should be alert to the physical findings of child abuse. Guidelines are available to help clinicians interview children who are potential victims of sexual abuse.[10,11] Suspected cases of child abuse or neglect must be reported to local child protective services agencies. Both children and adults who present with multiple injuries and an implausible explanation should be evaluated with attention to possible abuse or neglect. Specific guidelines are available for the evaluation of suspected victims of spouse abuse.[6] Injured pregnant women and elderly patients should receive special consideration for this problem. Suspected cases of abuse should receive proper documentation of the incident and physical findings (e.g., photographs, body maps); treatment of physical injuries; arrangements for counseling by a skilled mental health professional; and the telephone numbers of local crisis centers, shelters, and protective service agencies. The safety of children of victims of abuse should also be ensured.

Clinicians should ask adolescent and young adult males (aged 15–24) to discuss previous violent behavior, current alcohol and drug use, and the availability of handguns, shotguns, and rifles. Patients with evidence of violent behavior should be counseled regarding nonviolent alternatives to conflict resolution and about the risks of violent injury associated with easy access to firearms and intoxication with alcohol or other drugs.

Note: See also the relevant U.S. Preventive Services Task Force background paper: Stolley P. Preventing homicide. In: Goldbloom RB, Lawrence RS, eds. Preventing disease: beyond the rhetoric. New York: Springer-Verlag (in press).

REFERENCES

1. Federal Bureau of Investigation. Uniform crime reports for the United States, 1986. Washington D.C.: Government Printing Office, 1987.
2. Rosenberg ML, Gelles RJ, Holinger PC, et al. Violence: homicide, assault, and suicide. In: Amler RW, Dull HB, eds. Closing the gap: the burden of unnecessary illness. New York: Oxford University Press, 1987:164–78.
3. National Institute of Mental Health. The evaluation and management of rape and sexual abuse: a physician's guide. National Center for Prevention and Control of Rape. Rockville, Md.: National Institute of Mental Health, 1985. (Publication no. DHHS (ADM) 85–1409.)
4. Department of Health and Human Services. Report of the Secretary's Task Force on Black and Minority Health. Volume V: Homicide, suicide, and unintentional injuries. Washington D.C.: Government Printing Office, 1986.
5. Silverman MM, Lalley TL, Rosenberg ML, et al. Control of stress and violent behavior: mid-course review of the 1990 health objectives. Public Health Rep 1988; 103:38–49.
6. Stark E, Flitcraft A, Zuckerman D, et al. Wife abuse in the medical setting: an introduction for health personnel. Monograph Series No. 7. Rockville, Md.: National Clearinghouse on Domestic Violence, 1981.
7. McLeer SV, Anwar R. A study of battered women presenting in an emergency department. Am J Public Health 1989; 79:65–6.

8. Mehta P, Dandrea LA. The battered woman. Am Fam Physician 1988; 37:193–9.
9. Cupoli JM. Is it child abuse? Patient Care 1988; April:28–51.
10. American Medical Association. AMA diagnostic and treatment guidelines concerning child abuse and neglect. Chicago, Ill.: American Medical Association, 1985.
11. Schuh SE, Ralston ME. Medical interview of sexually abused children. South Med J 1985; 78:245–51.
12. Council on Scientific Affairs. Elder abuse and neglect. JAMA 1987; 257:966–71.
13. Centers for Disease Control. Years of potential life lost before age 65–United States, 1987. MMWR 1989; 38:27–9.
14. Police Foundation. Domestic violence and the police: studies in Detroit and Kansas City. Washington, D.C.: Police Foundation, 1977.
15. Milner JS, Gold RG, Ayoub C, et al. Predictive validity of the Child Abuse Potential Inventory. J Consult Clin Psychol 1984; 62:879–84.
16. Milner JS, Gold RG, Wimberley RC. Prediction and explanation of child abuse: cross-validation of the Child Abuse Potential Inventory. J Consult Clin Psychol 1986; 54: 865–6.
17. Raymond C. Campaign alerts physicians to identify, assist victims of domestic violence. JAMA 1989; 261:963–4.

47

Screening for Alcohol and Other Drug Abuse

Recommendation: All adolescents and adults should be asked to describe their use of alcohol and other drugs. Routine measurement of biochemical markers and drug testing are not recommended as the primary method of detecting alcohol and other drug abuse in asymptomatic persons. Persons in whom alcohol or other drug abuse or dependence is confirmed should receive appropriate counseling, treatment, and referrals (see *Clinical Intervention*). All persons who use alcohol, especially pregnant women, should be encouraged to limit their consumption, and all persons who use alcohol or other intoxicating drugs should be counseled about the dangers of operating a motor vehicle or performing other potentially dangerous activities while intoxicated.

Burden of Suffering

Although the exact prevalence of alcohol and other drug abuse is difficult to measure with certainty, it has been estimated from population surveys that over 11 million Americans meet the diagnostic criteria for abuse or dependence.[1] Commonly abused drugs in the United States include ethyl alcohol and illicit drugs (e.g., cocaine, heroin, marijuana, phencyclidine, and methaqualone, as well as amphetamines, benzodiazepines, and barbiturates not prescribed by a physician). The prevalence and consequences of abuse vary with each drug. Tobacco use is discussed in Chapter 48.

Alcohol is used by over half of all American adults, but reliable data on the percentage who abuse alcohol are lacking.[2] National surveys indicate that 11% of American drinkers use alcohol daily; 10% report losing control while drinking or admit to dependence on alcohol during the past year; and 8% report recent binge drinking (five or more drinks).[2,3] It has been estimated that alcohol accounted for over 69,000 deaths in 1980.[1] About half of all deaths from motor vehicle crashes, fires, drownings, homicides, and suicides are the result of alcohol intoxication.[4] In 1987, an estimated 23,630 persons were killed in alcohol-related motor vehicle crashes, accounting for nearly 7% of all years of potential life lost in the United States in that year.[5] Chronic alcohol abuse often leads to dependence, alcohol withdrawal syndrome, serious medical complications (e.g., hepatitis, cirrhosis, pancreatitis, thiamine deficiency, gastrointestinal bleeding, cardiomyopathy), and certain forms of cancer.[4] Over 560,000 hospital admissions in 1982 were for alcohol-related conditions.[2] A common complication, cirrhosis, was the ninth leading cause of death in the United States in 1986.[6] Excessive use of alcohol during pregnancy can produce the fetal alcohol syndrome,[7] which has been estimated to affect about 1 out of every 750 newborns.[8] Social consequences of alcohol and other drug dependence include divorce, unemployment, and poverty. It has been estimated that the economic costs of alcohol abuse,.including medical treatment, lost productivity, and property damage, exceeded $115 billion in 1983.[1] An estimated 27 million American children are at risk for abnormal psychosocial development due to the abuse of alcohol by their parents.[9]

Between 1 and 3 million Americans are thought to be regular users of **cocaine**.[10] Self-administration of this drug can produce sudden death due to cerebral hemorrhage, seizures, arrhythmias, myocardial infarction, or respiratory arrest.[10] Regular intranasal administration can cause sinus disease and nasal septal perforation; respiratory complications may occur in those who smoke the drug.[10] Intravenous use of cocaine is a risk factor for the acquired immunodeficiency syndrome (AIDS) and other medical complications of intravenous drug use (see below). Chronic use can lead to psychological dependence, and users of "crack," a popular smokeable form of cocaine, can become addicted with their first session.[11] Dependence on cocaine produces behavioral effects such as diminished motivation, psychomotor retardation, irregular sleep patterns, and other symptoms of depression.[12] Use of cocaine during pregnancy may increase the risk of premature labor, placental abruption, intrapartum fetal distress, and neonatal complications.[13]

About 500,000 Americans are addicted to **heroin**, and more than 2 million use the drug occasionally.[14] Mortality among heroin addicts is high (about 10 per 1000 annually) due to overdose, suicide, violence, and medical complications such as infectious hepatitis, bacterial endocarditis, and pulmonary emboli.[14] Infants born of women using narcotics often experience withdrawal symptoms and are possibly at risk for long-term psychological and behavioral effects.[15] Intravenous use of heroin and other drugs is an important risk factor for developing AIDS; transmission of the human immunodeficiency virus (HIV) through contaminated needles accounts for about 25% of all AIDS cases.[16] There are a total of about 900,000 intravenous drug users in the United States, and it is estimated that in some cities half are infected with the HIV virus (see Chapter 24).[16]

Marijuana is smoked regularly by over 10 million Americans.[17] As with alcohol and other psychoactive drugs, safe operation of a motor vehicle is compromised when the driver is intoxicated with marijuana.[18] In addition, marijuana smoke may contain more carcinogens and tar than tobacco smoke, and thus there may be an increased risk of pulmonary disease in chronic smokers of cannabis.[17,18] Other complications of regular use include amotivational syndrome and physical dependence.[17,18]

The use of drugs by adolescents and young adults is an increasingly serious problem. The leading causes of death at this age—motor vehicle and other unintentional injuries, homicides, and suicides—are associated with alcohol or other drug intoxication in about half of the cases.[19] Driving under the influence of alcohol is more than twice as common in adolescents as in adults.[20] A 1987 survey found that one out of four high school seniors has used an illicit drug other than marijuana in the past year.[21] Over 3% smoke marijuana and 5% drink alcohol daily; 37% admit to binge drinking in the past two weeks. Over 4% have used cocaine in the past month, and nearly 6% admit to having experimented with "crack." In addition to the risk of unintentional injuries and medical complications produced by these agents, drug abuse during adolescence and young adulthood can lead to chemical dependence, the use of more dangerous drugs, diminished academic performance, and limited opportunities for professional and personal growth.[22]

Efficacy of Screening Tests

The most meaningful indicators of substance abuse (e.g., patterns of drug use, impact on personal relationships, work performance) are difficult to assess accurately during the clinical encounter. Physical findings, such as hepatomegaly and eye signs, cannot be relied on; they are often late manifestations of drug abuse and, even when present, are not pathognomonic.[23] The detection of alcohol and drug abuse by clinicians is often possible only through indirect methods. These include patient descriptions of drug use, screening questionnaires, and laboratory analysis of body fluids.

Asking the patient about the quantity and frequency of alcohol and other drug consumption is often an important means of detecting abuse and dependence. There are, however, both limitations and variations in the accuracy of patient responses to such questions. While some studies have shown that patient descriptions of alcohol use are accurate,[24] such self-reported estimates are not always reliable. Patients may underestimate drug-using behavior because of denial or forgetfulness. Others may wish to conceal the information for fear of the associated social stigma[25] or punitive action by employers and law-enforcement officials. In one study, the questions, "How much do you drink?" and "How often do you drink?" had a sensitivity of less than 50% in detecting persons with a drinking problem, when compared with the Michigan Alcoholism Screening Test (see below).[26] Others estimate the sensitivity of historical inquiry to be as low as 10–15%.[27] Such studies, by relying on data from questionnaires examining both past and present drinking behavior as the reference criterion for defining a "true positive," may provide misleading information about the usefulness of historical questions in assessing current problems. Most agree that the accuracy and clinical value of asking patients about their use of alcohol and other drugs is highly variable and dependent on the patient, the clinician, and other individual circumstances.[28,29] There are special difficulties in obtaining an accurate drug history from certain patients, such as adolescents. It is common at this age to distrust authority figures such as clinicians, and young persons may be especially concerned about disclosure of the information to family members, school officials, or the police.[30]

A second screening method is the questionnaire, which has been most extensively evaluated as a means of detecting alcohol abuse. Examples include the Michigan Alcoholism Screening Test (MAST),[31] the CAGE questionnaire,[32] and the Self-Administered Alcoholism Screening Test (SAAST).[33] Of these, the most extensively validated instrument is the MAST, which has a reported sensitivity and specificity of 84–100% and 87–95%, respectively.[31,34,35] This instrument is too lengthy for routine use in primary care settings, however, and shorter questionnaires have been developed. These include the Brief MAST (BMAST) and a questionnaire addressing trauma history,[36] but the four-question CAGE instrument (see *Clinical Intervention*) is the most popular for use in primary care.[32] Some studies of this questionnaire have reported excellent sensitivity and specificity (85–89% and 79–95%, respectively),[25,37-39] but in other studies the reported sensitivity is as low as 49–68%.[40] Inconsistent reports for this and other questionnaires reflect, in part, different study populations, varying reference criteria for defining problem drinking or alcohol abuse, and confounding variables in published validation studies.[41,42] In addition, some questionnaires may be effective in identifying persons with established drinking disorders but may not serve as useful early detection tests because of an inability to detect problem drinking before the development of significant behavioral changes.[43] Although there are few reliable questionnaires for the primary detection of abuse of drugs other than alcohol, questionnaires such as the Addiction Severity Index[44] are available to help evaluate the treatment needs of patients with signs of drug/alcohol abuse or dependence.

A third screening method for alcohol and other drug abuse is the laboratory analysis of body fluids. Chronic abuse of alcohol, for example, is often as sociated with elevations in hepatic enzymes and the erythrocyte mean corpuscular volume. These abnormalities do not occur consistently, however, and therefore such biochemical markers serve as poor screening tests.[40] The sensitivity of the best marker for alcohol abuse, serum gamma-glutamyl transferase (GGT), has in some studies been reported to be as high as 60%.[39] In most research, however, estimates range between 30% and 50%.[27,37,45] GGT also has poor specificity, because it can be elevated by certain medications, trauma, diabetes, and heart or kidney disease.[46] Thus, the reported false-positive rate is high, ranging between 13% and 50%.[37,39,47] Through sophisticated statistical analysis, it may be possible to combine the results of more than one biochemical test or to combine biochemical information with interview and questionnaire data to predict alcoholism with greater accuracy, but these techniques remain research tools at this time.[40,48,49]

Biological tests for evidence of drugs other than alcohol often only provide evidence of recent drug exposure and thus are of limited value in determining whether the drug is being used chronically or during potentially dangerous activities.[50] Since the metabolites of such drugs as cocaine and marijuana can be present in the urine for days to weeks following a single exposure,[10,50-52] it is often impossible to determine retrospectively the regularity of drug use, the level of intoxication, or whether other persons, such as coworkers or motorists, were endangered by the patient at the time of its use. Depending on the drug, the method of analysis, and the population being tested, between 5% and 30% of positive results are false positives,[50,51] owing to sample contamination, cross-reactivity with other drugs, and laboratory error.[52] Also, a negative test does not rule out drug abuse, since the metabolites may have been excreted or, if custody of the sample has not been monitored, the specimen may have been subject to tampering.[52] The results may create personal difficulties for patients. A positive drug screen can affect employment, legal action, insurance coverage, and personal relationships.[50]

Effectiveness of Early Detection

Although early medical intervention is important in treating the systemic complications of acute drug intoxication or chronic abuse, there is less rigorous evidence that early intervention in asymptomatic persons is of benefit. Specifically, it has not been demonstrated in a controlled setting that the detection and treatment of alcohol and other drug abuse through screening asymptomatic persons can produce a better outcome than conventional treatment after signs and symptoms become apparent. There are, however, studies supporting the efficacy of counseling once the signs or symptoms of problem drinking or alcohol abuse are detected. A randomized controlled trial has shown that identification of heavy drinkers followed by counseling and repeated feedback of GGT results can lower the rate of sick absences, hospitalization, and mortality from alcohol abuse.[53-55] Another randomized trial found that problem drinkers on a medical ward who received counseling by a nurse had lower alcohol consumption than controls when evaluated 12 months later.[56] Early intervention for excessive drinking during pregnancy has been shown to be effective in lowering alcohol consumption and neonatal complications.[7,57]

Alcohol treatment programs and other approaches, such as psychotherapy and disulfiram treatment, can be equally effective in at least some patients.[40,58,59] It has been reported that over 60% of persons completing organized alcohol treatment programs remain abstinent after leaving them.[40,60] However, much of the data on the effectiveness of alcohol treatment programs suffers from important methodologic limitations. Many studies lack proper control groups, and the duration of follow-up is often inadequate to reveal subsequent relapse from abstinence to problem drinking. Participants in voluntary treatment programs often have unique personality characteristics,[61-63] and thus the outcome for subjects in studies lacking control groups or randomization may not be generalizable to persons unable or unwilling to join. Finally, since spontaneous remission occurs in as many as 30% of alcoholics,[64,65] reduced consumption may be inappropriately attributed to the clinical intervention. Surveys of recovered alcoholics suggest that while treatment is of some importance in the recovery process, social pressures represent the principal stimulus to changing drinking behavior.[66]

The evidence is more limited regarding the effectiveness of treatment for the abuse of drugs other than alcohol. Although successful results have been reported for persons addicted to cocaine and other drugs, the evidence is not conclusive.[67-69] More evidence is available regarding treatment of heroin dependence, primarily with methadone or naltrexone. Several studies, including a randomized controlled trial, have shown that heroin addicts who remain in methadone maintenance programs have reduced heroin consumption, lower rates of positive antibodies for the HIV virus, and decreased criminality and unemployment.[14,70] Over the short term, methadone treatment is associated with a 95% reduction in self-reported heroin use and a 57–68% reduction in self-reported cocaine use.[71] However, some persons may switch from heroin to other drugs while on treatment. One study found that among cocaine-using heroin addicts in long-term (greater than one year) methadone maintenance programs, 26% began and 6% increased the frequency of cocaine injection after beginning treatment.[71] Moreover, selection bias is possible, since many addicts drop out of programs when the methadone dose is lowered or discontinued,[14] and many studies rely on imprecise criteria, such as patient self-reports, to measure outcome.[72]

Recommendations of Others

There is a consensus among experts that clinicians should be alert to the signs and symptoms of alcohol and other drug abuse and should routinely discuss patterns of use with all patients. There are no guidelines, however, on the content of the patient interview, and there are no official recommendations for physicians to routinely use questionnaires or laboratory tests to detect alcohol and other drug abuse in asymptomatic persons. A workshop sponsored by the National Institute on Alcohol Abuse and Alcoholism recommended that clinicians routinely ask a neutral question about alcohol consumption, followed by completion of the CAGE questionnaire for patients who drink.[73] The American Medical Association (AMA) advises physicians to remain alert to the presenting signs and symptoms of alcoholism and drug abuse and to include an indepth history of substance abuse as part of a complete health examination.[74] The AMA also supports drug testing (in conjunction with rehabilitation and treatment) as part of preemployment examinations for jobs affecting the health and safety of others, or when there is reasonable suspicion of alcohol or other drug impairment.[75] There is a strong consensus among experts that once drug abuse is suspected, further evaluation of the patient and laboratory results is important to discriminate between true cases of abuse and false positives. Once the diagnosis is established, the clinician should either provide or arrange appropriate treatment and counseling for the patient and family.

Recommendations for children and adolescents have been issued by the American Academy of Pediatrics (AAP).[76] The AAP recommends careful discussion with all adolescents regarding the extent of drug use and regular counseling regarding abstinence from intoxicants when driving. Clinicians should advise parents and children to discuss the proper use of alcohol at teen parties and to recommend alternatives to driving while intoxicated or riding in a vehicle operated by an intoxicated driver. The AAP also advises physicians to counsel parents regarding their own use of alcohol in the home. If problem drinking is discovered in the child, appropriate counseling and referrals for treatment should be provided for the patient and family.[76]

The U.S. Surgeon General advises health professionals caring for pregnant women or those considering pregnancy to inquire routinely about alcohol consumption, to advise women to abstain from alcoholic beverages during pregnancy, and to be aware of the alcohol content of foods and drugs.[77] The American College of Obstetricians and Gynecologists recommends counseling pregnant women to avoid alcohol during pregnancy, noting that although moderate drinking may not be harmful to the fetus, the definition of moderate alcohol consumption during pregnancy has not been determined.[78]

Discussion

Clinical efforts to detect alcohol and other drug abuse in asymptomatic persons suffer from the lack of a sensitive and specific screening test for use in primary care. Conventional historical questions are not standardized and cannot be relied on to detect all cases of alcohol and other drug abuse. The MAST questionnaire is too lengthy for busy practices, and there are inconsistent results regarding the accuracy of shorter instruments such as the CAGE questionnaire. Laboratory tests lack sensitivity and specificity, and they often provide evidence only of a recent drug exposure, rather than of chronic drug abuse. Even if alcohol or other drug abuse is detected, further research is needed to establish the efficacy of various early treatment strategies in improving prognosis.

Nonetheless, clinicians should pursue this diagnosis because of the enormous burden of suffering associated with abuse and dependence and the central etiologic role of alcohol and other drug abuse in several leading causes of death in the United States. Even if treatment successes are infrequent, the benefits to the population as a whole may be substantial. This is especially the case in adolescents and adults below age 45, for whom motor vehicle and other injuries are the leading causes of death and years of potential life lost.

Clinical Intervention

Clinicians should routinely ask all adults and adolescents to describe their use of alcohol and other drugs. They should be asked to describe the quantity, frequency, and other characteristics of their use of wine, beer, liquor, and other drugs. Certain questionnaires may be helpful to clinicians in assessing important alcohol use patterns. An affirmative answer to at least two of the four questions* in the CAGE instrument,[32] for example, may

---

*C: "Have you ever felt you ought to Cut down on drinking?"
A: "Have people Annoyed you by criticizing your drinking?"
G: "Have you ever felt bad or Guilty about your drinking?"
E: "Have you ever had a drink first thing in the morning to steady your nerves or get rid of a hangover (Eye-opener)?"

provide useful information on the likelihood of a previous or current problem with alcohol abuse. Discussions with adolescents should be approached with discretion to establish a trusting relationship and to respect the patient's concerns about the confidentiality of disclosed information. Routine measurement of biochemical markers, such as serum GGT, and drug testing of urine or other body fluids are not recommended as the primary method of detecting alcohol or other drug abuse in asymptomatic persons. If drug testing is done for other reasons, positive results should be interpreted with an awareness of the pharmacokinetics of the drug and the limitations of the laboratory and analytic method. Persons in whom drug abuse or dependence is suspected should receive further evaluation to confirm the diagnosis and accuracy of test results and to rule out false positives. Once the diagnosis is confirmed, the clinician should inform the patient of the effects of the drug and should develop a treatment plan for the patient and family that is tailored to the drug of abuse and the needs of the patient. Many patients may benefit from referrals to appropriate consultants and community programs specializing in the treatment of alcohol and other drug dependencies.

All persons who use alcohol should be informed of the health and injury risks associated with alcohol consumption and should be encouraged to limit consumption to moderate intake levels (e.g., fewer than two drinks per day). One drink is defined as 12 ounces of beer, a 5-ounce glass of wine, or 1.5 fluid ounces (one jigger) of distilled spirits. Persons who use alcohol or other psychoactive drugs should also be counseled regarding the dangers of operating motor vehicles and engaging in other potentially dangerous activities when intoxicated, as well as the risks of riding in a vehicle in which the driver is intoxicated. Adolescents and young adults in particular should be encouraged to discuss with their families transportation alternatives for social activities where alcohol and other drugs are used. Pregnant women should be given information in the first trimester about the harmful effects of alcohol and other drugs on the fetus. They should be advised to drink moderately, if at all, during pregnancy. Intravenous drug users should be referred for treatment and warned against the use of contaminated needles, which can transmit the human immunodeficiency virus, hepatitis B, and other organisms (see also Chapter 53).

REFERENCES

1. Kamerow DB, Pincus HA, Macdonald DI. Alcohol abuse, other drug abuse, and mental disorders in medical practice. JAMA 1986; 255:2054–7.
2. Derkelman RL, Ralston M, Herndon J, et al. Patterns of alcohol consumption and alcohol-related morbidity and mortality. MMWR CDC Surveill Summ 1986; 35:1SS-5SS.
3. Clark WB, Midanik L. Alcohol use and alcohol problems among U.S. adults: results of the 1979 national survey. In: National Institute on Alcohol Abuse and Alcoholism. Alcohol consumption and related problems. Alcohol and Health Monograph 1. Rockville, Md.: National Institute on Alcohol Abuse and Alcoholism, 1982. (Publication no. DHHS (ADM) 82–1190.)
4. West LJ, Maxwell DS, Noble EP, et al. Alcoholism. Ann Intern Med 1984; 100:405–16.
5. Centers for Disease Control. Premature mortality due to alcohol-related motor vehicle traffic fatalities—United States, 1987. MMWR 1988; 37:753–5.
6. National Center for Health Statistics. Advance report of final mortality statistics, 1986. Monthly Vital Statistics Report [Suppl], vol. 37, no. 6. Hyattsville, Md.: Public Health Service, 1988. (Publication no. DHHS (PHS) 88–1120.)

7. Rosett HL, Weiner L, Edelin KC. Treatment experience with preg nant problem drinkers. JAMA 1983; 249:2029–33.

8. Hanson JW, Streissguth AP, Smith DW. The effects of moderate alcohol consumption during pregnancy on fetal growth and morphogenesis. J Pediatr 1978; 92:457–60.

9. Harrigan JA. Children of alcoholics. Am Fam Phys 1987; 35(1): 139–44.

10. Tarr JE, Macklin M. Cocaine. Pediatr Clin North Am 1987; 34:319–31.

11. Jekel JF, Allen DF. Trends in drug abuse in the mid-1980's. Yale J Biol Med 1987; 60:45–52.

12. Gold MS, Washton AM, Dackis CA. Cocaine abuse: neurochemistry, phenomenology, and treatment. Natl Inst Drug Abuse Res Monogr Ser 1985; 61:130–50.

13. Chasnoff IJ, Burns KA, Burns WJ. Cocaine use in pregnancy: perinatal morbidity and mortality. Neurotoxicol Teratol 1987; 9:291–3.

14. Greenstein RA, Resnick RB, Resnick E. Methadone and naltrexone in the treatment of heroin dependence. Psychiatr Clin North Am 1984; 7:671–9.

15. Hutchings DE. Methadone and heroin during pregnancy: a review of behavioral effects in human and animal offspring. Neurobehav Toxicol Teratol 1982; 4:429–34.

16. Booth W. AIDS and drug abuse: no quick fix. Science 1988; 239:717–9.

17. Jones RT. Marijuana: health and treatment issues. Psychiatr Clin North Am 1984; 7: 703–12.

18. Schwartz RH. Marijuana: an overview. Pediatr Clin North Am 1987; 34:305–17.

19. National Center for Health Statistics. Annual summary of births, marriages, divorces, and deaths, United States, 1987. Monthly Vital Statistics Report, vol. 36, no. 13. Hyattsville, Md.: Public Health Service, 1988. (Publication no. DHHS (PHS) 88–1120.)

20. Centers for Disease Control. Drinking and driving and binge drinking in selected states, 1982 and 1985: the behavioral risk factor surveys. MMWR 1987; 35:788–91.

21. Alcohol, Drug Abuse, and Mental Health Administration. ADAMHA update: facts from the 1987 National High School Senior Survey. Rockville, Md.: Alcohol, Drug Abuse, and Mental Health Administration, 1988.

22. Wheeler K, Malmquist J. Treatment approaches in adolescent chemical dependency. Pediatr Clin North Am 1987; 34:437–47.

23. Glaze LW, Coggan PG. Efficacy of an alcoholism self-report questionnaire in a residency clinic. J Fam Pract 1987; 25:60–4.

24. Sobell LC, Sobell MB. Outpatient alcoholics give valid self-reports. J Nerv Ment Dis 1975; 161:32–42.

25. Dean JC, Poremba GA. The alcoholic stigma and the disease concept. Int J Addict 1983; 18:739–51.

26. Cyr MG, Wartman SA. The effectiveness of routine screening questions in the detection of alcoholism. JAMA 1988; 259:51–4.

27. Persson J, Magnusson PH. Comparison between different methods of detecting patients with excessive consumption of alcohol. Acta Med Scand 1988; 223:101–9.

28. Magura S, Goldsmith D, Casriel C, et al. The validity of methadone clients' self-reported drug use. Int J Addict 1987; 22:727–49.

29. Babor TF, Stephens RS, Marlatt GA. Verbal report methods in clinical research on alcoholism: response bias and its minimization. J Stud Alcohol 1987; 48:410–24.

30. Cogswell BE. Cultivating the trust of adolescent patients. Fam Med 1985; 17:254–8.

31. Selzer ML. The Michigan Alcoholism Screening Test: the quest for a new diagnostic instrument. Am J Psychiat 1971; 127:1653–8.

32. Ewing JA. Detecting alcoholism: the CAGE questionnaire. JAMA 1984; 252:1905–7.

33. Hurt RD, Morse RM, Swenson WM. Diagnosis of alcoholism with a self-administered alcoholism screening test: results with 1002 consecutive patients receiving general examination. Mayo Clin Proc 1980; 55:365–70.

34. Pokorny AD, Miller BA, Kaplan HB. The brief MAST: a shortened version of the Michigan Alcoholism Screening Test. Am J Psychiat 1972; 129:342–5.

35. Moore RA. The diagnosis of alcoholism in a psychiatric hospital: a trial of the Michigan Alcoholism Screening Test (MAST). Am J Psychiat 1972; 128:1565–9.

36. Skinner HA, Holt S, Schuller R, et al. Identification of alcohol abuse using laboratory tests and a history of trauma. Ann Intern Med 1984; 101:847–51.

37. Bernadt MW, Mumford J, Taylor C, et al. Comparison of questionnaire and laboratory tests in the detection of excessive drinking and alcoholism. Lancet 1982; 1:325 8.
38. King M. At risk drinking among general practice attenders: validation of the CAGE questionnaire. Psychol Med 1986; 16:213–7.
39. Bush B, Shaw S, Cleary P, et al. Screening for alcohol abuse using the CAGE questionnaire. Am J Med 1987; 82:231–5.
40. Hays JT, Spickard WA. Alcoholism: early diagnosis and intervention. J Gen Intern Med 1987; 2:420–7.
41. Kaplan HB, Pokorny AD, Kanas T, et al. Screening tests and self-identification in the detection of alcoholism. J Health Soc Beh 1974; 15:51–6.
42. Babor TF, Kadden R. Screening for alcohol problems: conceptual issues and practical considerations. In: Chang NC, Chao HM, eds. Early identification of alcohol abuse. Research Monograph No. 17. Rockville, Md.: National Institute on Alcohol Abuse and Alcoholism, 1985:1–30. (Publication no. DHHS (ADM) 85–1258.)
43. Babor TF, Ritson EB, Hodgson RJ. Alcohol-related problems in the primary health care setting: a review of early intervention strategies. Br J Addict 1986; 81:23–46.
44. McLellan AT, Luborsky L, Woody GE, et al. An improved diagnostic evaluation instrument for substance abuse patients. The Addiction Severity Index. J Nerv Ment Dis 1980; 168:26–33.
45. Cushman P, Jacobson G, Barboriak JJ, et al. Biochemical markers for alcoholism: sensitivity problems. Alcohol Clin Exp Res 1984; 8:253–7.
46. Salaspuro M. Use of enzymes for the diagnosis of alcohol-related organ damage. Enzyme 1987; 37:87–107.
47. Chick J, Kreitman N, Plant M. Mean cell volume and gamma-glutamyl-transpeptidase as markers of drinking in working men. Lancet 1981; 1:1249–51.
48. Bernadt MW, Mumford J, Murray RM. A discriminant-function analysis of screening tests for excessive drinking and alcoholism. J Stud Alcohol 1984; 45:81–6.
49. Babor TF, Kranzler HR, Lauerman RJ, et al. Early detection of harmful alcohol consumption: comparison of clinical, laboratory and self-report screening procedures. Addict Behav 1989; 14:139–57.
50. Rosenstock L. Routine urine testing for evidence of drug abuse in workers: the scientific, ethical, and legal reasons not to do it. J Gen Intern Med 1987; 2:135–7.
51. American Medical Association, Council on Scientific Affairs. Scientific issues in drug testing. JAMA 1987; 257:3110–4.
52. Dougherty RJ. Controversies regarding urine testing. J Subst Abuse Treat 1987; 4: 115–7.
53. Kristenson H, Trell E, Hood B. Serum glutamyl-transferase in screening and continuous control of heavy drinking in middle-aged men. Am J Epidemiol 1981; 114:862–72.
54. Kristenson H, Ohlin H, Hulten-Nosslin M, et al. Identification and intervention of heavy drinkers in middle-aged men: results and follow-up of 24–60 months of long-term study with randomized controls. J Alcohol Clin Exp Res 1983; 203–9.
55. Kristenson H. Methods of intervention to modify drinking patterns in heavy drinkers. Recent Dev Alcohol 1987; 5:403–23.
56. Chick J, Lloyd G, Crombie E. Counselling problem drinkers in medical wards: a controlled study. Br Med J 1985; 290.905–7.
57. Allen CD, Ries CP. Smoking, alcohol, and dietary practices during pregnancy: comparison before and after prenatal education. J Am Diet Assoc 1985; 85:605–6.
58. Edwards G, Offord J, Egert S, et al. Alcoholism: a controlled trial of "treatment" and "advice." J Stud Alcohol 1977; 38:1004–31.
59. Polich JM, Armor DJ, Braiker HB. The course of alcoholism: four years after treatment. New York: Wiley, 1981.
60. Hoffmann NG, Harrison PA, Belille CA. Alcoholics Anonymous after treatment: attendance and abstinence. Int J Addict 1983; 18:311–8.
61. Thurstin AH, Alfano AM, Sherer M. Pretreatment MMPI profiles of A.A. members and nonmembers. J Stud Alcohol 1986; 47:468–71.
62. Hurlburt G, Gade E, Fuqua D. Personality differences between Alcoholics Anonymous members and nonmembers. J Stud Alcohol 1984; 45:170–1.

63. Emrick CD. Alcoholics Anonymous: affiliation processes and effectiveness as treatment. Alcohol Clin Exp Res 1987; 11:416–23.
64. Smart R. Spontaneous recovery in alcoholics: a review and analysis of the available research. Drug Alcohol Depend 1975/76; 1:277.
65. Saunders WM, Kershaw PW. Spontaneous remission from alcoholism: a community study. Br J Addict 1979; 74:251–65.
66. Nordstrom G, Berglund M. Successful adjustment in alcoholism: relationships between causes of improvement, personality, and social factors. J Nerv Ment Dis 1986; 174: 664–8.
67. Washton AM. Nonpharmacologic treatment of cocaine abuse. Psychiatr Clin North Am 1986; 9:563–71.
68. Gawin F, Kleber H. Pharmacologic treatments of cocaine abuse. Psychiatr Clin North Am 1986; 9:573–83.
69. Gawin FH, Kleber HD, Byck R, et al. Desipramine facilitation of initial cocaine abstinence. Arch Gen Psychiatry 1989; 46:117–21.
70. Gunne LM, Gronbladh L. The Swedish methadone maintenance program: a controlled study. Drug Alcohol Depend 1981; 7:249–56.
71. Chaisson RE, Bacchetti P, Osmond D, et al. Cocaine use and HIV infection in intravenous drug users in San Francisco. JAMA 1989; 261:561–5.
72. Klein DF. Evaluation methodology. Int J Addict 1977; 12:837–49.
73. National Institute on Alcohol Abuse and Alcoholism. Screening for alcoholism in primary care settings. U.S. Department of Health and Human Services. Rockville, Md.: Alcohol, Drug Abuse, and Mental Health Administration, 1987:37–9.
74. American Medical Association, Council on Scientific Affairs. Guidelines for alcoholism diagnosis, treatment and referral. Chicago, Ill.: American Medical Association, 1979.
75. American Medical Association. Drug abuse in the United States: a policy report. Report of the Board of Trustees. Chicago, Ill.: American Medical Association, 1988.
76. American Academy of Pediatrics, Committee on Adolescence. Alcohol use and abuse: a pediatric concern. Pediatrics 1987; 79:450–3.
77. Surgeon General's Advisory on alcohol and pregnancy. FDA Drug Bulletin 1981; 11(2): 9–10.
78. American College of Obstetricians and Gynecologists. Alcohol and pregnancy. Committee on Obstetrics: Maternal and Fetal Medicine. Committee Opinion No. 58. Washington, D.C.: American College of Obstetricians and Gynecologists, 1987.

II. Counseling

48

Counseling to Prevent Tobacco Use

Recommendation: Tobacco cessation counseling should be offered on a regular basis to all patients who smoke cigarettes, pipes, or cigars, and to those who use smokeless tobacco. The prescription of nicotine gum may be an appropriate adjunct for some patients. Adolescents and young adults who do not currently use tobacco products should be advised not to start (see *Clinical Intervention*).

Burden of Suffering

Smoking accounts for one out of every six deaths in the United States.[1] It is the most important modifiable cause of death.[2,3] Each year, 390,000 Americans die as a result of smoking.[3] Over 130,000 of these deaths are due to smoking-related cancers. In adult men, smoking accounts for 90% of all deaths from cancer of the lung, trachea, and bronchus; 92% of deaths from cancers of the lip, oral cavity, and pharynx; 80% of deaths from cancer of the larynx; 78% of deaths from esophageal cancer; 48% of deaths from cancer of the kidney; 47% of deaths from bladder cancer; 29% of deaths from pancreatic cancer; and 17% of deaths from stomach cancer.[1,3] Smoking is also responsible for over 115,000 deaths each year from coronary heart disease and 27,500 deaths due to cerebrovascular disease.[3] Smoking accounts for nearly 60,000 deaths per year from pulmonary diseases such as chronic airway obstruction.[3] Smoking during pregnancy is responsible for about 18% of all cases of low birthweight, shortened gestation, respiratory distress syndrome, and sudden infant death syndrome.[1] Involuntary, or passive, smoking accounts for an estimated 3800 nonsmoker deaths each year from lung cancer.[4] Cigarettes are also responsible for about 1500 fire-related deaths and 4000 injuries each year.[5,6] The total direct and indirect costs of smoking may be as high as $200 billion per year.[7]

Although smoking has become less common in recent years, nearly one-third of all adults in the United States continue to smoke.[8] Cigarette smoking is more common among blacks and persons of low socioeconomic status. Due to an increase in smoking by women during the period between 1940 and the early 1960s, lung cancer mortality in females has been rising steadily since the mid-1960s; lung cancer recently replaced breast cancer as the chief cause of cancer death in women.[9] Over three-quarters of smokers begin smoking as teenagers. Currently, one out of five high school seniors smokes on a daily basis, and one-third of persons aged 20–24 are current smokers.[8,10] Between 25% and 40% of female smokers do not quit smoking during pregnancy.[11,12] Smokeless tobacco, a leading cause of oral cancer, is used by over 10 million Americans.[13,14] Between

8% and 36% of male high school and college students are regular users of smoke-less tobacco.[15]

Efficacy of Risk Reduction

Beginning with early studies in the 1950s and 1960s, a large body of epide-miologic evidence has accumulated regarding the health effects of smoking. Major cohort studies, a large number of case-control studies, and other data sources have since provided consistent evidence linking the use of tobacco with a variety of serious pulmonary, cardiovascular, and neoplastic diseases. The scope of this report does not permit an examination of each study of the health effects of smoking, or the nature of the risk relationship (e.g., relative risk, dose-response relationship) between smoking and each disease. Detailed reviews of this literature have been published elsewhere.[1,3,7,16-18]

Several consistent findings from this body of evidence are well established. First, tobacco is one of the most potent of human carcinogens. The majority of all cancers of the lung, trachea, bronchus, larynx, pharynx, oral cavity, and esophagus are attributable to the use of smoked or smokeless tobacco. Smoking also accounts for a significant but smaller proportion of cancers of the pancreas, kidney, bladder, and stomach. Second, smoking promotes atherosclerosis. Along with hypertension and hypercholesterolemia, smoking is one of the leading risk factors for myocardial infarction and coronary artery disease, and it accounts for up to 30% of all coronary events. Smoking is also a risk factor for cerebrovascular disease and peripheral vascular disease. Third, smoking causes chronic obstructive pulmonary disease, and it is an important risk factor for other respiratory illnesses such as pneumonia and influenza. Fourth, smoking can affect the health of nonsmokers. Involuntary smoking can increase the risk of lung cancer in healthy nonsmokers and the frequency of respiratory illness among children. In utero exposure to maternal smoking increases the risk of miscarriage, stillbirth, low birthweight, and retarded growth. Finally, cigarettes are responsible for about 25% of deaths from residential fires.

There is also a large body of evidence from prospective studies that many of these health risks can be reduced by stopping smoking. Over a period of 15–20 years, the ex-smoker's risk of dying from lung cancer decreases gradually to a risk that is comparable to that of nonsmokers.[19,20] Similarly, a large number of cohort studies of persons with atherosclerotic heart disease have demonstrated that the risk of subsequent myocardial infarction is reduced significantly among persons who stop smoking. These cardiovascular benefits of smoking cessation have been well demonstrated among the young,[21] and recent evidence suggests that risk is also reduced even among persons who stop smoking after age 55.[22]

Effectiveness of Counseling

Clinicians have both the opportunity and the means to modify smoking behavior in patients. It has been estimated that about 38 million of the 53 million adult smokers in the United States could potentially be reached by physicians during the course of ongoing medical care.[23] Moreover, a number of clinical trials[24-29] have demonstrated the effectiveness of certain forms of physician counseling in changing the smoking behavior of patients. As many as 40 controlled clinical trials have examined different types of clinical smoking cessation techniques involving various combinations of counseling, distribution of literature, and nicotine replace-ment therapy.[30,31] These studies have found that effectiveness depends on a variety of factors, such as the number of contacts with the patient, the number of months of intervention, the use of personal face-to-face advice, and the type of counselor. Characteristics of the patient, such as level of nicotine dependence, personal motivation to stop smoking, and confidence in the ability to quit, are also critical variables.[32] Although some studies have reported a 40–50% increase in smoking cessation as a result of clinical intervention, a recent meta-analysis of 39 clinical trials found that differences in cessation rates of unselected patients who receive treatment average about 8% after six months and 6% after one year.[30] The most effective techniques are those involving more than one modality (e.g., physician advice, self-help materials), those that involve both physicians and non-physicians, and those that provide the greatest number of motivational messages for the longest period of time.[30] The key elements of effective counseling appear to be providing reinforcement through consistent and repeated advice to stop smoking, setting a specific "quit date," and scheduling a follow-up contact or visit.[30,33] Providing self-help materials along with counseling appears to further enhance the effectiveness of physician advice.[24,34]

In addition to counseling, the prescription of nicotine gum can facilitate smoking cessation. A number of randomized controlled trials support the efficacy of nicotine replacement therapy, especially for highly nicotine-dependent smokers.[25,26,31,32,35,36] The evidence suggests, however, that nicotine gum is not effective in isolation but rather as an adjunct to ongoing smoking cessation counseling.[37] When used correctly and when combined with physician advice to stop smoking, nicotine gum may increase long-term smoking cessation rates by about one-third.[38] It is contraindicated in pregnant and nursing women, in persons with recent myocardial infarction, and in those with temporomandibular joint disease. It may also have adverse effects in persons with peptic ulcer disease, claudication, hypertension, arrhythmias, and diabetes.[39] Some patients may use the gum without discontinuing smoking, thereby increasing the risk of nicotine toxicity, while others may continue to chew the gum for more than a year.[40] Clonidine is another drug of potential value as an adjunct in treating nicotine withdrawal,[41] but further studies are needed before smoking cessation becomes an approved indication for this drug. There are few studies supporting the adjunctive use of anxiolytics and antidepressants in the treatment of smoking cessation.

The primary prevention of tobacco use in adolescents who do not smoke or use smokeless tobacco is an increasingly important role for the clinician. The use of tobacco as a teenager is an important risk factor for long-term nicotine dependence.[42] The clinician has an opportunity to intervene by providing information on the health effects and addictive potential of tobacco and by providing the adolescent with incentives and skills to resist peer pressure to use tobacco. Early results from programs providing this form of counseling suggest that the use of tobacco can be prevented in at least some teenagers,[43,44] but there are no data from prospective studies regarding the effectiveness of physicians in achieving these outcomes.

Recommendations of Others:

Official recommendations for physicians to encourage smoking cessation have been made by the American College of Physicians,[45,46] the American Academy of Family Physicians,[47] the American Academy of Pediatrics,[48] the American College of Obstetricians and Gynecologists,[49] the National Heart, Lung, and Blood Institute,[50,51] the National Cancer Institute,[52] and many other medical organizations and agencies. Specific recommendations regarding the use of smokeless tobacco have been issued by the American Academy of Otolaryngology, Head and Neck

Surgery,[53] the American Academy of Oral Medicine, the American Medical Association, and the American Dental Association.[54]

Discussion

Although the significant health benefits of smoking cessation are well established, studies suggest that many physicians fail to advise smokers to quit.[55,56] This reluctance to intervene may be the result of a number of variables, including lack of confidence in the ability to provide adequate counseling, skepticism about the ability to achieve behavior change through counseling, and concerns about the effectiveness of devoting time to smoking cessation during the clinical encounter. As mentioned above, however, a number of studies have shown that physician counseling can change behavior, even when the advice consists of a relatively simple message. Moreover, even a modest effect on smoking rates can have significant public health implications when multiplied by the estimated 38 million smokers seen annually by U.S. physicians. Cost-effectiveness studies also support the clinical value of offering smoking cessation counseling during the routine office visit of patients who smoke.[57]

Clinical Intervention

A complete history of tobacco use should be obtained on all adolescent and adult patients. Smoking cessation counseling should be offered on a regular basis to all patients who smoke cigarettes, pipes, or cigars, or use smokeless tobacco. Persons who do not currently use tobacco but who are at increased risk of adopting such behavior (e.g., adolescents) should be advised to resist pressure to begin smoking or using smokeless tobacco. The optimal frequency for performing smoking cessation counseling has not been determined with certainty and is left to clinical discretion. Pregnant women and parents with young children should receive information on the potential harmful effects of smoking on fetal and child health. Certain strategies can increase the effectiveness of counseling regarding tobacco use:

- *Direct, face-to-face advice and suggestions*: The most effective physician message is a brief, unambiguous, and informative statement on the need to stop using tobacco. If possible, the clinician should also review the short- and long-term health, social, and economic benefits of quitting and foster the smoker's belief in the ability to stop. The message should address the patient's concerns and any barriers presented by age, social environment, nicotine dependence, and general health. The physician should try to get agreement on a specific "quit date" and should prepare the patient for withdrawal symptoms. Patients who have experienced a relapse after previously quitting should be reassured that most smokers achieve long-term cessation only after several unsuccessful attempts.
- *Scheduled reinforcement*: Scheduled "support visits" or follow-up telephone calls, especially during the first four to eight weeks, make cessation more effective. Use of a register system for smokers increases the probability that a smoking message is delivered at each visit.
- *Self-help materials*: Clinicians can dispense a variety of effective self-help packages to aid the majority of smokers who quit on their own. These materials are available from voluntary organizations in most communities.
- *Referral to community programs*: Local hospitals, health departments, community health centers, worksites, commercial services, and voluntary

organizations frequently offer smoking cessation programs to which patients can be referred. However, clinicians should not refer patients to programs providing treatment of unproven efficacy (e.g., electric shock therapy, chemical treatment).[58]

- *Drug therapy*: When coupled with other interventions, the prescription of nicotine gum may facilitate cessation by relieving withdrawal symptoms. Patients should be provided with information on the proper use of nicotine gum.[59] Specifically, smokers should be advised to stop smoking completely before starting to use the gum and should be instructed to chew the gum slowly and intermittently to allow proper absorption by the buccal mucosa. The gum should be used as needed for at least three months, when the risk of relapse is greatest, but it is not recommended for use beyond six months.

Note: See Appendix A for the U.S. Preventive Services Task Force Table of Ratings for this topic. See also the relevant Task Force background paper: Kottke TE, Battista RN, DeFriese GH, et al. Attributes of successful smoking cessation interventions in medical practice: a meta-analysis of 39 controlled trials. JAMA 1988; 259:2882–9.

REFERENCES

1. Centers for Disease Control. Smoking-attributable mortality and years of potential life lost—United States, 1984. MMWR 1987; 36:693–7.
2. Department of Health and Human Services. The health consequences of smoking:a report of the Surgeon General. Rockville, Md.: Department of Health and Human Services, 1982. (Publication no. DHHS (PHS) 82–50179.)
3. *Idem*. Reducing the health consequences of smoking: 25 years of progress. A report of the Surgeon General. Rockville, Md.: Department of Health and Human Services, 1989 (Publication no. DHHS (PHS) 89–0411.)
4. National Academy of Sciences. Environmental tobacco smoke: measuring exposures and assessing health effects (Appendix D). Washington, D.C.: National Academy Press, 1986.
5. Hall JR Jr. Expected changes in fire damages from reducing cigarette ignition propensity. Report no. 5, Technical Study Group, Cigarette Safety Act of 1984. Quincy, Mass.: National Fire Protection Association, Fire Analysis Division, 1987.
6. Federal Emergency Management Agency. Fire in the United States. Washington, D.C.: The National Fire Incidence Reporting System, 1982.
7. Fielding JE. Smoking: health effects and control. N Engl J Med 1985; 313:491–8, 555–61.
8. Fiore MC, Novotny TE, Pierce JP, et al. Trends in cigarette smoking in the United States: the changing influence of gender and race. JAMA 1989; 261:49–55.
9. American Cancer Society. Cancer statistics, 1988. CA 1988; 38:5–22.
10. Office on Smoking and Health. Smoking, tobacco and health: a fact book. Rockville, Md.: Department of Health and Human Services, 1987.
11. Kleinman JC, Kopstein A. Smoking during pregnancy, 1967–1980. Am J Public Health 1987; 77:823–5.
12. Williamson DF, Serdula MK, Kendrick JS, et al. Comparing the prevalence of smoking in pregnant and nonpregnant women, 1985 to 1986. JAMA 1989; 261:70–4.
13. Department of Health and Human Services. The health consequences of smokeless tobacco: a report of the advisory committee to the Surgeon General. Washington, D.C.: Government Printing Office, 1986. (Publication no. DHHS (PHS) 86–2874.)
14. National Institutes of Health. Consensus development conference statement: health implications of smokeless tobacco use. Bethesda, Md.: National Institutes of Health, 1986.

15. Connolly GN, Winn DM, Hecht SS, et al. The reemergence of smokeless tobacco. N Engl J Med 1986; 314:1020–7.
16. Department of Health and Human Services. The health consequences of smoking: a report of the Surgeon General. Rockville, Md.: Department of Health and Human Services, 1983. (Publication no. DHHS (PHS) 84–50204.)
17. Idem. The health consequences of involuntary smoking: a report of the Surgeon General. Rockville, Md.: Department of Health and Human Services, 1986. (Publication no. DHHS (CDC) 87–8398.)
18. Wynder EL. Tobacco and health: a review of the history and suggestions for public health policy. Public Health Rep 1988; 103:8–18.
19. Doll R, Peto R. Mortality in relation to smoking: 20 years' observations on male British doctors. Br Med J 1976; 2:1525–36.
20. Rogot E, Murray JL. Smoking and causes of death among U.S. veterans: 16 years of observation. Public Health Rep 1980; 95:213–22.
21. Vliestra RE, Kronmal RA, Oberman A, et al. Effect of cigarette smoking on survival of patients with angiographically documented coronary artery disease: report from the CASS registry. JAMA 1986; 255:1023–7.
22. Hermanson B, Omenn GS, Kronmal RA, et al. Beneficial six-year outcome of smoking cessation in older men and women with coronary artery disease: results from the CASS registry. N Engl J Med 1988; 319:1365–9.
23. Ockene JK. Smoking intervention: the expanding role of the physician. Am J Public Health 1987; 77:782–3.
24. Russell MAH, et al. Effect of general practitioners' advice against smoking. Br Med J 1979; 2:231–5.
25. Russell MAH, Merriman R, Stapleton J, et al. Effect of nicotine chewing gum as an adjunct to general practitioner's advice against smoking. Br Med J 1983; 287:1782–5.
26. Fagerstrom KO. Effects of nicotine chewing gum and follow-up appointments in physician-based smoking cessation. Prev Med 1984; 13:517–27.
27. Ewart CK, Li VC, Coates TC. Increasing physician antismoking influence by applying an inexpensive feedback technique. J Med Educ 1983; 58:517–27.
28. Wilson D, Wood G, Johnson N, et al. Randomized clinical trial of supportive follow-up for cigarette smokers in family practice. Can Med Assoc J 1982; 126:127–9.
29. Wilson DM, Taylor DW, Gilbert JR, et al. A randomized trial of a family physician intervention for smoking cessation. JAMA 1988; 260:1570–4.
30. Kottke TE, Battista RN, DeFriese GH, et al. Attributes of successful smoking cessation interventions in medical practice: a meta-analysis of 39 controlled trials. JAMA 1988; 259:2882–9.
31. Lam W, Sze PC, Sacks HS, et al. Meta-analysis of randomised controlled trials of nicotine chewing-gum. Lancet 1987; 2:27–30.
32. Jarvis MJ, Raw M, Russell MAH. Randomised controlled trial of nicotine chewing gum. Br Med J 1982; 285:537–40.
33. Cummings KM, Giovino G, Emont SL, et al. Factors influencing success in counseling patients to stop smoking. Patient Educ Counsel 1986; 8:189–200.
34. Janz NK, Becker MH, Kirscht MK, et al. Evaluation of a minimal contact smoking cessation intervention in an outpatient setting. Am J Public Health 1987; 77:805–8.
35. West RJ, Hajek P, Belcher M. Which smokers report most relief from craving when using nicotine chewing gum. Psychopharmacology 1986; 89:189–91.
36. Jackson P, Stapleton JA, Russell MAH, et al. Predictors of outcome in a general practitioner's intervention against smoking. Prev Med 1986; 15:244–53.
37. Schwartz JL. Review and evaluation of smoking cessation methods: the United States and Canada, 1978–1985. Bethesda, Md.: National Cancer Institute, 1987.
38. Oster G, Huse DM, Delea TE, et al. Cost-effectiveness of nicotine gum as an adjunct to physician's advice against cigarette smoking. JAMA 1986; 256:1315–8.
39. Benowitz NL. Toxicity of nicotine: implications with regard to nicotine replacement therapy. In: Pomerlau OF, Pomerlau CS, eds. Nicotine replacement: a critical evaluation. New York: Alan R. Liss, 1988:187–217.

40. Hajek P, Jackson P, Belcher M. Long-term use of nicotine chewing gum: occurrence, determinants, and effect on weight gain. JAMA 1988; 260;1593–6.

41. Glassman AH, Stetner F, Walsh T, et al. Heavy smokers, smoking cessation, and clonidine: results of a double-blind, randomized trial. JAMA 1988; 259:2863–6.

42. Department of Health and Human Services. The health consequences of smoking: nicotine addiction. A report of the Surgeon General. Washington, D.C.: Department of Health and Human Services, 1988. (Publication no. DHHS (PHS) 88–8406.)

43. Perry CL. Results of prevention programs with adolescents. Drug Alcohol Depend 1987; 20:13–9.

44. DuPont RL. Prevention of adolescent chemical dependency. Pediatr Clin North Am 1987; 34:495–505.

45. American College of Physicians, Health and Public Policy Committee. Methods for stopping cigarette smoking. Ann Intern Med 1986; 105:281–91.

46. American College of Physicians. Cigarette use epidemic (position paper). Philadelphia: American College of Physicians, 1986.

47. American Academy of Family Physicians. AAFP stop smoking program. Kansas City, Mo.: American Academy of Family Physicians, 1987.

48. American Academy of Pediatrics. Tobacco use by children and adolescents. Pediatrics 1987; 79:479–81.

49. American College of Obstetricians and Gynecologists. Statement on smoking. Policy statement of the Executive Board. Washington, D.C.: American College of Obstetricians and Gynecologists, 1986.

50. National Institutes of Health. Clinical opportunities for smoking intervention: a guide for the busy physician. Bethesda, Md.: National Institutes of Health, 1986. (Publication no. DHHS (NIH) 86–2178.)

51. Idem. How to help your hypertensive patients stop smoking: the physician's guide. Bethesda, Md.: National Institutes of Health, 1983. (Publication no. DHHS (NIH) 83–1271.)

52. Idem. How to help your patients stop smoking: a National Cancer Institute manual for physicians. Bethesda, Md.: National Institutes of Health, 1989, (Publication no. DHHS (NIH) 89-3064.)

53. American Academy of Otolaryngology, Head and Neck Surgery. Smokeless tobacco. Washington, D.C.: American Academy of Otolaryngology, Head and Neck Surgery, 1988.

54. Eskow RN. Hazards of smokeless tobacco. N Engl J Med 1987; 317:1229.

55. Wechsler H, Levine S, Idelson RK, et al. The physician's role in health promotion: a survey of primary-care practitioners. N Engl J Med 1983; 308:97–100.

56. Anda RF, Remington PL, Sienko DG, et al. Are physicians advising smokers to quit? The patient's perspective. JAMA 1987; 257:1916–9.

57. Cummings SR, Rubin SM, Oster G. The cost-effectiveness of counseling smokers to quit. JAMA 1989; 261:75–9.

58. Orleans CT. Understanding and promoting smoking cessation: overview and guidelines for physician intervention. Ann Rev Med 1985; 36:51–61.

59. Schneider N. How to use nicotine gum and other strategies to help quit. New York: Pocket Books, 1988.

49

Exercise Counseling

Recommendation: Clinicians should counsel all patients to engage in a program of regular physical activity, tailored to their health status and personal lifestyle.

Burden of Suffering

Physical inactivity has been associated with a number of debilitating medical conditions in the United States, including coronary artery disease (CAD), hypertension, noninsulin-dependent diabetes mellitus (NIDDM), and osteoporosis. CAD is the leading cause of death in the United States, accounting for about 1.5 million myocardial infarctions and over 520,000 deaths each year.[1,2] About 400,000 Americans are victims of sudden death each year, due primarily to underlying atherosclerotic disease. Hypertension, which occurs in up to 58 million Americans,[3] is a leading risk factor for CAD, as well as for other serious diseases such as renal disease, retinopathy, and stroke. Cerebrovascular disease alone accounts for about 150,000 deaths each year and is the third leading cause of death in the United States.[1] NIDDM is an important risk factor for CAD, cerebrovascular disease, retinopathy, and hypertension. Nearly 6 million Americans suffer from NIDDM.[4] Osteoporosis is responsible for an estimated 1.3 million fractures each year.[5] About one-quarter of all women over age 60 have spinal compression fractures, and about 15% of women sustain hip fractures during their lifetime.[6,7] There is a 15–20% reduction in expected survival in the first year following a hip fracture.[8] Hip fractures cost the United States over $7 billion each year in direct and indirect costs.[9]

Efficacy of Risk Reduction

Studies have shown that men who are physically active on a regular basis have a lower overall mortality than those who are physically inactive.[10,11] Exercise appears to be especially effective in improving health status in six disease-specific areas: CAD, hypertension, obesity, NIDDM, osteoporosis, and diminished psychological well-being.

Physically inactive persons are twice as likely to develop CAD as are persons who engage in regular physical activity.[12] Evidence from cohort studies has shown a consistent association between physical activity and reduced incidence of CAD.[11,13,14] Similar benefits from exercise have been reported in older men (up to age 75);[15,16] efficacy in women is presumed on the basis of extrapolation. Studies have also shown that exercise may have a beneficial effect on plasma lipoprotein concentrations.[17] A possible criticism of the apparent benefits of exercise is that those who are physically active are at decreased risk for CAD by virtue of self-selection—that is, persons who choose to exercise may be inherently more healthy and have fewer overall risk factors for CAD. However, studies controlling for such confounding variables have found that the effects of exercise are independent of other CAD risk factors, and that the cardiovascular benefits may even be augmented in the presence of other risk factors for CAD.[16,18] It has also been shown that the type of individual who adopts athletic behavior is not protected from CAD if regular exercise is discontinued. A study of former college athletes who had become physically inactive found that CAD risk in this cohort was similar to that of inactive alumni who had not been college athletes.[19]

Regular exercise is an important means of improving caloric balance and preventing obesity. A large body of epidemiologic evidence supports an association between physical activity and weight control, even after controlling for dietary factors.[20] The contribution of physical activity to daily caloric expenditure is often relatively small. For example, a daily one-mile walk may amount to only a 4% contribution to total daily expenditure. However, weight gain often occurs as a result of small differences between caloric intake and expenditures, and therefore it is possible through regular exercise to achieve a caloric balance that prevents progressive increases in weight. Although exercise may increase caloric intake, it is accompanied by an even greater increase in caloric expenditure, so that a negative caloric balance is maintained.[21]

Exercise may reduce the risk of developing hypertension and NIDDM. Cohort studies suggest that physically inactive persons have a 35–52% greater risk of developing hypertension than those who exercise; this effect appears to be independent of other risk factors for hypertension.[22,23] The average reduction in blood pressure achieved through regular exercise has been estimated to be about 10 mm Hg.[24] Physical activity is also associated with increased insulin sensitivity and glucose clearance, and epidemiologic studies of South Pacific natives suggest that differences in physical activity may have contributed to the increased prevalence of NIDDM in this population.[25,26] Further evidence is needed, however, to prove that exercise improves glucose tolerance or that it reduces the risk of developing NIDDM.[27]

Weight-bearing physical activity may also reduce bone loss in postmenopausal women.[28-34] Further research is needed to prove that bone mineral content is improved sufficiently to reduce the incidence of osteoporosis-related fractures. Although studies suggest the risk of hip fractures is lower in persons who exercise regularly,[35,36] prospective evidence is necessary to prove that this effect is due specifically to exercise. Additional studies are also needed to determine whether the risk of fall-related fractures during exercise offsets the intended benefits of preventing osteoporosis.

A commonly mentioned benefit of regular exercise is improved affect (positive mood, reduced depression, lowered anxiety).[37,38] The nature of the relationship between exercise and mental health is poorly understood. It is known that physically active persons report higher levels of self-esteem, perhaps in response to improved personal appearance and self-image. No well-designed studies have shown that the incidence of clinically confirmed psychiatric disorders can be reduced through exercise.[39]

Most studies have used different definitions for physical activity,[40] and therefore it is not clear from the evidence exactly what form of exercise is most beneficial. To improve cardiovascular fitness, it is known that exercise cannot be performed occasionally or seasonally,[41] nor can one expect protection from CAD by having exercised regularly in the past.[19] The cardiovascular effects at increasing levels of exercise intensity appear to operate in a dose-response relationship, with modest benefits at low energy expenditures (150–500 kcal/week) and maximal benefits at higher levels (2000–3500 kcal/week).[10,10] Small increases in activity among the most inactive persons appear to be associated with the largest magnitudes of risk reduction. It has traditionally been thought that an improvement in cardiovascular fitness requires a threshold level of aerobic intensity during an exercise session and a minimum frequency of sessions, and this has served as the basis for a number of similar exercise criteria. Three of these include: (1) dynamic movement of large muscle groups for at least 20 minutes, three or more days per week, performed at an intensity of at least 60% of cardiorespiratory capacity; (2) intensity of 50–100% of cardiorespiratory capacity, frequency of two to four times per week, duration of 15–45 minutes, program length of 5–11 weeks; and (3) achieving and maintaining a pulse rate equal to the formula: (220 − age) x 70%.[42,43]

It has also become clear that many of the health benefits of exercise may be obtained even at lower intensity and frequency levels. Furthermore, vigorous exercise may not be advisable in some individuals, especially those who are at increased risk of injury or cardiovascular complications from vigorous physical activity (e.g., the elderly). A number of studies suggest that the threshold intensity for improving cardiovascular fitness may be lower than previously thought and that activities such as brisk walking, climbing stairs, and gardening can be beneficial.[11,18,40,41,44] These benefits have been validated in studies of low intensity activity in elderly persons[44-47] and those with poor baseline fitness.[43] Inactive persons, as well as those who are hypertensive or obese, can benefit significantly from even modest increases in physical activity. In addition, as described above, persons who engage in low intensity exercise may also enjoy the benefits of exercise other than those relating to CAD; these include improved strength and flexibility (which may reduce the risk of falls in the elderly; see Chapter 52), increased bone density, and improved mood.

The benefits of exercise must be weighed against its potential adverse effects, which include injury, osteoarthritis, and, rarely, sudden death. Although injuries are commonly reported in competitive sports, there are few reliable data on the incidence of injuries during typical noncontact exercises.[48,49] It is currently thought that most injuries during exercise are preventable. They often occur as a result of excessive levels of physical activity, dramatic incremental changes in activity level (especially in persons with poor baseline fitness), and improper exercise techniques or equipment. A second concern is that long-term physical activity may accelerate the development of osteoarthritis in major weight-bearing joints (e.g., hips, knees). Cross-sectional studies in long-distance runners, however, have been unable to demonstrate a strong association between exercise and osteoarthritis.[50-52] A third concern is the risk of sudden death, which is known to be increased during vigorous physical activity.[53] Studies suggest that sedentary persons who engage in vigorous activity are at greater risk for sudden death than are those who are regularly active.[54] In fact, due to the cardiovascular benefits of exercise, the overall risk of sudden death (both during and not during exercise) in men who engage regularly in high levels of physical activity is considerably lower than in sedentary men.[54]

Effectiveness of Counseling

At least 40% of the U.S. population is considered sedentary, and as many as 80–94% fail to exercise at an adequate level to obtain cardiorespiratory benefit.[55,56] Thus, the majority of patients seen by physicians could potentially benefit from encouragement to increase physical activity levels. There is, however, a limited amount of information regarding the ability of physicians to influence the exercise behavior of patients. Studies that have demonstrated benefits from counseling provide little information about long-term compliance and are of limited generalizability, because the form of counseling, type of patients, or clinical setting have not been representative of typical primary care physician counseling of healthy patients.[57-63] It is known from surveys, however, that negative perceptions of exercise activity (e.g., inconvenience, cost of equipment, discomfort) can often act as powerful disincentives.[64,65] In particular, high-intensity activities and greater perceived exertion are major barriers to adherence to physical activity programs, especially in sedentary persons over the age of 35. Persons most likely to adopt vigorous exercise programs are those already exercising at a moderate level.[65]

Recommendations of Others

Although counseling patients to exercise is widely recognized as clinically prudent, there are few official recommendations for physicians to include exercise counseling in the periodic health examination. The American College of Sports Medicine has issued specific guidelines on the medical contraindications to exercise.[66]

Discussion

Despite the absence of direct evidence that physician counseling can increase the physical activity of asymptomatic patients, the intervention is warranted because of the numerous potential health benefits associated with physical activity. Physical inactivity results in a slightly lower relative risk for CAD than the commonly accepted risk factors of hypertension, hypercholesterolemia, and cigarette smoking, but it is a much more common cardiac risk factor in the U.S. population.[67] Physical inactivity is also a risk factor for other serious diseases, such as hypertension and obesity. Thus, from a population perspective, even modest increases in physical activity levels could have large public health implications.[67]

Nonetheless, it is important for clinicians to use discretion in recommending appropriate forms of physical activity for patients. In addition to considering potential contraindications in persons with underlying medical disorders, it is also necessary to design an exercise program with an awareness of potential barriers to compliance in the patient's personal lifestyle. Since some patients will be unable or unwilling to engage in any high intensity activities, recommending low intensity exercise for certain individuals may ultimately achieve greater health benefits than urging vigorous exercise activities. Brisk walking, for example, offers improved cardiovascular fitness along with the compliance-enhancing features of convenience, lower perceived discomfort, and safety. The addition of a strong arm swing (aerobic or "pace" walking), although slightly more difficult technically, is a simple measure to increase the aerobic activity of walking.

Clinical Intervention

Clinicians should provide all patients with information on the role of physical activity in disease prevention and assist in selecting an appropriate type of exercise. Factors that should be considered in designing a program include medical limitations and activity characteristics that both improve health (e.g., weight-bearing, increased caloric expenditure, enhanced cardiovascular fitness, low potential adverse effects) and enhance compliance (e.g., low perceived exertion, cost, inconvenience). The patient should also be given instructions on how to perform the exercise safely to reduce the risk

of injuries. The patient should be encouraged to set at least one specific exercise goal; the Initial target should be only a small increment above baseline status. Beginners should emphasize regular, rather than vigorous, exercise; an appropriate short-term goal is to engage in regular walking at least three times per week for at least 30 minutes. Ultimately, over a period of several months, the patient should progress to a level that achieves increased cardiovascular fitness (e.g., 30 minutes of daily brisk walking). For most healthy persons, maximum cardiovascular fitness can be achieved by a program of vigorous aerobic exercise for 15–45 minutes, two to four times per week, during which a pulse rate of about (220 – age) x 70% is reached and maintained. Clinicians who are unable to design an effective exercise program may wish to refer patients to an accredited fitness center or exercise specialist.

Note: See Appendix A for the U.S. Preventive Services Task Force Table of Ratings for this topic. See also the relevant Task Force background paper: Harris SS, Caspersen CJ, DeFriese GH, et al. Physical activity counseling for healthy adults as a primary preventive intervention in the clinical setting; report for the US Preventive Services Task Force. JAMA 1989; 261:3590–8.

REFERENCES

1. National Center for Health Statistics. Advance report of final mortality statistics, 1986. Monthly Vital Statistics Report [Suppl], vol. 37, no. 6. Hyattsville, Md.: Public Health Service, 1988. (Publication no. DHHS (PHS) 88–1120.)
2. American Heart Association. 1989 heart facts. Dallas, Tex.: American Heart Association, 1988.
3. 1988 Joint National Committee. The 1988 report of the Joint National Committee on Detection, Evaluation, and Treatment of High Blood Pressure. Arch Intern Med 1988; 148:1023–38.
4. National Center for Health Statistics. Current estimates from the National Health Interview Survey, United States, 1982. Vital and Health Statistics, series 10, no. 150. Washington, D.C.: Government Printing Office, 1985. (Publication no. DHHS (PHS) 85–1578.)
5. Consensus conference statement: osteoporosis. JAMA 1984; 252:799–802.
6. Melton LJ III. Epidemiology of fractures. In: Riggs BL, Melton LJ III. Osteoporosis: etiology, diagnosis, and management. New York: Raven Press, 1988.
7. Cummings SR, Kelsey JL, Nevitt MC, et al. Epidemiology of osteoporosis and osteoporotic fractures. Epidemiol Rev 1985; 7:178–208.
8. Jensen GF, Christiansen C, Boesen J, et al. Epidemiology of postmenopausal spinal and long bone fractures: a unifying approach to postmenopausal osteoporosis. Clin Orthoped 1982; 166:75–81.
9. Holbrook TL, Grazier K, Kelsey JL, et al. The frequency of occurrence, impact, and cost of selected musculoskeletal conditions in the United States. Chicago, Ill.: American Academy of Orthopedic Surgeons, 1984.
10. Paffenbarger RS Jr, Hyde RT, Wing AL, et al. Physical activity, all-cause mortality, and longevity of college alumni. N Engl J Med 1986; 314:605–13.
11. Leon AS, Connett J, Jacobs DR, et al. Leisure-time physical activity levels and risk of coronary heart disease and death. The Multiple Risk Factor Intervention Trial. JAMA 1987; 258:2388–95.
12. Powell KE, Thompson PD, Caspersen CJ, et al. Physical activity and the incidence of coronary heart disease. Ann Rev Public Health 1987; 8:253–87.
13. Kannel WB, Wilson P, Blair SN. Epidemiological assessment of the role of physical activity and fitness in the development of cardiovascular disease. Am Heart J 1985; 109:876–85.
14. Donahue RP, Abbott RD, Reed DM, et al. Physical activity and coronary heart disease

in middle-aged and elderly men: the Honolulu Heart Program. Am J Public Health 1988; 78:683–5.

15. Morris JN, Pollard R, Everitt MG, et al. Vigorous exercise in leisure-time: protection against coronary events. Lancet 1980; 8206:1207–10.

16. Siscovick DS, Weiss NS, Fletcher RH, et al. Habitual vigorous exercise and primary cardiac arrest: effect of other risk factors on the relationship. J Chronic Dis 1984; 37: 625–31.

17. Wood PD, Haskell WL, Blair SN, et al. Increased exercise level and plasma lipoprotein concentrations: a one-year, randomized, controlled study in sedentary, middle-aged men. Metabolism 1983; 32:31–9.

18. Paffenbarger RS Jr, Wing AL, Hyde RT. Physical activity as an index of heart risk in college alumni. Am J Epidemiol 1978; 108:161–75.

19. Paffenbarger RS Jr, Hyde RT, Wing AL, et al. A natural history of athleticism and cardiovascular health. JAMA 1984; 252:491–5.

20. Epstein LH, Wing RR. Aerobic exercise and weight. Addict Behav 1980; 5:371–8.

21. Wood PD, Terry RB, Haskell WL. Metabolism of substrates: diet, lipoprotein metabolism, and exercise. Federation Proc 1985; 44: 358–63.

22. Paffenbarger RS Jr, Wing AL, Hyde RT, et al. Physical activity and the incidence of hypertension in college alumni. Am J Epidemiol 1983; 117:245–6.

23. Blair SN, Goodyear NN, Gibbons LW, et al. Physical fitness and incidence of hypertension in healthy normotensive men and women. JAMA 1984; 252:487–90.

24. Bouchard C, Shephard RJ, Stephens T, et al., eds. Exercise, fitness, and health: research and consensus. Proceedings of the International Conference on Exercise, Fitness, and Health. Champaign, Ill.: Human Kinetics Publishers (in press).

25. King H, Taylor R, Zimmet P, et al. Non-insulin-dependent diabetes in a newly independent Pacific nation: the Republic of Kiribati. Diabetes Care 1984; 7:409–15.

26. Zimmet P, Faaiuso S, Ainuu J, et al. The prevalence of diabetes in the rural and urban Polynesian population of Western Samoa. Diabetes 1981; 30:45–51.

27. Rauramaa R. Relationship of physical activity, glucose tolerance and weight management. Prev Med 1984; 13:37–46.

28. Mazess RB, Wheedon GD. Immobilization and bone. Calcif Tissue Int 1983; 35:265–7.

29. Nilsson BE, Westlin NE. Bone density in athletes. Clin Orthop 1971; 77:179–82.

30. Dalen N, Olsson KE. Bone mineral content and physical activity. Acta Orthop Scand 1974; 45:170–4.

31. Smith EL, Reddan W, Smith PE. Physical activity and calcium modalities for bone mineral increase in aged women. Med Sci Sports Exerc 1981; 13:60–4.

32. Smith EL, Reddan W. Physical activity: a modality for bone accretion in the aged. Am J Roentgenol 1976; 126:1297.

33. Aloia JF, Conn SH, Ostani JA, et al. Prevention of involutional bone loss by exercise. Ann Intern Med 1978; 89:356–8.

34. Krolner B, Toft B, Nielson SP, et al. Physical exercise as prophylaxis against involutional vertebral bone loss: a controlled clinical trial. Clin Sci 1983; 541–6.

35. Paganini-Hill A, Ross RK, Gerkins JR, et al. Menopausal estrogen therapy and hip fractures. Ann Intern Med 1981; 95:28–31.

36. Chalmers J, Ho KC. Geographic variations in senile osteoporosis: the association of physical activity. J Bone Joint Surg 1970; 52:667–75.

37. Stephens T. Physical activity and mental health in the United States and Canada: evidence from four population surveys. Prev Med 1988; 17:35–47.

38. Folkins CH, Sime WE. Physical fitness training and mental health. Am Psychol 1981; 36:373–89.

39. Hughes JR. Psychological effects of habitual aerobic exercise: a critical review. Prev Med 1984; 13:66–78.

40. LaPorte RE, Adams LL, Savage DD, et al. The spectrum of physical activity, cardiovascular disease and health: an epidemiologic perspective. Am J Epidemiol 1984; 120: 507–17.

41. Magnus K, Matroos A, Strackee J. Walking, cycling, gardening with or without seasonal interruption in relation to acute coronary events. Am J Epidemiol 1979; 110:724–33.

42. American College of Sports Medicine. Position statement on the recommended quantity and quality of exercise for developing and maintaining fitness in healthy adults. Med Sci Sports Exerc 1978, 10.7-10.
43. Wenger HA, Bell GJ. The interactions of intensity, frequency and duration of exercise training in altering cardiorespiratory fitness. Sports Med 1986; 3:346-56.
44. Haskell WL, Montoye HJ, Orenstein D. Physical activity and exercise to achieve health-related physical fitness components. Public Health Rep 1985; 100:202-12.
45. Badenhop DT, Cleary P, Schaal SF, et al. Physiologic adjustments to higher- or lower-intensity exercise in elders. Med Sci Sports Exerc 1983; 15:496-502.
46. DeVries HA. Exercise intensity threshold for improvement of cardiovascular-respiratory function in older men. Geriatrics 1971; 26:94-101.
47. Emes CG. The effects of a regular program of light exercise on seniors. J Sports Med Phys Fitness 1979; 19:185-9.
48. Kraus JF, Conroy C. Mortality and morbidity from injuries in sports and recreation. Ann Rev Public Health 1984; 5:163-92.
49. Koplan JP, Siscovick DS, Goldbaum GM. The risks of exercise: a public health view of injuries and hazards. Public Health Rep 1985; 101:189-94.
50. Sohn RS, Michel LJ. The effects of running on the pathogenesis of osteoarthritis of the hips and knees. Clin Orthop Rel Res 1985; 198:106-9.
51. Panish RS, Schmidt C, Caldwell JR, et al. Is running associated with degenerative joint disease? JAMA 1986; 255:1152-4.
52. Lane NE, Bioch DA, Jones HH, et al. Long distance running, bone density and osteoarthritis. JAMA 1986; 255:1147-51.
53. Thompson PD, Fink EJ, Carleton RA, et al. Incidence of death through jogging in Rhode Island from 1975 through 1980. JAMA 1982; 247:2535-8.
54. Siscovick DS, Weiss NS, Fletcher RH, et al. The incidence of primary cardiac arrest during vigorous exercise. N Engl J Med 1984; 311:874-7.
55. Caspersen CJ, Christenson GM, Pollard RA. Status of the 1990 physical fitness objectives: evidence from NHIS 1985. Public Health Rep 1986; 101:587-92.
56. Stephens T, Jacobs DR Jr, White CC. A descriptive epidemiology of leisure time physical activity. Public Health Rep 1985; 100:147-58.
57. Mulder JA. Prescription home exercise therapy for cardiovascular fitness. J Fam Pract 1981; 13:345-8.
58. Campbell MJ, Browne D, Waters WE. Can general practitioners influence exercise habits? Controlled trial. Br Med J 1985; 290:1044-6.
59. Dishman RK. Compliance/adherence in health-related exercise. Health Psychol 1982; 1:237-67.
60. Blair SN. Physical activity leads to fitness and pays off. Physician Sports Med 1985; 13:153-7.
61. Kriska AM, Bayles JA, Cauley RE, et al. A randomized exercise trial in older women: increased activity over two years and the factors associated with compliance. Med Sci Sports Exerc 1986; 18:557-62.
62. Iverson DC, Fielding JE, Crow RS, et al. The promotion of physical activity in the United States population: the status of programs in medical, worksite community, and school settings. Public Health Rep 1985; 100:212-24.
63. Blair SN, Piserchia PV, Wilbur CS, et al. A public health intervention model for work-site health promotion. JAMA 1986; 255:921-6.
64. Dishman RK, Sallis JF, Orenstein DR. The determinants of physical activity and exercise. Public Health Rep 1985; 100:158-71.
65. Sallis JF, Haskell WL, Fortmann SP, et al. Predictors of adoption and maintenance of physical activity in a community sample. Prev Med 1986; 15:331-41.
66. American College of Sports Medicine. Guidelines for graded exercise testing and exercise prescription. Philadelphia: Lea and Febiger, 1975.
67. Centers for Disease Control. Protective effect of physical activity on coronary heart disease. MMWR 1987; 36:426-30.

50

Nutritional Counseling

Recommendation: Clinicians should provide periodic counseling regarding dietary intake of calories, fat (especially saturated fat), cholesterol, complex carbohydrates (starches), fiber, and sodium. Women and adolescent girls should receive counseling on calcium and iron intake, and pregnant women should receive specific information on nutritional guidelines during pregnancy. Parents should also be counseled about the nutritional requirements of infancy and early childhood (see *Clinical Intervention*). Counseling regarding alcohol consumption is discussed in Chapter 47.

Burden of Suffering

Diseases associated with dietary excess and imbalance rank among the leading causes of illness and death in the United States. Major diseases in which diet plays a role include coronary artery disease, some types of cancer, and stroke. Coronary artery disease is the leading cause of death in the United States,[1] and it accounts for about 1.5 million myocardial infarctions and over 520,000 deaths each year.[1,2] Cancer of the colon, breast, and prostate, the three forms of cancer most closely associated epidemiologically with nutritional risk factors, together cause over 130,000 deaths annually.[3] Cerebrovascular disease, the third leading cause of death, accounted for about 150,000 deaths in 1986.[1] Hypertension, another disease with nutritional risk factors, occurs in up to 58 million Americans.[4] Caloric intake, when it exceeds energy expenditures, can also lead to obesity, which affects about 32 million American adults aged 25–74.[5] Obesity is a risk factor for a number of serious disorders (see Chapter 18), including both hypertension and adult-onset diabetes mellitus. The latter is present in about 11 million persons in the United States, causes or contributes to over 130,000 deaths each year, and is a leading cause of neuropathy, peripheral vascular disease, renal failure, and blindness.[6-8]

Nutritional factors have also been linked to osteoporosis, constipation, diverticular disease, and dental disease. An estimated 1.3 million osteoporosis-related fractures occur each year in the United States.[9] Hip fractures in particular are associated with significant pain and disability, decreased functional independence, and high mortality; there is a 15–20% reduction in expected survival in the first year following a hip fracture.[10] Frequent constipation is a complaint of over 3.5 million Americans, and intestinal diverticular disease is reported by nearly 1.5 million persons.[11] Dental caries are present in most children by age 9, and an average of eight cavities are present by age 17.[12,13] The average adult in the

United States has 10–17 decayed, missing, or filled permanent teeth and 1 untreated decayed permanent tooth.[14,15]

Efficacy of Risk Reduction

Eating habits can have a significant impact on the incidence and severity of many health disorders. The complete body of literature regarding the health effects of foods is beyond the scope of this report and has recently been the subject of extensive reviews.[16,17] In summary, it is clear that a direct relationship exists between nutritional risk factors and certain key diseases. It is well established, for example, that caloric imbalance (intake exceeding expenditure) can lead to obesity. Persons who are significantly overweight are at increased risk for glucose intolerance, hypertension, hypercholesterolemia, and other disorders (see Chapter 18); reduction of body weight has been shown to reduce these risks.[18-21] The average person is likely to benefit from dietary practices and exercise activities (see Chapter 49) that keep caloric intake equal to or below the level of daily energy expenditures. In addition to the overall objective of caloric balance, modified intake of specific dietary factors may also help prevent certain diseases.

Reduced intake of **dietary fat**, especially saturated fat, can reduce the risk of developing coronary artery disease. A large body of epidemiologic evidence links serum cholesterol levels to the development of coronary atherosclerosis.[22-24] Serum cholesterol levels can in turn be modified by dietary measures. Controlled clinical trials in which diets low in saturated fat were given to asymptomatic middle-aged men with selected cardiac risk factors have reported a 10–15% reduction in serum cholesterol levels[25-33] and, in most trials, a decrease in the incidence of cardiac events such as myocardial infarction and sudden death.[25,26,29-31,33] More recently, the WHO Cooperative Trial,[34-36] the Lipid Research Clinics Coronary Primary Prevention Trial,[37,38] and the Helsinki Heart Study[39] have found that serum cholesterol-lowering drugs can reduce the incidence of coronary artery disease in asymptomatic middle-aged men with hyperlipidemia. These studies found that the incidence of cardiac events in such men is decreased by an average of 2% for every 1% reduction in serum cholesterol (see Chapter 2). A reduction in all-cause mortality was not observed, however. **Dietary cholesterol** intake may also influence serum cholesterol levels, especially low-density-lipoprotein (LDL) cholesterol levels, but the association appears to be weaker and more variable than that of dietary fat intake.[16]

The association between dietary fat and certain forms of cancer is currently under investigation. An effect of dietary fat on carcinogenesis has been demonstrated in animal research. Furthermore, international comparisons of cancer incidence and case-control studies have revealed an epidemiologic correlation between dietary fat consumption and the incidence of cancer of the breast, colon, and prostate.[40-44] Within more homogenous populations, however, cohort studies to date have been unable to provide consistent evidence of a causal relationship between increased dietary fat consumption and the incidence of breast cancer or other cancers.[45-48]

A diet emphasizing the consumption of foods high in **complex carbohydrates** and fiber (e.g., whole grain foods and cereal products, vegetables [including dried beans and peas], and fruits) is an important means of lowering dietary fat consumption. There are other health benefits associated with the replacement of foods high in simple carbohydrates (e.g., table sugar, honey, corn sweeteners) with those containing starch and fiber. Foods high in complex carbohydrates and fiber have lower average caloric density, and they are therefore preferred for maintaining caloric balance and healthful body weight.[16] Reduced intake and less frequent consumption of refined sugars may also lower the risk of developing dental caries[49,50] (see Chapter 55).

Increased intake of **dietary fiber** improves gastrointestinal motility.[51] Certain types of dietary fiber may also be helpful in the treatment of glucose intolerance, weight reduction, and the control of lipid disorders.[51] A high-fiber diet may be effective in reducing intracolonic pressure and preventing diverticular disease.[52] The risk of developing colorectal cancer may also be influenced by dietary fiber intake. At least 15 cross-cultural studies have shown an inverse relationship between dietary fiber consumption and the incidence of colon cancer.[53,54] Such studies do not, however, provide direct evidence that high dietary fiber intake, rather than other population dietary characteristics (e.g., low fat intake), is directly responsible for the lower cancer incidence rate. Case-control studies have produced inconsistent results regarding the association between dietary fiber and colon cancer.[55-57] Cohort studies to date have also produced inconsistent results and suffer from methodologic limitations.[58-60] Data from ongoing cohort studies examining this issue are expected in the future.

Reduced intake of **dietary sodium** may be of clinical benefit to persons who either have hypertension or are likely to develop it in the future. A number of clinical trials have demonstrated the ability of dietary sodium restriction to lower blood pressure by at least several millimeters of mercury in some hypertensive and normotensive individuals.[61-68] In addition, cross-cultural studies have shown a correlation between the sodium intake of different populations and the incidence of hypertension.[69-71] A recent multi-national study involving 52 sites also demonstrated an association between sodium excretion and the rate of change of blood pressure with age.[72] However, controlled prospective studies will ultimately be necessary to provide definitive evidence that normotensive persons who practice dietary sodium restriction are at lower risk of developing hypertension over time than are those with more typical sodium consumption. Nonetheless, there is at least suggestive evidence of potential benefit and no known harm associated with moderate sodium restriction. The typical American consumes significantly more dietary sodium (about 4–6 g/day)[16] than is considered necessary by the National Research Council (1.1–3.3 g/day).[73]

Many American women and adolescent girls consume less **dietary calcium** than the daily allowance recommended by the National Research Council (adults: 800 mg/day; adolescent, pregnant, or lactating women: 1200 mg/day).[73,74] The clinical implications of reduced dietary calcium intake remain uncertain, however. Population studies suggest that reduced calcium intake among women may be an important risk factor for bone mineral loss and postmenopausal osteoporosis. However, prospective studies of asymptomatic postmenopausal women have produced inconsistent results about the efficacy of increasing dietary calcium intake as a means of slowing bone loss. Although some studies have reported that a daily intake of 750–1040 mg/day can reduce significantly the rate of bone loss in asymptomatic postmenopausal women,[75,76] other controlled studies have shown either no effect or an effect only on compact bone with doses as high as 1800–2000 mg/day.[77-80] It is also unclear from current evidence whether women who have already developed clinical evidence of postmenopausal osteoporosis benefit from calcium supplementation.[81-83] Postmenopausal estrogen replacement therapy may be a more effective form of chemoprophylaxis than calcium supplementation (see Chapter 59). Nonetheless, there is little significant risk to women who moderately increase their consumption of dietary calcium. Under unusual circumstances, gross and prolonged use of calcium supplements can result in milk alkali syndrome and may contribute to an increased occurrence of renal stones.

Adequate **dietary iron** intake is important for menstruating women and for young children to maintain iron stores and prevent iron deficiency anemia. This topic is discussed in detail in Chapter 28. Iron deficiency anemia during infancy has been associated with impaired infant behavior and development, and infants therefore require iron-fortified foods to replace depleted iron stores. There is little evidence from prospective studies of older children and menstruating women that mild anemia in the absence of symptoms is a direct cause of increased morbidity or mortality (Chapter 28). It is clinically prudent, however, to recommend diets including iron-rich foods (e.g., lean meats, certain beans, iron-enriched cereals and whole grain products) for these groups as well.

Nutritional status is especially important during pregnancy. Studies have shown that low birthweight and neonatal mortality are more common in pregnant women with very poor nutritional status[84,85] and in those who fail to gain adequate weight during pregnancy.[86,87] Prenatal programs providing nutritional support for pregnant women have been associated with improved perinatal outcomes.[88] Pregnancy brings increased requirements for energy and specific nutrients, such as protein, calcium, phosphorus, folic acid, and iron.[89] Oral iron supplements may be beneficial in preventing iron-deficiency anemia in pregnancy, and they are often prescribed routinely as part of prenatal health care. Some authors have suggested, however, that routine iron supplementation is not necessary during pregnancy and that iron tablets need be prescribed only to women with documented iron deficiency.[90-92]

Other population groups also have special nutritional needs. Infants require breast milk or appropriate alternatives (e.g., infant formulas) to provide adequate nutrition.[93] Nutritional status remains important throughout childhood to facilitate normal growth and development.[94] The elderly can also have special nutritional requirements.[95] Depending on the patient's nutritional status, underlying medical disorders, and therapeutic drug regimens, it can be important to modify recommended daily intake levels of calories, sodium, dietary fat, fiber, protein, and other nutrients.[95]

Effectiveness of Counseling

The effectiveness of nutritional counseling in changing the dietary habits of patients has been demonstrated in a number of clinical trials.[96] In most of these studies, however, the counselor was not a physician, but rather a nurse, nutritionist, registered dietitian, health educator, or psychologist. Since many of the interventions tested in these studies were highly specialized or community-wide programs, they are not easily reproduced in the typical physician-patient clinical encounter. Although physicians can often provide general guidelines on proper nutrition, many lack the time and the skills to obtain a thorough dietary history, to address potential barriers to changes in eating habits, and to offer specific guidance on food selection.[97,98] Patients may also have difficulty with long-term compliance if food selection and preparation for weight reduction and healthy diets are perceived as unappealing or inconvenient. It is possible, however, that physicians can overcome many of these limitations by expanding the content of the nutritional information they provide to patients, by emphasizing to the patient the health benefits of good nutrition, and by referring those requiring help with dietary changes to qualified nutritionists, registered dietitians, health educators, nurses, or other providers with greater nutrition expertise.

Recommendations of Others

Dietary guidelines for the general population have been issued by the U.S. Department of Agriculture and the U.S. Department of Health and Human Services[99] and reaffirmed recently by the U.S. Surgeon General.[16] The Food and Nutrition Board of the National Research Council has published Recommended Dietary Allowances (RDAs) for specific nutrients,[73] and it has recently released an extensive report on diet and health.[17] Specific recommendations for physicians to offer nutritional counseling to patients have been issued by the American Medical Association,[100-102] the American College of Physicians,[103] and the American Heart Association.[94,104,105] Guidelines for dietary practices to reduce the risk of cancer have been issued by the National Research Council,[106] the American Cancer Society,[107] and the National Cancer Institute.[108] Recommendations on nutritional counseling to reduce cardiac risk factors have been issued by a panel convened by the National Heart, Lung, and Blood Institute.[109] The National Cholesterol Education Program has issued guidelines on dietary measures to lower serum cholesterol.[110] Dietary recommendations for pregnant women have been issued by the American College of Obstetricians and Gynecologists.[111]

Clinical Intervention

Clinicians should provide periodic counseling regarding dietary intake of calories, fat (especially saturated fat), cholesterol, complex carbohydrates and fiber, and sodium. Specifically, patients should receive a diet and exercise prescription designed to achieve and maintain a desirable weight by keeping caloric intake balanced with energy expenditures. Adolescents and adults, in particular, should be given dietary guidance on how to reduce total fat intake to less than 30% of total calories and dietary cholesterol to less than 300 mg/day. Saturated fat consumption should be reduced to less than 10% of total calories. To achieve these goals, patients should emphasize consumption of fish, poultry prepared without skin, lean meats, and low-fat dairy products. More detailed food selection guidelines to lower total fat, saturated fat, and cholesterol consumption have been published elsewhere.[110,112]

Patients should be encouraged to eat a variety of foods, with emphasis on the consumption of whole grain products and cereals, vegetables, and fruits. Those who are at increased risk for dental caries, especially children, should limit their consumption of foods high in refined sugars. It is also reasonable to recommend eating foods low in sodium and limiting the amount of salt added in food preparation and at the table. Adolescent girls and women should receive counseling on methods to ensure adequate calcium and iron intake; parents should be encouraged to include iron-enriched foods in the diet of infants and young children; and pregnant women should receive specific nutritional guidelines to enhance fetal and maternal health. Counseling regarding alcohol consumption is discussed in Chapter 47.

Clinicians who lack the time or skills to perform a complete dietary history, to address potential barriers to changes in eating habits, and to offer specific guidance on food selection and preparation, should either have patients seen by other trained providers in the office or clinic or should refer patients to a registered dietitian or qualified nutritionist for further counseling.

Note: See Appendix A for the U.S. Preventive Services Task Force Table of Ratings for this topic. See also the relevant Task Force background papers: Weise WH, Hutchins S. Dietary fat and cancers of the breast, colon and prostate: a causal relation?; and Kushi LH, Kottke TE. Dietary lipids and coronary heart disease: evidence for a causal relation? In: Goldbloom RB, Lawrence RS, eds. Preventing disease: beyond the rhetoric. New York: Springer-Verlag (in press).

REFERENCES

1. National Center for Health Statistics. Advance report of final mortality statistics, 1986. Monthly Vital Statistics Report, vol. 37, no. 6. Hyattsville, Md.: Public Health Service, 1988. (Publication no. DHHS (PHS) 88–1120.)

2. American Heart Association. 1989 heart facts. Dallas, Tex.: American Heart Association, 1988.

3. American Cancer Society. Cancer statistics, 1989. CA 1989; 39:3–20.

4. 1988 Joint National Committee. The 1988 report of the Joint National Committee on Detection, Evaluation, and Treatment of High Blood Pressure. Arch Intern Med 1988; 148:1023–38.

5. Department of Health and Human Services, Department of Agriculture. Nutrition monitoring in the United States. Washington, D.C.: Government Printing Office, 1986:2,54, 59–62.

6. American Diabetes Association. Diabetes facts and figures. Alexandria, Va.: American Diabetes Association, 1986.

7. Harris MI. Prevalence of non-insulin-dependent diabetes and impaired glucose tolerance. In: National Diabetes Data Group. Diabetes in America: diabetes data compiled 1984. Washington, D.C.: Department of Health and Human Services, 1985:VI-1 to VI-31.(Publication no. DHHS (NIH) 85–1468.)

8. Kovar MG, Harris MI, Hadden WC. The scope of diabetes in the United States population. Am J Public Health 1987; 77:1549–50.

9. Consensus Conference Statement. JAMA 1984; 252:799–802.

10. Jensen GF, Christiansen C, Boesen J, et al. Epidemiology of postmenopausal spinal and long bone fractures: a unifying approach to postmenopausal osteoporosis. Clin Orthoped 1982; 166:75–81.

11. National Center for Health Statistics. Prevalence of selected chronic conditions, United States, 1979–81. Vital and Health Statistics, series 10, no. 155. Washington, D.C.: Government Printing Office, 1986. (Publication no. DHHS (PHS) 86–1583.)

12. National Institute of Dental Research. The Prevalence of Dental Caries in United States Children 1979–80. The National Dental Caries Prevalence Survey. Bethesda, Md.: National Institute of Dental Research, 1981. (Publication no. DHHS (NIH) 82–2245.)

13. Idem. Survey shows dramatic decline in tooth decay among U.S. children. NIDR Research News, June 21, 1988.

14. National Center for Health Statistics. Decayed, missing, and filled teeth among persons 1–74 years, United States. Data from the National Health Survey. Vital and Health Statistics, series 11, no. 223. Hyattsville, Md.: National Center for Health Statistics, 1981. (Publication no. DHHS (PHS) 81–1673.)

15. National Institute of Dental Research. Oral health of United States adults, the National Survey of Oral Health in U.S. Employed Adults and Seniors: 1985–86. Bethesda, Md.: National Institute of Dental Research, 1987. (Publication no. DHHS (NIH) 88–2868.)

16. Department of Health and Human Services. The Surgeon General's report on nutrition and health. Washington, D.C.: Government Printing Office, 1988. (Publication no. DHHS (PHS) 88–50210.)

17. Food and Nutrition Board, National Research Council. Diet and health; implications for reducing chronic disease. Washington, D.C.: National Academy Press, 1989.

18. Henry RR, Schaeffer L, Olefsky, JM. Glycemic effects of intensive caloric restriction and isocaloric refeeding in noninsulin-dependent diabetes mellitus. J Clin Endocrinol Metab 1985; 61:917–25.

19. Henry RR, Wiest-Kent TA, Schaeffer L, et al. Metabolic consequences of very-low-calorie diet therapy in obese noninsulin-dependent diabetic and nondiabetic subjects. Diabetes 1986; 35:155–64.

20. MacMahon S, Cutler J, Brittain E, et al. Obesity and hypertension: epidemiological and clinical issues. Eur Heart J [Suppl B] 1987; 8:57–70.

21. Rifkind BM, Goor R, Schucker B. Compliance and cholesterol-lowering in clinical trials: efficacy of diet. In: Schettler FG, Gotto AM, Middelhoff G, et al., eds. Atherosclerosis

VI. Proceedings of the Sixth International Symposium. New York: Springer-Verlag, 1983. 306 10.

22. Stamler J. Lifestyles, major risk factors, proof and public policy. Circulation 1978; 58: 3–19.

23. Stallones RA. Ischemic heart disease and lipids in blood and diet. Ann Rev Nutr 1983; 3:155–85.

24. Grundy SM. Cholesterol and coronary heart disease: a new era. JAMA 1986; 256: 2849–58.

25. Dayton S, Pearce ML, Goldman H, et al. Controlled trial of a diet high in unsaturated fat for prevention of atherosclerotic complications. Lancet 1968; 2:1060–2.

26. Hjermann I, Holme I, Velve Byre K, et al. Effect of diet and smoking intervention on the incidence of coronary heart disease. Report from the Oslo Study Group of a randomized trial in healthy men. Lancet 1981; 2:1303–10.

27. Multiple Risk Factor Intervention Trial Research Group. Multiple Risk Factor Intervention Trial: risk factor changes and mortality results. JAMA 1982; 248:1465–77.

28. World Health Organization European Collaborative Group. European collaborative trial of multifactorial prevention of coronary heart disease: final report on the 6–year results. Lancet 1986; 1:869–72.

29. Rinzler S. Primary prevention of coronary heart disease by diet. Bull NY Acad Med 1968; 44:936–49.

30. Turpeinen O, Karvonen MJ, Pekkarinen M, et al. Dietary prevention of coronary heart disease: the Finnish Mental Hospital Study. Int J Epidem 1979; 8:99–118.

31. Miettinen M, Turpeinen O, Karvonen MJ, et al. Effect of cholesterol-lowering diet on mortality from coronary heart disease and other causes: a twelve-year clinical trial in men and women.Lancet 1972; 2:835–8.

32. Stamler J. Acute myocardial infarction, progress in primary prevention. Br Heart J 1971; 33:145–64.

33. Frantz ID, Dawson EA, Kuba K. The Minnesota Coronary Survey: effect of diet on cardiovascular events and deaths. Circulation [Suppl II] 1975; 52:II-4.

34. Report from the Committee of Principal Investigators. A cooperative trial in the primary prevention of ischaemic heart disease using clofibrate. Br Heart J 1978; 40:1069–118.

35. Report of the Committee of Principal Investigators. W.H.O. cooperative trial on primary prevention of ischaemic heart disease using clofibrate to lower serum cholesterol: mortality follow-up. Lancet 1980; 2:379–85.

36. Idem. W.H.O. cooperative trial on primary prevention of ischaemic heart disease with clofibrate to lower serum cholesterol: final mortality follow-up. Lancet 1984; 2:600–4.

37. The Lipid Research Clinics Coronary Primary Prevention Trial Results. I. Reduction in incidence of coronary heart disease. JAMA 1984; 251:351–64.

38. The Lipid Research Clinics Coronary Primary Prevention Trial Results. II. The relationship of reduction in incidence of coronary heart disease to cholesterol lowering. JAMA 1984; 251:365–74.

39. Frick MH, Elo O, Haapa K, et al. Helsinki Heart Study: primary prevention trial with gemfibrozil in middle-aged men with dyslipidemia. Safety of treatment, changes in risk factors, and incidence of coronary heart disease. N Engl J Med 1987; 317:1237–45.

40. Kakar F, Henderson M. Diet and breast cancer. Clin Nutr 1985; 4:119–30.

41. Kolonel LN, Hankin JH, Nomura AM. Multiethnic studies of diet, nutrition, and cancer in Hawaii. In: Hayashi Y, ed. Diet, nutrition, and cancer. Tokyo: Japan Science Society Press, 1986:29–40.

42. Rose DP. The biochemical epidemiology of prostatic carcinoma. In: Ip C, Birt DF, Rogers AE, et al., eds. Dietary fat and cancer. New York: Alan R. Liss, 1986:11–48.

43. Wynder EL, McCoy GD, Reddy BS, et al. Nutrition and metabolic epidemiology of cancers of the oral cavity, esophagus, colon, breast, prostate, and stomach. In: Newell GR, Ellison NM, eds. Nutrition and cancer: etiology and treatment. New York: Raven Press, 1981.

44. Toniolo P, Riboli E, Protta F, et al. Calorie-providing nutrients and risk of breast cancer. JNCI 1989; 81:278–86.

45. Hirayama T. Epidemiology of breast cancer with special reference to the role of diet. Prev Med 1978; 7:173–95.
46. Phillips RL, Snowden DA. Association of meat and coffee use with cancers of the large bowel, breast, and prostate among Seventh-day Adventists: preliminary results. Cancer Res [Suppl 5] 1983; 43:2403S-8S.
47. Willett WC, Stampfer MJ, Colditz GA, et al. Dietary fat and the risk of breast cancer. New Engl J Med 1987; 316:22–8.
48. Jones DY, Schatzkin A, Green SB, et al. Dietary fat and breast cancer in the National Health and Nutrition Examination Survey. I. Epidemiological follow-up study. JNCI 1987; 79:465–71.
49. Gustafsson BE, Quensel CE, Lanke LS, et al. The Vipeholm dental caries study: the effect of different levels of carbohydrate intake on caries activity in 436 individuals observed for 5 years. Acta Odontol Scand 1954; 11:232–364.
50. Harris R. Biology of the children of Hopewood House, Bowral, Australia. IV. Observations of dental caries experience extending over five years (1957–1961). J Dent Res 1963; 42:1387–98.
51. Federation of American Societies for Experimental Biology. Physiological effects and health consequences of dietary fiber. Report to the Food and Drug Administration. Bethesda, Md.: Federation of American Societies for Experimental Biology, 1987.
52. Painter N. Diverticular disease of the colon. In: Trowell H, Burkitt D, Heaton K, eds. Dietary fibre, fibre-depleted foods and disease. New York: Academic Press, 1985: 145–60.
53. Irving D, Drasar BS. Fibre and cancer of the colon. Br J Cancer 1973; 28:462–3.
54. McKeown-Eyssen GE, Bright-See E. Dietary factors in colon cancer: international relationships. Nutr Cancer 1984; 6:160–70.
55. Modan B, Barrell V, Lubin F, et al. Low-fiber intake as an etiologic factor in cancer of the colon. JNCI 1975; 55:15–8.
56. Jain M, Cook GM, Davis FG, et al. A case-control study of diet and colo-rectal cancer. Int J Cancer 1980; 26:757–68.
57. Potter JD, McMichael AJ. Diet and cancer of the colon and rectum: a case-control study. JNCI 1986; 76:557–69.
58. Hirayama T. A large-scale cohort study on the relationship between diet and selected cancers of the digestive organs. In: Bruce WR, Correa P, Lipkin M, et al., eds. Banbury Report 7. Gastrointestinal cancer: endogenous factors. Cold Spring Harbor, NY: Cold Spring Harbor Laboratory, 1981:409–29.
59. Kromhout D, Bosschieter EB, de Lezenne Coulander C. Dietary fibre and 10–year mortality from coronary heart disease, cancer, and all causes: the Zutphen Study. Lancet 1982; 2:518–22.
60. Phillips RL, Snowden DA. Dietary relationships with fatal colorectal cancer among Seventh-Day Adventists. JNCI 1985; 74:307–17.
61. Grobbee DE, Hofman A. Does sodium restriction lower blood pressure? Br Med J 1986; 293:27–9.
62. Parijs J, Joosens JV, Van der Linden L, et al. Moderate sodium restriction and diuretics in the treatment of hypertension. Am Heart J 1973; 85:22–34.
63. MacGregor GA, Markandu N, Best F, et al. Double-blind, randomized, crossover trial of moderate sodium restriction in essential hypertension. Lancet 1982; 1:351–5.
64. Langford HG, Blaufox MD, Oberman A, et al. Dietary therapy slows the return of hypertension after stopping prolonged medication. JAMA 1985; 253:657–64.
65. Morgan T, Adams W, Gillies A, et al. Hypertension treated by salt restriction. Lancet 1978; 1:227–30.
66. Beard TC, Cooke HM, Gray WR, et al. Randomized, controlled trial of a no-added-sodium diet for mild hypertension. Lancet 1982; 2:455–8.
67. Weinberger MH, Cohen SJ, Miller JZ, et al. Dietary sodium restriction as adjunctive treatment of hypertension. JAMA 1988; 259:2561–5.
68. Miller JZ, Daugherty SA, Weinberger MH, et al. Blood pressure response to dietary sodium restriction in normotensive adults. Hypertension 1983; 5:790–5.

69. Page LB, Damon A, Moellering RC Jr. Antecedents of cardiovascular disease in six Solomon Island societies. Circulation 1974; 49: 1132–46.

70. Kaminer B, Lutz WPW. Blood pressure in bushmen of the Kalahari Desert. Circulation 1960; 22:289–95.

71. Saunders GM, Bancroft H. Blood pressure studies on negro and white men and women living in the Virgin Islands of the United States. Am Heart J 1942; 23:410–23.

72. Intersalt Cooperative Research Group. Intersalt: an international study of electrolyte excretion and blood pressure. Results for 24 hour urinary sodium and potassium excretion. Br Med J 1988; 297:319–28.

73. National Research Council, Food and Nutrition Board. Recommended Dietary Allowances, ninth revised edition. Committee on Dietary Allowances. Washington, D.C.: National Academy of Sciences, 1980.

74. National Center for Health Statistics, Carroll MD, Abraham S, Dresser CM. Dietary intake source data: United States, 1976–80. Vital and Health Statistics, series 11, no. 231. Washington, D.C.: Government Printing Office, 1983. (Publication no. DHHS (PHS) 83–1681.)

75. Horsman A, Gallagher JC, Simpson M, et al. Prospective trial of oestrogen and calcium in postmenopausal women. Br Med J 1977; 2:789–92.

76. Recker RR, Saville PD, Heaney RP. Effect of estrogens and calcium carbonate on bone loss in postmenopausal women. Ann Intern Med 1977; 87:649–55.

77. Ettinger B, Genant HK, Cann CE. Postmenopausal bone loss is prevented by treatment with low-dosage estrogen with calcium. Ann Intern Med 1987; 106:40–5.

78. Riis B, Thomsen K, Christiansen C. Does calcium supplementation prevent postmenopausal bone loss? A double-blind, controlled clinical study. N Engl J Med 1987; 316:173–7.

79. Nilas L, Christiansen C, Rodbro P. Calcium supplementation and postmenopausal bone loss. Br Med J 1984; 289:1103–6.

80. Stevenson JC, Whitehead MI, Padwick M, et al. Dietary intake of calcium and postmenopausal bone loss. Br Med J 1988; 297:15–7.

81. Nordin BEC, Horsman A, Crilly RG, et al. Treatment of spinal osteoporosis in postmenopausal women. Br Med J 1980; 280:451–4.

82. Riggs BL, Seeman E, Hodgson SF, et al. Effect of the fluoride/ calcium regimen on vertebral fracture occurrence in postmenopausal women: comparison with conventional therapy. N Engl J Med 1982; 306:446–50.

83. Resnick NM, Greenspan SL. "Senile" osteoporosis reconsidered. JAMA 1989; 261: 1025–9.

84. Antonov AN. Children born during the siege of Leningrad in 1942. J Pediatr 1947; 30:250–95.

85. Stein A, Susser M, Saenger G, et al. Famine and human development: the Dutch hunger winter of 1944/45. New York: Oxford University Press, 1974.

86. Singer JE, Westphal M, Niswander K. Relationship of weight gain during pregnancy to birthweight and infant growth and development in the first year of life: a report from the collaborative study of cerebral palsy. Obstet Gynecol 1968; 31:417.

87. Abrams BF, Laros RD. Prepregnancy weight, weight gain, and birthweight. Am J Obstet Gynecol 1986; 154:503.

88. Rush D, Leighton J, Sloan NL, et al. The National WIC evaluation: evaluation of the Special Supplemental Food Program for Women, Infants, and Children. II. Review of past studies of WIC. Am J Clin Nutr 1988; 48:394–411.

89. Institute of Medicine. Preventing low birthweight. Washington, D.C.: National Academy Press, 1985.

90. Goodlin RC. Why treat "physiologic" anemias of pregnancy? J Reprod Med 1982; 27:639–46.

91. Do all pregnant women need iron? Br Med J 1978; 2:1317.

92. Lind T. Nutrient requirements during pregnancy. Am J Clin Nutr 1981; 34:669–78.

93. South-Paul JE. Infant nutrition. Am Fam Physician 1987; 36:173–8.

94. American Heart Association. Diet in the healthy child: Task Force Committee of the

Nutrition Committee and the Cardiovascular Disease in the Young Council. Circulation 1983; 67:1411A-4A.

95. Chen LH, ed. Nutritional aspects of aging, vols. 1 and 2. Boca Raton, Fla.: CRC Press, Inc., 1986.

96. Glanz K. Nutrition education for risk factor reduction and patient education: a review. Prev Med 1985; 14:721–52.

97. Wechsler H, Levine S, Idelson RK, et al. The physician's role in health promotion: a survey of primary-care practitioners. N Engl J Med 1983; 308:97–100.

98. Cooper-Stephenson C, Theologides A. Nutrition in cancer: physicians' knowledge, opinions, and educational needs. J Am Diet Assoc 1981; 78:472–6.

99. Department of Agriculture, Department of Health and Human Services. Dietary guidelines for Americans. Bulletin no. 232. Washington, D.C.: Department of Agriculture, 1985.

100. Council on Scientific Affairs. Medical evaluation of healthy persons. Chicago, Ill.: American Medical Association, 1983.

101. Idem. Sodium in processed foods. JAMA 1983; 249:784–9.

102. Idem. American Medical Association concepts of nutrition and health. JAMA 1979; 242:2335–8.

103. American College of Physicians. Nutrition: position paper. Washington, D.C.: American College of Physicians, 1985.

104. American Heart Association. Dietary guidelines for healthy American adults: a statement for physicians and health professionals by the Nutrition Committee, American Heart Association. Circulation 1988; 77:721A-4A.

105. Grundy SM, Greenland P, Herd A, et al. Cardiovascular and risk factor evaluation of healthy American adults. Circulation 1987; 75:1340A-62A.

106. National Research Council, Committee on Diet, Nutrition, and Cancer. Diet, nutrition, and cancer. Washington, D.C.: National Academy Press, 1982.

107. American Cancer Society. Nutrition and cancer: cause and prevention. An American Cancer Society special report. CA 1984; 34:121–6.

108. National Cancer Institute. Diet, nutrition, and cancer prevention: the good news. Washington, D.C.: Government Printing Office, 1986. (Publication no. DHHS (NIH) 87–2878.)

109. National Heart, Lung, and Blood Institute. Heart to heart: a manual on nutritional counseling for the reduction of cardiovascular disease risk factors. Bethesda, Md.: National Heart, Lung, and Blood Institute, 1983. (Publication no. DHHS (NIH) 85–1528.)

110. Report of the National Cholesterol Education Program Expert Panel on Detection, Evaluation, and Treatment of High Blood Cholesterol in Adults. Arch Intern Med 1988; 148:36–69.

111. American College of Obstetricians and Gynecologists. Food, pregnancy, and health. Washington, D.C.: American College of Obstetricians and Gynecologists, 1982.

112. American Heart Association. The American Heart Association diet: an eating plan for healthy Americans. Dallas, Tex.: American Heart Association, 1987.

51

Counseling to Prevent
Motor Vehicle Injuries

Recommendation: All patients should be urged to use occupant restraints (safety belts and child safety seats) for themselves and others, to wear safety helmets when riding motorcycles, and to refrain from driving while under the influence of alcohol or other drugs (see *Clinical Intervention*). The prevention of bicycle injuries is discussed in Chapter 52.

Burden of Suffering

Injuries are the fourth leading cause of death in the United States and the leading cause of death in persons under age 45. Motor vehicle injuries account for about half of these deaths.[1] In 1986, nearly 48,000 Americans died in motor vehicle crashes, and each year several million suffer nonfatal injuries.[1-3] Over 3100 children under age 15 died in motor vehicle crashes in 1986.[4] Motor vehicle injuries occur most commonly in males and in persons aged 15–24.[5] This age group has the highest mortality rate and accounts for one-third of all deaths from motor vehicle crashes in the United States.[1] Motor vehicles crashes are the leading cause of death in persons aged 5–24; in 1986 they accounted for 38% of all deaths in young persons aged 15–24.[1] The risk of motor vehicle crashes is also increased for persons over age 60, but elderly motorists account for only 10% of fatal crashes, primarily because they drive less than younger persons.[6]

Only 46% of Americans use seat belts[7] and, in 1986, 1.7 million persons were arrested for alcohol-impaired driving.[4] About 40% of persons killed in motor vehicle crashes are intoxicated by alcohol.[4] In 1987, an estimated 23,630 persons were killed in alcohol-related motor vehicle crashes, accounting for about 7% of the total years of potential life lost before age 65 in the United States during that year.[8] The proportion of fatally injured drivers having illegally high blood alcohol concentrations (BAC) is highest for those aged 20–34.[9,10]

Efficacy of Risk Reduction

Driving while intoxicated and failing to use occupant protection (e.g., safety belts, child safety seats) are two important personal behaviors that increase the risk of motor vehicle injury. Several crash studies have found that about half of fatally injured drivers have BACs of 0.10% by weight (the legal limit in most states) or higher.[3,11] Controlled studies have shown that fatally injured drivers are more likely to have a BAC of at least 0.10% than are drivers who are not killed.[12,13] In addition to its role as a risk factor for causing motor vehicle crashes, alcohol intoxication increases the risk of death or serious injury during and after a crash,[14,15] and it can limit the ability of the victim to escape from the vehicle.[11,14] Alcohol-intoxicated survivors with severe brain injuries appear to have longer hospitalizations and more persistent neurologic impairment than those who are not intoxicated.[16] Intoxication by drugs other than alcohol, such as benzodiazepines, narcotics, amphetamines, barbiturates, cocaine, and marijuana, has also been documented in motor vehicle crash victims, but most studies have been unable to separate the effects of these drugs from those of alcohol.[17] It has been estimated, however, that about 10–20% of motor vehicle crashes are associated with drugs other than alcohol.[18]

Use of occupant protection systems has been shown to reduce the risk of motor vehicle injury by about 40–50%. The effectiveness of safety belts has been demonstrated in a variety of study designs that include laboratory experiments (using human volunteers, cadavers, and anthropomorphic crash dummies), postcrash comparisons of injuries sustained by restrained and unrestrained occupants, and postcrash judgments by crash analysts regarding the probable effects of restraints had they been used.[19] It has been estimated on the basis of such evidence that the proper use of lap and shoulder belts can decrease the risk of moderate to serious injury to front seat occupants by 45–55%[20,21] and can reduce crash mortality by 40–50%.[20] When brought to the hospital, crash victims who are wearing safety belts at the time of the crash have less severe injuries, are less likely to require admission, and have lower hospital charges.[22]

Child safety seats also appear to be effective. It has been reported that unrestrained children are over 10 times as likely to die in a motor vehicle crash than are restrained children,[23,24] although these data come from studies with important design limitations. Other studies suggest that child safety seats can reduce serious injury by 67% and mortality by 71%.[25] A 20–25% decline in head and extremity injuries for children under age 4 has been reported in states with mandatory child restraint legislation.[26] Child restraints may also reduce noncrash injuries to child passengers by preventing falls both within and out of the vehicle.[27]

By wearing safety helmets, persons who operate or ride on motorcycles can reduce their risk of injury or death from head trauma in the event of a crash. In states where their use is required by law, such helmets have been shown to reduce mortality by about 30%.[2] Head injury rates are reduced by about 75% among motorcyclists who wear safety helmets.[28] States that have repealed mandatory motorcycle helmet laws have experienced significant increases in motorcycle fatalities.[29]

Effectiveness of Counseling

The use of occupant protection systems has increased in recent years. From 1978 to 1988, the overall use of seat belts rose from under 13% to about 46%.[7] Nonetheless, most Americans, and presumably most patients seen by physicians, do not use occupant protection systems when driving or riding in a motor vehicle. Similarly, although the rate of alcohol-related driver fatalities has decreased slightly in recent years, as many as 1.7 million persons continue to be arrested annually for alcohol-impaired driving.[4] Thus, it is likely that many patients seen by clinicians could potentially benefit from counseling to modify their behaviors as drivers and passengers in motor vehicles. Since motor vehicle crashes represent a leading cause of death and nonfatal injury in the United States, even modest successes through clinical interventions could have major public health value.

In actual practice, however, it is not known how effectively clinicians can alter these behaviors. Although there is some evidence that persons involved in motor vehicle crashes while intoxicated demonstrate lower recidivism in alcohol treatment interventions[30] and that community interventions to reduce alcohol-impaired driving may be effective,[31] there is generally little information from clinical studies on the ability of physicians to influence patients to refrain from driving while intoxicated. Similarly, there have been few studies examining the effectiveness of physician counseling to use safety belts. In one questionnaire survey, patients claimed to have increased their use of safety belts as a result of a brief statement by their physician during a routine office visit,[32] but the study lacked controls and the patients were carefully selected. Other measures that have been proved successful in motivating persons to use safety belts, such as community educational programs and intensive psychological strategies, may not be generalizable to the clinical practice setting.[33]

The strongest evidence that clinician counseling can be effective comes from programs that encouraged parents to use infant safety seats before this practice became widely mandated by state law. Results from such programs suggest that significant short-term improvements are possible immediately after newborns are discharged, but the effect is rarely maintained for more than a few months.[34-37] A nonrandomized controlled trial found that the combined intervention of pediatrician counseling, a prescription for an infant restraint, and a pamphlet on crash protection was associated with increased correct use when compared with controls for the first two monthly well-baby visits.[37] A study in which nurses conducted educational sessions in the prenatal period, postpartum period, and at two-month intervals after discharge found that proper use of child safety seats had improved compared with rates in the previous year.[38] A small randomized study demonstrated that a loaner seat and instruction by a nurse resulted in increased correct use at discharge, but no difference in use after two to four weeks.[39] The same researchers in a subsequent trial found that a comprehensive hospital program combined with recent state legislation was effective in improving correct usage, but intensive counseling from pediatricians and nurses was of no additional benefit.[40] Another controlled study found that personal discussion was of limited value; a subgroup receiving free infant restraints and literature demonstrated slightly higher correct usage at discharge, but there was no significant difference between the groups in two to four months.[41] A randomized controlled trial involving parents of children aged 1 to 17 found no difference in the use of occupant protection in groups receiving various combinations of pamphlets, pediatrician counseling, and a slide show.[42] Finally, a study found that pediatrician counseling resulted in an immediate increase in safety belt use, but there was no difference in usage rates between the study group and controls at a one-year follow-up.[43]

Recommendations of Others

The use of safety belts and child safety seats is widely recommended by organizations and agencies concerned with injury prevention. Child safety seat use is required by law in all 50 states. Mandatory safety belt laws are in effect in 31 states and the District of Columbia.[44] Recommendations specifically urging physicians to counsel patients to use occupant restraints have been issued by a number of organizations, including the American Medical Association,[45] the American College of Physicians,[46] and the American Academy of Family Physicians.[47] The National Highway Traffic Safety Administration has also urged physicians and other health care providers to routinely advise patients about the importance of safety belts and the use of child safety seats.[44] The American Academy of Pediatrics (AAP) recommends counseling parents of infants and preschool children to use child safety seats and safety belts[48] and has instituted special parent-oriented educational programs ("Make Every Ride A Safe Ride") in which pediatricians encourage the use of child occupant protection beginning with the ride home from the hospital and continuing throughout childhood. The AAP also recommends counseling adolescents to abstain from intoxicants when driving; advising parents and children to discuss the proper use of alcohol at teen parties; and suggesting alternatives to driving while intoxicated or riding in a vehicle operated by an intoxicated driver.[49] In addition, most states prohibit the purchase or possession of alcohol by persons under the age of 21.[50] Recommendations for the use of passenger restraints by both children and pregnant women have been issued by the American College of Obstetricians and Gynecologists.[51]

Discussion

In summary, there is good evidence that persons who use occupant protection or avoid driving while intoxicated are at significantly decreased risk of injury or death from motor vehicle crashes. The evidence is less extensive that counseling by clinicians to adopt these practices is effective in changing the behavior of motorists or passengers. However, since motor vehicle injury represents one of the leading causes of death in the United States and years of potential life lost, interventions of even modest effectiveness are likely to have enormous public health implications.

Clinical Intervention

Clinicians should regularly urge their patients to use safety belts whenever driving or riding in an automobile. Operators of vehicles carrying infants and toddlers should be urged to install and regularly use federally approved child safety seats in accordance with the manufacturer's instructions and the child's size. Vehicle operators should be urged to use safety belts for children who have outgrown safety seats. Children should not be permitted to ride in the cargo area of station wagons, vans, or pickup trucks. Those who operate or ride on motorcycles should be counseled to wear safety helmets (recommendations for bicyclists appear in Chapter 52). All patients should be counseled regarding the dangers of operating a motor vehicle while under the influence of alcohol or other drugs, as well as on the risks of riding in a vehicle operated by someone who is under the influence of these substances. Adolescents and young adults in particular should be encouraged to avoid using alcohol or other drugs when driving is anticipated and to discuss with their families transportation alternatives for social activities where alcohol and other drugs are used. The optimal frequency for counseling patients about motor vehicle injury has not been determined and is left to clinical discretion. Counseling is most important for those at increased risk of motor vehicle injury, such as adolescents and young adults, persons who use alcohol or other drugs, and patients with medical conditions that may impair motor vehicle safety.

Note: See Appendix A for the U.S. Preventive Services Task Force Table of Ratings for this topic. See also the relevant Task Force background paper: Polen MR, Friedman GD. Automobile injury: selected risk factors and prevention in the health care setting. JAMA 1988; 259:76–80.

REFERENCES

1. National Center for Health Statistics. Advance report of final mortality statistics. Monthly Vital Statistics Report [Suppl], vol. 37, no. 6. Hyattsville, Md.: Public Health Service, 1988. (Publication no. DHHS (PHS) 88–1120.)
2. Centers for Disease Control. Deaths from motor vehicle-related injuries, 1978–1984. MMWR CDC Surv Summ 1988; 37:5–12.
3. Baker SP, O'Neill B, Karpf R. The injury fact book. Lexington, Mass.: DC Heath, 1984.
4. Centers for Disease Control. Progress toward achieving the national 1990 objectives for injury prevention and control. MMWR 1988; 37:138–40,145–9.
5. Department of Transportation Fatal Accident Reporting System (FARS). Table 8–2. All involved and fatally injured occupants and non-occupants, by age group. Washington, D.C.: Department of Transportation, 1988. (Publication no. DOT HS 807–245.)
6. Williams AF, Carsten O. Driver age and crash involvement. Am J Public Health 1989; 79:326–7.
7. National Highway Traffic Safety Administration. Nineteen-city safety belt and child safety seat use observational survey. Washington, D.C.: Department of Transportation, February 1989.
8. Centers for Disease Control. Premature mortality due to alcohol-related motor vehicle traffic fatalities—United States, 1987. MMWR 1988; 37:753–5.
9. Department of Transportation Fatal Accident Reporting System (FARS). Table 2–4. Percentage of drivers involved in fatal crashes, by age group and by estimated alcohol level. Washington, D.C.: Department of Transportation, 1988. (Publication no. DOT HS 807–245.)
10. Centers for Disease Control. Drinking and driving and binge drinking in selected states, 1982 and 1985: the behavioral risk factor surveys. MMWR 1987; 35:788–91.
11. Waller JA. Injury control: a guide to causes and prevention of trauma. Lexington, Mass.: DC Heath, 1985.
12. McCarroll JR, Haddon W Jr. A controlled study of fatal automobile accidents in New York City. J Chronic Dis 1962; 15:811–26.
13. National Highway Traffic Safety Administration. Alcohol and traffic safety: a review of the state of knowledge, 1978. Washington, D.C.: Department of Transportation, 1979. (Publication no. DOT HS 805–172.)
14. Council on Scientific Affairs. Alcohol and the driver. JAMA 1986; 255:522–7.
15. Waller PF, Stewart JR, Hansen AR, et al. The potentiating effects of alcohol on driver injury. JAMA 1986; 256:1461–6.
16. Kraus JF, Morgenstern H, Fife D, et al. Blood alcohol tests, prevalence of involvement, and outcomes following brain injury. Am J Public Health 1989; 79:294–9.
17. Williams AF, Peat MA, Crouch DJ, et al. Drugs in fatally injured young male drivers. Public Health Rep 1985; 100:19–25.
18. Department of Transportation, National Highway Traffic Safety Administration. Use of controlled substances and highway safety: a report to Congress, March 1988. Washington, D.C.: Government Printing Office, 1988. (Publication no. DOT HS 807–261 NRD-42.)
19. Newman RJ. A prospective evaluation of the protective effect of car seatbelts. J Trauma 1986; 561–4.
20. Department of Transportation. Final regulatory impact assessment on amendments to Federal Motor Vehicle Safety Standard 208, Front Seat Occupant Protection. Washington, D.C.: Department of Transportation, 1984. (Publication no. DOT HS 806–572.)
21. Campbell BJ. Safety belt injury reduction related to crash severity and front seated position. J Trauma 1987; 27:733–9.
22. Orsay EM, Turnbull TL, Dunne M, et al. Prospective study of the effect of safety belts on morbidity and health care costs in motor vehicle accidents. JAMA 1988; 260:3598–603.
23. Decker MD, Dewey MJ, Hutcheson RH, et al. The use and efficacy of child restraint devices: the Tennessee experience, 1982 and 1983. JAMA 1984; 252:2571–5.

24. Scherz R. Fatal motor vehicle accidents of child passengers from birth through 4 years of age in Washington State. Pediatrics 1981; 68:572–5.
25. Kahane C. An evaluation of child passenger safety: the effectiveness and benefits of safety seats. Washington, D.C.: Department of Transportation, 1986. (Publication no. DOT HS 806–890.)
26. Margolis LH, Wagenaar AC, Liu W, et al. The effects of mandatory child restraint law on injuries requiring hospitalization. Am J Dis Child 1988; 142:1099–103.
27. Agran PF, Dunkle DE, Winn DG. Motor vehicle childhood injuries caused by noncrash falls or ejections. JAMA 1985; 253:2530–3.
28. National Highway Traffic Safety Administration. A report to the Congress on the effect of motorcycle helmet use repeal—a case report for helmet use. Washington, D.C.: Department of Transportation, 1980. (Publication no. DOT HS 805–312.)
29. Chenier TC, Evans L. Motorcyclist fatalities and the repeal of mandatory helmet wearing laws. Accid Anal Prev 1987; 19:133–9.
30. Colquitt M, Fielding JE, Cronan JF. Drunk drivers and medical and social injury. N Engl J Med 1987; 317:1262–6.
31. Worden JK, Flynn BS, Merrill DG, et al. Preventing alcohol-impaired driving through community self-regulation training. Am J Public Health 1989; 79:287–90.
32. Kelly RB. Effect of a brief physician intervention on seat belt use. J Fam Pract 1987; 24:630–2.
33. Weinstein ND, Grubb PD, Vautier JS. Increasing automobile seat belt use: an intervention emphasizing risk susceptibility. J Appl Psychol 1986; 71:285–90.
34. Allen DB, Bergman AB. Social learning approaches to health education: utilization of infant auto restraint devices. Pediatrics 1976; 58:323–8.
35. Kanthor HA. Car safety for infants: effectiveness of prenatal counseling. Pediatrics 1976; 58:320–2.
36. Scherz RG. Restraint systems for the prevention of injury to children in automobile accidents. Am J Public Health 1976; 66:451–5.
37. Reisinger KS, Williams AF, Wells JK, et al. Effect of pediatricians' counseling on infant restraint use. Pediatrics 1981; 67:201–6.
38. Berger LR, Saunders S, Armitage K, et al. Promoting the use of car safety devices for infants: an intensive health education approach. Pediatrics 1984; 74:16–9.
39. Christophersen ER, Sullivan MA. Increasing the protection of newborn infants in cars. Pediatrics 1982; 70:21–5.
40. Christophersen ER, Sosland-Edelman D, LeClaire S. Evaluation of two comprehensive infant car seat loaner programs with one-year follow-up. Pediatrics 1985; 76:36–42.
41. Reisinger KS, Williams AF. Evaluation of programs to increase the protection of infants in cars. Pediatrics 1978; 62:280–7.
42. Miller JR, Pless IB. Child automobile restraints: evaluation of health education. Pediatrics 1977; 59:907–11.
43. Macknin ML, Gustafson C, Gassman J, et al. Office edcuation by pediatricians to increase seat belt use. Am J Dis Child 1987; 141:1305–7.
44. Steed D. The case for safety belt use. JAMA 1988; 260:3651.
45. American Medical Association. Resolution no.62 (A-84): seat belts and survival in auto accidents. Chicago, Ill.: American Medical Association, 1984.
46. American College of Physicians. Health promotion/disease prevention: seat belt use. Philadelphia: American College of Physicians, 1984.
47. American Academy of Family Physicians. AAFP positions on selected health issues: safety. Kansas City, Mo.: American Academy of Family Physicians, 1983.
48. American Academy of Pediatrics. Policy statement: injury prevention. Elk Grove, Ill.: American Academy of Pediatrics, 1987.
49. American Academy of Pediatrics, Committee on Adolescence. Alcohol use and abuse: a pediatric concern. Pediatrics 1987; 79:450–3.
50. Decker MD, Graitcer PL, Schaffner W. Reduction in motor vehicle fatalities associated with an increase in the minimum drinking age. JAMA 1988; 260:3604–10.
51. American College of Obstetricians and Gynecologists. Automobile passenger restraints for children and pregnant women. ACOG Technical Bulletin No. 74. Washington, D.C.: American College of Obstetricians and Gynecologists, 1983.

52

Counseling to Prevent Household and Environmental Injuries

Recommendation: Patients who use alcohol or other drugs should be warned against engaging in potentially dangerous activities while intoxicated. It may also be clinically prudent to provide counseling on other measures to reduce the risk of unintentional household or environmental injuries from falls, drownings, fires or burns, poisoning, and firearms (see *Clinical Intervention*). Counseling to prevent motor vehicle injuries is discussed in Chapter 51.

Burden of Suffering

Unintentional injuries accounted for over 95,000 deaths in the United States in 1986, making it the fourth leading cause of death.[1] Injury is the leading cause of death in persons aged 1–44.[1] There are an estimated 60 million nonfatal injuries each year in the United States.[2] About half of all injury-related deaths occur in motor vehicle crashes.[1] (This injury category is discussed separately in Chapter 51.) The other half of unintentional injury-related deaths, or about 47,000 per year,[1] are household and environmental injuries: falls, drownings, fires, poisonings, suffocation, and firearm mishaps. Each year about 12,000 Americans, primarily older persons, die as a result of falls.[3] Falls are the second leading cause of injury death in the United States and the leading cause of nonfatal injuries.[3] There are 172,000 hip fractures each year in the United States,[4] resulting in an estimated cost of over $7 billion per year.[5] Hip fractures are an especially serious complication of falls in the elderly, since there is a 15–20% reduction in expected survival in the first year following a hip fracture.[6,7] Roughly half of survivors never recover normal function.[7] About 7700 Americans die each year by drowning, including 1200 boating-related drownings.[3,8] In adolescents, drowning is the second leading cause of death.[8] Fires are the third leading cause of unintentional injury death in the United States. Each year, residential fires are responsible for about 5000 deaths, 19,000 injuries, and $3.4 billion in property damage.[3] Unintentional poisonings account for 3300 deaths per year.[9] Firearm injuries result in about 1800 unintentional deaths each year (5% of all firearm fatalities) and five times as many nonfatal injuries.[3]

Efficacy of Risk Reduction

Intoxication with alcohol or other drugs is a consistent risk factor for injuries. In addition to its role in motor vehicle crashes, which has been most thoroughly studied, alcohol intoxication is involved in 40% of all fatal fires and burns and 50% of all deaths from drowning, boating mishaps, and shootings.[3,10] The large body of evidence linking alcohol to injuries argues strongly for counseling on the safe use of alcohol as an important preventive measure (see Chapter 47). In addition, certain injury-specific risk factors have been identified for household and environmental injuries. These are discussed below. In general, injury control strategies based on these risk factors are derived from evidence of association observed in retrospective studies rather than from prospective studies demonstrating efficacy. There have been few cohort studies or clinical trials measuring the impact on injury rates of eliminating risk factors for household and environmental injuries.

Falls are the leading cause of nonfatal injuries in the United States.[3] Over 70% of deaths due to falls occur in persons aged 65 and over, making falls the leading cause of unintentional injury death in this age group.[11] Although falls are a regular occurrence for some older persons,[12] about a third of those who have fallen in the past three months are unable to recall the event.[13] The death rate due to falls in the general population is 5.1 per 100,000 persons. In the elderly, in whom complications such as hip fracture can be severe, the death rate per 100,000 increases with age, from 10.2 for those aged 65–74 to 147.0 for persons aged 85 and over.[3] Physiological changes and environmental agents are the principal risk factors for falls in older persons. Physiological risk factors include postural instability, gait disturbances, diminished muscle strength and proprioception, poor vision, and medications.[14-16] Environmental risk factors include stairs, pavement irregularities, slippery surfaces, inadequate lighting, unexpected objects, low chairs, and incorrect footwear.[17] Hard surfaces such as concrete increase the risk of fracture when a fall occurs. These risk factors serve as the basis for recommended interventions to prevent falls: exercise to enhance muscle strength, monitoring of medications, balance and gait training, and counseling to correct environmental hazards. The efficacy of these measures has not been fully evaluated. There is evidence, however, that some interventions can reduce fall rates in the institutional setting.[12,18] Community-based studies are currently under way.

In addition to falls in the elderly, falls also occur in younger persons, especially children under age 5. These injuries often involve falls from stairs or furniture;[19] collapsible gates have been advocated as a means of protecting children from stairways.[19] Although the efficacy of stairway gates has not been studied, there is evidence that window guards can reduce child falls from apartment windows.[20]

Nearly half of all Americans ride **bicycles**.[21] Bicycle injuries account for nearly 550,000 emergency room visits and about 1000 deaths each year, mostly in children and adolescents.[22,23] Potential interventions for the clinician include counseling bicyclists and the parents of children who ride bicycles about the importance of wearing safety helmets and avoiding riding near motor vehicle traffic. Between 50% and 75% of bicycle fatalities and hospitalizations are the result of head trauma;[22,24] central nervous system injury is the primary cause of death in 90% of childhood fatalities from bicycle or pedestrian collisions with a motor vehicle.[25] There are few controlled studies examining the efficacy of safety helmets in preventing head injuries while riding bicycles,[21,22] but recent data from a case-control study provide evidence that the risk of head injury among bicyclists might be reduced by as much as 80%.[26] It is also known that safety helmets can reduce head injury rates among motorcyclists by 76%.[27] States that have repealed mandatory motorcycle helmet laws have experienced significant increases in motorcycle fatalities.[28] The second potential intervention, counseling bicyclists to avoid riding near motor vehicle traffic, is based on evidence that nearly 95% of bicycle fatalities occur as a result of a collision with a motor vehicle.[22] Community efforts to separate bicyclists from motor vehicle traffic, such as designated bicycle lanes and paths, have met with success in preventing bicycle accidents,[29] but the effectiveness of counseling bicyclists to use these routes remains unstudied.

The patients at greatest risk for **drowning** are small children (aged 1–3) and young males aged 15–24.[1] Drowning is the second leading cause of death in adolescents.[8] The causes of drowning, and thus preventive strategies, differ with the age of the patient. In small children, about 60–80% of drownings occur in swimming pools, usually located in the back yard of the victim's home.[30-33] In about two-thirds of these cases, adult caretakers are unaware that the toddler has wandered near the pool or entered the water.[31] Several studies suggest that about 80% of such drownings can be prevented by using four-foot fences with latchgates to protect children from wandering into the swimming pool area.[31,34-36] Clinicians could advise swimming pool owners to install fences, although the impact of this form of counseling on drowning rates is unknown. In some states, pool gates and cover alarm systems are required by law. Some recommend toddler swimming lessons as a means of improving survival after submersion. The effectiveness of lessons at this age has never been proved convincingly, however;[37] their safety has been questioned on the basis of case reports of water intoxication and hyponatremia.[8]

Drownings of adolescents and adults occur under different circumstances.[38] Most drownings occur in lakes, rivers, and ponds in association with such water activities as swimming, wading, diving, boating, rafting, and fishing.[38,39] Intoxication by alcohol or other drugs is common in both drownings and boating mishaps; about half of all victims have a significant blood alcohol level, and about 10% have evidence of other drugs with central nervous system effects.[38,40] Discouraging swimming or boating while intoxicated would therefore appear to be appropriate, but there has been little research on the impact of such a clinical intervention. About 82% of boating-related drownings are associated with nonuse or inappropriate use of personal flotation devices,[41] but there are few data on the impact of promoting the use of these devices. Swimming lessons may offer some protection against drowning, but this has also never been proved convincingly.

Fires and burns are the third leading cause of unintentional injury-related death. Most injuries and 75–90% of deaths from fires occur in residential fires.[42,43] Smoke detectors provide the most efficacious means of preventing deaths in residential fires. Fire department statistics indicate that death in a residential fire is two to three times more likely in homes without smoke detectors than in those with such devices.[44,45] However, there is no evidence of the magnitude of reduction in fire injuries achieved by advising patients to install and test smoke detectors. It is known, for example, that smoke detectors often fail to operate due to incorrect installation or inadequate testing, and some occupants (very young children and the handicapped) may be unable to hear or respond to the alarm signal.[43,46] For these reasons, it is important that smoke alarm counseling emphasize the importance of correct installation and periodic testing to ensure proper operation.

Cigarette smoking causes about 25% of residential fires, usually through unintentional ignition of bedding or upholstery, and many advocate counseling regarding careless smoking practices and the promotion of self-extinguishing cigarettes. In children, flame-retardant clothing is effective in reducing injury from clothing ignition.[3,47,48] Since residential fires occur more frequently in the winter, some attention has been given to the hazards of certain stoves and heaters,[49] but the feasibility of clinical intervention in such matters is limited. Counseling regarding hot water heaters is appropriate, however, since hot tap water burns, which account for 2600 hospitalizations each year, are preventable by setting household water heaters at 120° F.[3,50,51]

Childhood **poisoning** can be prevented by placing medications in child-resistant containers. Federal legislation requiring such containers for aspirin, acetaminophen, prescription drugs, and household chemicals has been associated with a subsequent decrease in childhood poisoning from these substances.[52-54] Poisoning with children's aspirin has also been reduced by limiting the number of tablets packaged in each bottle.[52,55] In contrast, poison-warning labels designed for children do not appear to be efficacious. Controlled trials have demonstrated that poison warning stickers (such as the "Mr. Yuk" series) do not deter children from playing with medication containers[56] or reduce the rate of childhood poisoning.[57] Intentional self-poisoning by adolescents and adults is discussed in Chapter 45.

Most unintentional injuries from **firearms** involve adolescent and young adult males, and about 65–78% of these injuries occur in or around the home.[3] Over 90% of firearm incidents involving children occur at home; a study in children aged 0–14 found that 40% involved a firearm stored in the room where the shooting occurred.[58] Potential preventive strategies to prevent firearm injuries (e.g., counseling firearm owners to store weapons unloaded and in a locked compartment, gun control legislation) would appear to be effective but have been inadequately studied.

After the home, the second most common location for unintentional firearm injuries is the hunting site: These incidents often involve members of the same hunting party and often result from accidental discharge of the firearm, unsafe handling of the firearm, and the victim being out of sight or mistaken for game.[37,59] A recent study found that 40% of shooters in hunting accidents were less than 20 years of age and fewer than half were supervised by adults; unsafe hunting practices such as carrying the firearm incorrectly were significantly more common in shooters who were 8–19 years of age.[59] The investigators suggested that hunting firearm injuries might be reduced by adult supervision of child and adolescent hunters, particularly those who have not had formal instruction in the safe use of firearms, and by wearing fluorescent orange clothing while hunting to increase visibility. The effectiveness of these measures has not been studied, however. Hunter education programs have had mixed results in changing fatality rates.[37]

Effectiveness of Counseling

The most effective measures to control injuries are passive interventions, those that do not rely on the potential victim to adopt new behaviors voluntarily. Examples of passive interventions include revised building codes to prevent falls and child-resistant containers to prevent poisoning. Since injury prevention advice from clinicians usually requires active cooperation from patients (e.g., changing smoking practices in bed, inspecting batteries in smoke detectors), the effectiveness of this form of counseling faces inherent limitations. It is therefore not surprising to find in injury control research that counseling is most effective in combination with other measures that promote compliance, such as safety regulations.[20,60]

Clinical counseling by itself appears to be of some benefit when offered to parents. Studies suggest an association between counseling and improved knowledge and fewer home hazards, but it is unclear whether this results in lower injury rates. Education has been shown to motivate parents to obtain syrup of ipecac, to display poison control center telephone numbers, and to learn more about the proper use of ipecac.[61,62] A randomized controlled trial found that parents who received an individualized course on child safety during well-baby visits demonstrated greater knowledge about home hazards and had fewer hazards in the home when tested one month after the last visit, but there was no difference in the rate of injuries reported by the parents or recorded in hospital records.[63] Another study found that infants of mothers who received counseling on fall prevention had fewer falls over the course of a year than did those whose mothers were not counseled.[64] A randomized controlled trial found that couples who received information on burn prevention during well-child care classes were more likely to have their hot water heaters set at 130° F or lower when checked by investigators during a home visit.[65]

Other studies have found counseling to be ineffective in promoting safety: A controlled trial found that a program providing mothers with counseling on household hazards, a safety booklet, and free safety devices was unsuccessful in changing either the knowledge of the subjects or the number of home hazards detected in an unannounced home visit.[66] Controlled studies of counseling parents to prevent childhood poisoning have not shown a significant effect on poison injury rates.[67] There is even concern that injury control counseling may be harmful in some patients, such as adolescents.[37] Several investigators have hypothesized that adolescents who favor risk-taking behavior may respond to counseling by performing dangerous activities.[68-70]

Some researchers have attempted to prevent injuries through free distribution of injury control devices during the clinic visit. When smoke detectors were made available in one program, 92% of the recipients installed the devices in their home.[71] A study providing parents with poison-warning labels designed for children was unsuccessful, however, in part because parents failed to apply the labels to all poisons in the home.[57] In another study, free distribution of cabinet locks and electrical outlet covers resulted in increased use of outlet covers, which are easy to apply, but no increase in the installation of cabinet locks, a more inconvenient task.[72]

Recommendations of Others

Although experts agree on the importance of counseling by clinicians to prevent injuries, there are few guidelines on the specific injury control measures clinicians should encourage their patients to adopt. Recommendations for pediatricians on specific safety topics have been issued periodically by the American Academy of Pediatrics (AAP). In addition, as part of its Injury Prevention Program (TIPP), the AAP recommends that pediatricians distribute safety surveys to parents and integrate age-specific safety counseling into the well-child examination. All physicians caring for children are advised by the AAP to encourage parents to acquire smoke detectors for the child's sleeping area, window and stairway guards/gates, and syrup of ipecac, and to ensure safe hot water temperatures at the tap.[73]

Discussion

Although there are few injury control measures for which there is conclusive evidence of efficacy, and the effectiveness of injury control counseling is largely unstudied, counseling by physicians on these matters may be justified because of the enormous burden of suffering associated with injuries. Unintentional injuries are the leading cause of years of potential life lost in the United States.[74] Thus, even minor reductions in their incidence can have large public health implications. In addition, there is little cost associated with this form of counseling when included in the clinical encounter. The cost of physician time may, however, be kept to a minimum by focusing attention during injury control counseling on specific injuries for which the patient is at greatest risk and on those preventive strategies for which the strongest evidence of efficacy is available. Of these, intoxication by alcohol and other drugs appears to be most strongly associated with the risk of unintentional injury or death.

Clinical Intervention

Clinicians should urge adolescents and adults who use *alcohol or other drugs* to avoid engaging in potentially dangerous activities (e.g., operation of a motor vehicle, swimming, boating, handling of firearms, smoking in bed, bicycling) while intoxicated. It may also be clinically prudent for clinicians to recommend specific injury control measures for persons at increased risk for certain types of household or environmental injuries. *Smokers* who cannot discontinue the use of tobacco (see Chapter 48) should be advised against smoking near bedding or upholstery. *Homeowners* should be advised to install smoke detectors in appropriate locations and to test the devices periodically to ensure proper operation. Hot water heaters should be set at 120° F, and firearms should be kept unloaded in a locked compartment. *Parents*, grandparents, or other patients with children in the home should be advised to keep a 1 oz bottle of syrup of ipecac, to display the telephone number of the local poison control center, and to place all medications, toxic substances, matches, and firearms in child-resistant containers. Collapsible gates or other barriers should be placed at stairway entrances, a four-foot latchgate installed around swimming pools, and window guards installed in high-rise buildings to prevent falls in children. *Bicyclists* and parents of children who ride bicycles should be counseled about the importance of wearing safety helmets and avoiding riding in motor vehicle traffic. *Boaters* should be encouraged to observe safe boating practices and to wear personal flotation devices. Clinical interventions to prevent motor vehicle injuries are discussed in Chapter 51.

Elderly patients or those responsible for older persons should be advised to inspect the home for adequate lighting, to remove or repair floor structures (e.g., loose rugs, electrical cords, toys) that predispose to tripping, and to install handrails and traction strips in stairways and bathtubs. Clinicians caring for older persons should periodically test visual acuity (see Chapter 31), counsel patients with medical conditions affecting mobility, and monitor the use of drugs associated with falls. Older patients who lack medical contraindications should be counseled to engage in exercise programs to maintain and improve mobility and flexibility (see Chapter 49).

The need to prevent household or environmental injuries should be discussed regularly with patients, especially those who are at increased risk for certain types of injuries. The optimal frequency for such counseling has not been determined, however, and is left to clinical discretion.

Note: See Appendix A for the U.S. Preventive Services Task Force Table of Ratings for this topic. See also the relevant Task Force background paper: Hindmarsh J, Estes EH Jr. Falls in older persons: causes and prevention. In: Goldbloom RB, Lawrence RS, eds. Preventing disease: beyond the rhetoric. New York: Springer-Verlag (in press).

REFERENCES

1. National Center for Health Statistics. Advance report of final mortality statistics, 1986. Monthly Vital Statistics Report [Suppl], vol. 37, no. 6. Hyattsville, Md.: Public Health Service, 1988. (Publication no. DHHS (PHS) 88–1120.)
2. *Idem.* Current estimates from the National Health Interview Survey, United States, 1982. Vital and Health Statistics, series 10, no. 150. Washington, D.C.: Government Printing Office, 1985. (Publication no. DHHS (PHS) 85–1578.)
3. Centers for Disease Control. Public health surveillance of 1990 injury control objectives for the nation. MMWR CDC Surveillance Summary, vol. 37, no. SS-1, 1988.

4. Baker SP, Harvey AH. Fall injuries in the elderly. Clin Geriatr Med 1985; 1:501–12.
5. American Academy of Orthopedic Surgeons. The frequency of occurrence, impact, and cost of musculoskeletal conditions in the United States. Chicago, Ill.: American Academy of Orthopedic Surgeons, 1984.
6. Jensen GF, Christiansen C, Boesen J, et al. Epidemiology of postmenopausal spinal and long bone fractures: a unifying approach to postmenopausal osteoporosis. Clin Orthoped 1982; 166:75–81.
7. Cummings SR, Kelsey J, Nevitt M, et al. Epidemiology of osteoporosis and osteoporotic fractures. Epidemiol Rev 1985; 7:178–208.
8. Spyker DA. Submersion injury: epidemiology, prevention, and management. Pediatr Clin North Am 1985; 32:113–23.
9. National Safety Council. Accident facts, 1985 ed. Chicago, Ill.: National Safety Council, 1985.
10. Brodzka W, Thornhill HL, Howard S. Burns: causes and risk factors. Arch Phys Med Rehabil 1985; 66:746–52.
11. Baker SP, O'Neill B, Karpf RS. The injury fact book. Lexington, Mass.: DC Heath, 1984.
12. Wolf-Klein GP, Silverstone FA, Basavaraju N, et al. Prevention of falls in the elderly population. Arch Phys Med Rehabil 1988; 69:689–91.
13. Cummings SR, Nevitt MC, Kidd S. Forgetting falls: the limited accuracy of recall of falls in the elderly. J Am Geriatr Soc 1988; 36:613–6.
14. Isaacs B. Clinical and laboratory studies of falls in old people: prospects in prevention. Clin Geriatr Med 1985; 1:513–20.
15. Wolfson LO, Whipple R, Ammerman P, et al. Falls and the elderly: gait and balance in the elderly, two functional capacities that link sensory and motor ability to falls. Clin Geriatr Med 1985; 1:649–59.
16. MacDonald J. Falls in the elderly: the role of drugs in the elderly. Clin Geriatr Med 1985; 1:621–36.
17. Archea J. Falls in the elderly: environmental risk factors associated with stair accidents by the elderly. Clin Geriatr Med 1985; 1:555–69.
18. Kellogg International Work Group on the Prevention of Falls in the Elderly. The prevention of falls in later life. Dan Med Bull [Suppl 4] 1987; 34:1–24.
19. Garrettson LK, Gallagher SS. Falls in children and youth. Pediatr Clin North Am 1985; 32:153–62.
20. Spiegel CN, Lindaman FC. Children can't fly: a program to prevent childhood morbidity and mortality from window falls. Am J Public Health 1977; 67:1143.
21. Rivara FP. Traumatic deaths of children in the United States: currently available prevention strategies. Pediatrics 1985; 75:456–62.
22. Friede AM, Azzara CV, Gallagher SS, et al. The epidemiology of injuries to bicycle riders. Pediatr Clin North Am 1985; 32:141–51.
23. Consumer Product Safety Commission. NEISS data highlights, vol. 6, no. 3. Washington, D.C.: Consumer Product Safety Commission, 1982.
24. Guichon DMP, Mules JT. Bicycle injuries: one-year sample in Calgary. J Trauma 1975; 15:504–6.
25. Rivara FP, Maier RV, Mueller BA, et al. Evaluation of potentially preventable deaths among pedestrian and bicyclist fatalities. JAMA 1989; 261:566–70.
26. Thompson RS, Rivara FP, Thompson DC. Prevention of head injury by bicycle helmets: a field study of efficacy. Am J Dis Child 1988; 142:386. abstract.
27. National Highway Traffic Safety Administration. A report to the Congress on the effect of motorcycle helmet use repeal—a case report for helmet use. Washington, D.C.: Department of Transportation, 1980. (Publication no. DOT HF-805-312.)
28. Chenier TC, Evans L. Motorcyclist fatalities and the repeal of mandatory helmet wearing laws. Accid Anal Prev 1987; 19:133–9.
29. Organization for Economic Cooperation and Development. Traffic safety of children. Report of OECD Scientific Expert Group. Paris, France: Organization for Economic Cooperation and Development, 1983.
30. Centers for Disease Control. Aquatic deaths and injuries—United States. MMWR 1982; 31:417–9.

31. Pitt WR. Increasing incidence of childhood immersion injury in Brisbane. Med J Aust 1986; 144:683–5.
32. Pearn J, Nixon J, Wilkey I. Freshwater drowning and near-drowning accidents involving children. Med J Aust 1976; 2:942–6.
33. Wintemute GJ, Kraus JF, Teret SP, et al. Drowning in childhood and adolescence: a population-based study. Am J Public Health 1987; 77:830–2.
34. Pearn JH, Wong RYK, Brown J III, et al. Drowning and near-drowning involving children: a five-year population study from the city and county of Honolulu. Am J Public Health 1979; 69:450–4.
35. Pearn J, Brown J III, Hsia EY. Swimming pool drownings and near-drownings involving children: a total population study from Hawaii. Milit Med 1980; 145:15–8.
36. Milner N, Pearn J, Guard R. Will fenced pools save lives? A 10–year study from Mulgrave Shire, Queensland. Med J Aust 1980; 2:510–1.
37. Halperin SF, Bass JL, Mehta KA, et al. Unintentional injuries among adolescents and young adults: a review and analysis. J Adol Health Care 1983; 4:275–81.
38. Wintemute GJ, Kraus JF, Teret SP, et al. The epidemiology of drowning in adulthood: implications for prevention. Am J Prev Med 1988; 4:343–8.
39. Press E, Walker J, Crawford I. An interstate drowning study. Am J Public Health 1968; 12:2275–89.
40. Dietz PE, Baker SP. Drowning: epidemiology and prevention. Am J Public Health 1974; 64:303–12.
41. Coast Guard. Boating statistics, 1985. Technical Report COMDITINST M16754.1g. Washington, D.C.: Department of Transportation, 1986.
42. Federal Emergency Management Agency. Preliminary fire statistics for 1983. Washington, D.C.: Fire Administration, National Fire Information Council, 1983.
43. Centers for Disease Control. Regional distribution of deaths from residential fires—United States, 1978–1984. JAMA 1987; 258:2355–6.
44. Budnick EK. Estimating effectiveness of state-of-the-art detectors and automatic sprinklers on life safety in residential occupancies. Washington, D.C.: Department of Commerce, National Bureau of Standards, National Engineering Laboratory, Center for Fire Research, 1984. (Publication no. NBSIR 84–2819.)
45. Hall JR Jr. A decade of detectors: measuring the effect. Fire 1985; 79:37–43.
46. Council on Scientific Affairs. Preventing death and injury from fires with automatic sprinklers and smoke detectors. JAMA 1987; 257:1618–20.
47. Anonymous. Accident prevention in childhood. Lancet 1979; 2:564–5.
48. McLoughlin E, Clarke N, Stahl K, et al. One pediatric burn unit's experiences with sleepware-related injuries. Pediatrics 1977; 60:405–9.
49. Harwood B, Kluge P. Hazards associated with the use of wood- or coal-burning stoves or free-standing fireplaces. Washington, D.C.: Consumer Product Safety Commission, 1985.
50. Katcher ML. Prevention of tap water scald burns: evaluation of a multi-media injury control program. Am J Public Health 1987; 77:1195–7.
51. Feldman KW, Schaller RT, Feldman JA, et al. Tap water scald burns in children. Pediatrics 1978; 62:1–7.
52. Centers for Disease Control. Unintentional poisoning among young children—United States. MMWR 1983; 32:117–8.
53. Palmisano P. Targeted intervention in the control of accidental overdoses in children. Public Health Rep 1981; 96:150–6.
54. Walton WW. An evaluation of the Poison Prevention Packaging Act. Pediatrics 1982; 69:363–70.
55. Clarke A, Walton WW. Effect of safety packaging on aspirin ingestion by children. Pediatrics 1979; 63:687–93.
56. Vernberg K, Culver-Dickinson P, Spyker DA. The deterrent effect of poison-warning stickers. Am J Dis Child 1984; 138:1018–20.
57. Fergusson DM, Horwood LJ, Beautrais AL, et al. A controlled field trial of a poisoning prevention method. Pediatrics 1982; 69:515–20.

58. Wintemute GJ, Teret SP, Kraus JF, et al. When children shoot children: 88 unintended deaths. JAMA 1987; 257:3107–9.
59. Cole TB, Patotta MJ. Hunting firearm injuries, North Carolina. Am J Public Health 1988; 78:1585–6.
60. Gallagher SS, Hunter P, Guyer B. A home injury prevention program for children. Pediatr Clin North Am 1985; 32:95–112.
61. Woolf A, Lewander W, Fillipone G, et al. Prevention of childhood poisoning: efficacy of an educational program carried out in an emergency clinic. Pediatrics 1987; 80: 359–63.
62. Dershewitz RA, Posner M, Paichel W. The effectiveness of health education on home use of ipecac. Clin Pediatr 1983; 22:268–70.
63. Kelly B, Sein C, McCarthy PL. Safety education in a pediatric primary care setting. Pediatrics 1987; 79:818–24.
64. Kravitz H, Grove M. Prevention of accidental falls in infancy by counseling mothers. IMJ 1973; 144:570–3.
65. Thomas KA, Hassanein RS, Christophersen ER. Evaluation of group well-child care for improving burn prevention practices in the home. Pediatrics 1984; 74:879–82.
66. Dershewitz RA, Williamson JW. Prevention of childhood household injuries: a controlled clinical trial. Am J Public Health 1977; 67:1148–53.
67. Steele P, Spyker DA. Poisonings. Pediatr Clin North Am 1985; 32:77–86.
68. Stuart RB. Teaching facts about drugs: pushing or preventing? J Educ Psych 1974; 66:189–201.
69. Tennant FS, Weaver SC, Lewis CE. Outcomes of drug education: four case studies. Pediatrics 1973; 52:246–51.
70. Chilton LA. Potential benefit vs. risks of current attempts in health education among adolescents. J Pediatr 1977; 90:163–4.
71. Gorman R, Holtzman N, Charney E, et al. Evaluation of a smoke detector giveaway program: will a high-risk population install free smoke detectors? Am J Dis Child 1983; 137:528.
72. Dershewitz RA. Will mothers use free household safety devices? Am J Dis Child 1979; 133:61–4.
73. Krassner L. TIPP usage. Pediatrics 1984; 74(5 pt 2):976–80.
74. Centers for Disease Control. Years of potential life lost before age 65—United States, 1987. MMWR 1989; 38:27–9.

53

Counseling to Prevent Human Immunodeficiency Virus Infection and Other Sexually Transmitted Diseases

Recommendation: Clinicians should take a complete sexual and drug use history on all adolescent and adult patients. Sexually active patients should be advised that abstaining from sex or maintaining a mutually faithful monogamous sexual relationship with a partner known to be uninfected are the most effective strategies to prevent infection with human immunodeficiency virus or other sexually transmitted diseases (see *Clinical Intervention*). Patients should also receive counseling about the indications and proper methods for using condoms and spermicides in sexual intercourse and about the health risks associated with anal intercourse. Intravenous drug users should be encouraged to enroll in a drug treatment program and should be warned against sharing drug equipment or using unsterilized needles and syringes. All patients should be offered testing in accordance with recommendations on screening for syphilis, gonorrhea, chlamydia, genital herpes, hepatitis B, and infection with human immunodeficiency virus (see Chapters 20, 22–26).

Burden of Suffering

Each year in the United States, there are about 3–4 million cases of chlamydial infection,[1] 2 million cases of gonorrhea,[2] and over 35,000 cases of primary and secondary syphilis.[3] Primary episodes of genital herpes occur each year in approximately 270,000 Americans,[4] and nearly 20 million persons are already infected and suffering recurrent episodes.[5] These diseases are associated with considerable morbidity. Chlamydia and gonorrhea produce urethritis, epididymitis, and proctitis in men and mucopurulent cervicitis and painful pelvic inflammatory disease (PID) in women.[1,6,7] PID is an important risk factor for ectopic pregnancy and infertility,[8] and about 1 million cases are reported annually in the United States.[7] Syphilis produces ulcers of the genitalia, pharynx, and rectum, and it can progress to secondary syphilis (with skin lesions, lymphadenopathy, and condyloma lata) and the severe complications of tertiary syphilis (cardiovascular and neurologic disorders) if left untreated.[9] Persons with genital herpes suffer painful vesicular and ulcerative lesions and recurrent episodes due to latent infection.[10]

Hepatitis B and acquired immunodeficiency syndrome (AIDS) are sexually transmitted diseases that are also transmitted through the exchange of blood or blood products. An estimated 500,000 to 1 million persons in the United States have been infected with hepatitis B virus (HBV),[11] and an estimated 1–1.5 million persons are infected with the human immunodeficiency virus (HIV).[12,13] Chronic carriers of HBV are at risk for developing chronic active hepatitis, cirrhosis, and primary hepatocellular carcinoma, and nearly 5000 die each year as a result of these complications.[11] Within 10 years of infection with HIV, about 50% of persons develop AIDS and another 40% or more develop other clinical illnesses associated with HIV infection.[14] Over 82,000 cases of AIDS had been reported by the end of 1988.[15] Persons with AIDS can develop severe opportunistic infections, Kaposi's sarcoma, and multiple-system medical complications. Many also experience social ostracism and discrimination. Although some antimicrobial agents may extend survival,[16] there is currently no available treatment to prevent death in persons with AIDS. In a study performed before the licensure of AZT (azidothymidine, zidovudine), the five-year survival rate was only 15%.[17] AIDS has become the seventh leading cause of years of potential life lost in the United States,[18] and it is the leading cause of death in intravenous (IV) drug abusers and hemophiliacs.[19] By the end of 1992, a projected total of 365,000 cases of AIDS will have been diagnosed in the United States, and 260,000 persons will have died from this disease.[13]

Pregnant women with sexually transmitted diseases can transmit the organisms to their children. Congenital syphilis often results in fetal or perinatal death or serious neonatal complications. Active gonococcal or chlamydial infection can produce obstetrical complications and neonatal infections such as ophthalmia neonatorum.[6] Transmission of genital herpes to the newborn is fatal in 65% of untreated cases, and less than 10% of survivors with central nervous system infection have normal development.[10] Infants who become infected with HBV usually develop chronic carrier status,[20,21] and more than 25% of these children will die eventually from primary hepatocellular carcinoma or cirrhosis of the liver.[22-24] Pregnant women with HIV infection may be at increased risk of developing AIDS,[25,26] and about 30–35% of them transmit the virus to their children.[27] Three-quarters of AIDS cases in children under age 13 result from perinatal transmission.[28]

The economic consequences of sexually transmitted diseases are enormous. The estimated costs per year in the United States include $500 million for genital herpes,[29] $1 billion for chlamydial infection,[7] and $2.2 billion for AIDS.[30] Costs for AIDS are expected to climb to as high as $13 billion per year by 1992.[13]

Sexually transmitted diseases are most common in young persons, those with multiple sexual contacts, prostitutes, homosexual and bisexual men, and persons with infected sexual partners.[6,7,31] Additional risk factors for infection with HBV or HIV include intravenous drug use, a history of blood transfusion between 1978 and 1985, hemophilia, and being born to an infected mother.[28,32] The incidence of syphilis has been increasing steadily in recent years,[3] and there is evidence that this and other genital ulcer diseases (e.g., genital herpes) may be associated with infection with HIV.[33,34]

Efficacy of Risk Reduction

The most efficacious means of reducing the risk of acquiring AIDS or other sexually transmitted diseases through sexual contact is either abstinence from sexual relations or maintenance of a mutually monogamous sexual relationship with an uninfected partner. If the infection status of the partner is uncertain, sexual relations should be avoided, particularly with persons at increased risk for HIV infection (e.g., homosexual and bisexual men, IV drug users). The prevalence of HIV infection in heterosexual partners of persons in high-risk categories may be as high as 11%, and as many as 60% of heterosexual partners of HIV-infected individuals may be seropositive.[12] Risk is directly related to the number of sexual partners,[25] in part because of the difficulty of obtaining adequate information on risk status from each partner.[35]

Certain sexual practices may also influence the risk of infection. Among homosexual men, for example, receptive anal intercourse has been repeatedly implicated as a principal risk factor for HIV infection,[36,37] and other practices that increase rectal trauma may have a similar role.[25] Conversely, some sexual practices, such as using latex condoms and spermicides, may reduce the risk of infection. Condoms have been shown in the laboratory to prevent transmission of *Chlamydia trachomatis*, herpes simplex virus,[38,39] trichomonas,[40] cytomegalovirus, and HIV.[41] Although further data are needed on the efficacy of latex condoms in actual practice, there is epidemiologic evidence that persons who use condoms correctly are at decreased risk of acquiring gonococcal and nongonococcal urethritis[40,42,43] and HIV infection.[44,45] Even under optimal conditions, however, condoms are not always efficacious in preventing transmission. Condom failures occur at an estimated rate of 10–15%,[46-48] either as a result of product failure (e.g., breakage) or as a result of incorrect or inconsistent use. Natural membrane condoms may be more permeable than latex condoms to passage of HIV[49] and other sexually transmitted organisms such as herpes virus, and they are less uniform than latex condoms.[50] Errors on the part of users, however, are thought to be the most likely cause of condom failure.[51] Incorrect use has been shown to limit the effectiveness of condoms in preventing gonorrhea[43] and presumably also permits passage of more dangerous organisms such as HIV.

The use of spermicides, along with condoms, has been proposed as a means of further reducing the risk of infection. One of the spermicidal agents that has been investigated, nonoxynol 9, has been shown to have *in vitro* activity against herpes simplex virus,[52] hepatitis B,[53] and HIV.[54,55] It also has clinical efficacy in reducing the risk of gonorrhea[56-60] and chlamydial infection in women.[60] In many clinical studies, however, spermicides were used in combination with condoms or diaphragms, and therefore it is unclear which intervention or combination of interventions was directly responsible for the outcome. There is also inadequate information on the effectiveness of spermicides inserted in condoms if the condoms rupture; subinhibitory concentrations of spermicide would presumably be more likely if condom rupture occurs in the rectum (or in the vagina in the absence of supplemental vaginal application of spermicide).[55]

Additional measures to reduce the risk of infection with HIV and hepatitis B include avoiding the use of intravenous drugs or unsterilized needles and syringes. The characteristics of drug addiction often make prompt discontinuation of IV drug abuse difficult. Drug treatment programs, such as methadone maintenance clinics, can be effective in some patients, but many drug addicts lack access to such facilities or return to their habit following treatment (see Chapter 47). Even in persons who continue to use IV drugs, morbidity and mortality from HIV, hepatitis B, and bacterial endocarditis could be reduced by using sterilized needles and syringes. AIDS is the leading cause of death in this population,[19] and even a modest reduction in risk could have significant public health implications. Methods for obtaining uncontaminated drug equipment include purchasing sterilized equipment, obtaining free products through distribution programs, and cleaning used equipment with a bleach solution.

Effectiveness of Counseling

There have been few studies examining the effectiveness of physicians in influencing the sexual behavior of patients. Studies of clinic-based educational programs, which in some cases have included physician counseling as a component, have reported increased rate of return for test-of-cure[61,62] and reduced incidence of certain sexually transmitted diseases,[63] but these studies involved select populations and provided little evidence of change in sexual behavior. Other successful measures have included distribution of free condoms to inner-city male adolescents[64] and of bleach products to clean drug injection equipment,[65] but these items were not distributed by physicians. Sexual behavior appears to have changed significantly in recent years as a result of increased public awareness of AIDS. Homosexual and bisexual men report fewer high-risk sexual practices.[66-71] Behavior may also be changing in heterosexual populations living in high-risk areas[72,73] and in some intravenous drug users.[74-78] Surveys in New York City have found that the proportion of patients taking methadone who reported some form of behavioral change to reduce the risk of acquiring HIV infection increased from 59% in 1984 to 75% in 1986 and to 85% in 1987.[76,77]

There is also evidence from recent surveys that behavior is not changing dramatically in certain population groups, such as adolescents[79,80] and college students,[81] despite increased knowledge of the health risks associated with high-risk sexual practices. A number of factors may account for this reluctance to change behavior. Compliance with the proper use of condoms and spermicides can be affected by perceptions of inconvenience, concerns about sexual spontaneity, and cultural attitudes.[48,62,82] Prostitutes and drug addicts, who have special dependency on high-risk behaviors, face added difficulties in changing behavior. Only 4% of female prostitutes report condom use with each vaginal exposure,[83] and an unknown number of IV drug users continue to use contaminated injection equipment. Sterilized needles and syringes are frequently unavailable or prohibitively expensive, and access to health care for substance abuse counseling and medical treatment is often poor.

Clinicians may provide ineffective counseling or no counseling if they have inadequate historical data on the patient's sexual and drug use behavior. A complete sexual history is therefore especially important as a prelude to any form of effective counseling to prevent sexually transmitted diseases. Many clinicians do not, however, take an adequate sexual history. A recent survey of primary care physicians found that only 10% asked new patients questions specific enough to identify those at risk of exposure to HIV.[84]

Recommendations of Others

Recommendations for physicians to counsel patients on measures to prevent sexually transmitted diseases have been issued by a number of authorities, including the U.S. Surgeon General,[85] the Food and Drug Administration (FDA),[50] the American Medical Association,[86] the American College of Physicians,[87] and the American College of Obstetricians and Gynecologists.[88] The key elements of such counseling have been outlined by the U.S. Public Health Service and include the following: abstain from sex or maintain a mutually faithful monogamous sexual relationship with an uninfected partner; abstain from sex with individuals who are not known with certainty to be seronegative and who have not been the sole partner for six months prior to or any time after the test; do not practice anal intercourse; do not use unsterilized syringes, needles, or drugs; and always use a condom if there are any doubts about the status of the sexual partner. Detailed instructions for patients on the proper use of condoms have been published by the Centers for Disease Control (CDC)[51] and the FDA.[50] The CDC recommends that condoms be made more widely available by health care providers in clinics for sexually transmitted diseases, family planning, and drug treatment.[51]

The CDC, in collaboration with a number of other groups, has also recommended that seronegative pregnant women and women of childbearing age who are at increased risk of becoming infected with HIV receive additional counseling regarding the maternal and fetal risks associated with pregnancy should they become infected, and that they should be advised to consider delaying pregnancy.[26]

Discussion

Although it has not been proved that physicians can change the sexual behavior of patients, there is evidence that the frequency of high-risk behaviors can be reduced in response to information provided through public education. While clinicians are principally involved in the treatment of infected persons with clinical illness, they can also play an important role in asymptomatic persons by reinforcing and clarifying educational messages, providing literature and community resource references for additional information, and dispelling misconceptions about unproven modes of transmission. In addition, physicians treating the medical problems of certain high-risk groups (e.g., IV drug users, prostitutes) have special access to persons who may receive little information through public media about preventive measures and thus may continue to practice high-risk behavior. IV drug users account for the largest proportion of new cases of hepatitis B and, in some areas, AIDS.[28,32] Physicians are also an important source of information about and encouragement to use drug treatment centers; clinics for sexually transmitted diseases and family planning; and community programs offering free condoms, sterilized drug equipment, and cleaning solutions for needles.

Clinical Intervention

Clinicians should take a complete sexual and drug use history on all adolescent and adult patients. Sexually active patients should receive complete information on their risk for acquiring sexually transmitted diseases. They should be advised that abstaining from sex or maintaining a mutually faithful monogamous sexual relationship with a partner known to be uninfected are the most effective strategies to prevent infection with HIV or other sexually transmitted diseases. Patients should be advised against sexual activity with individuals whose infection status is uncertain. A nonreactive HIV test does not rule out infection if the sexual partner has not been monogamous for at least six months before the test. Patients who choose to engage in sexual activity with multiple partners or with persons who may be infected should be advised to use a condom at each encounter and to avoid anal intercourse. Women should be informed of the potential risks of HIV infection during pregnancy. Persons who use intravenous drugs should be encouraged to enroll in a drug treatment program, warned against sharing drug equipment and using unsterilized syringes and needles, and given sources for uncontaminated injection equipment or referred to community programs with this information. Patients should be offered testing in accordance with recommendations on screening for syphilis, gonorrhea, chlamydia, genital herpes, hepatitis B, and infection with HIV (see Chapters 20–26).

Condoms need not be recommended to prevent infection in long-standing mutually monogamous relationships in which neither partner uses IV drugs or is infected with HIV. Those patients who need to use condoms should be

informed that they do not provide complete protection against infection and must be used in accordance with the following guidelines to be effective:

- Latex condoms, rather than natural membrane condoms, should be used. Torn condoms, those in damaged packages, or those with signs of age (brittle, sticky, discolored) should not be used.
- The condom should be put on an erect penis, before any intimate contact, and should be unrolled completely to the base.
- A space should be left at the tip of the condom to collect semen; air pockets in the space should be removed by pressing the air out towards the base.
- Water-based lubricants should be used. Those made with petroleum jelly, mineral oil, cold cream, and other oil-based lubricants should not be applied because they may damage the condom.
- Insertion of nonoxynol 9 in the condom increases protection, but vaginal application in addition to condom use is likely to provide greater protection.
- If a condom breaks, it should be replaced immediately.
- After ejaculation and while the penis is still erect, the penis should be withdrawn while carefully holding the condom against the base of the penis so that the condom remains in place.
- Condoms should not be reused.

Note: See Appendix A for the U.S. Preventive Services Task Force Table of Ratings for this topic. See also the relevant Task Force background paper: Horsburgh CR Jr, Douglas JM, LaForce FM. Preventive strategies in sexually transmitted diseases for the primary care physician. JAMA 1987; 258:814–21.

REFERENCES

1. National Institutes of Health. NIAID Study Group on Sexually Transmitted Diseases: 1980 status report. Summaries and panel recommendations. Washington, D.C.: Government Printing Office, 1981:215–64.
2. Cates W Jr. Epidemiology and control of sexually transmitted diseases: strategic evolution. Infect Dis Clin North Am 1987; 1:1–23.
3. Centers for Disease Control. Syphilis and congenital syphilis, United States, 1985–1988. MMWR 1988; 37:486–9.
4. Chuang TY, Su WPD, Perry HO, et al. Incidence and trend of herpes progenitals: a 15–year population study. Mayo Clinic Proc 1983; 58:436–41.
5. Guinan ME, Wolinsky SM, Reichman RC. Epidemiology of genital herpes simplex virus infection. Epidemiol Rev 1985; 7:127–46.
6. Hook EW, Holmes KK. Gonococcal infections. Ann Intern Med 1985; 102:229–43.
7. Centers for Disease Control. *Chlamydia trachomatis* infections: policy guidelines for prevention and control. MMWR [Suppl 3] 1985; 34:53S-74S.
8. Westrom L. Effect of acute pelvic inflammatory disease on fertility. Am J Obstet Gynecol 1975; 121:707–13.
9. Clark EG, Danbolt N. The Oslo study of the natural course of untreated syphilis: an epidemiologic investigation based on a restudy of the Boeck-Bruusgaard material. Med Clin North Am 1964; 48:613–23.
10. Corey L, Spear PG. Infections with herpes simplex viruses. N Engl J Med 1986; 314: 749–57.
11. Immunization Practices Advisory Committee. Recommendations for protection against viral hepatitis. MMWR 1985; 34:313–35.
12. Centers for Disease Control. Human immunodeficiency virus infection in the United States: a review of current knowledge. MMWR [Suppl 6] 1987; 36:1–20.

13. *Idem*. Quarterly report to the Domestic Policy Council on the prevalence and rate of spread of HIV and AIDS, United States. MMWR 1988; 37:551–9.
14. Hessol NA, Rutherford GW, Lifson AR, et al. The natural history of HIV infection in a cohort of homosexual and bisexual men: a decade of follow-up. Proceedings of IV International Conference on AIDS, Stockholm, Sweden, June 14, 1988. abstract 4096.
15. Centers for Disease Control. AIDS weekly surveillance report—United States. January 2, 1989.
16. Broder S, Fauci AS. Progress in drug therapies for HIV infection. Public Health Rep 1988; 103:224–9.
17. Rothenberg R, Woelfel M, Stoneburner R, et al. Survival with the acquired immuno-deficiency syndrome: experience with 5833 cases in New York City. N Engl J Med 1987; 317:1297–1302.
18. Centers for Disease Control. Years of potential life lost before age 65—United States, 1987. MMWR 1989; 38:27–9.
19. Curran JW, Jaffe HW, Hardy AM, et al. Epidemiology of HIV infection and AIDS in the United States. Science 1988; 239:610–6.
20. Stevens CE, Beasley RP, Tsui J, et al. Vertical transmission of hepatitis B antigen in Taiwan. N Engl J Med 1975; 292:771–4.
21. Stevens CE, Toy PT, Tong MJ, et al. Perinatal hepatitis B virus transmission in the United States: prevention by passive-active immunization. JAMA 1985; 253:1740–5.
22. Beasley RP, Hwang LY. Epidemiology of hepatocellular carcinoma. In: Vyas GN, Dienstag JL, Hoofnagle JH, eds. Viral hepatitis and liver disease. Orlando, Fla.: Grune and Stratton, 1984:209–24.
23. Beasley RP. Hepatitis B virus as the etiologic agent in hepatocellular carcinoma: epidemiologic considerations. Hepatology 1982; 2:21S-26S.
24. Beasley RP, Hwang LY, Lin CC, et al. Hepatocellular carcinoma and HBV: a prospective study of 22,707 men in Taiwan. Lancet 1981; 2:1129–33.
25. Allen JR, Curran JW. Prevention of AIDS and HIV infection: needs and priorities for epidemiologic research. Am J Public Health 1988; 78:381–6.
26. Centers for Disease Control. Recommendations for assisting in the prevention of perinatal transmission of human T-lymphotrophic virus Type III/lymphadonopathy associated virus and acquired immunodeficiency syndrome. MMWR 1985; 34:721–6,731.
27. *Idem*. Public Health Service guidelines for counseling and antibody testing to prevent HIV infection and AIDS. MMWR 1987; 36:509–14.
28. *Idem*. Quarterly report to the Domestic Policy Council on the prevalence and rate of spread of HIV and AIDS in the United States. MMWR 1988; 37:223–6.
29. Nahmias AJ, Keyserling HL, Kerrick GM. Herpes simplex. In: Remington JS, Klein JO, eds. Infectious diseases of the fetus and newborn infant. Philadelphia: WB Saunders, 1983:636–78.
30. Hellinger FJ. Forecasting the personal medical care costs of AIDS from 1988 through 1991. Public Health Rep 1988; 103:309–19.
31. Handsfield HH, Jasman LL, Roberts PL, et al. Criteria for selective screening of *Chlamydia trachomatis* infection in women attending family planning clinics. JAMA 1986; 255:1730–4.
32. Centers for Disease Control. Changing patterns of groups at high risk for hepatitis B in the United States. MMWR 1988; 37:429–32,437.
33. Cates W Jr. The "other STDs": do they really matter? JAMA 1988; 259:3606–8.
34. Stamm WE, Handsfield HH, Rompalo AM, et al. The association between genital ulcer disease and acquisition of HIV infection in homosexual men. JAMA 1988; 260:1429–33.
35. Hearst N, Hulley SB. Preventing the heterosexual spread of AIDS: are we giving our patients the best advice? JAMA 1988; 259:2428–32.
36. Darrow WW, Echenberg DF, Jaffe HW, et al. Risk factors for human immunodeficiency virus (HIV) infection in homosexual men. Am J Public Health 1987; 77:479–83.
37. Winkelstein W, Lyman DM, Padian N, et al. Sexual practices and risk of infection by the human immunodeficiency virus—the San Francisco men's health study. JAMA 1987; 257:321–5.

38. Conant MA, Spicer DW, Smith CD. Herpes simplex virus transmission: condom studies. Sex Transm Dis 1984; 11:94–5.
39. Kish LS, McMahon JT, Bergfeld WF, et al. An ancient method and a modern scourge: the condom as a barrier against herpes. J Am Acad Dermatol 1983; 9:769–70.
40. Hart G. Role of preventive methods in the control of venereal disease. Clin Obstet Gynecol 1975; 18:243–53.
41. Conant M, Hardy D, Sernatinger J, et al. Condoms prevent transmission of AIDS-associated retrovirus. JAMA 1986; 255:1706.
42. Hart G. Factors influencing venereal infection in a war environment. Br J Vener Dis 1973; 49:107–15.
43. Barlow D. The condom and gonorrhea. Lancet 1977; 2:811–3.
44. Fischl MA, Dickinson GM, Scott GB, et al. Evaluation of heterosexual partners, children, and household contacts of adults with AIDS. JAMA 1987; 257:640–4.
45. Mann J, Quinn TC, Piot P, et al. Condom use and HIV infection among prostitutes in Zaire. N Engl J Med 1987; 316:345.
46. Pritchard JA, MacDonald PC. Family planning. In: Pritchard JA, MacDonald PC, eds. Williams obstetrics, 16th ed. New York: Appleton-Century-Crofts, 1980:1011.
47. Katchadourian HA, Lunde DT. Fundamentals of human sexuality. New York: Holt, Rinehart, and Winston, 1972.
48. Goldsmith MF. Sex in the age of AIDS calls for common sense and "condom sense." JAMA 1987; 257:2261–6.
49. Van de Perre P, Jacobs D, Sprecher-Goldberger S. The latex condom, an efficient barrier against sexual transmission of AIDS-related viruses. AIDS 1987; 1:49–52.
50. Food and Drug Administration. Counseling patients about prevention. FDA Drug Bull 1987; Sept:17–19.
51. Centers for Disease Control. Condoms for prevention of sexually transmitted diseases. MMWR 1988; 37:7,9.
52. Singh B, Postic B, Cutler JC. Virucidal effect of certain chemical contraceptives on type 2 herpes virus. Am J Obstet Gynecol 1976; 126:422–5.
53. Minuk GY, Bohme CE, Bowen TJ. Condoms and hepatitis B virus infection. Ann Intern Med 1986; 104:584.
54. Hicks DR, Martin LS, Getchell JP, et al. Inactivation of HTLV-III/LAV-infected culture of normal human lymphocytes by nonoxynol-9 in vitro. Lancet 1985; 2:1422–3.
55. Rietmeijer CAM, Krebs JW, Feorino PM, et al. Condoms as physical and chemical barriers against human immunodeficiency virus. JAMA 1988; 259:1851–3.
56. Jick H, Hannan MT, Stergachis A, et al. Vaginal spermicides and gonorrhea. JAMA 1982; 248:1619–21.
57. Austin H, Louv WC, Alexander J. A case-control study of spermicides and gonorrhea. JAMA 1984; 251:2822–4.
58. Rendon AL, Covarrubias J, McCarney KE, et al. A controlled, comparative study of phenylmercuric acetate, nonoxynol-9, and placebo vaginal suppositories as prophylactic agents against gonorrhea. Curr Ther Res 1980; 27:780–3.
59. Cole CH, Lacher TG, Bailey JC, et al. Vaginal chemoprophylaxis in the reduction of reinfection in women with gonorrhea: clinical evaluation of the effectiveness of a vaginal contraceptive. Br J Vener Dis 1980; 56:314–8.
60. Rosenberg MJ, Rojanapithayakorn W, Feldblum PJ, et al. Effect of the contraceptive sponge on chlamydial infection, gonorrhea, and candidiasis: a comparative clinical trial. JAMA 1987; 257:2308–12.
61. Kroger F. Compliance strategies in a clinic for treatment of sexually transmitted diseases. Sex Transm Dis 1980; 7:178–82.
62. Solomon MZ, DeJong W. Recent sexually transmitted disease prevention efforts and their implications for AIDS health education. Health Educ Q 1986; 13:301–16.
63. Vaughn CL, Freiberg AD. A pilot study of the navy's educational program on venereal disease. Am J Syph 1950; 34:476–80.
64. Arnold CB, Cogswell BE. A condom distribution program for adolescents: the key findings of a feasibility study. Am J Public Health 1971; 61:739–50.
65. Chaisson RE, Moss AR, Onishi R, et al. Human immunodeficiency virus infection in heterosexual intravenous drug users in San Francisco. Am J Public Health 1987; 77:169–72.

66. Winkelstein W Jr, Samuel M, Padian NS, et al. The San Francisco Men's Health Study. III. Reduction in immunodeficiency virus transmission among homosexual/bisexual men, 1982–86. Am J Public Health 1987; 7C:COC 0.
67. McKusick L, Wiley JA, Coates TJ, et al. Reported changes in the sexual behavior of men at risk for AIDS, San Francisco, 1982–84: the AIDS Behavioral Research Project. Public Health Rep 1985; 100:622–9.
68. Winkelstein W Jr, Wiley JA, Padian NS, et al. The San Francisco Men's Health Study: continued decline in HIV seroconversion rates among homosexual/bisexual men. Am J Public Health 1988; 78:1472–4.
69. Martin JL. The impact of AIDS on gay male sexual behavior patterns in New York City. Am J Public Health 1987; 77:578–81.
70. Centers for Disease Control. Self-reported changes in sexual behavior among homosexual and bisexual men from the San Francisco Clinic cohort. MMWR 1987; 36: 187–9.
71. Schechter MT, Craib KJP, Willoughby B, et al. Patterns of sexual behavior and condom use in a cohort of homosexual men. Am J Public Health 1988; 78:1535–8.
72. Keeter S, Bradford JB. Knowledge of AIDS and related behavior change among unmarried adults in a low-prevalence city. Am J Prev Med 1988; 4:146–52.
73. Winkelstein W, Samuel M, Padian NS, et al. Selected sexual practices of San Francisco heterosexual men and risk of infection by the human immunodeficiency virus. JAMA 1987; 257:1470–1.
74. Friedman SR, Des Jarlais DC, Sotheran JL. AIDS health education for intravenous drug users. Health Educ Q 1986; 13:383–93.
75. Des Jarlais DC, Friedman SR, Hopkins W. Risk reduction for the acquired immunodeficiency syndrome among intravenous drug users. Ann Intern Med 1985; 103:755–9.
76. Friedman SR, Des Jarlais DC, Sotheran JL, et al. AIDS and self-organization among intravenous drug users. Int J Addict 1987; 22:201–20.
77. Des Jarlais DC, Friedman SR, Novick DM, et al. HIV-1 infection among intravenous drug users in Manhattan, New York City, from 1977 through 1987. JAMA 1989; 261: 1008–12.
78. Selwyn PA, Feiner C, Cox CP, et al. Knowledge about AIDS and high-risk behavior among intravenous drug abusers in New York City. AIDS 1987; 1:247–54.
79. Kegeles SM, Adler NE, Irwin CE. Sexually active adolescents and condoms: changes over one year in knowledge, attitudes and use. Am J Public Health 1988; 78:460–1.
80. Strunin L, Hingson R. Acquired immunodeficiency syndrome and adolescents: knowledge, beliefs, attitudes, and behaviors. Pediatrics 1987; 79:825–8.
81. Landenfeld CS, Chren MM, Shega J, et al. Students' sexual behavior, knowledge, and attitudes relating to the acquired immunodeficiency syndrome. J Gen Intern Med 1988; 3:161–5.
82. Darrow WW. Attitudes toward condom use and the acceptance of venereal disease prophylactics. In: Redford MH, Duncan MH, Prager DJ, et al., eds. The condom: increasing utilization in the United States. San Francisco, Calif.: San Francisco Press, 1974:173–85.
83. Centers for Disease Control. Antibody to human immunodeficiency virus in female prostitutes. MMWR 1987; 36:157–61.
84. Lewis CE, Freeman HE. The sexual history-taking and counseling practices of primary care physicians. West J Med 1987; 147:165–7.
85. Koop CE. Physician leadership in preventing AIDS. JAMA 1987; 258:2111.
86. American Medical Association. Board of Trustees Report. Prevention and control of acquired immunodeficiency syndrome: an interim report. JAMA 1987; 258:2097–103.
87. American College of Physicians. Acquired immunodeficiency syndrome. Ann Intern Med 1986; 104:575–81.
88. American College of Obstetricians and Gynecologists. Prevention of human immune deficiency virus infection and acquired immune deficiency syndrome. ACOG Committee Statement of Committee on Obstetrics: Maternal and Fetal Medicine and Gynecologic Practice. Washington, D.C.: American College of Obstetricians and Gynecologists, 1987.

54

Counseling to Prevent
Unintended Pregnancy

Recommendation: Clinicians should obtain a complete sexual history from all adolescent and adult patients. Sexually active women who do not want to become pregnant and men who do not want to have a child should receive detailed counseling on methods to prevent unintended pregnancy (see *Clinical Intervention*). Sexually active patients should also receive information on measures to prevent sexually transmitted diseases (see Chapter 53).

Burden of Suffering

The exact prevalence of unwanted pregnancies in the United States is uncertain due to difficulties in data collection, but it is thought to represent a significant proportion of pregnancies, especially among adolescent and young adult parents. Unwanted pregnancies represent a subset of unintended pregnancies. It has been estimated that about 37% of births among women aged 15–44 are unintended (i.e., came sooner than wanted or were not wanted ever) and just over one-quarter of these (10% of births) are thought to be unwanted.[1] Over 18% of births to women aged 35–44 are thought to be unwanted.[1] Each year there are about 1.5 million induced abortions performed in the United States, primarily as an elective procedure to terminate unwanted pregnancies.[2] The rate of unintended pregnancies occurring among adolescents is higher in the United States than in most other developed nations.[1] Each year in the United States, about 1 million adolescent females aged 15–19 (about 8–10% of this age group) and nearly 30,000 girls under age 15 become pregnant.[2,3] About 40% of pregnant females aged 15–19 choose to undergo induced abortion.[2] Female teenagers account for 27% of all induced abortions in the United States; the abortion rate in women aged 18–19 is higher than at any other age.[2] Nearly 490,000 females aged 15–19 give birth each year, and a third of these mothers are age 17 or younger.[2,3] Nearly one-third of pregnant girls under age 15 carry their fetuses to term, resulting in 10,000 live births per year in this age group.[2]

Unintended pregnancies can have adverse effects on both children and their parents. Unwanted pregnancy is a risk factor for child abuse and neglect, and many children born of unwanted pregnancies have behavioral and/or educational problems at later ages.[4,5] When pregnancy occurs during adolescence, there may be increased risk of maternal and neonatal complications (such as low birthweight).[6] This is in part because adolescents often fail to obtain adequate antenatal care and often fail to modify behavioral risk factors (e.g., smoking, poor nutrition) during pregnancy. Adolescents and young adults who bear children often must postpone or abandon educational and employment opportunities to care for their children. About half of adolescents who bear children are unmarried at the time of birth.[7,8] Those who are married often face intense marital pressures that can lead to divorce or separation while the child is still young. It has been estimated that first births to adolescents in 1979 cost the United States at least $8.3 billion,[9] and current estimates are in the range of $11–13 billion per year.

Initiation of sexual activity at a young age, a primary risk factor for unintended pregnancy, is common in the United States. Over half of unmarried American adolescents in the United States report having had sexual intercourse by age 18.[10] Teenagers account for one-third of patients attending family planning clinics in the United States.[11] The proportion of unmarried female teenagers who are sexually active increases with age: 18% at age 15, 29% at age 16, 40% at age 17, 54% at age 18, and 66% by age 19.[10] In a survey of urban black high school males, 87% of the respondents reported having had sexual intercourse.[12] Sexual activity is reported in about 75% of never married women aged 20–24.[13] Sexual activity at younger ages is more common among blacks and families of low socioeconomic status and among adolescents who smoke, use alcohol or other drugs, and have evidence of delinquency.[13-16]

Efficacy of Risk Reduction

Without contraception, 89% of heterosexual couples who engage in regular sexual intercourse will conceive within one year.[17,18] There are several approaches to preventing unintended pregnancy. Complete sexual abstinence is the most effective form of contraception, and it is seen by many as the most appropriate behavior for unmarried adolescents. In persons who are sexually active, available methods to prevent conception include those that work either temporarily (contraceptive hormones, barrier methods, spermicides, coitus interruptus, periodic abstinence, intrauterine devices) or permanently (sterilization). Selection of an appropriate method of birth control must take into consideration the personal preferences, religious beliefs, and abilities of the patient, the nature of the relationship with the partner(s), and the attitudes and legal restrictions of society. It is clear from a medical and scientific perspective, however, that certain methods are more effective than others in preventing unintended pregnancy.

Contraceptive hormones include oral contraceptives (combined preparations and progestin-only pills), postcoital preparations, and injectable contraceptives. Combination oral contraceptives are the most effective and popular method of reversible contraception; they are used by an estimated 10 million American women.[19] "The pill" is generally taken daily for 21 days, followed by either placebo or no pills for 7 days. The failure rate (proportion of women who conceive during first year of use) is about 3% under typical usage conditions and as low as 0.1% when used correctly and consistently.[17,18] Women who take oral contraceptives also may experience noncontraceptive benefits, such as a reduction in certain menstrual disorders (e.g., primary dysmenorrhea, menorrhagia), and reduced risk of benign breast disease, functional ovarian cysts, leiomyomata, and some gynecologic cancers.[20]

Some women taking oral contraceptives experience unpleasant side effects, such as breakthrough bleeding and breast tenderness, but these have been minimized in recent years by lowering the dose of estrogen to less than 50 mcg and by adopting multiphasic regimens that alter the dose during the menstrual cycle.[21] Some epidemiologic studies have shown an association between the use of oral contraceptives and certain diseases, including myocardial infarction, hypertension, strokes, thromboembolic disorders, hepatocellular and perhaps breast cancer, and gallbladder disease.[22-29] Definitive evidence regarding the strength of these associations, independent of other risk factors for these diseases, is lacking due to the logistical problems of performing appropriate long-term prospective studies.[30] Moreover, the probability of such complications from oral contraceptives is relatively small (especially in the absence of known contraindications). The probability of a fatal complication is 1 in 63,000 for nonsmoking women who take oral contraceptives for one year, whereas the risk is 1 in 10,000 for women who carry a fetus to term.[17] Women informed of the low level of risk and potential noncontraceptive benefits associated with oral contraceptives may find this a more acceptable and safer method than using alternative techniques or risking the consequences of unintended pregnancy.

Other contraceptive hormone preparations include the progestin-only pill, postcoital administration, and injectable progestins. The progestin-only pill, which has a failure rate of 0.5–3.0%,[17] is somewhat less effective than combination oral contraceptives and is used infrequently in the United States. Postcoital administration of oral contraceptives can be of some value after unprotected intercourse.[17,18] These agents, which usually consist of ethinyl estradiol and levonorgestrel, are taken within 72 hours of intercourse. Prominent side effects include irregular bleeding and nausea and vomiting; the latter occurs in about half of recipients.[31] Injectable progestins (medroxyprogesterone) are administered two to four times a year and have a failure rate of only 0.3%.[17,18] They require intramuscular injections, however, and have not yet been licensed for routine use in the United States. Neither oral nor injectable contraceptives offer protection against sexually transmitted diseases.

Barrier contraceptive methods include the condom, diaphragm, cervical cap, and vaginal sponge. Barrier methods have the advantage of fewer side effects than oral contraceptives, but they are highly dependent on patient compliance to ensure proper use. When used correctly, condoms have a 2% failure rate in preventing pregnancy, but the rate may be as high as 12% under conditions of typical usage.[17,18] Diaphragms, in combination with spermicides, have a failure rate of about 3% when used correctly but the rate may be as high as 18% when used incorrectly or inconsistently.[17,18] The corresponding failure rates for the cervical cap are 5% and 18%, respectively.[17,18] Failures of condoms and diaphragms are occasionally the result of product deficiencies (e.g., condom rupture), but more often they are due to user error. Spermicides (e.g., foams, creams, jellies) improve the effectiveness of barrier methods by providing protection in the event of product or user failure.

The vaginal sponge, which is impregnated with spermicide, is less effective than other barrier methods, with failure rates as high as 18–28% under typical usage conditions.[17,18] When used correctly, the failure rate is about 5–8%. It provides protection for up to 24 hours following insertion and should remain in place for at least six hours after the last act of intercourse. Cases of toxic shock syndrome (TSS) have been reported in women using the vaginal sponge, but the risk of this complication appears to be very low.[32] It has been estimated that only 10 cases of TSS can be expected for every 100,000 women who use the vaginal sponge;[33] the risk of death in persons with TSS is about 3%.[17] Spermicides can be used alone as a contraceptive, but must be inserted deep into the vagina before each act of coitus to be effective. Failure rates range from 3%, when used correctly, to as high as 21% under typical usage conditions.[17,18]

Barrier methods and spermicides are the only birth control techniques (other than sexual abstinence) that are also effective in reducing the risk of acquiring sexually transmitted diseases. In particular, latex condoms combined with spermicides containing nonoxynol 9 have been shown to reduce the transmission of human immunodeficiency virus (HIV) and a number of other important sexually transmitted organisms (see Chapter 53). It is therefore important for clinicians to consider both the risks of infection as well as those of pregnancy when recommending specific contraceptive techniques.

Modified coital behaviors, such as coitus interruptus (withdrawal) or fertility awareness methods (e.g., periodic abstinence or natural family planning), offer less protection against pregnancy than do the most commonly used contraceptive techniques. However, they may be more acceptable alternatives for persons with religious restrictions,[34] those concerned about the long-term use of oral contraceptives, and those who find insertion of contraceptive devices unacceptable. It is often difficult to perform these methods correctly. Fertility awareness methods require monitoring the calendar dates of the last menstrual period, body temperature, or cervical mucus characteristics. Coitus interruptus can fail if withdrawal is not timed properly or if preejaculatory fluid is released before withdrawal. Due to these difficulties with compliance, withdrawal and periodic abstinence both carry failure rates as high as 18–20%.[17,18] Effectiveness may be improved by combining these with other contraceptive methods, such as barrier methods during the fertile days of the menstrual cycle.

Intrauterine devices (IUD) are effective contraceptives (1–6% failure rate) and have the added convenience of needing infrequent replacement.[17,18] However, most IUD devices were withdrawn from the U.S. market in the early 1980s due to medicolegal concerns about a possible association with pelvic inflammatory disease and subsequent tubal infertility. Aside from an expensive progesterone-releasing IUD[35] and a new copper IUD that has only recently been introduced,[36] this form of contraception is largely unavailable in the United States. This has led many women uncomfortable with oral contraceptives and barrier methods to turn to less effective contraceptive alternatives.[35] In contrast to barrier methods, the IUD does not offer protection against sexually transmitted diseases.

Sterilization is the most common method of contraception in the United States.[37] The failure rate is 0.1–0.2% for male sterilization (vasectomy) and 0.2–0.4% for female sterilization (tubal ligation).[17,18] Both methods are associated with occasional surgical complications. About 0.3–1.6% of vasectomies are complicated by acute side effects (e.g., hematoma, infection, epididymitis).[17]The risk of surgical or anesthesia-related complications from tubal ligation depends on the center and the type of procedure (e.g., mini-laparotomy, laparoscopy, colpotomy), but the complication rate is often less than 1%.[17] Suggested long-term effects of sterilization, such as endocrinologic changes, effects on atherosclerosis in men, and abnormal menstrual patterns in women have not been demonstrated convincingly in clinical studies.[17] Sterilization does not offer protection against sexually transmitted diseases, but it may reduce the risk of pelvic inflammatory disease.[38]

Effectiveness of Counseling

Many patients of childbearing age seen by clinicians are at risk for unintended pregnancy and do not practice effective contraceptive techniques. About 30% of unmarried teens aged 15–19 practice unprotected sexual intercourse.[37] A survey of sexually active black high school males found that only 60% had used a contraceptive at their last sexual encounter, and most lacked accurate knowledge about the relative effectiveness and availability of various birth control methods.[12] Inconsistent or incorrect use of contraceptives is reported in at least half of pregnant women receiving counseling for abortion.[39]

Thus, many of the patients seen by primary care clinicians are in need of better information about contraceptive methods and the prescription of appropriate products. The need for clinicians to provide this type of counseling is not restricted to family planning clinics; family planning counseling is often indicated in the primary care setting. Many women in the United States do not have access to family planning clinics or they seek their care elsewhere.[40] About 70% of women who sought medical family planning between 1979 and 1982 visited an obstetrician-gynecologist or a family practitioner.[41] Of the estimated 5 million adolescents in the United States at risk for unintended pregnancy, 1.4 million visit private physicians.[11] Men who require counseling are also seen frequently in the primary care setting.

Since clinicians have access to a large proportion of persons at risk for unintended pregnancy, counseling regarding the use of contraceptive methods could have a significant public health impact if performed effectively. It has been estimated that as many as one-third of all unintended pregnancies and 500,000 abortions could be prevented if the proportion of women not using contraception were reduced by half.[42]

There is only limited information, however, on the effectiveness of clinician counseling in altering sexual behavior. Clearly, the effectiveness of counseling depends on the age, level of maturity, sex, parity, and medical history of the patient, as well as on the level of training, clinical practice setting, and counseling skills of the provider. However, the effectiveness of counseling has been studied primarily in the context of sex education in schools and family planning clinics. Such studies have found that young women who attend a sex education course in school use contraceptives more effectively,[43-45] but the designs of these studies do not permit the conclusion that sex education itself is responsible for the outcome or that sex education performed by clinicians is equally as effective. Clinical interventions in family planning clinics appear to be beneficial in preventing unintended adolescent pregnancy. Studies in family planning clinics have demonstrated a correlation between levels of contraceptive compliance and certain characteristics of the patient-provider relationship.[46] Adolescents living in communities with subsidized family planning services are less likely to become pregnant than those living elsewhere.[47] Teenage attendance at family planning clinics has been associated with increased use of oral contraceptives, decreased use of barrier and rhythm methods, and dramatic reductions in unprotected sexual intercourse.[48] Pregnancy rates have also been shown to decrease for adolescents attending schools adjacent to adolescent health clinics (see below).[49] In general, however, clinic attenders are self-selected, and in many the effects of counseling are short-lived. In one study, only 66% of adolescents attending a family planning clinic were compliant at a three-month follow-up visit, and less than one-half were compliant after a year.[50] Attempts by family planning clinics to improve compliance through family counseling and increased telephone contact with patients have met with limited success.[51]

Since the causes of unintended pregnancy are complex, it has been suggested that only limited effectiveness can be achieved by providing information or prescribing contraceptives without also providing patients with the psychological tools to use these methods. To help adolescents confront social pressures, it may be important to expand counseling beyond sex education to emphasize "life option" skills in decisionmaking, assertiveness, and interpersonal communication with peers.[52] Another strategy directed at unintended teenage pregnancy is the emergence of the adolescent health clinic, in which family planning services are provided as a component of a comprehensive program of health care and psychological support for teens.[53] The establishment of such clinics in secondary schools has been associated with a decrease in local fertility rates.[54] One program, with two clinics adjacent to a high school and a middle school, reported a 30% decline in conceptions, despite a 58% increase in adolescent pregnancies at control schools.[49] Organized community-wide initiatives have also proved highly successful in preventing unintended adolescent pregnancy.[55]

Recommendations of Others

The Canadian Task Force and many other groups recommend the inclusion of counseling to prevent unwanted pregnancy in the periodic health examination of adolescents.[56] The American College of Obstetricians and Gynecologists[57] and the Society for Adolescent Medicine[58] have issued specific recommendations for counseling adolescents on contraceptive techniques to prevent unwanted pregnancy. These groups also encourage physicians to protect the confidentiality of the doctor-adolescent relationship within the confines of local legal requirements regarding parental consent. The subject of unwanted adolescent pregnancy also has been the subject of an extensive report by the National Research Council.[59] Finally, the American Academy of Pediatrics has recently issued guidelines for counseling adolescents about contraception and pregnancy.[60]

Discussion

The effectiveness of the clinician in preventing unintended pregnancy depends in part on the clinician's sensitivity to the personal concerns and privacy of the patient. These issues are especially important when addressing issues of sexuality with adolescents. The presentation of a nonjudgmental and understanding attitude and the performance of the physical examination without the parents present are cornerstones of this approach. Many physicians, especially pediatricians and general practitioners, are reluctant to prescribe contraceptives for adolescents without parental consent.[61] Legislation in some states requires parental notification before treating a minor. At the same time, physicians have a professional obligation to protect the well-being of the adolescent and the confidentiality of the doctor-patient relationship.[62] A practice of informing parents may act as a disincentive for sexually active adolescents in need of professional assistance. After the cost of an office visit, concern that a physician will inform parents is the most common reason adolescents cite for choosing family planning clinics over private physicians to obtain contraceptive care,[63] and presumably many more choose not to contact any facility. Family planning services are obtained from private physicians by 73% of women aged 29 and older, but by only 48% of teenagers.[64] For these reasons, some states specifically exempt contraception and pregnancy-related care from notification requirements. It is important for clinicians to give careful consideration to each of these factors when making decisions about the notification of parents.

Clinical Intervention

Clinicians should obtain a detailed sexual history from all adolescent and adult patients, male and female. For sexually active patients, the interview should include a discussion of the sexual practices and feelings of the patient and partner(s), as well as an assessment of the level of patient concern about the risk of unintended pregnancy. Based on this information, the clinician should provide appropriate counseling on the level of risk associated with the patient's current contraceptive techniques and, when indicated, available alternatives for more effective prevention. Clear instructions should be provided for the proper use of recommended contraceptive techniques. Oral contraceptives and barrier methods (with spermicides) should be recommended as the most effective means of reducing risk in sexually active persons, and complete sexual abstinence as the most effective method overall. Sexual abstinence and the maintenance of a mutually faithful monogamous sexual relationship should be emphasized as two important measures to reduce the risk of sexually transmitted diseases (see Chapter 53). Patients who engage in sexual activity with multiple partners or with persons who may be infected with sexually transmitted organisms should be advised to use condoms and instructed in their proper use (see Chapter 53).

Empathy, confidentiality, and a nonjudgmental supportive attitude are especially important when discussing issues of sexuality with adolescents. Clinicians should involve young pubertal patients and, where appropriate, their parents in early, open discussion of sexual development and effective methods to prevent unintended pregnancy and sexually transmitted diseases. Sexually abstinent adolescents should be encouraged to remain abstinent, and they should also be given support in asserting themselves in the event of an unwelcome or coercive sexual relationship. They should be encouraged to obtain counseling on the proper use of contraceptives if they plan to begin engaging in sexual intercourse. Adolescents should be examined without their parent(s) present. Clinicians providing birth control services for minors should take into consideration both the confidentiality of the doctor-patient relationship as well as local legal restrictions when making decisions pertaining to the notification of parents. The optimal frequency of counseling to prevent unintended pregnancy has not been determined and is left to clinical discretion.

Note: See Appendix A for the U.S. Preventive Services Task Force Table of Ratings for this topic. See also the relevant Task Force background paper: Fielding JE, Williams CA. Preventing unwanted teenage pregnancy in the United States. In: Goldbloom RB, Lawrence RS, eds. Preventing disease: beyond the rhetoric. New York: Springer-Verlag (in press).

REFERENCES

1. Jones EF, Forrest JD, Henshaw SK, et al. Unintended pregnancy, contraceptive practice and family planning services in developed countries. Fam Plann Perspect 1988; 20: 53–67.
2. Ventura SJ, Taffel SM, Mosher WD. Estimates of pregnancies and pregnancy rates for the United States, 1976–1985. Am J Public Health 1988; 78:504–11.
3. Maciak BJ, Spitz AM, Strauss LT, et al. Pregnancy and birth rates among sexually experienced U.S. teenagers—1974, 1980, and 1983. JAMA 1987; 258:2069–71.
4. Myhrman A. Family relation and social competence of children unwanted at birth: a follow-up study at the age of 16. Acta Psychiatr Scand 1988; 77:181–7.
5. Furstenberg FF Jr, Brooks-Gunn J, Morgan SP. Adolescent mothers and their children in later life. Fam Plann Perspect 1987; 19:142–51.
6. Zuckerman BS, Walker DK, Frank DA, et al. Adolescent pregnancy: biobehavioral determinants of outcome. J Pediatr 1984; 105:857–63.
7. Bureau of the Census. 1983 marital status and living arrangements, current population reports. Series P-20 (389), 1984.
8. Ventura SJ. Trends in teenage childbearing: United States, 1970–1981. Vital and Health Statistics, series 21, no. 41. Hyattsville, Md.: National Center for Health Statistics, 1984.
9. SRI International. An analysis of government expenditures consequent on teenage childbirth. Menlo Park, Calif.: SRI International, 1979.
10. Pratt WF, Mosher WD, Bachrach CA, et al. Understanding U.S. fertility: findings from the National Survey of Family Growth, Cycle III. Popul Bull 1984; 39:1–42.

11. Torres A, Forrest JD. Family planning clinic services in the United States, 1981. Fam Plann Perspect 1983; 15:272–8.
12. Clark SD Jr, Zabin LS, Hardy JB. Sex, contraception and parenthood: experience and attitudes among urban black young men. Fam Plann Perspect 1984; 16:77–82.
13. National Center for Health Statistics. Married and unmarried couples: United States, 1982. Vital and Health Statistics, series 23, no. 15. Washington, D.C.: Government Printing Office, 1987.
14. Zabin LS. The association between smoking and sexual behavior among teens in U.S. contraceptive clinics. Am J Public Health 1984; 74:261–3.
15. Zabin LS, Hardy JB, Smith EA, et al. Substance use and its relation to sexual activity among inner-city adolescents. J Adolesc Health Care 1986; 7:320–31.
16. Jessor R, Costa F, Jessor SL, et al. Time of first intercourse: a prospective study. J Person Soc Psychol 1983; 44:608–26.
17. Hatcher RA, Guest F, Stewart F, et al. Contraceptive technology, 1988–1989. Atlanta, Ga.: Printed Matter, Inc., 1988.
18. Trussell J, Kost K. Contraceptive failure in the United States: a critical review of the literature. Stud Fam Plann 1987; 18:237–83.
19. Curran DL, Campbell BF. Contraception update: improvements in safety, convenience, and benefits. Consultant 1987; 27:23–32.
20. Derman R. Oral contraceptives: assessment of benefits. J Reprod Med 1986; 31:879–86.
21. Hale RW. Phasic approach to oral contraceptives. Am J Obstet Gynecol 1987; 157:1052–8.
22. Beral V. Cardiovascular disease mortality trends and oral contraceptive use in young women. Lancet 1976; 2:1047–52.
23. Collaborative Group for the Study of Stroke in Young Women. Oral contraceptives and stroke in young women: associated risk factors. JAMA 1975; 231:718–22.
24. Royal College of General Practitioners. Oral contraceptives and health: an interim report from the oral contraception study of the Royal College of General Practitioners. New York: Pitman Medical, 1974.
25. Vessey M, Doll R, Peto R, et al. A long-term follow-up study of women using different methods of contraception: an interim report. J Biosoc Sci 1976; 8:373–427.
26. Pike MC, Henderson BE, Krailo MD, et al. Breast cancer in young women and the use of oral contraceptives: possible modifying effect of formulation and age at use. Lancet 1983; 2:926–30.
27. McPherson K, Neil A, Vessey MP, et al. Oral contraceptives and breast cancer. Lancet 1983; 2:1414–5.
28. The Cancer and Steroid Hormone Study of the Centers for Disease Control and the National Institute of Child Health and Human Development. Oral contraceptive use and the risk of breast cancer. N Engl J Med 1986; 315:405–11.
29. Miller DR, Rosenberg L, Kaufman DW, et al. Breast cancer before age 45 and oral contraceptive use: new findings. Am J Epidemiol 1989; 129:269–80.
30. Doll R, Vessey MP. Evaluation of rare adverse effects of systemic contraceptives. Br Med Bull 1970; 26:33–8.
31. Percival-Smith RK, Abercrombie B. Postcoital contraception with dl-norgestrel/ethinyl estradiol combination: six years experience in a student medical clinic. Contraception 1987; 36:287–93.
32. Faich G, Pearson K, Fleming D, et al. Toxic shock syndrome and the vaginal contraceptive sponge. JAMA 1986; 255:216–8.
33. Centers for Disease Control. Toxic shock syndrome and the vaginal contraceptive sponge. MMWR 1984; 33:43–8.
34. Notzer N, Levran D, Mashiach S, et al. Effect of religiosity on sex attitudes, experience and contraception among university students. J Sex Marital Ther 1984; 10:57–62.
35. Rapkin AJ, Alcalay R, Mitchell J. Non-availability of the IUD and contraceptive choice. Contraception 1988; 37:383–90.
36. New copper IUD. Med Lett Drugs Ther 1988; 30:25–6.
37. Bachrach CA, Mosher W. Use of contraception in the United States, 1982. Advance

Data from Vital and Health Statistics, no. 102. Hyattsville, Md.: National Center for Health Statistics, 1984.

38. Phillips AJ, D'Ablaing G. Acute salpingitis subsequent to tubal ligation. Obstet Gynecol 1986; 67:55S-8S.
39. Sophocles AM Jr, Brozovich EM. Birth control failure among patients with unwanted pregnancies: 1982–1984. J Fam Pract 1986; 22:45–8.
40. Torres A, Forrest JD. Family planning clinic services in U.S. counties, 1983. Fam Plann Perspect 1987; 19:54–8.
41. Orr MT, Forrest JD. The availability of reproductive health services from U.S. private physicians. Fam Plann Persp 1985; 17:63–9.
42. Mosher W. Fertility and family planning in the United States: insights from the National Survey of Family Growth. Fam Plann Perspect 1988; 20:207–17.
43. Zelnik M, Kim YJ. Sex education and its association with teenage sexual activity, pregnancy and contraceptive use. Fam Plann Perspect 1982; 14:117–26.
44. Dawson DA. The effects of sex education on adolescent behavior. Fam Plann Perspect 1986; 18:162–70.
45. Mott FL, Marsiglio W. Early childbearing and completion of high school. Fam Plann Perspect 1985; 17:234–7.
46. Nathanson CA, Becker MH. The influence of client-provider relationships on teenage women's subsequent use of contraception. Am J Public Health 1985; 75:33–8.
47. Moore KA, Caldwell SB. The effect of government policies on out-of-wedlock sex and pregnancy. Fam Plann Perspect 1977; 9:164–9.
48. Forrest JD, Hermalin A, Henshaw SK. The impact of family planning clinic programs on adolescent pregnancy. Fam Plann Perspect 1981; 13:109–16.
49. Zabin LS, Hirsch MB, Smith EA, et al. Evaluation of a pregnancy prevention program for urban teenagers. Fam Plann Perspect 1986; 18:119–26.
50. Emans SJ, Grace E, Woods E, et al. Adolescents' compliance with the use of oral contraceptives. JAMA 1987; 257:3377–81.
51. Herceg-Baron R, Furstenberg FF Jr, Shea J, et al. Supporting teenagers' use of contraceptives: a comparison of clinic services. Fam Plann Perspect 1986; 18:61–6.
52. Schinke SP, Blythe B, Gilchrist L. Cognitive, behavioral prevention of adolescent pregnancy. J Couns Psychol 1981; 28:451–4.
53. Klerman LV. Evaluating comprehensive service programs for pregnant adolescents. Eval Health Prof 1979; 2:55–70.
54. Edwards L, Steinman M, Arnold K, et al. Adolescent pregnancy services in high school clinics. Fam Plann Perspect 1980; 12:6–14.
55. Vincent ML, Clearie AR, Schluchter MD. Reducing adolescent pregnancy through school and community-based education. JAMA 1987; 257:3382–6.
56. Canadian Task Force on the Periodic Health Examination. The periodic health examination. 2. 1987 update. Can Med Assoc J 1988; 138:618–26.
57. American College of Obstetricians and Gynecologists. The adolescent obstetric-gynecologic patient. ACOG Technical Bulletin No. 94. Washington, D.C.: American College of Obstetricians and Gynecologists, 1986.
58. Society for Adolescent Medicine. Position papers on reproductive health care for adolescents. J Adoles Health Care 1983; 4:208–10.
59. National Research Council. Risking the future: adolescent sexuality, pregnancy, and childbearing. Washington, D.C.: National Academy Press, 1987.
60. American Academy of Pediatrics. Counseling the adolescent about pregnancy options. Pediatrics 1989; 83:135–7.
61. Orr M. Private physicians and the provision of contraceptives to adolescents. Fam Plann Perspect 1984; 16:83–6.
62. Committee on Education in Family Life, American College of Obstetricians and Gynecologists. The management of sexual crises in the minor female. Washington, D.C.: American College of Obstetricians and Gynecologists, 1982.
63. Chamie M, Eisman S, Forrest JD, et al. Factors affecting adolescents' use of family planning clinics. Fam Plann Perspect 1982; 14:126–39.
64. Forrest JD. The delivery of family planning services in the United States. Fam Plann Persp 1988; 20:88–95.

55

Counseling to Prevent Dental Disease

Recommendation: All patients should be encouraged to visit a dental care provider on a regular basis. Primary care clinicians should counsel patients regarding daily tooth brushing and dental flossing, the appropriate use of fluoride for caries prevention, avoiding sugary foods, and risk factors for developing baby bottle tooth decay. Children living in communities with inadequate water fluoridation should receive appropriate dietary fluoride supplements. While examining the mouth, clinicians should be alert for obvious signs of oral disease (see *Clinical Intervention*). Oral cancer is discussed in Chapter 15.

Burden of Suffering

A large proportion of the population of the United States suffers from dental caries (tooth decay) and periodontal (gum and bone) disease. Although the prevalence of dental caries among school-aged children has declined in recent years, the average schoolchild has at least 1 cavity in permanent teeth by age 9, 2.6 cavities by age 12, and 8 by age 17.[1,2] About one-quarter have five or more decayed, missing, or filled teeth. The average adult in the United States has 10–17 decayed, missing, or filled permanent teeth.[3,4] Nearly half of all employed adults have gingivitis (gum inflammation), and periodontitis (inflammation of the gums and bone supporting the teeth) has been experienced to some degree by 80%.[4] Ninety-five percent of the elderly have periodontitis, with more than one-third experiencing moderate to severe periodontal disease (i.e., 6 mm attachment loss).[4] It has been estimated that as many as 4–15% of American adults, and over 40% of the elderly, are edentulous.[4,5] Each year in the United States, dental conditions account for about 11 million days of restricted activity, 4 million days of bed disability, 2 million lost workdays, and over 1 million days of lost school.[6] Dental expenditures in the United States approached $30 billion in 1986.[7] Dental disease is more common in persons whose personal behaviors (e.g., smoking, alcohol abuse), medications, or coexisting medical illnesses (e.g., diabetes mellitus, xerostomia) increase the risk of oral pathology. With the aging of the population, a growing number of older Americans are experiencing medical disorders and taking medications that affect their oral health.[8]

Efficacy of Risk Reduction

Personal oral disease prevention practices can reduce the risk of developing caries and periodontal disease. These measures include regular use of fluoride, reduced dietary intake of foods containing refined sugars, and tooth brushing and flossing. The incidence of caries has been reduced significantly by the fluoridation of community water supplies.[9] However, only 87% of the U.S. population is served by community water supplies, and only 64% of these communities have optimally fluoridated water.[10] In locations where adequate community water fluoridation is not available, the risk of caries can be reduced by providing alternate sources of fluoride.[11-14] These include systemic (e.g., school water fluoridation, fluoride tablets, drops) and topical (e.g., fluoridated mouth rinses, professional fluoride treatment) forms. Also, virtually all toothpastes sold in the United States contain fluoride that has been proved to be effective in reducing the incidence of caries by about 20–40%.[15-17]

Reduced intake of certain dietary carbohydrates, especially refined sugars, may lower the risk of developing caries. Studies in the 1950s and 1960s conducted in institutionalized settings suggest that diets containing large amounts of sucrose and other sugary foods are associated with a higher incidence of caries.[18,19] The correlation has been more difficult to demonstrate in more recent studies, in which dietary intake was less carefully controlled,[20,21] but it is widely held that the consumption of sugary foods, especially between meals, is cariogenic. For ethical reasons, definitive studies to prove a causal relationship between diet and carious lesions are unlikely to be performed in the future.

Improper infant feeding practices are another source of caries in young children, especially in those who regularly fall asleep sucking the nipple of a baby bottle containing an acidic or cariogenic beverage (fruit juice, milk, formula). Prolonged pooling of these liquids around the anterior primary teeth (baby incisors) can cause extensive destruction, particularly of the primary incisors but also of molars.[22,23] Education to curb the practice of putting children to bed with a bottle may decrease the risk of nursing bottle tooth decay.

It is mainly the fluoride contained in toothpastes, rather than tooth brushing and flossing per se, that reduces tooth decay.[24] It has been established, however, that brushing and flossing can prevent the development and progression of periodontal disease by removing bacterial plaque deposits.[25-27] Their efficacy, however, depends on the ability of the patient to keep teeth adequately plaque-free, and this necessitates thorough daily tooth brushing and cleaning between teeth with dental floss or other mechanical devices. Due to the difficulty many patients have in adopting and maintaining these habits, personal oral hygiene measures often fail to adequately remove plaque and prevent gingivitis. For this reason, it is also important for patients to receive regular professional dental care.

Among the most important measures performed by dentists and dental hygienists are primary preventive measures, such as prophylactic cleaning, scaling, and root planing of teeth, and secondary preventive maneuvers, such as careful oral and dental examination for the early detection of dental disease. Other preventive interventions include the application of topical fluoride[28] and occlusal sealants[29,30] to prevent caries, placement of orthodontic space-maintaining appliances to prevent malocclusion, and the early detection of oral cancer (see Chapter 15). Experimental studies have demonstrated that meticulous and very frequent dental prophylaxis can reduce the incidence of caries in schoolchildren,[31-36] but these studies required an intense program of professional dental care that would not be feasible under typical dental practice conditions in the United States. Professional tooth cleaning can also delay progression of periodontal disease because the dentist or dental hygienist can remove plaque and tartar from subgingival areas generally not reached by the patient. Dental care alone, however, is inadequate to prevent periodontal disease. Failure by the patient to regularly remove plaque deposits between dental visits can lead to extension of supragingival plaque beneath the gum, bacterial recolonization of the gingival crevice, accumulation of calculus, and recurrent periodontitis.[07] Thus, programs combining personal oral hygiene with professional prophylaxis are most effective in the prevention of periodontal disease.[25,38]

Although dental examinations and prophylaxis are widely recommended every year or six months, there is little scientific evidence that this frequency is necessary on a routine basis for the maintenance of oral health in asymptomatic persons.[39] It is clear that regular examinations are necessary to detect and treat disease processes before they threaten the viability of the teeth, gums, and other oral soft tissues; in addition, more frequent visits are necessary for persons at increased risk by virtue of their age, risk factors (e.g., pregnancy, smoking, alcohol abuse), state of periodontal health, rate of accumulation of tartar, personal oral hygiene practices, and medical and dental history (e.g., diabetes mellitus, xerostomia, infection with human immunodeficiency virus).

Effectiveness of Counseling

There is little information on the effectiveness of physician advice in changing oral hygiene habits, increasing the optimal use of fluoride supplements, or increasing patient visits to dentists. It is well known among dentists, however, that patients frequently face difficulties in complying with guidelines for proper tooth brushing and dental flossing without repeated reinforcement. Recommendations to limit intake of foods containing refined sugars and between-meal sweet snacks are especially problematic for children. There is little information regarding the willingness or ability of patients to comply with physician advice to visit the dentist for a routine checkup.

In communities with inadequate water fluoridation, primary care physicians are an important source of supplemental fluoride drops or tablets to prevent dental caries in children. There is little information on patient compliance with such prescriptions. Studies have shown, however, that physicians often fail to prescribe dietary fluoride supplements in accordance with existing guidelines.[40]

Recommendations of Others

The Canadian Task Force recommends an annual examination for caries, orthodontic conditions, and periodontal disease and annual counseling to perform daily oral hygiene beginning at age 12; the dental examination should include visual and tactile inspection and, when appropriate, dental x-rays.[41] The American Dental Association (ADA) advises that the frequency of dental examinations be tailored to the individual.[42] Both the ADA[43] and the American Academy of Pediatrics[44] have issued guidelines on the prescription of dietary fluoride supplements for children in areas with inadequate water fluoridation.

Discussion

Although there is little scientific evidence that physician counseling can reduce the incidence of dental diseases such as caries and periodontal disease, it is reasonable to provide patients with information about proven methods to reduce the risk of developing these potentially painful and disfiguring conditions. There is sufficient evidence of benefit to justify efforts by physicians and other health care professionals to encourage frequent tooth brushing, daily dental flossing, appropriate use of fluorides, and periodic visits to the dentist. There is, however, little evidence that this form of counseling must be performed frequently, or that annual or semiannual dental checkups are necessary for persons without clinical evidence of dental disease. Although it is likely that consuming fewer foods containing refined sugars or avoiding between-meal sweets will reduce the incidence of dental caries, this has not been demonstrated in a controlled prospective study. Nonetheless, it is clinically prudent to recommend these dietary changes. Finally, clinicians can offer advice regarding effective measures to reduce the risk of developing oral cancer, such as discontinuing the use of tobacco products and reducing the consumption of alcoholic beverages (see Chapter 15).

Clinical Intervention

All patients should be encouraged to visit the dentist on a regular basis. The optimal frequency of visits should be determined by the patient's dentist; for most healthy patients, a dental checkup once every one to two years is sufficient. All patients should also be encouraged to brush their teeth daily with a fluoride-containing toothpaste. Adolescents and adults should be advised to clean thoroughly between the teeth with dental floss each day. Those persons with a history of frequent caries may benefit from reduced intake of foods containing refined sugars and by avoiding sugary between-meal snacks. Pregnant women, parents, and caregivers of young children should be counseled to put children to bed without a bottle and to substitute a cup for the bottle when the child reaches 1 year of age. If the child must have a bottle, it should be filled with water.

In accordance with existing guidelines,[43,44] children living in an area with inadequate water fluoridation (less than 0.7 parts per million [ppm]) should be prescribed daily fluoride drops or tablets. Fluoride tablets should be prescribed for children over age 3; the recommended dose is 1 mg/day if the community water fluoride concentration is less than 0.3 ppm, and 0.50 mg/day if the concentration is 0.3–0.7 ppm. For children 2 to 3 years of age, the corresponding doses are 0.50 mg/day and 0.25 mg/day, respectively, and either drops or tablets are appropriate. Children under age 2 should be treated with fluoride drops if the water concentration is less than 0.3 ppm; the recommended dose is 0.25 mg/day.

When examining the mouth, clinicians should be alert for obvious signs of untreated tooth decay, inflamed or cyanotic gingiva, loose teeth, and severe halitosis. Screening for oral cancer should be performed for high-risk groups (see Chapter 15), and all patients should be counseled regarding the use of tobacco products (Chapter 48). Children should also be examined for evidence of baby bottle tooth decay, mismatching of upper and lower dental arches, crowding or malalignment of the teeth, premature loss of primary posterior teeth (baby molars), and obvious mouth breathing. Patients with these or other suspected abnormalities should be referred to their dentist for further evaluation.

Note: See Appendix A for the U.S. Preventive Services Task Force Table of Ratings for this topic. See also the relevant Task Force background paper: Greene JC, Louie R, Wycoff SJ. Preventive dentistry. In: Goldbloom RB, Lawrence RS, eds. Preventing disease: beyond the rhetoric. New York: Springer-Verlag (in press).

REFERENCES

1. National Institute of Dental Research. The prevalence of dental caries in United States children 1979–80. The National Dental Caries Prevalence Survey. Bethesda, Md.: National Institute of Dental Research, 1981. (Publication no. DHHS (NIH) 82–2245.)

2. *Idem.* Survey shows dramatic decline in tooth decay among U.S. children. NIDR Research News, June 21, 1988.
3. National Center for Health Statistics. Decayed, missing, and filled teeth among persons 1–74 years, United States. Data from the National Health Survey. Vital and Health Statistics, series 11, no. 223. Hyattsville, Md.: National Center for Health Statistics, 1981. (Publication no. DHHS (PHS) 81–1673.)
4. National Institute of Dental Research. Oral health of United States adults, the national survey of oral health in U.S. employed adults and seniors: 1985–86. Bethesda, Md.: National Institute of Dental Research, 1987. (Publication no. DHHS (NIH) 87–2868.)
5. National Center for Health Statistics. Basic data on dental examination findings of persons 1–74 years, U.S. 1971–1974. Vital and Health Statistics, series 11, no. 214. Hyattsville, Md.: National Center for Health Statistics, 1979. (Publication no. DHEW (PHS) 79–1662.)
6. *Idem.* Current estimates from the National Health Interview Survey, United States, 1982. Vital and Health Statistics, series 10, no. 150. Hyattsville, Md.: National Center for Health Statistics, 1985. (Publication no. DHHS (PHS) 85–1578.)
7. Health Care Financing Administration. Health care financing review. VIII (4). Washington, D.C.: Health Care Financing Administration, 1987.
8. Hunt RJ, Beck JD, Lemke JH, et al. Edentulism and oral health problems among elderly rural Iowans: the Iowa 65+ rural health study. Am J Public Health 1985; 75:1177–81.
9. Dunning JM. Principles of dental public health. Cambridge, Mass.: Harvard University Press, 1986:409–14.
10. Centers for Disease Control. Fluoridation census, 1985. U.S. Department of Health and Human Services. Washington, D.C.: Public Health Service, 1988.
11. Driscoll WS. The use of fluoride tablets for the prevention of dental caries. In: Forrester DJ, Schulz EM Jr, eds. International Workshop on Fluorides and Dental Caries Reductions. Baltimore, Md.: School of Dentistry, University of Maryland, 1974:25–93.
12. Carlos JP. Fluoride mouthrinses. In: Wei S, ed. Clinical uses of fluorides. Philadelphia: Lea and Febiger, 1985:75–82.
13. Heifetz SB, Meyers RJ, Kingman A. A comparison of the anticaries effectiveness of daily and weekly rinsing with sodium-fluoride: final results after three years. Pediatr Dent 1982; 4:300–3.
14. Driscoll WS, Swango PA, Horowitz AM, et al. Caries-preventive effects of daily and weekly fluoride mouthrinsing in a fluoridated community: final results after 30 months. J Am Dent Assoc 1982; 105:1010–3.
15. Newburn E, ed. Fluorides and dental caries, 3rd ed. Springfield, Ill.: CC Thomas, 1986.
16. Stookey GH. Are all fluoride dentifrices the same? In: Wei S, ed. Clinical uses of fluorides. Philadelphia: Lea and Febiger, 1985:105–31.
17. Mellberg JM, Ripa LW. Fluoride dentifrices. In: Mellberg JM, Ripa LW, eds. Fluoride in preventive dentistry: theory and clinical application. Chicago, Ill.: Quintessence, 1983: 215–41.
18. Gustafsson BE, Quensel CE, Lanke LS, et al. The Vipeholm dental caries study: the effect of different levels of carbohydrate intake on caries activity in 436 individuals observed for 5 years. Acta Odontol Scand 1954; 11:232–364.
19. Harris R. Biology of the children of Hopewood House, Bowral, Australia. IV. Observations of dental caries experience extending over five years (1957–1961). J Dent Res 1963; 42:1387–98.
20. Burt RA, Eklund SA, Morgan KJ, et al. The effect of diet on the development of dental caries. Final report, contract DE-22438. Bethesda, Md.: National Institute of Dental Research, 1987.
21. Rugg-Gunn AJ, Hackett AF, Appleton DR, et al. Relationship between dietary habits and caries increments assessed over two years in 405 English adolescent schoolchildren. Arch Oral Biol 1984; 29:983–92.
22. Loesche WJ. Nutrition and dental decay in infants. Am J Clin Nutr 1985; 41:423–35.
23. Ripa LW. Nursing habits and dental decay in infants: "nursing bottle caries." J Dent Child 1978; 45:274–5.
24. Andlaw RJ. Oral hygiene and dental caries: a review. Int Dent J 1978; 28:1–6.

25. Suomi JD, Greene JC, Vermillion JR, et al. The effect of controlled oral hygiene procedures on the progression of periodontal disease in adults: results after third and final year. J Periodontol 1971; 42:152–60.
26. Horowitz AM, Suomi JD, Peterson JK, et al. Effects of supervised daily dental plaque removal by children after 3 years. Community Dent Oral Epidemiol 1980; 8:171–6.
27. Lang NP, Cumming BR, Loe H. Toothbrush frequency as it is related to plaque development and gingival health. J Periodontol 1973; 44:398–405.
28. Ripa LW. Professionally (operator) applied topical fluoride therapy: a critique. Clin Prev Dent 1982; 4:3–10.
29. Idem. The current status of pit and fissure sealants: a review. Can Dent Assoc J 1985; 5:367–80.
30. Mertz-Fairhurst EJ, Fairhurst CW, Williams JE, et al. A comparative clinical study of two pit and fissure sealants: 7–year results in Augusta, Georgia. J Am Dent Assoc 1984; 109:252–5.
31. Axelsson P, Lindhe J. The effect of a preventive program on dental plaque, gingivitis and caries in school children: results after one and two years. J Clin Periodontol 1974; 1:126–38.
32. Idem. The effect of various plaque control measures on gingivitis and caries in school children. Community Dent Oral Epidemiol 1976; 4:232–9.
33. Agerback N, De Paola PF, Brudevold F. Effects of professional toothcleaning every third week on gingivitis and dental caries in children. Community Dent Oral Epidemiol 1978; 6:40–1.
34. Ashley FP, Sainsbury RH. The effect of a school-based plaque control programme on caries and gingivitis. Br Dent J 1981; 150:41–5.
35. Badersten A, Egelberg J, Koch G. Effect of monthly prophylaxis on caries and gingivitis in schoolchildren. Community Dent Oral Epidemiol 1975; 3:1–4.
36. Hamp SE, Lindhe J, Fornell LA, et al. Effect of a field program based on systematic plaque control on caries and gingivitis in schoolchildren after 3 years. Community Dent Oral Epidemiol 1978; 6:17–23.
37. Loe H, Kleinman DV. Dental plaque control measures and oral hygiene practices. Proceedings from a state-of-the-science workshop. Washington, D.C.: IRL Press, 1986.
38. Axelsson P, Lindhe J. Effect of controlled oral hygiene procedures on caries and periodontal disease in adults: results after six years. J Clin Periodontol 1981; 8:239–48.
39. Sheiham A. Is there a scientific basis for six-monthly dental examinations? Lancet 1977; 2:442–4.
40. Margolis FJ, Burt BA, Schork MA, et al. Fluoride supplements for children: a survey of physicians' prescription practices. Am J Dis Child 1980; 134:865–8.
41. Canadian Task Force on the Periodic Health Examination. The periodic health examination. Can Med Assoc J 1979; 121:1–45.
42. American Dental Association. The importance of professional teeth cleaning. Chicago, Ill.: American Dental Association, 1985.
43. Idem. Prescribing fluoride supplements. In: Accepted Dental Therapeutics, 39th ed. Chicago, Ill.: American Dental Association, 1982.
44. American Academy of Pediatrics. Fluoride supplementation: revised dosage schedule. Pediatrics 1979; 63:150.

III. Immunizations/
Chemoprophylaxis

56

Childhood Immunizations

Recommendation: All children without established contraindications should receive diphtheria-tetanus-pertussis (DTP), oral poliovirus (OPV), measles-mumps-rubella (MMR), and conjugate *Haemophilus influenzae* type b vaccines in accordance with recommended schedules (see *Clinical Intervention*). A tetanus-diphtheria (Td) booster should be administered at age 14–16 years and every 10 years thereafter.

Burden of Suffering

A number of infectious diseases are almost completely preventable through routine childhood immunizations. These include diphtheria, pertussis, tetanus, poliomyelitis, *Haemophilus influenzae* type b infection, measles, mumps, and rubella. Largely as a result of widespread childhood vaccination, these diseases have become considerably less common in the United States than in prevaccination years. A comparison of the total number of reported cases in the United States in 1987 and in the years preceding vaccination reveals an impressive decrease in reported cases of measles (from 481,530 [1962] to 3655 cases), pertussis (from 74,715 [1948] to 2823 cases), diphtheria (from 9493 [1948] to 3 cases), tetanus (from 601 [1948] to 48 cases), and paralytic poliomyelitis (from 18,308 [1954] to 5 cases).[1] Before the introduction of poliovirus vaccine in 1955, this disease occurred in epidemic waves of increasing magnitude, reaching a peak incidence of more than 20,000 paralytic cases in 1952.[2] The last outbreak in 1979, however, totaled only 10 paralytic cases.[3] Systemic illness from *Haemophilus influenzae* type b occurs before age 5 in about 1 out of every 200 children born in the United States.[4] Severe systemic complications include meningitis, the most common clinical presentation in children, as well as pneumonia, arthritis, epiglottitis, and cellulitis.

Efficacy of Vaccines

The efficacy of the DTP and MMR vaccines are well established on the basis of clinical studies and decades of experience with universal childhood immunization.[5-7] Although a single dose of MMR is highly protective, a two-stage vaccination protocol against measles may be necessary in areas with recurrent measles transmission.[8] The MMR vaccine is associated with rare adverse effects. Approximately one case of encephalitis or encephalopathy has been reported in temporal association with vaccination for every million doses of measles-containing vaccines distributed.[9] Increased attention has focused in recent years on the safety of the pertussis vaccine.[10] The whole-cell preparation, which confers 80–90% protection after three doses, produces serious adverse events such as seizures and hypotonic/hyporesponsive episodes in 1 out of 1750 doses.[11] The risk of seizures may be higher in certain children, such as those with a personal history or family history of seizures.[12] However, limited follow-up of such cases suggests most if not all are associated with benign outcomes.[13] Very rarely (1/140,000 doses), pertussis-containing vaccines have been associated with more severe neurologic illnesses, including encephalopathy, which may result in permanent brain damage (1/330,000 doses).[14] The incidence of serious neurologic disorders following DTP administration is substantially less than that following pertussis disease.[14] Acellular forms of pertussis vaccine with fewer side effects are being evaluated as alternatives, but it is currently not known if they are as effective as whole cell vaccines.[15,16]

The oral attenuated live poliomyelitis vaccine (OPV) offers 95–100% protection against poliovirus. As a result, disease caused by wild poliovirus has been virtually eliminated in the United States. However, 1 out of every 2.6 million vaccine doses results in paralytic poliomyelitis.[3] Most cases of endemic disease in the United States since 1981 (about eight cases per year) have been associated with the vaccine.[3] The development and recent licensing of enhanced-potency inactivated poliomyelitis vaccine (IPV), which is not known to carry this risk and appears to have comparable immunogenicity,[17,18] has led some to recommend replacement of the live vaccine with this product. IPV may be less effective, however, in limiting transmission of wild poliovirus among susceptible members of the population.[3] To take advantage of the properties of both vaccines, the Institute of Medicine has recently recommended consideration of a schedule consisting of two or more doses of IPV followed by OPV, once a combined preparation of DTP and IPV becomes available.[19]

The efficacy of a capsular polysaccharide vaccine in preventing infection with Haemophilus influenzae type b in children over age 2 was first demonstrated in Finland in 1984.[20] The polysaccharide vaccine had limited efficacy in children under 18 months of age and questionable efficacy in those aged 18–24 months. Subsequent studies in the United States have produced inconsistent and occasionally conflicting results in attempts to confirm the efficacy of the polysaccharide vaccine and the optimal age for its administration.[21-26] The uncertain performance characteristics of the vaccine in children under 2 years of age is of significance because three-quarters of all systemic illnesses occur in this age group. A more immunogenic conjugate vaccine recently has been demonstrated in Finland to have 87% efficacy in children less than 12 months of age.[27] Based on its superior immunogenicity, the conjugate vaccine has been licensed in the United States for use in children 18 months of age or older.[28,29] Its use in American infants will have to await the results of confirmatory studies.

Recommendations of Others

Detailed recommendations on the administration of childhood vaccines are issued regularly by the Immunization Practices Advisory Committee[30] and the American Academy of Pediatrics.[9] In recent years, the Immunization Practices Advisory Committee has also issued specific updates on the use of DTP vaccine;[6,31] IPV;[18] measles vaccine;[7,8] and Haemophilus influenzae type b polysaccharide and conjugate vaccines.[28-29,32-33] These recommendations have recently been combined in one report.[34]

Clinical Intervention

The recommended childhood immunization schedule[30] includes DTP vaccine along with trivalent OPV at ages 2 months, 4 months, 6 months (DTP only), 15 months, and finally between ages 4 and 6 years just prior to school entry. MMR vaccine should be administered at age 15 months, and *Haemophilus influenzae* type b conjugate vaccine should be given at 18 months of age. In areas with recurrent measles transmission, such as counties or cities reporting more than five cases among preschool-aged children during each of the previous five years, monovalent measles vaccine should be administered at 9 months of age (or first visit thereafter) in addition to administering MMR vaccine at age 15 months. A Td booster should be administered at age 14–16 years and every 10 years thereafter. Clinicians are referred to published guidelines for details on vaccine contraindications, instructions for immunizing children with medical disorders, and modified protocols recommended during community outbreaks or epidemics.[9,30]

Note: See Appendix A for the U.S. Preventive Services Task Force Table of Ratings for this topic. See also the relevant Task Force background paper: LaForce FM. Immunizations, immunoprophylaxis, and chemoprophylaxis to prevent selected infections. JAMA 1987; 257:2464–70.

REFERENCES

1. Centers for Disease Control. Summary of notifiable diseases, United States, 1987. MMWR 1988; 36:1–59.
2. Langmuir AD. Inactivated virus vaccines: protective efficacy. In: International Poliomyelitis Congress. Poliomyelitis. Philadelphia: JB Lippincott, 1961:240–56.
3. Hinman AR, Koplan JP, Orenstein WA, et al. Live or inactivated poliovirus vaccine: an analysis of benefits and risks. Am J Public Health 1988; 78:291–5.
4. Cochi SL, Broome CV, Hightower AW. Immunization of children with *Haemophilus influenzae* type b vaccine: a cost-effectiveness model of strategy assessment. JAMA 1985; 253:521–9.
5. Edsall G. Specific prophylaxis of tetanus. JAMA 1959; 171:417–27.
6. Immunization Practices Advisory Committee. Diphtheria, tetanus, and pertussis: guidelines for vaccine prophylaxis and other preventive measures. MMWR 1985; 34:405–14,419–26.
7. *Idem.* Measles prevention. MMWR 1987; 36:409–18,423–5.
8. *Idem.* Measles prevention: supplementary statement. MMWR 1989; 38:11–4.
9. Peter G, Giebink GS, Hall CB, et al., eds. Report of the Committee on Infectious Diseases, 20th ed. Elk Grove, Ill.: American Academy of Pediatrics, 1986:266–75.
10. Hinman AR, Koplan JP. Pertussis and pertussis vaccine: reanalysis of benefits, risks, and costs. JAMA 1984; 251:3109–13.
11. Cody CL, Baraff LJ, Cherry JD, et al. Nature and rates of adverse reactions associated with DTP and DT immunizations in infants and children. Pediatrics 1981; 68:650–60.
12. Stetler HC, Orenstein WA, Bart KJ, et al. History of convulsions and use of pertussis vaccine. J Pediatr 1985; 107:175–9.
13. Baraff LJ, Shields WD, Beckwith L, et al. Infants and children with convulsions and hypotonic-hyporesponsive episodes following diphtheria-tetanus-pertussis immunization: follow-up evaluation. Pediatrics 1988; 81:789–94.
14. Miller D, Wadsworth J, Diamond J, et al. Pertussis vaccine and whooping cough as risk factors in acute neurological illness and death in young children. Dev Biol Stand 1985; 61:389–94.
15. Aoyama T, Murase Y, Kato T, et al. Efficacy of an acellular pertussis vaccine in Japan. J Pediatr 1985; 107:180–3.
16. Ad Hoc Group for the Study of Pertussis Vaccines. Placebo controlled trial of two acellular

pertussis vaccines in Sweden: protective efficacy and adverse events. Lancet 1988; 1:955–60.

17. McBean AM, Thomas MI, Johnson RH, et al. A comparison of the serological responses to oral and injectable trivalent poliovirus vaccine. Rev Infect Dis 1984; 6:S552–5.

18. Centers for Disease Control. Poliomyelitis prevention: enhanced-potency inactivated poliomyelitis vaccine—supplementary statement. MMWR 1987; 36:795–8.

19. Institute of Medicine. An evaluation of poliomyelitis vaccine policy options. Washington, D.C.: National Academy Press, 1988.

20. Peltola H, Kayhty H, Virtanen M, et al. Prevention of *Haemophilus influenzae* type b bacteremic infection with the capsular polysaccharide vaccine. N Engl J Med 1984; 310:1561–6.

21. Daum RS, Granoff DM, Gilsdorf J, et al. *Haemophilus influenzae* type b infections in day care attendees: implications for management. Rev Infect Dis 1986; 8:558–67.

22. Granoff DM, Schackelford PG, Suarez BK, et al. *Haemophilus influenzae* type b disease in children vaccinated with type b polysaccharide vaccine. N Engl J Med 1986; 315: 1584–90.

23. Shapiro ED, Murphy TD, Wald ER, et al. The protective efficacy of *Haemophilus* b polysaccharide vaccine. JAMA 1988; 260:1419–22.

24. Harrison LH, Broome CV, Hightower AW, et al. A day care-based study of the efficacy of *Haemophilus* b polysaccharide vaccine. JAMA 1988; 260:1413–8.

25. Osterholm MT, Rambeck JH, White KE, et al. Lack of efficacy of *Haemophilus* b polysaccharide vaccination in Minnesota. JAMA 1988; 260:1423–8.

26. Black SB, Shinefield HR, Hiatt RA, et al. Efficacy of *Haemophilus influenzae* type b capsular polysaccharide vaccine. Pediatr Infect Dis 1988; 7:149–56.

27. Eskola J, Peltola H, Takala AK, et al. Efficacy of *Haemophilus influenzae* type b polysaccharide-diphtheria toxoid conjugate vaccine in infancy. N Engl J Med 1987; 317: 717–22.

28. Immunization Practices Advisory Committee. Update: prevention of *Haemophilus influenzae* type b disease. MMWR 1988; 37:13–6.

29. Centers for Disease Control. Update: *Haemophilus influenzae* type b vaccine. MMWR 1989; 38:14.

30. Immunization Practices Advisory Committee. New recommended schedule for active immunization of normal infants and children. MMWR 1986; 35:577–9.

31. *Idem.* Pertussis immunization: family history of convulsions and use of antipyretics—supplementary ACIP statement. MMWR 1987; 36:281–2.

32. *Idem.* Polysaccharide vaccine for prevention of *Haemophilus influenzae* type b disease. MMWR 1985; 34:201–5.

33. *Idem.* Update: prevention of *Haemophilus influenzae* type b disease. MMWR 1986; 35:170–4,179–80.

34. *Idem.* General recommendations on immunization. MMWR 1989; 38:205–14,219–27.

57

Adult Immunizations

Recommendation: Pneumococcal vaccine should be administered at least once and influenza vaccine should be administered annually to all persons aged 65 and older and to persons in selected high-risk groups (see *Clinical Intervention*). Hepatitis B vaccine should be offered to homosexually active men, intravenous drug users, and others at high risk for infection (see *Clinical Intervention*). Recommendations for persons with possible percutaneous or sexual exposure to persons infected with hepatitis B virus are in Chapter 58 (see also Chapter 20). All adults should receive tetanus-diphtheria toxoid boosters at least once every 10 years. Vaccination against measles and mumps should be provided to all adults who lack evidence of immunity. Recommendations for rubella immunization are provided in Chapter 36.

Burden of Suffering

Pneumococcal disease and influenza are significant causes of morbidity and mortality in the United States. Pneumococcal disease accounts for about 40,000 deaths each year,[1] and pneumococcal pneumonia is fatal in 5% of patients.[2-4] Bacteremia occurs in 20% of patients with pneumococcal pneumonia and has a mortality of 20–40%.[2,3,5,6] Influenza, which frequently causes incapacitating malaise for several days, is responsible for significant morbidity and decreased productivity during epidemics. Ten thousand or more excess deaths have been documented in 19 different epidemics during 1957–1986; more than 40,000 excess deaths occurred in each of several recent influenza epidemics.[7] During severe pandemics (e.g., 1957 and 1968), there are often high attack rates across all age groups, and mortality is usually markedly increased. Elderly persons and persons with underlying medical disorders are at increased risk for complications from both pneumococcal and influenza infections. About 80–90% of all reported deaths from influenza occur among persons aged 65 and older.[7]

Measles, a childhood illness, occurred in 486 American adults (aged 20 or older) in 1987.[8] Adult cases accounted for nearly 15% of all reported cases.[8] About 40% of adult infections occur among persons aged 20–24,[8] often in places where young adults congregate, such as college campuses.[9]

Over 300,000 persons become infected with hepatitis B virus each year, and more than 10,000 require hospitalization.[10,11] An estimated 500,000 to 1 million persons in the United States are chronic carriers of hepatitis B virus.[11] About one-quarter of them develop chronic active hepatitis, and this often progresses to cirrhosis.[11] An estimated 4000 hepatitis B-related deaths occur each year as a result of cirrhosis, and more than 1000 occur as a result of liver cancer.[1,11]

Largely as a result of routine immunization, tetanus and diphtheria have become uncommon diseases in the United States; only 48 cases of tetanus and 3 cases of diphtheria were reported in 1987.[8] In 1948, before tetanus and diphtheria toxoids were widely introduced, there were over 600 cases of tetanus and about 9500 cases of diphtheria in the United States. Although uncommon, tetanus remains a serious infection, with death occurring in 26–31% of cases.[12] The case-fatality ratio (proportion of cases resulting in death) is greater than 30% for persons aged 50 and older, who account for over two-thirds of all cases.

Efficacy of Vaccines

The 14-valent polysaccharide pneumococcal vaccine, which was licensed in 1977, was replaced in 1983 by a 23-valent polysaccharide vaccine.[2] The latter contains purified capsular materials from 88% of the strains of *Streptococcus pneumoniae* causing bacteremic pneumococcal disease reported in the United States.[13] The efficacy of pneumococcal vaccine in the U.S. population has not been determined with certainty. Although it appeared to be effective in controlled trials during the 1970s involving high-risk populations in other countries,[14,15] controlled trials in the United States involving older adults have failed to demonstrate protective efficacy.[16] The relatively low incidence of pneumococcal infection in healthy U.S. adults makes efficacy difficult to establish in a prospective clinical trial. Case-control studies and studies comparing the distribution of pneumococcal serotypes in the blood of vaccinated and unvaccinated persons, which have been much more feasible to perform, support the protective value of pneumococcal vaccine, with estimates of 60–70% efficacy reported in immunocompetent recipients.[17-20] Other studies, including a randomized placebo-controlled trial, have found the vaccine to have more limited efficacy.[21,22] Additional research is needed to obtain more definitive data on the efficacy of pneumococcal vaccine. There is, however, little evidence of serious adverse effects from this vaccine, although erythema and pain at the injection site occur in about half of patients. Fever, myalgias, and severe reactions occur in no more than 1% of patients.[13,23] The total duration of antibody protection is unknown; elevated titers appear to persist in adults for at least 5 years after immunization but, in some persons, they may fall to prevaccination levels within 10 years.[13]

Influenza vaccine containing antigens identical or similar to currently circulating influenza A and B viruses has been shown in controlled studies to be 70–80% effective.[24] Although no controlled clinical trials have studied the vaccine in the high-risk groups for whom it is generally recommended, retrospective studies support its efficacy in elderly high-risk populations.[25,26] Because of frequent seasonal variation in the hemagglutinin and neuraminidase antigens of circulating viruses, it is necessary to administer the vaccine annually in the fall so that it can include antigens known from recent surveillance data to be circulating during the season. Although allergic reactions have been described in patients with sensitivity to eggs, adverse effects from influenza vaccine are quite uncommon.[27]

Amantadine is 70–90% effective in preventing illness caused by naturally occurring strains of influenza A.[7,26,28] Since it does not prevent influenza B infection, it is appropriate only in presumed influenza A epidemics. It is most useful as short-term prophylaxis for high-risk persons who have not received the vaccine or are vaccinated late, when the vaccine may be ineffective due to major antigenic changes in the virus; for unvaccinated persons who provide home care for high-risk persons;

or to supplement protection provided by vaccine in persons who are expected to have a poor antibody response,[7,29] It may also be useful throughout the epidemic period for some high-risk patients In whom the vaccine is contraindicated. Amantadine occasionally produces insomnia, nausea, dizziness, and impaired concentration, and it has been associated with falls in the elderly.[7,29]

A single dose of measles vaccine is 95% effective in producing long-term immunity, presumably for the life of the patient.[30] Recent vaccine failures have been associated primarily with the timing of vaccination during infancy and early childhood.[31] As childhood measles vaccination has become more common, the age distribution of new cases has shifted to older age groups, with increased incidence in older adolescents and young adults, primarily college students. Adult infections are more likely in persons who have not been naturally infected or properly vaccinated in the past. Vaccination of young adults in settings such as colleges and the workplace is likely to be most effective. Persons born before 1957 are likely to have been naturally infected and need not be considered susceptible.[32] Administration of combined measles-mumps-rubella (MMR) vaccine is not associated with adverse effects for persons already immune to any of these diseases, and thus the combined MMR vaccine is preferable to measles vaccine since many recipients may also be susceptible to mumps or rubella. Although susceptible adolescent and young adults should be vaccinated against mumps, routine mumps vaccination is not necessary for persons in these age groups since most are likely already to have been infected naturally.[33] Rubella immunization is discussed in Chapter 36.

Plasma-derived hepatitis B vaccine, which became available in 1982, has 85–95% protective efficacy when administered in three intramuscular doses to immunocompetent patients.[34-37] A newer vaccine, produced by recombinant DNA technology, was licensed in 1986 and appears to induce protective antibodies in more than 95% of young adult (aged 20–39) vaccinees. Older adults generate a somewhat lower antibody response to both vaccines.[10,11] Injection at the buttocks has been associated with a suboptimal immune response, and therefore the deltoid muscle is the preferred injection site. Local soreness at the injection site is a common side effect. Immunity from hepatitis B vaccine appears to last at least seven years. The possible need for booster doses after longer intervals will be assessed as additional data become available.

Tetanus-diphtheria toxoid (Td) is highly effective in producing protective antibody titers, but it requires a primary series of three doses, followed by booster doses every 10 years.[38] Td often produces mild local inflammation and occasionally Arthus-type reactions.

Recommendations of Others:

Detailed physician guidelines on adult immunizations have been published by the American College of Physicians[29] and the Immunization Practices Advisory Committee.[30] These groups have also issued recent, updated recommendations on the use of tetanus and diphtheria toxoids[39] and pneumococcal,[13,40] influenza,[7,27] hepatitis B,[10,11] and measles[32] vaccines. These recommendations are not universally accepted, however; for example, some authors argue against routine vaccination of the elderly against influenza and pneumococcal disease in the absence of known risk factors.[41] The use of amantadine to prevent influenza was recommended in 1980 by a National Institutes of Health consensus development conference[42] and has recently been the subject of recommendations by the Immunization Practices Advisory Committee.[7] The American College of Obstetricians and Gynecologists has issued detailed guidelines on the use of vaccines during pregnancy.[43]

Discussion

Most adults have not been immunized in accordance with existing immunization guidelines.[1] The cost of vaccines is one possible barrier to widespread immunization, but studies have shown that the prevention of morbidity and mortality from infectious diseases makes immunization cost effective. For example, routine pneumococcal vaccination of persons aged 65 and older has been estimated to cost about $6000 (1983 dollars) for every year of healthy life gained.[44] Hepatitis B vaccination of high-risk groups has also proved to be cost-effective.[45,46]

Clinical Intervention

Pneumococcal vaccination should be provided at least once to all persons aged 65 and older and to those with medical conditions that increase the risk of pneumococcal infection (e.g., chronic cardiac or pulmonary disease, sickle cell disease, nephrotic syndrome, Hodgkin's disease, asplenia, diabetes mellitus, alcoholism, cirrhosis, multiple myeloma, renal disease, and conditions associated with immunosuppression). Patients living in special environments or social settings with an identified increased risk of pneumococcal disease should also be vaccinated. Although routine revaccination is not recommended, it may be appropriate to consider revaccination in high-risk persons who have not been vaccinated for six or more years or in those who received the older 14-valent vaccine. Influenza vaccine should be administered annually to all persons aged 65 and older, residents of chronic care facilities, and persons suffering from chronic cardiopulmonary disorders, metabolic diseases (including diabetes mellitus), hemoglobinopathies, immunosuppression, or renal dysfunction. Health care providers for high-risk patients should also receive influenza vaccine. In persons at high risk for influenza A, amantadine prophylaxis (100 mg orally per day) may be started at the time of vaccination and continued for two weeks. If vaccine is contraindicated, amantadine should be started at the beginning of the influenza season and continued daily for the duration of influenza activity in the community.

Hepatitis B vaccine should be offered to susceptible individuals in high-risk groups, including homosexually active men, intravenous drug users, recipients of certain blood products, and persons in health-related jobs with frequent exposure to blood or blood products. The recommended regimen for both the plasma-derived and recombinant hepatitis B vaccine is to administer 10 mcg IM in the deltoid muscle at the time of exposure and at 1 and 6 months following exposure. Infants born to mothers who are positive for hepatitis B surface antigen should be immunized beginning at birth (see Chapter 20). Immunization recommendations for persons with possible percutaneous or sexual exposure to individuals infected with hepatitis B virus are in Chapter 58.

All adults should receive a Td booster at least once every 10 years. The complete series of combined tetanus-diphtheria toxoids should be given to patients who have not received a primary series.

MMR vaccine should be administered to all persons born after 1956 who lack evidence of immunity to measles (receipt of live vaccine on or after the first birthday, laboratory evidence of immunity, or a history of physician-

diagnosed measles). **The MMR vaccine should not be administered during pregnancy. Susceptible individuals should be vaccinated against mumps. See also Chapter 36 regarding rubella vaccination of susceptible women of childbearing age.**

Note: See Appendix A for the U.S. Preventive Services Task Force Table of Ratings for this topic. See also the relevant Task Force background paper: LaForce MF. Immunizations, immunoprophylaxis, and chemoprophylaxis to prevent selected infections. JAMA 1987; 257:2464–70.

REFERENCES

1. Williams WW, Hickson MA, Kane MA, et al. Immunization policies and vaccine coverage among adults: the risk for missed opportunities. Ann Intern Med 1988; 108:616–25.
2. Centers for Disease Control. Update: pneumococcal polysaccharide vaccine usage— United States. MMWR 1984; 33:273–6,281.
3. Schwartz JS. Pneumococcal vaccine: clinical efficacy and effectiveness. Ann Intern Med 1982; 96:208–20.
4. Foy HM, Wentworth B, Kenny GE, et al. Pneumococcal isolations from patients with pneumonia and control subjects in a prepaid medical care group. Am Rev Respir Dis 1975; 3:595–603.
5. Austrian R, Gold J. Pneumococcal bacteremia with special reference to bacteremic pneumococcal pneumonia. Ann Intern Med 1964; 60:759–76.
6. Mufson MA, Kruss DM, Wasil RE, et al. Capsular types and outcome of bacteremic pneumococcal disease in the antibiotic era. Arch Intern Med 1974; 134:505–10.
7. Immunization Practices Advisory Committee. Prevention and control of influenza. MMWR 1988; 37:361–4.
8. Centers for Disease Control. Summary of notifiable diseases, United States. MMWR 1988; 36:1–59.
9. Idem. Measles on college campus—United States, 1985. MMWR 1985; 254:445–9.
10. Immunization Practices Advisory Committee. Update on hepatitis B prevention. Ann Intern Med 1987; 107:353–7.
11. Idem. Recommendations for protection against viral hepatitis. MMWR 1985; 34:313–24,329–35.
12. Centers for Disease Control. Tetanus—United States, 1985–1986. MMWR 1987; 36: 477–81.
13. Immunization Practices Advisory Committee. Pneumococcal polysaccharide vaccine. MMWR 1989; 38:64–8,73–5.
14. Austrian R, Douglas RM, Schiffman G, et al. Prevention of pneumococcal pneumonia by vaccination. Trans Assoc Am Physicians 1976; 89:184–94.
15. Riley ID, Tarr PI, Andrews M, et al. Immunisation with a polyvalent pneumococcal vaccine: reduction of adult respiratory mortality in a New Guinea Highlands community. Lancet 1977; 1:1338–41.
16. Austrian R. Surveillance of pneumococcal infection for field trials of polyvalent pneumococcal vaccines. Report DAB-VDP-12–84. Bethesda, Md.: National Institutes of Health, 1980.
17. Shapiro ED, Clemens JD. A controlled evaluation of the protective efficacy of pneumococcal vaccine for patients at high risk of serious pneumococcal infections. Ann Intern Med 1984; 101:325–30.
18. Shapiro ED, Austrian R, Adair RK, et al. The protective efficacy of pneumococcal vaccine. Clin Res 1988; 36:470A. abstract.
19. Bolan G, Broome CV, Facklam RR, et al. Pneumococcal vaccine efficacy in selected populations in the United States. Ann Intern Med 1986; 104:1–6.
20. Sims RV, Steinmann WC, McConville JH, et al. The clinical effectiveness of pneumococcal vaccine in the elderly. Ann Intern Med 1988; 108:653–7.
21. Simberkoff MS, Cross AP, Al-Ibrahim M, et al. Efficacy of pneumococcal vaccine in high-

risk patients: results of a Veterans Administration cooperative study. N Engl J Med 1986; 315:318–27.

22. Forrester HL, Jahnigen DW, LaForce FM. Inefficacy of pneumococcal vaccine in a high-risk population. Am J Med 1987; 83:425–30.

23. Semel JD, Seskind C. Severe febrile reaction to pneumococcal vaccine. JAMA 1979; 241:1792.

24. Meiklejohn G. Effectiveness of monovalent influenza A-prime vaccine during the 1957 influenza A-prime epidemic. Am J Hyg 1958; 67:237–49.

25. Barker WH, Mullooly JP. Influenza vaccination of elderly persons: reduction in pneumonia and influenza hospitalizations and deaths. JAMA 1980; 244:2547–9.

26. Rubin FL. Prevention of influenza in the elderly. J Am Geriatr Soc 1982; 30:577–80.

27. Immunization Practices Advisory Committee. Prevention and control of influenza. MMWR 1985; 34:261–75.

28. Oker-Blom N, Houi T, Leinikki P, et al. Protection of man from natural infection with influenza Hong Kong virus by amantadine: a controlled study. Br Med J 1970; 3: 676–8.

29. American College of Physicians. Guide for adult immunization, 1985. Philadelphia: American College of Physicians, 1985.

30. Immunization Practices Advisory Committee. Adult immunization: recommendations of the Immunization Practices Advisory Committee (ACIP). MMWR 1984; 33:1S-68S.

31. Centers for Disease Control. Measles—United States, 1987. MMWR 1988; 37:527–31.

32. Immunization Practices Advisory Committee. Measles prevention. MMWR 1987; 36:409–18,423–5.

33. Idem. Mumps vaccine. MMWR 1982; 31:617–25.

34. Szmuness W, Stevens CE, Harley EJ, et al. Hepatitis B vaccine: demonstration of efficacy in a controlled clinical trial in a high-risk population in the United States. N Engl J Med 1980; 303:833–41.

35. Szmuness W, Stevens CE, Zang EA, et al. A controlled clinical trial of the efficacy of hepatitis B vaccine (Heptavax B): a final report. Hepatology 1981; 1:377–85.

36. Francis DP, Hadler SC, Thompson SE, et al. The prevention of hepatitis B with vaccine: report of the Centers for Disease Control multi-center efficacy trial among homosexual men. Ann Intern Med 1982; 97:362–6.

37. Krugman S. The newly licensed hepatitis B vaccine. JAMA 1982; 247:2012–5.

38. Edsall G. Specific prophylaxis of tetanus. JAMA 1959; 171:417–27.

39. Immunization Practices Advisory Committee. Diphtheria, tetanus, and pertussis: guidelines for vaccine prophylaxis and other preventive measures. MMWR 1985; 34:405–14,419–26.

40. American College of Physicians, Health and Public Policy Committee. Pneumococcal vaccine. Ann Intern Med 1986; 104:118–20.

41. Frame PS. A critical review of adult health maintenance. Part 2. Prevention of infectious diseases. J Fam Pract 1986; 22:417–22.

42. National Institutes of Health Consensus Development Conference. Amantadine: does it have a role in the prevention and treatment of influenza? Ann Intern Med 1980; 92: 256–8.

43. American College of Obstetricians and Gynecologists. Immunization during pregnancy. ACOG Technical Bulletin No. 64. Washington, D.C.: American College of Obstetricians and Gynecologists, 1982.

44. Sisk JE, Riegelman RK. Cost effectiveness of vaccination against pneumococcal pneumonia: an update. Ann Intern Med 1986; 104:79–86.

45. Jonsson B. Cost-benefit analysis of hepatitis B vaccination. Postgrad Med J [Suppl 2] 1987; 63:27–32.

46. Mulley AG, Silverstein MD, Dienstag JL. Indications for use of hepatitis B vaccine, based on cost-effectiveness analysis. N Engl J Med 1982; 307:644–52.

58

Postexposure Prophylaxis

Recommendation: Postexposure prophylaxis should be provided to selected persons with exposures to *Haemophilus influenzae* type b disease, meningococcal infection, hepatitis A, hepatitis B, tuberculosis, and rabies (see *Clinical Intervention*).

Burden of Suffering

Secondary infection following exposure to persons with certain infectious diseases may be preventable through the prompt administration of prophylactic antibiotics or immunobiologics. Although a complete discussion of each of these diseases is beyond the scope of this report, certain exposures deserve special emphasis. These include *Haemophilus influenzae* type b disease, infection with *Neisseria meningitidis*, hepatitis A and B, tuberculosis, and rabies.

Systemic *Haemophilus influenzae* type b occurs in about 1 out of every 200 children born in the United States.[1] Most cases occur during infancy,[2,3] but children remain susceptible to infection until age 5. Children are at especially increased risk if they are exposed to infected persons at home or at day-care centers.[2-4] Meningococcal infections were reported in nearly 3000 persons in 1987.[5] Infection with *Neisseria meningitidis* can lead to severe meningitis and septicemia.[6] Hepatitis A and hepatitis B each accounted for over 25,000 new cases in 1987, and over 22,000 new cases of tuberculosis were reported in the same year.[5] Human rabies remains an uncommon disease in the United States, with only nine cases diagnosed since 1980.[7] In the absence of adequate postexposure prophylaxis, however, infected persons often die from rabies encephalitis.[8]

Efficacy of Prophylaxis

Rifampin prophylaxis can reduce the risk of secondary infection in persons exposed to *Haemophilus influenzae* type b (Hib) and *Neisseria meningitidis*. Studies have shown that a four-day antibiotic regimen can reduce both the rate of asymptomatic carriage of Hib and the incidence of secondary infection in household and day-care contacts of infected persons.[3,9-11] Rifampin may also be effective in reducing secondary infection in children exposed at day-care centers to Hib-infected children.[4,12] Similarly, rifampin prophylaxis in contacts of patients with meningococcal infection can reduce the rate of colonization and secondary infection.[13] Sulfonamides are preferred over rifampin if the strain of *Neisseria meningitidis* is known to be sensitive.[14]

Since the 1940s, passive immunization with immune globulin has been shown to be an effective means of preventing infection with hepatitis A in persons exposed to active disease.[15] Standard immunoglobulin (IG) must be administered within two weeks of exposure. Hepatitis B immune globulin (HBIG) is about 75% effective when administered promptly to susceptible persons with percutaneous, sexual, or mucosal exposure to hepatitis B.[16-18] Combined HBIG plus hepatitis B vaccine is over 90% effective in preventing perinatal transmission (see Chapter 20) and is likely to be equally effective in other circumstances. For passive prophylaxis, a second HBIG dose is generally necessary after one month. This second dose can be obviated through active immunization with hepatitis B vaccine at the time of the first dose of HBIG. Active-passive immunization has the advantage of providing long-term protection against future exposure.[19] Recombinant DNA hepatitis B vaccine has recently become available in the United States and appears to be more immunogenic (see Chapter 57).

Bacille Calmette-Guerin (BCG), a live vaccine derived from attenuated *Mycobacterium bovis*, has been used worldwide for more than 50 years to prevent tuberculosis (TB). Clinical trials of the efficacy of BCG have yielded inconsistent results since the early 1930s, however, with reported levels of protection ranging from -56% to 80%.[20] In a recent report, a large controlled trial in India reported no significant reduction in the risk of sputum-positive pulmonary TB in 15 years of follow-up.[21] Observational studies have shown that the incidence of the disease is lower in vaccinated children than in unvaccinated controls.[22-27] Factors contributing to the wide variation in results in BCG vaccine efficacy include genetic changes in the bacterial strains as well as differences in production techniques, methods of administration, and the populations and environments in which the vaccine has been studied.[28] In the United States, where the risk of becoming infected with TB is relatively low, the disease can be controlled most successfully by periodic tuberculin skin testing of high-risk groups and the administration of preventive chemotherapy to those whose skin tests convert from negative to positive (see Chapter 21). However, BCG vaccination may have a role in the United States for persons with special exposures to individuals with active TB, such as uninfected children who are at high risk for continuous or repeated exposure to infectious persons who remain undetected or untreated.[28]

Combined active-passive immunization provides effective postexposure prophylaxis against exposure to rabies. Two vaccine preparations, human diploid cell vaccine and rabies vaccine adsorbed, are licensed in the United States, but only the former is widely available.[29] All persons treated with at least five doses of human diploid cell vaccine (or rabies vaccine, adsorbed) and human rabies immune globulin have developed adequate antibody titers.[29] Since human rabies is a rare disease, with less than five cases per year having occurred in the United States since 1960,[30] it is difficult to measure the efficacy of postexposure prophylaxis by the incidence of actual cases. No cases of rabies were reported in over 500 persons given postexposure therapy (human diploid cell vaccine and rabies immune globulin) for bite exposures to rabid animals.[31,32] Very rarely, cases of fatal encephalitis have been reported in individuals given human diploid cell vaccine; in one case immune globulin was not administered, and in the other, rabies vaccine was not administered as directed.[14,33] Rabies vaccination is also recommended for preexposure prophylaxis in persons at high risk of contact with rabies virus, such as animal handlers, veterinarians, cave explorers, and hunters exposed to rabid animals.[31,34] A three-dose series of human diploid cell vaccine (1 mL IM or 0.1 mL ID) on days 0, 7, and 28 provides adequate antibody response in virtually all recipients.[35,36]

Recommendations of Others

The Immunization Practices Advisory Committee of the Centers for Disease Control (CDC) and/or the American College of Physicians have issued recommendations on postexposure prophylaxis for *Haemophilus influenzae* type b disease,[37] meningococcal infection,[38] hepatitis A and B,[39,40] rabies,[36,41] and tuberculosis.[28] The American College of Obstetricians and Gynecologists has issued detailed guidelines on the use of vaccines during pregnancy.[42]

Clinical Intervention

Oral rifampin prophylaxis should be prescribed promptly for all household contacts of patients with *Haemophilus influenzae* type b, if at least one of the contacts is a child less than 4 years old. Prophylaxis of infants and young children (less than 2 years old) with day-care exposure to infected cases may also be appropriate. The dosage is 20 mg/kg, with a maximum of 600 mg, daily for four days for children and adults. Infants less than 1 month old should receive 10 mg/kg.

Oral rifampin prophylaxis is also indicated for household or day-care contacts of persons with meningococcal infection, as well as for those with direct exposure to oral secretions (e.g., kissing). Dosage is 600 mg for adults, 10 mg/kg for children 1 month of age or older, and 5 mg/kg for children under 1 month of age, all given twice daily for two days. Rifampin is contraindicated during pregnancy. Sulfonamides should be used if the meningococcus is adequately sensitive.

Hepatitis A immune globulin (0.02 mL/kg intramuscularly) should be administered to close household and sexual contacts of persons with hepatitis A, staff and children at day-care centers where hepatitis A is occurring, staff and patients of custodial institutions in which hepatitis A is occurring, and co-workers of food handlers with hepatitis A. Immune globulin should be given within two weeks of exposure.

The recommended protocol for postexposure prophylaxis against hepatitis B depends on the nature of the exposure and the HB vaccination status of the exposed person. For unvaccinated persons with percutaneous or mucous membrane exposure to blood known to be hepatitis B surface antigen (HBsAg) positive, or those bitten by a known carrier, a single intramuscular dose of HBIG (0.06 mL/kg) should be administered immediately, and a three-dose series of hepatitis B vaccine should be initiated. The first dose should accompany the dose of HBIG; the second and third doses should be given one and six months later. If vaccine is not administered, a second dose of HBIG should be given after one month. The three-dose vaccine series should also be initiated for persons with percutaneous or mucosal exposure to bodily fluids of persons at high risk of being infected. However, serologic confirmation of the HBsAg status of the suspected person should be obtained within seven days of exposure before administering HBIG. For percutaneous exposure to bodily fluids of persons at low risk, a three-dose vaccine series should be administered; testing of the source person and HBIG administration are not necessary.

Previously vaccinated persons exposed to infected bodily fluids should receive serologic testing. If the exposed person has inadequate antibody, one dose of HBIG should be given along with a vaccine booster dose (1 mL or 20 mcg) at a different site. If the source is at high risk of HB infection but

HBsAg status is unknown, serologic testing of the source is indicated only if the exposed person is a known vaccine nonresponder. If the source is HBsAg-positive, the exposed person should receive one dose of HBIG and a vaccine booster dose.

Persons with sexual exposure to HBsAg-positive persons should receive serologic screening before treatment, unless it will delay intervention to more than 14 days after exposure. Seronegative persons should receive a single dose of HBIG within 14 days of the last sexual contact. A second dose should be given if the source remains HBsAg-positive at three months and exposure continues. If the source becomes a carrier (HBsAg-positive for six months), the contact should receive a complete vaccine series. For exposures among homosexual men, the HB vaccine series should be initiated at the time HBIG is given; for exposures among heterosexuals, the HB vaccine is optional. If HB vaccine is given, additional doses of HBIG are unnecessary.

See Chapter 20 for recommendations on prenatal screening and neonatal vaccination against hepatitis B, as well as for general information about HB vaccine. More details on postexposure prophylaxis for HB are available from CDC publications.[39-40]

Postexposure prophylaxis against rabies should be instituted if a possible exposure to rabies virus has occurred. Criteria for making this assessment, which include the type of animal (e.g., carnivorous wild animals, bats), the circumstances of the incident (e.g., unprovoked attack), and the type of exposure (e.g., bite), are available in published guidelines[14] and from local health departments. Rabies immune globulin is given at a dose of 20 IU/kg; half of the dose is infiltrated around the wound, and the remainder is given intramuscularly at another site. Rabies vaccine is administered in the deltoid area in five 1 mL intramuscular injections: days 0, 3, 7, 14, and 28. Persons who were immunized before the incident require only two 1 mL doses of vaccine (day of exposure and day 3) and do not require immune globulin. Rabies vaccination is also recommended for preexposure prophylaxis in persons at high risk of contact with rabies virus, such as veterinarians, animal handlers, cave explorers, and hunters exposed to rabid animals.

BCG vaccination against TB should be considered only in tuberculin-negative children who cannot be placed on isoniazid (INH) and who have continuous exposure to persons with active disease, those with continuous exposure to patients with organisms resistant to INH or rifampin, and those belonging to groups with a rate of new infections greater than 1% per year and for whom the usual surveillance and treatment programs may not be operationally feasible. These groups may also include persons with limited access to or willingness to use health care services.

Note: See Appendix A for the U.S. Preventive Services Task Force Table of Ratings for this topic. See also the relevant Task Force background paper: LaForce MF. Immunizations, immunoprophylaxis, and chemoprophylaxis to prevent selected infections. JAMA 1987; 257:2464–70.

REFERENCES

1. Cochi SL, Broome CV, Hightower AW. Immunization of children with *Haemophilus influenzae* type b vaccine: a cost-effectiveness model of strategy assessment. JAMA 1985; 253:521–9.
2. Redmond SR, Pichichero ME. *Hemophilus influenzae* type b disease: an epidemiologic study with special reference to day-care centers. JAMA 1984; 252:2581–4.

3. Casto DT, Edwards DL. Preventing *Haemophilus influenzae* type b disease. Clin Pharm 1985; 4:637–48.

4. Fleming DW, Leibenhuaut MH, Albanes D, et al. Secondary *Haemophilus influenzae* type b in day-care facilities: risk factors and prevention. JAMA 1985; 254:509–14.

5. Centers for Disease Control. Summary of notifiable diseases, United States. MMWR 1988; 36:1–59.

6. Stephens DS. *Neisseria meningitidis*. Infect Control 1985; 6:37–40.

7. Centers for Disease Control. Human rabies—California, 1987. MMWR 1988; 37: 305–8.

8. Kauffman FH, Goldmann BJ. Rabies. Am J Emerg Med 1986; 4:525–31.

9. Glode MP, Daum RS, Boies EG, et al. Effect of rifampin chemoprophylaxis on carriage eradication and new acquisition of *Haemophilus influenzae* type b in contacts. Pediatrics 1985; 76:537–42.

10. Band JD, Fraser DW, Ajello G. Prevention of *Hemophilus influenzae* type b disease. JAMA 1984; 251:2381–6.

11. Murphy TV, Chrane DF, McCracken GH Jr, et al. Rifampin prophylaxis for household contacts of children with *Hemophilus influenzae* type b disease. Am J Dis Child 1983; 137:627–32.

12. Makintubee S, Istre GR, Ward JI. Transmission of invasive *Haemophilus influenzae* type b disease in day care settings. J Pediatr 1987; 111:180–6.

13. Guttler RB, Counts GW, Avent CK, et al. Effect of rifampin and minocycline on meningococcal carrier rates. J Infect Dis 1971; 124:199–204.

14. American College of Physicians. Guide for adult immunization, 1985. Philadelphia: American College of Physicians, 1985.

15. Stokes J, Neefe JR. The prevention and attenuation of infectious hepatitis by gamma globulin. JAMA 1945; 127:144–5.

16. Maynard JE. Passive immunization against hepatitis B: a review of recent studies and comment on current aspects of control. Am J Epidemiol 1978; 107:77–86.

17. Hoofnagle JH, Seeff LB, Bales ZB, et al. Passive-active immunity from hepatitis B immune globulin: reanalysis of a Veterans Administration cooperative study of needlestick hepatitis. The Veterans Administration Cooperative Study Group. Ann Intern Med 1979; 91.813–8.

18. Perrillo RP, Campbell CR, Strang S, et al. Immune globulin and hepatitis B immune globulin: prophylactic measures for intimate contacts exposed to acute type B hepatitis. Arch Intern Med 1984; 144:81–5.

19. Palmovic D. Prevention of hepatitis B infection in health care workers after accidental exposure. J Infect 1987; 15:221–4.

20. Clemens JD, Chuong JJH, Feinstein AR. The BCG controversy: a methodological and statistical reappraisal. JAMA 1983; 249:2362–9.

21. Tripathy SP. Fifteen-year follow-up of the Indian BCG prevention trial. In: International Union Against Tuberculosis. Proceedings of the XXVIth IUAT World Conference on Tuberculosis and Respiratory Diseases. Singapore: Professional Postgraduate Services International, 1987:69–72.

22. Romanus V. Tuberculosis in *Bacillus Calmette-Guerin*-immunized children in Sweden: a ten-year evaluation following the cessation of general *Bacillus Calmette-Guerrin* immunization of the newborn in 1975. Pediatr Infect Dis 1987; 6:272–80.

23. Smith PG. Case-control studies of the efficacy of BCG against tuberculosis. In: International Union Against Tuberculosis. Proceedings of the XXVIth IUAT World Conference on Tuberculosis and Respiratory Diseases. Singapore: Professional Postgraduate Services International, 1987:73–9.

24. Padungchan S, Konjanart S, Kasiratta S, et al. The effectiveness of BCG vaccination of the newborn against childhood tuberculosis in Bangkok. Bull WHO 1986; 64:247–58.

25. Tidjani O, Amedome A, ten Dam HG. The protective effect of BCG vaccination of the newborn against childhood tuberculosis in an African community. Tubercle 1986; 67: 269–81.

26. Centers for Disease Control. Tuberculosis, final data—United States, 1986. MMWR 1987; 36:817–20.

27. Slutkin G. Management of tuberculosis in urban homeless indigents. Public Health Rep 1986; 101:481–5.
28. Immunization Practices Advisory Committee. Use of BCG vaccines in the control of tuberculosis: a joint statement by the ACIP and the Advisory Committee for Elimination of Tuberculosis. MMWR 1988; 37:663–4,669–75.
29. Centers for Disease Control. Rabies vaccine, adsorbed: a new rabies vaccine for use in humans. MMWR 1988; 37:217–18,223.
30. *Idem.* Rabies surveillance, United States, 1987. MMWR 1988; 37:1–17.
31. Bernard KW, Mallonee J, Wright JC, et al. Preexposure immunization with intradermal human diploid cell rabies vaccine: risks and benefits of primary and booster vaccination. JAMA 1987; 257:1059–63.
32. Helmick C. The epidemiology of human rabies postexposure prophylaxis, 1980–1981. JAMA 1983; 250:1990–6.
33. Centers for Disease Control. Human rabies despite treatment with rabies immune globulin and human diploid cell rabies vaccine—Thailand. MMWR 1987; 36:759–60,765.
34. Immunization Practices Advisory Committee. Adult immunization: recommendations of the Immunization Practices Advisory Committee (ACIP). MMWR 1984; 33:1S-68S.
35. Turner GS, Nicholson KG, Tyrrell DAJ, et al. Evaluation of a human diploid cell strain rabies vaccine: final report of a three year study of pre-exposure immunization. J Hyg 1982; 89:101–10.
36. Immunization Practices Advisory Committee. Rabies prevention: supplemental statement on the preexposure use of human diploid cell rabies vaccine by the intradermal route. MMWR 1986; 35:767–8.
37. *Idem.* Update: prevention of *Haemophilus influenzae* type b disease. MMWR 1986; 35:170–80.
38. *Idem.* Meningococcal vaccines. MMWR 1985; 34:255–9.
39. *Idem.* Recommendations for protection against viral hepatitis. MMWR 1985; 34:313–24,329–35.
40. *Idem.* Update on hepatitis B prevention. MMWR 1987; 36:353–60,366.
41. *Idem.* Rabies prevention—United States, 1984. MMWR 1984; 33:393–402,407–8.
42. American College of Obstetricians and Gynecologists. Immunization during pregnancy. ACOG Technical Bulletin No. 64. Washington, D.C.: American College of Obstetricians and Gynecologists, 1982.

59

Estrogen Prophylaxis

Recommendation: Although routine postmenopausal estrogen replacement is not recommended, estrogen therapy should be considered for asymptomatic women who are at increased risk for osteoporosis, who lack known contraindications, and who have received adequate counseling about potential benefits and risks (see *Clinical Intervention*). The role of exercise and dietary calcium supplementation in preventing osteoporosis is discussed in Chapters 49 and 50; see Chapter 40 regarding screening for low bone mineral content.

Burden of Suffering

It is estimated that 1.3 million osteoporosis-related fractures occur each year in the United States.[1] Most of these injuries occur in postmenopausal women. It has been estimated that about one-quarter of all women over age 60 have spinal compression fractures and about 15% of women sustain hip fractures during their lifetime.[2,3] Hip fractures are associated with significant pain and disability, decreased functional independence, and high mortality. There is a 15–20% reduction in expected survival in the first year following a hip fracture.[4] Hip fractures cost the United States over $7 billion each year in direct and indirect costs.[5] Important risk factors for osteoporosis include advanced age, female sex, Caucasian or Asian race, slender build, bilateral oophorectomy prior to natural menopause, smoking, and alcohol abuse.

Efficacy of Chemoprophylaxis

There is good evidence from retrospective studies[6-9] and clinical trials[10-17] that estrogen replacement can reduce the rate of bone loss in postmenopausal women. Although it is likely that this physiological effect on bone mineral content can reduce the incidence of fractures and other clinical measures of osteoporosis, prospective evidence linking estrogen to fracture rates has been difficult to obtain because of the long interval between the onset of osteoporosis and the occurrence of symptoms. There is, however, a large body of evidence from retrospective studies,[6,8,9,18] cross-sectional studies,[19] cohort studies, and nonrandomized clinical trials[20,21] that estrogen replacement is associated with a decreased rate of fractures. These findings do not provide conclusive evidence of efficacy, due to the potential influence of selection bias, recall bias, and confounding in many of these studies. It may be impractical, however, to carry out randomized controlled trials of sufficient duration to provide definitive evidence that estrogen replacement can lower fracture rates.

The use of estrogen to prevent osteoporosis can also have other benefits. Estrogen can reduce the incidence of vasomotor flushes and vaginal atrophy. Perhaps the most important benefit of estrogen, however, is its ability to improve lipoprotein profiles; many studies in recent years have demonstrated an association between the use of estrogen and reduced mortality from coronary artery disease.[22-28] At the same time, there are potentially important side effects associated with long-term use of unopposed estrogen. Prolonged use of unopposed, conjugated estrogens increases the risk of endometrial hyperplasia and endometrial cancer.[29-33] Although these tumors are usually early-stage and minimally invasive at diagnosis, an increased risk of disseminated endometrial cancer has been documented.[29,30] Combining estrogen with cycled progestins may reduce the risk of cancer,[34] but conclusive evidence of an effect on endometrial cancer mortality is lacking.[35] In addition, some women may dislike the menstrual bleeding produced by progestins and discontinue use of the drug. There is inconsistent evidence regarding the reported association between estrogen therapy and such diseases as breast cancer and gallbladder disease.[35-40]

Effectiveness of Counseling

Few studies have examined the effectiveness of physician counseling to use estrogen. There is evidence, however, that compliance with estrogen therapy is generally poor among postmenopausal women, in part because of the perceived risk of developing cancer and unpleasant side effects. One author, citing personal communications from the investigators, reported that 20–30% of women in the Massachusetts Women's Health Survey never had their prescriptions filled because they were not convinced of the benefits and safety of therapy; of those who began therapy, 20% discontinued the drug within nine months.[41] Compliance with estrogen replacement is often limited by the inconvenience associated with daily administration. The availability of transdermal estrogen and new dosage regimens may offer potential means of reducing inconvenience, but the effectiveness of alternative routes of administration in enhancing long-term compliance has yet to be proved.[41]

Recommendations of Others

The American College of Obstetricians and Gynecologists recommends consideration of estrogen therapy in all hypoestrogenic (including postmenopausal) women.[42] A 1984 National Institutes of Health consensus development conference recommended that estrogen therapy after menopause should be considered in high-risk women who have no medical contraindications and who are willing to adhere to a program of careful follow-up.[1] The Canadian Task Force advises against widespread use of estrogen to prevent osteoporosis, but recommends offering therapy to women who appear to be at increased risk on an individual basis.[43]

Discussion

Although there is good evidence that estrogen therapy can reduce bone loss in postmenopausal women, there is insufficient evidence to recommend its routine prescription. Definitive evidence that estrogen replacement therapy can prevent bone fractures or other clinical measures of osteoporosis requires a lengthy randomized controlled trial that may be difficult to perform in the future for logistical roacono. In the absence of such evidence, It Is difficult to determine with certainty whether the benefits of estrogen replacement (e.g., preservation of bone mass, improved lipoprotein profiles and cardiovascular mortality reduction, reduced menopausal symptoms) outweigh its potential risks (e.g., endometrial cancer) and inconvenience (e.g., vaginal bleeding, daily administration) in all postmenopausal women. In some asymptomatic women, however, such as those at increased risk and those with early indications of low peak bone mass (see Chapter 40), the benefit-risk ratio is likely to be more favorable. It is especially important for such women to receive counseling about potential benefits and risks so that they can make an informed decision about therapy. The perimenopausal period is an important time for such decisions; the evidence is less clear regarding the benefits of beginning estrogen treatment at older ages.[44]

Clinical Intervention

Although estrogen replacement is not recommended for all postmenopausal women, estrogen therapy should be considered in asymptomatic women who are at increased risk for osteoporosis (e.g., Caucasian or Asian women, women with low bone mineral content, those with a slender build, and those with a history of early menopause or bilateral oophorectomy prior to menopause) and who are without known contraindications (e.g., history of undiagnosed vaginal bleeding, active liver disease, thromboembolic disorders, or hormone-dependent cancer). These patients should receive information on the risks and consequences of osteoporotic fractures and the risks and benefits of hormonal therapy. All women should receive information about potential alternatives for osteoporosis prevention such as weight-bearing exercise (see Chapter 49) and dietary calcium supplementation (see Chapter 50). Women consenting to estrogen therapy should be counseled about the various estrogen and progestin preparations and routes of administration that are available. One common regimen is 0.625 mg conjugated equine estrogen on days 1–25 (or daily) with the addition of 5–10 mg medroxyprogesterone acetate during the last 12 days of the cycle. Dosages should be modified to reduce side effects such as nausea, headache, breakthrough bleeding, weight gain, and breast tenderness.

Note: See the relevant U.S. Preventive Services Task Force background paper: Mann K, Wiese WH, Stachencko S. Preventing postmenopausal osteoporosis and related fractures. In: Goldbloom RB, Lawrence RS, eds. Preventing disease: beyond the rhetoric. New York: Springer-Verlag (in press).

REFERENCES

1. Consensus conference: osteoporosis. JAMA 1984; 252:799–802.
2. Melton LJ III. Epidemiology of fractures. In: Riggs BL, Melton LJ III, eds. Osteoporosis: etiology, diagnosis, and management. New York: Raven Press, 1988.
3. Cummings SR, Kelsey JL, Nevitt MC, et al. Epidemiology of osteoporosis and osteoporotic fractures. Epidemiol Rev 1985; 7:178–208.
4. Jensen GF, Christiansen C, Boesen J, et al. Epidemiology of postmenopausal spinal and long bone fractures: a unifying approach to postmenopausal osteoporosis. Clin Orthoped 1982; 166:75–81.
5. Holbrook TL, Grazier K, Kelsey JL, et al. The frequency of occurrence, impact, and cost of selected musculoskeletal conditions in the United States. Chicago, Ill.: American Academy of Orthopedic Surgeons, 1984.

6. Weiss NS, Ure CL, Ballard JH, et al. Decreased risk of fractures of the hip and lower forearm with postmenopausal use of estrogen. N Engl J Med 1980; 303:1195–8.
7. Kreiger N, Kelsey JL, Holford TR, et al. An epidemiologic study of hip fracture in post-menopausal women. Am J Epidemiol 1982; 116:141–8.
8. Hutchinson TA, Polansky SM, Feinstein AR. Post-menopausal oestrogens protect against fractures of hip and distal radius: a case-control study. Lancet 1979; 2:705–9.
9. Paganini-Hill A, Ross RK, Gerkins VR, et al. Menopausal estrogen therapy and hip fractures. Ann Intern Med 1981; 95:28–31.
10. Nachtigall LE, Nachtigall RH, Nachtigall RD, et al. Estrogen replacement therapy I: a 10–year prospective study in the relationship to osteoporosis. Obstet Gynecol 1979; 53:277–81.
11. Jensen GF, Christiansen CV, Transbol I. Treatment of postmenopausal osteoporosis: a controlled therapeutic trial comparing oestrogen/gestagen, 1,25–dihydroxy-vitamin D3 and calcium. Clin Endocrinol 1982; 16:515–24.
12. Horsman A, Gallagher JC, Simpson M, et al. Prospective trial of oestrogen and calcium in postmenopausal women. Br Med J 1977; 2:789–92.
13. Christiansen C, Christensen MS, Transbol I. Bone mass in postmenopausal women after withdrawal of oestrogen/gestagen replacement therapy. Lancet 1981; 1:459–61.
14. Riis B, Thomsen K, Christiansen C. Does calcium supplementation prevent postmen-opausal bone loss? A double-blind, controlled clinical study. N Engl J Med 1987; 316: 173–7.
15. Christiansen C, Rodbro P. Does menopausal bone loss respond to estrogen therapy independent of bone loss rate? Calcif Tissue Int 1983; 35:720–2.
16. Lindsay R, Hart DM, Clark DM. The minimum effective dose of estrogen for prevention of post-menopausal bone loss. Obstet Gynecol 1984; 63:759–63.
17. Recker RR, Saville PD, Heaney RP. Effect of estrogens and calcium carbonate on bone loss in post-menopausal women. Ann Intern Med 1977; 87:649–55.
18. Ettinger B, Genant HK, Cann CE. Long-term estrogen replacement therapy prevents bone loss and fractures. Ann Intern Med 1985; 102:319–24.
19. Wasnich R, Yano K, Vogel J. Postmenopausal bone loss at multiple sites: relationship to estrogen use. J Chron Dis 1983; 36:781–90.
20. Kiel DP, Felson DT, Anderson JJ, et al. Hip fracture and the use of estrogens in post-menopausal women: the Framingham Study. N Engl J Med 1987; 317:1169–74.
21. Lindsay R, Hart DM, Forrest C, et al. Prevention of spinal osteoporosis in oopherec-tomised women. Lancet 1980; 2:1151–4.
22. Ross RK, Paganini-Hill A, Mack TM, et al. Menopausal oestrogen therapy and protection from death from ischaemic heart disease. Lancet 1981; 1:858–60.
23. Stampfer MJ, Willett WC, Colditz GA, et al. A prospective study of postmenopausal estrogen therapy and coronary heart disease. N Engl J Med 1985; 313:1044–9.
24. Wilson PWF, Garrison RJ, Castelli WP. Postmenopausal estrogen use, cigarette smok-ing, and cardiovascular morbidity in women over 50: the Framingham Study. N Engl J Med 1985; 313:1038–43.
25. Bain C, Willett W, Hennekens CH, et al. Use of postmenopausal hormones and risk of myocardial infarction. Circulation 1981; 64:42–6.
26. Bush TL, Barrett-Connor E, Cowan LD, et al. Cardiovascular mortality and noncontra-ceptive use of estrogen in women: results from the Lipid Research Clinics Program follow-up study. Circulation 1987; 75:1102–9.
27. Colditz GA, Willett WC, Stampfer MJ, et al. Menopause and the risk of coronary heart disease in women. N Engl J Med 1987; 316:1105–10.
28. Sullivan JM, Vander Zwagg R, Lemp GF, et al. Postmenopausal estrogen use and coronary atherosclerosis. Ann Intern Med 1988; 108:358–63.
29. Shapiro S, Kelly JP, Rosenberg L, et al. Risk of localized and widespread endometrial cancer in relation to recent and discontinued use of conjugated estrogens. N Engl J Med 1985; 313:969–72.
30. Antunes CMF, Stolley PD, Rosenshein NB, et al. Endometrial cancer and estrogen use: report of a large case-control study. N Engl J Med 1979; 300:9–13.

31. Buring JE, Bain CJ, Ehrmann RL. Conjugated estrogen use and risk of endometrial cancer. Am J Epidemiol 1986; 124:434–41.

32. Spengler RF, Clarke EA, Woolever CA, et al. Exogenous estrogens and endometrial cancer: a case-control study and assessment of potential biases. Am J Epidemiol 1981; 114:497–506.

33. Cali RW. Estrogen replacement therapy—boon or bane? Postgrad Med 1984; 75:279–86.

34. American College of Obstetricians and Gynecologists. Estrogen replacement therapy. Technical Bulletin No. 93. Washington, D.C.: American College of Obstetricians and Gynecologists, 1986.

35. Gambrell RD. The menopause: benefits and risks of estrogen-progestogen replacement therapy. Fertil Steril 1982; 37:457–74.

36. Hunt K. Long-term effects of postmenopausal hormone therapy. Br J Hosp Med 1987; 38:450–60.

37. Sherman B, Wallace R, Bean J. Estrogen use and breast cancer: interaction with body mass. Cancer 1983; 51:1527–31.

38. Brinton LA, Hoover R, Fraumeni JF. Menopausal oestrogens and breast cancer risk: an expanded case-control study. Br J Cancer 1986; 54:825–32.

39. Nomura AMY, Lolonel LN, Hirohata T, et al. The association of replacement estrogens with breast cancer. Int J Cancer 1986; 37:49–53.

40. Ross RK, Paganini-Hill A, Gerkins VR, et al. A case-control study of menopausal estrogen therapy and breast cancer. JAMA 1980; 243:1635–9.

41. Ravnikar VA. Compliance with hormone therapy. Am J Obstet Gynecol 1987; 156:1332–4.

42. American College of Obstetricians and Gynecologists. Osteoporosis. Technical Bulletin No. 118. Washington, D.C.: American College of Obstetricians and Gynecologists, 1988.

43. Canadian Task Force on the Periodic Health Examination. The periodic health examination, 1987 update. Can Med Assoc J 1988; 137:618–26.

44. Resnick NM, Greenspan SL. Senile osteoporosis reconsidered. JAMA 1989; 261:1025–9.

60

Aspirin Prophylaxis

Recommendation: Low-dose aspirin therapy should be considered for men aged 40 and over who are at significantly increased risk for myocardial infarction and who lack contraindications to the drug (see *Clinical Intervention*). Patients should understand the potential benefits and risks of aspirin therapy before beginning treatment.

Burden of Suffering

Coronary artery disease is the leading cause of death in the United States, accounting for about 1.5 million myocardial infarctions and over 520,000 deaths each year.[1,2] About 400,000 Americans are victims of sudden death each year, due primarily to underlying atherosclerotic disease. Myocardial infarction is associated with significant mortality, morbidity, and disability. The cost to the United States of medical care and lost productivity due to cardiovascular diseases was nearly $80 billion in 1986.[2] Myocardial infarction and sudden death often occur without warning in persons without a history of angina pectoris or other clinical symptoms. The principal risk factors for coronary artery disease are smoking, hypertension, elevated serum cholesterol, obesity, and family history.

Efficacy of Chemoprophylaxis

The platelet-inhibitory effect of aspirin prevents the formation of arterial thrombi on atherosclerotic plaques.[3] A number of secondary prevention trials have shown that daily aspirin ingestion can lower the risk of nonfatal strokes and myocardial infarctions (MI) in persons at increased risk for atherosclerosis and thrombogenesis (persons with unstable angina, previous MI, transient ischemic attacks, and post-coronary artery bypass graft surgery and thrombolysis).[4,5] Few studies, however, have examined the efficacy of using aspirin as a primary prevention tool in asymptomatic persons without such a history, who are thus at much lower risk of developing myocardial infarctions. The use of aspirin in preventing stroke in persons without neurologic symptoms has been proposed for persons at risk for thromboembolic events (e.g., those with carotid bruits, valvular heart disease, atrial fibrillation),[6] but convincing data to support its efficacy even in these populations is lacking.

Two recent randomized controlled trials, in the United States and Britain, have examined the efficacy of aspirin in preventing myocardial infarction in healthy men. In the American trial, over 22,000 asymptomatic male physicians received either

325 mg of aspirin every other day or placebo.[7] The study was terminated prematurely after 4.5 years when a statistically significant 47% reduction in the incidence of fatal and nonfatal MI was noted in the group receiving aspirin. The British trial, with a smaller sample size (5139 male physicians) and a higher dose (500 mg daily), found no significant reduction in MI.[8] Although the absence of an apparent reduction in MI may have been due to lack of efficacy, the British trial may have failed to demonstrate a significant effect on MI due to its inadequate sample size and other differences in study design (e.g., higher dose, no placebo).[9] Neither study had sufficient statistical power to demonstrate a reduction in overall cardiovascular mortality.[9]

Both trials observed an increase in the incidence of stroke among persons taking aspirin, but in neither study was the difference statistically significant.[7,8] In the preliminary results of the American trial, a statistically significant increase in the incidence of moderate and severe hemorrhagic strokes was reported among men taking aspirin.[7] In a more recent analysis of the final data, however, the investigators determined that this difference was not statistically significant.[10]

Other side effects of aspirin therapy must also be considered in evaluating its long-term safety. Aspirin can produce unpleasant gastrointestinal symptoms such as stomach pain, heartburn, nausea and constipation, as well as occult gastrointestinal blood loss, hematemesis, and melena.[5] The likelihood of such side effects in otherwise healthy persons is directly related to the dose of the drug. In the British trial, in which the dose was 500 mg daily, 20% of the doctors taking aspirin had to discontinue the drug due to dyspepsia and constipation, 3.6% experienced bleeding or bruising, and 2.2% had gastrointestinal blood loss.[8] In the American trial, in which the dose was 325 mg every other day, there was less than a 1% difference in gastrointestinal complaints between the aspirin and placebo groups, and only one case of fatal gastrointestinal hemorrhage was reported in 4.5 years of treatment.[7,10] Similarly, a large secondary prevention trial also reported little difference in epigastric discomfort, decreased hemoglobin concentration, or occult blood in stool in persons receiving 324 mg per day.[11]

In addition to reducing the risk of side effects, low-dose therapy appears to have comparable (if not greater) platelet-inhibitory action when compared with higher doses. A review of 25 secondary prevention trials with a total of 29,000 patients found little difference in outcome in dosages ranging from 300 to 1200 mg per day.[4] In one study, a dose of only 60 mg daily was effective in reducing the incidence of pregnancy-induced hypertension.[12] It is possible that high-dose therapy may even have less platelet-inhibitory effect, by inhibiting vessel wall synthesis of prostacyclin along with platelet production of thromboxane A_2. Doses as low as 30–40 mg daily may be necessary to achieve an optimal balance.[13] The probability of adverse effects at such low doses is likely to be small, but further studies of aspirin therapy are needed to provide definitive evidence regarding both the clinical efficacy of low-dose regimens and the safety of long-term administration.

Effectiveness of Counseling

There is little information on whether asymptomatic patients will comply with physician advice to take aspirin for an extended period of time. Aspirin is the most consumed drug in the United States, with an estimated 20–30 billion tablets ingested each year,[5] but most users are suffering from pain, fever, or other forms of discomfort when they choose to use the drug. It is not known whether healthy individuals would be able or willing to comply with a lifelong daily (or alternate day) regimen, especially if it produces unpleasant side effects. As noted above, over the course of six years, 20% of the doctors participating in the British trial were forced to discontinue a daily 500 mg aspirin regimen because of dyspepsia and constipation.[8]

Recommendations of Others

The American Heart Association has recently advised physicians to exercise care before starting a patient on lifelong aspirin therapy; efforts should first be directed at modifying primary risk factors for heart disease and stroke, assessing potential contraindications to aspirin, and counseling patients about potential side effects and symptoms requiring medical attention.[14] Investigators in the U.S. and British trials have recommended that physicians prescribing aspirin to asymptomatic persons first consider the cardiovascular risk profile of the patient and balance the known hazards of aspirin (e.g., gastrointestinal discomfort and bleeding, cerebral hemorrhage) against the benefit of reducing the risk of a first myocardial infarction.[9]

Discussion

Although data from a large trial have provided evidence that low-dose aspirin therapy can reduce the risk of myocardial infarction in asymptomatic men,[7] it is premature to recommend routine use of aspirin for this purpose in the general population. These benefits were demonstrated in a select population: male doctors between the ages of 40 and 84 in exceptionally good health, who were then prescreened to eliminate persons unable to tolerate aspirin. In addition, the study was terminated prematurely; therefore, it is not known with certainty whether the long term complications of aspirin therapy might have ultimately exceeded its benefits.[15] Some patients might judge the reduced risk of MI inadequate to justify the unpleasant side effects or increased risk of gastrointestinal bleeding. Moreover, in both the U.S. and British studies, strokes may have been more common in men taking aspirin. Although the differences were not statistically significant, the consistency of the findings suggests that further study of the relationship between aspirin therapy and cerebral hemorrhage is warranted. Hypertensives, a population at increased risk for both coronary artery and cerebrovascular disease, may be more likely to experience hemorrhagic stroke while taking this drug.[5,16]

Clinical Intervention

Low-dose aspirin therapy (325 mg every other day) should be considered for primary prevention in men aged 40 and over who have risk factors for myocardial infarction (e.g., hypercholesterolemia, smoking, diabetes mellitus, family history of early-onset coronary artery disease) and who lack a history of uncontrolled hypertension, liver or kidney disease, peptic ulcer disease, a history of gastrointestinal or other bleeding problems, or other risk factors for bleeding or cerebral hemorrhage. Patients should understand the potential benefits and risks associated with aspirin therapy before beginning treatment, and they should be encouraged to focus their efforts on modifying primary risk factors such as smoking (see Chapter 48), elevated cholesterol (Chapters 2 and 50), and hypertension (Chapter 3).

REFERENCES

1. National Center for Health Statistics. Advance report of final mortality statistics, 1986. Monthly Vital Statistics Report [Suppl], vol. 37, no. 6. Hyattsville, Md.: Public Health Service, 1988. (Publication no. DHHS (PHS) 88–1120.)
2. American Heart Association. 1989 heart facts. Dallas, Tex.: American Heart Association, 1988.
3. Fuster V, Adams PC, Badimon JJ, et al. Platelet-inhibitor drugs' role in coronary artery disease. Prog Cardiovasc Dis 1987; 29:325–46.
4. Anti-Platelet Trialists Collaboration. Secondary prevention of vascular disease by prolonged antiplatelet treatment. Br Med J 1988; 296:320–31.
5. Fuster V, Cohen M, Chesebro JH. Usefulness of aspirin for coronary artery disease. Am J Cardiol 1988; 61:637–40.
6. Foster JW, Hart RG. Antithrombotic therapy for cerebrovascular disease: prevention and treatment of stroke. Postgrad Med 1986; 80:199–206.
7. The Steering Committee of the Physicians' Health Study Research Group. Preliminary report: findings from the aspirin component of the ongoing Physicians' Health Study. N Engl J Med 1988; 318:262–4.
8. Peto R, Gray R, Collins R, et al. Randomised trial of prophylactic daily aspirin in British male doctors. Br Med J 1988; 296:313–6.
9. Hennekens CH, Peto R, Hutchison GB, et al. An overview of the British and American aspirin studies. N Engl J Med 1988; 318:923–4.
10. Hennekens CH. Personal communication, November 1988.
11. Lewis HD, Davis JW, Archibald DG, et al. Protective effects of aspirin against acute myocardial infarction and death in men with unstable angina: results of a Veterans Administration cooperative study. N Engl J Med 1983; 309:396–403.
12. Wallenburg HCS, Dekker GA, Makovitz JW, et al. Low-dose aspirin prevents pregnancy-induced hypertension and preeclampsia in angiotensin-sensitive primigravidae. Lancet 1986; 1:1–3.
13. Anonymous. Aspirin: what dose? Lancet 1986; 1:592–3.
14. American Heart Association. Physicians' Health Study report on aspirin. Circulation 1988; 77:1447A.
15. Rimm AA. (letter). N Engl J Med 1988; 318:926.
16. Shapiro S. The Physicians' Health Study: aspirin for the primary prevention of myocardial infarction (letter). N Engl J Med 1988; 318:924.

Appendices

Appendix A
Task Force Ratings

The tables of ratings on the following pages were developed by the U.S. Preventive Services Task Force between July 1984 and February 1988 using a methodology adapted from the Canadian Task Force on the Periodic Health Examination.* They do not reflect more recently published evidence. The U.S. Task Force did not develop ratings for all the topics examined in the *Guide*. In addition, some of the interventions listed in these tables (and indicated by a caret [˄]) were rated during Task Force deliberations but are not discussed in the text of the *Guide*.

The Task Force graded the *strength of recommendations* for or against preventive interventions as follows:

Strength of Recommendations

A: There is good evidence to support the recommendation that the condition be specifically considered in a periodic health examination.
B: There is fair evidence to support the recommendation that the condition be specifically considered in a periodic health examination.
C: There is poor evidence regarding the inclusion of the condition in a periodic health examination, but recommendations may be made on other grounds.
D: There is fair evidence to support the recommendation that the condition be excluded from consideration in a periodic health examination.
E: There is good evidence to support the recommendation that the condition be excluded from consideration in a periodic health examination.

Determination of the quality of evidence (i.e., "good," "fair," "poor") in the strength of recommendations above was based on a systematic consideration of three sets of criteria: the burden of suffering from the target condition, the characteristics of the intervention, and the effectiveness of the intervention as demonstrated in published research. Effectiveness of the intervention received special emphasis. In reviewing clinical studies, the Task Force used strict criteria for selecting admissible evidence and placed special emphasis on the quality of study designs. In grading the *quality of evidence*, the Task Force gave special weight to those study designs that, for methodologic reasons, are less subject to bias and inferential error. The following rating system was used:

---

*Canadian Task Force on the Periodic Health Examination. The periodic health examination. Can Med Assoc J 1979; 121:1193–254.

Quality of Evidence

I: Evidence obtained from at least one properly-designed randomized controlled trial.

II-1: Evidence obtained from well-designed controlled trials without randomization.

II-2: Evidence obtained from well-designed cohort or case-control analytic studies, preferably from more than one center or research group.

II-3: Evidence obtained from multiple time series with or without the intervention. Dramatic results in uncontrolled experiments (such as the results of the introduction of penicillin treatment in the 1940's) could also be regarded as this type of evidence.

III: Opinions of respected authorities, based on clinical experience, descriptive studies, or reports of expert committees.

See Chapter ii for further information about the methodology used to develop the body of this report.

Table A-1.
Breast Cancer Screening

Age Group, y	Preventive Intervention	Quality of Evidence	Strength of Recommendations
40–49	Annual CBE*	III	C
50–59	Annual mammogram and CBE	I	A
60+	Annual mammogram and CBE	II-2	B
40+	Teaching BSE*	III	C

*CBE indicates clinical breast examinations; BSE, breast self-examination.

Table A-2.
Screening for Diabetes Mellitus

Preventive Intervention	Quality of Evidence	Strength of Recommendations
Gestational Diabetes Mellitus		
Glucose screening test (GST) for all pregnant women, followed by oral glucose tolerance test (OGTT) for plasma glucose >140 mg/dL (7.8 mmol/L)	I	B
Type I and Type II Diabetes Mellitus		
Screening of non-pregnant adults	I	D

Table A-3.
Colorectal Cancer Screening

Preventive Intervention	Quality of Evidence	Strength of Recommendations
Fecal Occult Blood Screening		
Fecal occult blood screening	III	C
Sigmoidoscopic Screening in Persons with No Known Risk Factors		
Periodic sigmoidoscopy	III	
Persons aged < 40 y		D
Persons aged 40 + y		C
Sigmoidoscopic Screening in Persons with a Questionably Increased Risk		
Periodic sigmoidoscopy	III	
Persons with one first-degree relative with colorectal cancer developing after age 40 y		C
Women with a personal history of endometrial, ovarian, or breast cancer		C
Endoscopic Surveillance in Persons at High Risk		
Periodic sigmoidoscopy in families with hereditary polyposis syndromes (beginning at ages 10–15 y)	III	A
Periodic colonoscopy	III	
Families with hereditary nonpolyposis syndromes (beginning at age 30 y)		A
Persons with ulcerative colitis (after 10 y of disease)		B
Persons with history of colorectal cancer or adenomatous polyps*		B
Persons with two or more first-degree relatives with colorectal cancer** (beginning at age 40 y)		B

*Particularly if polyps are greater than 10 mm in diameter.
**Particularly if age of onset in relatives is early (e.g., < 40 y).

Table A-4.
Prevention of Sexually Transmitted Diseases

Disease	Preventive Intervention	Quality of Evidence	Strength of Recommendations
	General Recommendations		
	Epidemiologic treatment^	I	A
	Contact tracing	II-2	B
	Disease reporting	III	B
	Barrier methods	II-3	B
	Patient education	III	C
	Gonorrhea		
Gonorrhea	Culture of high-risk group members	II-1	A
Gonococcal ophthalmia neonatorum	Erythromycin ophthalmic ointment postpartum	I	A
Gonococcal ophthalmia neonatorum	Culture of pregnant women	III	C
	Syphilis		
Syphilis	Epidemiologic treatment of sexual contacts of established infection	I	A
Syphilis	VDRL testing of high-risk group members	II-3	B
Congenital syphilis	VDRL testing of pregnant women	II-3	Risk group: B No-risk group: C
	Human Immunodeficiency Virus (HIV)		
HIV infection	HIV antibody testing	III	Risk group: B Pregnant women: B No-risk group: C
HIV infection	Use of heat-treated blood products^	II	A
HIV infection	Blood and needle precautions for persons exposed to infected secretions^	II	A
	Sexually Transmitted Infections Caused by Enteric Pathogens		
Hepatitis A	Immune serum globulin	I	A

Table A-4. (continued).

Disease	Preventive Intervention	Quality of Evidence	Strength of Recommendations
	Sexually Transmitted Human Papillomavirus Infection		
Genital warts	Physical examination of risk group members^	III	C
	Sexually Transmitted Herpes Simplex Virus Infection		
Neonatal herpes	Cesarean section in women with active genital herpes during labor^	III	B
	Sexually Transmitted Chlamydia trachomatis Infection		
Ophthalmia neonatorum	Erythromycin eye ointment	I	A
Neonatal chlamydia infection	Culture screening of pregnant women	III	Risk group: B

^Examined by Task Force but not discussed in *Guide*.

Table A-5.
Automobile Occupant Protection Counseling

Preventive Intervention	Quality of Evidence	Strength of Recommendations
Use of lap/shoulder safety belts and child safety seats to reduce morbidity and mortality in automobile crashes	II	A
Reducing automobile injury and death by:		
Advising parents to use infant car seats	II	B
Advising patients to use occupant restraints for themselves and others; discussing other risk factors for motor vehicle injuries	III	C

Table A-6.
Dipstick Urinalysis

Preventive Intervention	Quality of Evidence	Strength of Recommendations
Dipstick urinalysis for hematuria		
Adults aged <60 y	II-2	D
Adults aged 60+ y	II-2	C
Dipstick urinalysis for proteinuria		
Adults aged <60 y	II-2	D
Adults aged 60+ y	III	D
Leukocyte esterase/nitrite test for bacteriuria		
High prevalence/treatment efficacious		
Pregnant women*	I	C
High prevalence/treatment not fully evaluated		
Women aged 60+ y	I	C
Diabetic women	III	C
High prevalence/treatment not efficacious		
Women aged <60 y	I	E
Men aged 60+ y	III	D
Institutionalized elderly	II-2	D
Low prevalence		
Men aged <60 y	II-2	E
Leukocyte esterase test for pyuria		
Low prevalence		
Men aged <60 y	II-2	D
Other populations	III	D

*Screening for bacteriuria in pregnant women with the more sensitive urine culture is given an A recommendation based on grade I quality of evidence.

Table A-7.
Smoking Cessation Counseling

Preventive Intervention	Quality of Evidence	Strength of Recommendations
Smoking cessation to reduce the risk of lung and other cancers, cardiovascular and lung disease, and complications of pregnancy	II-2	A
Reducing tobacco use by issuing repeated smoking cessation messages from multiple sources over an extended period of time	I	A

Table A-8.
Physical Activity Counseling

Target Condition or Preventive Intervention	Quality of Evidence	Strength of Recommendations
Efficacy of Physical Activity in Primary Prevention		
Coronary artery disease		
Adult males	II-2	A
Adult females	II-2	C
Hypertension (all adults)	II-2	A
Noninsulin-dependent diabetes mellitus (all adults)	III	C
Osteoporosis		
Prevention of bone loss		
Postmenopausal females	I	A
Premenopausal females	III	C
Prevention of hip fracture		
Postmenopausal females	III	C
Obesity (all adults)	I	A
Mental health (all adults)		
Affect	I	C
Self-esteem	I	B
Effectiveness of Preventive Interventions		
Exercise ECG to identify individuals at risk for cardiac arrest during physical activity	II-2	D
Physical activity counseling by physicians as a primary preventive intervention to increase physical activity levels	II-2	B

Table A-9.
Dietary Fat Counseling

Preventive Intervention	Category of Evidence	Strength of Recommendations
Reduction of Coronary Artery Disease		
Low-fat diet in all adults aged 18–59 y	II-1	B
Low-fat diet in persons younger than 18 y and older than 60 y that maintains appropriate caloric intake	III	C
Reduction of Cancer (Breast, Colon, Prostate)		
Lowering dietary fat	III	C
Counseling to Reduce Dietary Fat Consumption		
Issuing repeated dietary change messages from multiple sources over an extended period of time	I	A

Table A-10.
Fall Prevention Among Older Persons

Preventive Intervention	Quality of Evidence	Strength of Recommendations
Identifying intrinsic and extrinsic risk factors for falls among older patients to reduce falls and resulting injuries	III	C
Reducing falls and fall injury by:		
Identifying at office visit persons who have fallen: evaluate for underlying disease, effect of medications, and unsteady gait or balance	III	C
Advising patients or family to check home for environmental hazards and whenever possible make needed improvements	III	C
Advising patients, when appropriate, to maintain regular physical activity and/or to participate in an exercise program to provide the protective effects of increased muscle strength and tone and rapid response time	III	C

Table A-11.
Prevention of Unwanted Adolescent Pregnancy

Preventive Intervention	Quality of Evidence	Strength of Recommendations
Using contraceptives to reduce pregnancy in sexually active individuals	II-2	A*
Reducing unwanted pregnancies by having primary care clinicians provide contraceptive services (teaching, counseling, and contraceptive agents) to sexually active adolescents	II-3	B**

*Despite the fact that the evidence establishing the effectiveness of oral contraceptives has come from field and clinical studies rather than randomized clinical trials and studies not specifically directed to adolescents, the personal and financial burden of unwanted teenage pregnancy is so great that an A recommendation is warranted.
**While the quality of evidence supporting the effectiveness of sexual education by primary care clinicians is limited, based on expert opinion, education is an important component of the services that should be offered by clinicians. Further, such education should be provided at an early enough time that it can be incorporated into personal decisions about sexual matters.

Table A-12.
Preventive Dentistry

Preventive Intervention	Quality of Evidence	Strength of Recommendations
Caries		
Fluoride		
Systemic—water fluoridation, dietary supplements	I	A
Topical—self-applied (dentifrice, mouthrinse), professionally applied	I	A
Occlusal sealants	I	A
Dietary control		
Limit sweets	II-1	A
Avoid bedtime baby bottle containing cariogenic liquid	III	B
Personal oral hygiene (tooth brushing without fluoride, flossing)	III	C
Periodic dental examination	III	C

Table A-12. (continued).

Preventive Intervention	Quality of Evidence	Strength of Recommendations
Periodontal Disease		
Plaque and calculus control		
Personal oral hygiene	I	A
Professional care scaling and root planing, prophylaxis in combination with personal oral hygiene	I	A
Chlorhexidine (antiplaque agent) (high-risk groups only)^	I	A
Periodic dental examination	III	C
Malocclusion		
Space maintenance after loss of deciduous teeth^	II-2	B
Ceasing of finger- and thumb-sucking habits by age 6 y^	III	C
Maintenance of open airway while orofacial area is developing^	III	C
Trauma		
Mouthguards with contact sports^	II-3	A
Shoulder and lap safety belts in cars	II-3	A
Helmets and face shields while riding motorcycles	III	C
Helmets and mouthguards with skateboards^	III	C
Oral Cancer		
Avoidance of tobacco		
Smoking	II-2	A
Smokeless	II-2	A
Annual oral examination to detect premalignant and malignant lesions and to assess risk factors and provide counseling	III	C

^Examined by Task Force but not discussed in *Guide*.

Table A-13.
Immunizations, Immunoprophylaxis, and Chemoprophylaxis to Prevent
Selected Infections

Disease	Preventive Intervention	Quality of Evidence	Strength of Recommendations
Childhood Immunizations			
Diphtheria Pertussis Tetanus Poliomyelitis Measles Rubella Mumps	Vaccine (for all)	I (for all)	A (for all)
H. influenzae type b	Vaccine	I	A
	Chemoprophylaxis	I	A
Adult Immunizations			
Tetanus	Vaccine	I	A
Diphtheria	Vaccine	I	A
Influenza A & B	Vaccine	I for efficacy of vaccine; II-3 for efficacy in the elderly	A
Influenza A	Amantadine	I	A
Pneumococcal infection	Vaccine	II-1 for vaccine efficacy; II-2 for US population	B
Tuberculosis	Bacille Calmette-Guerin vaccine	I	A
	Isoniazid chemoprophylaxis	I	A
Hepatitis A	Immune globulin immunoprophylaxis	I	A
Hepatitis B	Vaccine	I	A
	Immune globulin immunoprophylaxis	I	A
Meningococcal infection	Vaccine^	I	A
	Rifampin and sulfadiazine chemoprophylaxis	II-1	
Rabies	Vaccine	II-1	A
	Rabies immune globulin	II-3	A
Malaria	Chloroquine prophylaxis ^	I	A

^Examined by Task Force but not discussed in *Guide.*

Appendix B
Reviewers

Listed below are the more than 300 Federal and non-Federal experts who reviewed Task Force draft background papers and recommendations during their various stages of preparation. In addition, the Senior Advisors to the Task Force, who are listed in the Acknowledgments, also served as reviewers for many recommendations.

It should be emphasized that while reviewer comments and suggestions were of substantial assistance, the Task Force is solely responsible for the final recommendations. Service as a reviewer does not necessarily reflect endorsement of any or all of the Task Force recommendations.

J. Gary Abulo, M.D.
Rhode Island Hospital
Providence, RI

Patricia Aiken-O'Neill, Esq.
American Academy of Ophthalmology
Washington, DC

Myron Allukian, Jr., D.D.S.
Boston City Hospital
Boston, MA

Marilena Amoni, M.S.
U.S. Department of Transportation
Washington, DC

Douglas J. Anderson, M.D., M.P.H.
University of Virginia
Richmond, VA

Geoffrey Anderson, M.D., Ph.D.
University of British Columbia
Vancouver, British Columbia, Canada

Robert Andres, Ph.D.
University of Massachusetts
Amherst, MA

Joseph Lee Annest, Ph.D.
Centers for Disease Control
Atlanta, GA

Katherine L. Armstrong, Dr.P.H.
Office of the Assistant Secretary for
    Health
Washington, DC

Constance W. Atwell, Ph.D.
National Institutes of Health
Bethesda, MD

Chris Bachrach, Ph.D.
National Institutes of Health
Bethesda, MD

Ernest Baden, D.D.S., M.D.
Fairleigh Dickinson University
Hackensack, NJ

Shirley P. Bagley
National Institutes of Health
Bethesda, MD

Susan Baker, M.P.H.
Johns Hopkins University
Baltimore, MD

Wendy Baldwin, Ph.D.
National Institutes of Health
Bethesda, MD

Thomas F. Babor, Ph.D.
University of Connecticut
Farmington, CT

Edward E. Bartlett, Dr.P.H.
International Patient Education
  Council
Rockville, MD

Robert C. Bast, Jr., M.D.
Duke University
Durham, NC

Renaldo N. Battista, M.D., Sc.D.
McGill University
Montreal, Quebec, Canada

Marie Dominique Beaulieu, M.D.,
  M.Sc.
University of Montreal
Montreal, Quebec, Canada

Peter H. Bennett, M.B.
National Institutes of Health
Phoenix, AZ

Ross S. Berkowitz, M.D.
Harvard Medical School
Boston, MA

Stuart M. Berman, M.D.
Centers for Disease Control
Atlanta, GA

Keith Berndtson, M.D.
The Portes Center
Chicago, IL

Fred H. Bess, Ph.D.
Vanderbilt University
Nashville, TN

Mohandas Bhat, D.D.S., Ph.D.
National Institutes of Health
Rockville, MD

Harrison G. Bloom, M.D.
Montefiore Medical Center
Bronx, NY

Bradley O. Boekeloo, Ph.D.
Prospect Associates
Rockville, MD

Linda Burnes Bolton, Dr.P.H., R.N.
Cedars-Sinai Medical Center
Los Angeles, CA

G. Stephen Bowen, M.D.
Centers for Disease Control
Atlanta, GA

John M. Bowman, M.D.
Women's Hospital
Winnipeg, Manitoba, Canada

Gail Boyd, Ph.D.
National Institutes of Health
Bethesda, MD

Edward W. Brink, M.D.
Centers for Disease Control
Atlanta, GA

Claire V. Broome, M.D.
Centers for Disease Control
Atlanta, GA

L. Jackson Brown, D.D.S., Ph.D.
National Institutes of Health
Rockville, MD

Stuart T. Brown, M.D.
Centers for Disease Control
Atlanta, GA

Philip B. Brunell, M.D.
University of Texas
San Antonio, TX

Bryan Burt, D.D.S.
University of Michigan
Ann Arbor, MI

Benjamin T. Burton, Ph.D.
National Institutes of Health
Bethesda, MD

Nabers Cabaniss
Office of the Assistant Secretary of
  Health
Washington, DC

James P. Carlos, D.D.S., M.P.H.
National Institutes of Health
Bethesda, MD

James R. Carlson, Ph.D.
University of California
Davis, CA

Jean Carmody, M.A.
National Center for Health Services
  Research and Health Care
  Technology Assessment
Rockville, MD

Carl J. Caspersen, Ph.D., M.P.H.
Centers for Disease Control
Atlanta, GA

Willard Cates, Jr., M.D., M.P.H.
Center for Disease Control
Atlanta, GA

Robert C. Cefalo, M.D., Ph.D.
University of North Carolina
Chapel Hill, NC

Martin K. Chen, Ed.D.
National Center for Health Services
   Research and Health Care
   Technology Assessment
Rockville, MD

Amoz I. Chernoff, M.D.
National Institutes of Health
Bethesda, MD

Leon C. Chesley, Ph.D.
State University of New York
Brooklyn, NY

James Chin, M.D.
California State Department of Health
   Services
Berkeley, CA

Gerald W. Chodak, M.D.
University of Chicago
Chicago, IL

Edward R. Christophersen, Ph.D.
University of Kansas
Kansas City, KS

Charles M. Clark, Jr., M.D.
Indiana University
Indianapolis, IN

James I. Cleeman, M.D.
National Institutes of Health
Bethesda, MD

Gene D. Cohen, M.D., M.P.H.
Alcohol, Drug Abuse, and Mental
   Health Administration
Rockville, MD

Lois K. Cohen, Ph.D.
National Institutes of Health
Rockville, MD

George Comstock, M.D.
Johns Hopkins University
Baltimore, MD

Stephen B. Corbin, D.D.S., M.P.H.
National Institutes of Health
Bethesda, MD

Lawrence Corey, M.D.
Children's Hospital
Seattle, WA

Joseph W. Cullen, Ph.D.
National Institutes of Health
Bethesda, MD

Larry Culpepper, M.D.
Memorial Hospital
Pawtucket, RI

Steven R. Cummings, M.D.
University of California
San Francisco, CA

James W. Curran, M.D.
Centers for Disease Control
Atlanta, GA

Jeffrey A. Cutler, M.D.
National Institutes of Health
Bethesda, MD

Peter R. Dallman, M.D.
University of California
San Francisco, CA

Darla Danford, D.Sc., M.P.H., R.D.
National Institutes of Health
Bethesda, MD

J. Gorman Daubs, O.D., M.D., Ph.D.
The Medical Research Consortium
Santo Domingo, Dominican Republic

Mayer B. Davidson, M.D.
Cedars-Sinai Medical Center
Los Angeles, CA

Michael P. Davis
National Institutes of Health
Bethesda, MD

Ronald M. Davis, M.D.
Centers for Disease Control
Rockville, MD

Felix de la Cruz, M.D.
National Institutes of Health
Bethesda, MD

Frank DeStefano, M.D., M.P.H.
Centers for Disease Control
Atlanta, GA

Eugene P. DiMagno, M.D.
Mayo Clinic and Mayo Foundation
Rochester, MN

Sharon L. Dorfman, Sc.M.
Focus Technologies, Inc.
Washington, DC

William S. Driscoll, M.D., M.P.H.
National Institutes of Health
Bethesda, MD

D. Peter Drotman, M.D., M.P.H.
Centers for Disease Control
Atlanta, GA

Thomas S. Drury, Ph.D.
National Institutes of Health
Rockville, MD

Lewis Drusin, M.D.
New York Hospital
New York, NY

George N. Eaves, M.D.
National Institutes of Health
Bethesda, MD

Michael Eckardt, Ph.D.
Alcohol, Drug Abuse, and Mental
   Health Administration
Bethesda, MD

David M. Eddy, M.D., Ph.D.
Duke University
Durham, NC

Theodore Eickhoff, M.D.
AMI Presbyterian-St. Luke's Medical
   Center
Denver, CO

Shirli Eilat-Greenberg, M.A.
University of Texas
Houston, TX

John M. Eisenberg, M.D.
University of Pennsylvania
Philadelphia, PA

Arnold E. Epstein, M.D.
Harvard School of Public Health
Boston, MA

Michael P. Eriksen, Sc.D.
University of Texas
Houston, TX

Nancy Ernst, M.S., R.D.
National Institutes of Health
Bethesda, MD

Abby G. Ershow, Ph.D.
National Institutes of Health
Bethesda, MD

Bruce Ettinger, M.D.
Kaiser Permanente Medical Center
San Francisco, CA

John W. Feightner, M.D.
McMaster University
Hamilton, Ontario, Canada

William Feldman, M.D.
University of Ottawa
Ottawa, Ontario, Canada

Allan Forbes, M.D.
Food and Drug Administration
Washington, DC

Judith E. Fradkin, M.D.
National Institutes of Health
Bethesda, MD

John W. Frank, M.D.
University of Toronto
Toronto, Ontario, Canada

Norbert Freinkel, M.D.
Northwestern University
Chicago, IL

William T. Friedewald, M.D.
National Institutes of Health
Bethesda, MD

Jay W. Friedman, D.D.S., M.P.H.
University of California
Los Angeles, CA

Lawrence M. Friedman, M.D.
National Institutes of Health
Bethesda, MD

Fredric D. Frigoletto, Jr., M.D.
Harvard Medical School
Boston, MA

Victor Froelicher, M.D.
Long Beach Veterans Administration
   Medical Center
Long Beach, CA

Jo Ann Gasper
Office of the Assistant Secretary for
   Health
Washington, DC

Lawrence A. Gavin, M.D.
University of California
San Francisco, CA

Saul Genuth, M.D.
Mount Sinai Medical Center
Cleveland, OH

Raymond W. Gifford, Jr., M.D.
Cleveland Clinic Foundation
Cleveland, OH

Helen C. Gift, Ph.D.
National Institutes of Health
Rockville, MD

Gary A. Giovino, Ph.D.
Centers for Disease Control
Rockville, MD

Mary Anne Glenday
University of Texas
Houston, TX

Thomas J. Glynn, Ph.D.
National Institutes of Health
Bethesda, MD

Howard K. Gogel, M.D.
University of New Mexico
Albuquerque, NM

Dorothy Gohdes, M.D.
Indian Health Service
Albuquerque, NM

Richard B. Goldbloom, M.D.
Dalhousie University
Halifax, Nova Scotia, Canada

John M. Goldenring, M.D.
Pediatric Medical Group
Redlands, CA

Donald E. Goldotono, M.D.
National Center for Health Services
  Research and Health Care
  Technology Assessment
Rockville, MD

Kathleen E. Grady, Ph.D.
University of Connecticut
Storrs, CT

Peter A. Greenwald, M.D., Dr.Ph.
National Institutes of Health
Bethesda, MD

David S. Greer, M.D.
Brown University
Providence, RI

Ellen R. Gritz, Ph.D.
Johnson Comprehensive Cancer
  Center
Los Angeles, CA

Stephen C. Hadler, M.D.
Centers for Disease Control
Atlanta, GA

Jeannie Haggerty, M.Sc.
Montreal General Hospital
Montreal, Quebec, Canada

Ferris M. Hall, M.D.
Beth Israel Hospital
Boston, MA

Margaret Hamburg, M.D.
National Institutes of Health
Bethesda, MD

H. Hunter Handsfield, M.D.
Harborview Medical Center
Seattle, WA

Maureen I. Harris, Ph.D., M.P.H.
National Institutes of Health
Bethesda, MD

Robert Hatcher, M.D.
Emory School of Medicine
Atlanta, GA

James Hedlund, Ph.D.
U.S. Department of Transportation
Washington, DC

D. Mark Hegsted, Ph.D.
Harvard School of Public Health
Southborough, MA

Fred Heidrich, M.D., M.P.H.
Group Health Cooperative of Puget
  Sound
Seattle, WA

Stan Heifitz, D.D.S., M.P.H.
Potomac, MD

William P. Hendee, Ph.D.
American Medical Association
Chicago, IL

Charles H. Hennekens, M.D.
Harvard Medical School
Brookline, MA

Stephen P. Heyse, M.D., M.P.H.
National Institutes of Health
Bethesda, MD

James G. Hill
National Institutes of Health
Bethesda, MD

Alan R. Hinman, M.D.
Centers for Disease Control
Atlanta, GA

Robert Hirschfeld, M.D.
Alcohol, Drug Abuse, and Mental
  Health Administration
Rockville, MD

W. Allen Hogge, M.D.
University of Virginia
Charlottesville, VA

Thomas Holohan, M.D.
Food and Drug Administration
Rockville, MD

Neil A. Holtzman, M.D., M.P.H.
Johns Hopkins University
Baltimore, MD

Michael J. Horan, M.D.
National Institutes of Health
Bethesda, MD

Alice M. Horowitz, R.D.H., M.A.
National Institutes of Health
Bethesda, MD

Herschel Horowitz, D.D.S., M.P.H.
Bethesda, MD

H. Dunbar Hoskins, Jr., M.D.
University of California
San Francisco, CA

Vernon N. Houck, M.D.
Centers for Disease Control
Atlanta, GA

Jan Howard, Ph.D.
National Institutes of Health
Bethesda, MD

Stephen B. Hulley, M.D., M.P.H.
University of California
San Francisco, CA

Donald C. Iverson, Ph.D.
University of Colorado
Denver, CO

Franklyn Judson, M.D.
Centers for Disease Control
Atlanta, GA

Henry S. Kahn, M.D.
Centers for Disease Control
Atlanta, GA

John T. Kalberer, Jr., Ph.D.
National Institutes of Health
Bethesda, MD

Mark A. Kane, M.D.
Centers for Disease Control
Atlanta, GA

William M. Kane, Ph.D.
American College of Preventive
  Medicine
Washington, DC

Edward H. Kass, M.D., Ph.D.
Harvard University
Boston, MA

Martha Katz
Centers for Disease Control
Atlanta, GA

Asta Kenny
Alan Guttmacher Institute
Washington, DC

Dushanka Kleinman, D.D.S., M.Sc.D.
National Institutes of Health
Bethesda, MD

Robert C. Knapp, M.D.
Harvard Medical School
Boston, MA

Ann Koontz, Dr.Ph., C.N.M.
Health Resources and Services
  Administration
Rockville, MD

Alfred W. Kopf, M.D.
New York University
New York, NY

Jeffrey P. Koplan, M.D., M.P.H.
Centers for Disease Control
Atlanta, GA

Calvin Kunin, M.D.
Ohio State University
Columbus, OH

Ronald LaPorte, Ph.D.
University of Pittsburgh
Pittsburgh, PA

Eric B. Larson, M.D.
University of Washington
Seattle, WA

Philip Lavin, Ph.D.
Harvard Medical School
Boston, MA

Ami Laws, M.D.
Stanford University
Stanford, CA

Kenneth J. Leveno, M.D.
University of Texas
Dallas, TX

Harvey L. Levy, M.D.
Massachusetts General Hospital
Boston, MA

Edward Lichtenstein, Ph.D.
Oregon Research Institute
Eugene, OR

Preston A. Littleton, D.D.S., Ph.D.
National Institutes of Health
Rockville, MD

Harold Loe, D.D.S.
National Institutes of Health
Bethesda, MD

Alexander Logan, M.D.
Mount Sinai Hospital
Toronto, Ontario, Canada

Joseph G. Lossick, D.O.
Centers for Disease Control
Atlanta, GA

Thomas L. Louden, D.D.S.
Health Resources and Services
   Administration
Rockville, MD

Richard R. Love, M.D., M.S.
University of Wisconsin
Madison, WI

Nathan Maccoby, Ph.D.
Stanford University
Stanford, CA

Kathleen MacPherson, R.N., Ph.D.
University of Southern Maine
Portland, ME

Audrey Manley, M.D., M.P.H.
Health Resources and Services
   Administration
Rockville, MD

Karen Mann, R.N., Ph.D.
Dalhousie University
Halifax, Nova Scotia, Canada

James S. Marks, M.D., M.P.H.
Centers for Disease Control
Atlanta, GA

John R. Marler, M.D.
National Institutes of Health
Bethesda, MD

James Marshall
American Dental Association
Chicago, IL

William J. Mayer, M.D.. M.P.H.
National Institutes of Health
Bethesda, MD

Donald McNellis, M.D.
National Institutes of Health
Bethesda, MD

Robert E. Mecklenburg, D.D.S.,
   M.P.H.
Health Resources and Services
   Administration
Rockville, MD

Myron R. Melamed, M.D.
Memorial Sloan-Kettering Cancer
   Center
New York, NY

L. Joseph Melton III, M.D.
Mayo Clinic
Rochester, MN

Walter Menniger, M.D.
Menniger Foundation
Topeka, KS

James Mercy, Ph.D.
Centers for Disease Control
Atlanta, GA

Linda D. Meyers, Ph.D.
Office of the Assistant Secretary for
   Health
Washington, DC

W. Phillip Mickelson, M.D.
Health and Welfare Canada
Ottawa, Ontario, Canada

Anthony B. Miller, M.B., F.R.C.P.(C)
University of Toronto
Toronto, Ontario, Canada

Herbert Miller
U.S. Department of Transportation
Washington, DC

Stephen C. Miller, O.D.
American Optometric Association
St. Louis, MO

David N. Mohr, M.D.
Mayo Clinic
Rochester, MN

Julian M. Morris
National Institutes of Health
Bethesda, MD

Brenda Morrison, Ph.D.
University of British Columbia
Vancouver, British Columbia, Canada

Eve Moscicki, Sc.D.
Alcohol, Drug Abuse, and Mental
  Health Administration
Rockville, MD

Patricia Dolan Mullen, Dr.P.H.
University of Texas at Houston
Houston, TX

George E. Murphy, M.D.
Washington University
St. Louis, MO

Alvin I. Mushlin, M.D.
University of Rochester
Rochester, NY

Ralph F. Naunton, M.D., F.A.C.S.
National Institutes of Health
Bethesda, MD

Herbert L. Needleman, M.D.
University of Pittsburgh
Pittsburgh, PA

Marion Nestle, Ph.D., M.P.H.
New York University
New York, NY

Susan Newcomer, Ph.D.
National Institutes of Health
Bethesda, MD

Guy R. Newell, M.D.
University of Texas
Houston, TX

Linda C. Niessen, D.M.D., M.P.H.
Veterans Administration
Perry Point, MD

Elena O. Nightingale, M.D., Ph.D.
Carnegie Corporation
Washington, DC

Stuart L. Nightingale, M.D.
Food and Drug Administration
Rockville, MD

Allan S. Noonan, M.D.
Health Resources and Services
  Administration
Rockville, MD

John W. Norris, M.D.
Sunnybrook Medical Centre
Toronto, Ontario, Canada

Thomas E. Novotny, M.D.
Centers for Disease Control
Rockville, MD

Leroy M. Nyberg, Jr., Ph.D., M.D.
National Institutes of Health
Bethesda, MD

Patrick O'Carroll, M.D.
Centers for Disease Control
Atlanta, GA

Daniel Offord, M.D.
McMaster University
Hamilton, Ontario, Canada

Michael F. Oliver, M.D.
University of Edinburgh
Edinburgh, Scotland

Robert E. Olson, M.D., Ph.D.
University of New York at Stony Brook
Stony Brook, NY

Walter A. Orenstein, M.D.
Centers for Disease Control
Atlanta, GA

Tracy Orleans, Ph.D.
Foxchase Cancer Center
Philadelphia, PA

Marian Osterweis, Ph.D.
Institute of Medicine
Washington, DC

Seymour Packman, M.D.
University of California
San Francisco, CA

Ralph Paffenbarger, M.D.
Standord University
Stanford, CA

Sushma Palmer, D.Sc.
Institute of Medicine
Washington, DC

Robert O. Pasnau, M.D.
University of California
Los Angeles, CA

Eugene R. Passamani, M.D.
National Institutes of Health
Bethesda, MD

Clifford H. Patrick, Ph.D.
Veterans Administration
Durham, NC

Christopher Patterson, M.D.
Chedoke McMaster Hospitals
Hamilton, Ontario, Canada

Terry Pechacek, Ph.D.
National Institutes of Health
Bethesda, MD

William Peck, M.D.
Jewish Hospital of St. Louis
St. Louis, MO

H.S. Pennypacker, Ph.D.
University of Florida
Gainesville, FL

Stanley Plotkin, M.D.
Children's Hospital
Philadelphia, PA

Ronald L. Poland, M.D.
Wayne State University
Detroit, MI

Kenneth E. Powell, M.D.
Centers for Disease Control
Atlanta, GA

Stephen R. Preblud, M.D.
Centers for Disease Control
Atlanta, GA

Jeffrey L. Probstfield, M.D.
National Institutes of Health
Bethesda, MD

Philip C. Prorok, Ph.D.
National Institutes of Health
Bethesda, MD

Milton Puziss, M.D.
National Institutes of Health
Bethesda, MD

Joan Quinlan, M.S.
U.S. Department of Transportation
Washington, DC

Clarice Reid, M.D.
National Institutes of Health
Bethesda, MD

Robert D. Reinecke, M.D.
Foerderer Eye Movement Center for
  Children
Philadelphia, PA

John Williams Richards, Jr., M.D.
Medical College of Georiga
Augusta, GA

Basil Rifkind, M.D.
National Institutes of Health
Bethesda, MD

Leon S. Robertson, Ph.D.
Yale University
New Haven, CT

Paul Robertson, D.D.S., M.S.
University of British Columbia
Vancouver, British Columbia, Canada

William Robinson, M.D.
Health Resources and Services
  Administration
Rockville, MD

Robert T. Rolfs, M.D.
Centers for Disease Control
Atlanta, GA

Mark L. Rosenberg, M.D.
Centers for Disease Control
Atlanta, GA

Kathryn Rost, Ph.D.
Washington University
St. Louis, MO

Richard Rothenberg, M.D.
New York State Department of Health
Albany, NY

Peter T. Rowley, M.D.
University of Rochester
Rochester, NY

Abraham Rudolph, M.D.
University of California
San Francisco, CA

Jonathan M. Samet, M.D., M.P.H.
University of New Mexico
Albuquerque, NM

Clyde B. Schechter, M.D.
Mount Sinai Medical Center
New York, NY

B. Thomas Scheib, M.A.
U.S. Department of Transportation
Washington, DC

George P. Schmid, M.D.
Centers for Disease Control
Atlanta, GA

Steven A. Schroeder, M.D.
University of California
San Francisco, CA

John A. Schuchmann, M.D.
Scott and White Clinic
Temple, TX

Herbert C. Schulberg, Ph.D.
Western Psychiatric Institute and
   Clinic
Pittsburgh, PA

Robert Selwitz, D.D.S., M.P.H.
National Institutes of Health
Bethesda, MD

Judith Senderowitz
Center for Population Options
Washington, DC

Ruby T. Senie, Ph.D.
Mount Sinai School of Medicine
New York, NY

Saleem A. Shah, Ph.D.
Alcohol, Drug Abuse, and Mental
   Health Administration
Rockville, MD

Donald Shopland
National Institutes of Health
Bethesda, MD

Morton Silverman, M.D.
Alcohol, Drug Abuse, and Mental
   Health Administration
Rockville, MD

Sol Silverman, Jr., D.D.S.
University of California
San Francisco, CA

Denise Simons-Morton, M.D., M.P.H.
University of Texas
Houston, TX

Daniel E. Singer, M.D.
Massachusetts General Hospital
Boston, MA

David Siscovick, M.D.
University of Washington
Seattle, WA

Jane E. Sisk, Ph.D.
Office of Technology Assessment
U.S. Congress
Washington, DC

Mary L. Skovron, Dr.P.H.
Mount Sinai Medical Center
New York, NY

Charles R. Smart, M.D.
National Institutes of Health
Bethesda, MD

Donald A. Smith, M.D., M.P.H.
Mount Sinai Medical Center
New York, NY

Michael Smith
U.S. Department of Transportation
Washington, DC

Dixie E. Snider, Jr., M.D., M.P.H.
Centers for Disease Control
Atlanta, GA

Frederic Solomon, M.D.
Institute of Medicine
Washington, DC

Katherine Bauer Sommers
Institute of Medicine
Washington, DC

Ann W. Sorenson, Ph.D.
National Institutes of Health
Bethesda, MD

George L. Spaeth, M.D.
Wills Eye Hospital
Philadelphia, PA

Walter O. Spitzer, M.D., M.P.H.
McGill University
Montreal, Quebec, Canada

Howard Spivak, M.D.
Massachusetts Department of Public
    Health
Boston, MA

Thomas Stephens, Ph.D.
Manotick, Ontario, Canada

Michael H. Stolar, Ph.D.
American Diabetes Association, Inc.
Alexandria, VA

Katherine M. Stone, M.D.
Centers for Disease Control
Atlanta, GA

D. Eugene Strandness, Jr., M.D.
University of Washington
Seattle, WA

Albert J. Stunkard, M.D.
University of Pennsylvania
Philadelphia, PA

Philip Swango, D.D.S., M.P.H.
National Institutes of Health
Bethesda, MD

Steven Teutsch, M.D., M.P.H.
Centers for Disease Control
Atlanta, GA

Stephen B. Thacker, M.D.
Centers for Disease Control
Atlanta, GA

Mary E. Tinetti, M.D.
Yale New Haven Hospital
New Haven, CT

Dennis D. Tolsma
Centers for Disease Control
Atlanta, GA

Theodore B. Van Italie, M.D.
St. Luke's-Roosevelt Hospital Center
New York, NY

Michael D. Walker, M.D.
National Institutes of Health
Bethesda, MD

Julian A. Waller, M.D., M.P.H.
University of Vermont
Burlington, VT

Elaine Wang, M.D., M.Sc.
Hospital for Sick Children
Toronto, Ontario, Canada

Kenneth E. Warner, Ph.D.
University of Michigan
Ann Arbor, MI

Galen Warren, D.D.S.
National Institutes of Health
Rockville, MD

Steven L. Warsof, M.D.
Kings Daughters Hospital
Norfolk, VA

Richard J. Waxweiler, Ph.D.
Centers for Disease Control
Atlanta, GA

Michael W. Werth
Chevy Chase, MD

Daniel Whiteside, D.D.S.
Health Resources and Services
    Administration
Rockville, MD

William L. Whittington
Centers for Disease Control
Atlanta, GA

Walter Willett, M.D.
Harvard University
Boston, MA

Allan F. Williams, Ph.D.
Insurance Institute for Highway Safety
Washington, DC

T. Franklin Williams, M.D.
National Institutes of Health
Bethesda, MD

Walter W. Williams, M.D., M.P.H.
Centers for Disease Control
Atlanta, GA

Sidney J. Winawer, M.D.
Memorial Sloan-Kettering Cancer
    Center
New York, NY

Peter D. Wood, D.Sc.
Stanford University
Palo Alto, CA

Ernst L. Wynder, M.D.
American Health Foundation
New York, NY

Robert C. Young, M.D.
National Institutes of Health
Bethesda, MD

Laurie Zabin, Ph.D.
Johns Hopkins University
Baltimore, MD

William J. Zukel, M.D.
National Institutes of Health
Bethesda, MD

Vincent R. Zurawski, Jr., Ph.D.
Centocor Corporation
Malvern, PA

Index*

*Page numbers followed by "t" refer to Task
Force rating tables in Appendix A.

411